Chest Imaging

Rotations in Radiology

Published and Forthcoming Books in the **Rotations in Radiology** Series

Pediatric Radiology
Janet Reid, Edward Lee, Angelisa Paladin, Caroline Carrico, and William Davros

Cardiac Imaging
Charles White, Linda Haramati, Joseph J.S. Chen, and Jeffrey Levsky

Gastrointestinal Imaging
Angela Levy, Koenraad Mortele, and Benjamin Yeh

Emergency Radiology
Hani H. Abujudeh

Neuroradiology
Zoran Rumboldt, Giulio Zuccoli, Clifford Eskey, Timothy Amrhein, and Benjamin Huang

Breast Imaging
Christoph I. Lee, Constance D. Lehman, and Lawrence W. Bassett

Musculoskeletal Imaging
Mihra S. Taljanovic, Imran Omer, Kevin Hoover, and Tyson Chadaz

Rotations in Radiology

Chest Imaging

Edited by

Melissa L. Rosado-de-Christenson, MD, FACR
Section Chief, Thoracic Imaging
Saint Luke's Hospital of Kansas City
Professor of Radiology
University of Missouri-Kansas City School of Medicine
Kansas City, Missouri

Sanjeev Bhalla, MD
Professor of Radiology
Chief, Cardiothoracic Imaging
Mallinckrodt Institute of Radiology
Washington University in St. Louis
St. Louis, Missouri

Santiago Martínez-Jiménez, MD
Saint Luke's Hospital of Kansas City
Professor of Radiology
University of Missouri-Kansas City School of Medicine
Kansas City, Missouri

Gerald F. Abbott, MD
Associate Professor of Radiology
Thoracic Imaging
Massachusetts General Hospital
Harvard University
Boston, Massachusetts

OXFORD
UNIVERSITY PRESS

OXFORD
UNIVERSITY PRESS

Oxford University Press is a department of the University of Oxford. It furthers the University's objective of excellence in research, scholarship, and education by publishing worldwide. Oxford is a registered trade mark of Oxford University Press in the UK and certain other countries.

Published in the United States of America by Oxford University Press
198 Madison Avenue, New York, NY 10016, United States of America.

Library of Congress Cataloging-in-Publication Data
Names: Rosado-de-Christenson, Melissa L., author. | Bhalla, Sanjeev, author. |
Abbott, Gerald F., author. | Martinez-Jiminez, Santiago, author.
Title: Chest imaging/Melissa L. Rosado-de-Christenson, Sanjeev Bhalla,
Gerald F. Abbott, and Santiago Martinez-Jiminez.
Other titles: Rotations in radiology.
Description: Oxford; New York : Oxford University Press, [2019] |
Series: Rotations in radiology | Includes bibliographical references and index.
Identifiers: LCCN 2015041342 | ISBN 9780199858064 (alk. paper)
Subjects: | MESH: Radiography, Thoracic. | Diagnostic Techniques, Respiratory System. | Respiratory Tract Diseases—radiography.
Classification: LCC RC941 | NLM WF 975 | DDC 617.5/40754—dc23
LC record available at http://lccn.loc.gov/2015041342

9 8 7 6 5 4 3 2 1

Printed by Sheridan Books, Inc., United States of America

Contents

Preface

Mastery of the skills of thoracic imaging is a daunting challenge for most radiologists and particularly for radiologists-in-training. Analysis of the chest radiograph involves identification, anatomic localization, and characterization of imaging abnormalities in order to formulate a reasonable differential diagnosis and recommend additional imaging and/or diagnostic testing. *Chest Imaging* is specifically tailored to provide a strong thoracic imaging knowledge base for diagnostic radiology residents but will also be useful to medical students, clinicians-in-training, and practicing radiologists and clinicians.

Content organization revolves around the analysis and interpretation of specific radiologic abnormalities and common diseases, including developmental, iatrogenic, and acquired conditions. Introductory chapters provide a description of the various thoracic imaging modalities, a basic review of imaging anatomy, a description of the radiologic report, and a review of basic signs encountered in chest radiography. Chapters are grouped into sections, each with a concise section introduction that provides a succinct illustrated overview of its contents. Each chapter presents a definition of a disease or process, the clinical presentation, and the relevant anatomic and physiologic considerations that are helpful for image interpretation. Differential diagnostic considerations and imaging findings are presented in a bulleted format for ease of use and rapid reference. In addition, each chapter provides helpful sections on how to approach the image, what not to miss, and a summary of key points. Common imaging manifestations of a disease are illustrated with radiographs, computed tomography, and magnetic resonance images.

Chest Imaging provides a succinct but comprehensive review of basic concepts in chest imaging. A reader's command of the content of this book will form a solid knowledge base in chest imaging and enable learners to build on that knowledge as they proceed to higher levels of competence in thoracic imaging.

Contributors

Joseph T. Azok, MD
Associate Staff
Thoracic Imaging
Cleveland Clinic
Assistant Clinical Professor of Radiology
Case Western Reserve University
Cleveland, Ohio

Ryo E. C. Benson, MD
Associate Staff
Thoracic Imaging
Cleveland Clinic
Cleveland, Ohio

Sonia L. Betancourt-Cuellar, MD
Associate Professor, Division of Diagnostic Imaging
Department of Diagnostic Radiology
The University of Texas MD Anderson Cancer Center
Houston, Texas

Andrew J. Bierhals, MD
Associate Professor of Radiology
Cardiothoracic Imaging Section
Mallinckrodt Institute of Radiology
Washington University in St. Louis
St. Louis, Missouri

Juliana Bueno, MD
Assistant Professor of Radiology
Cardiothoracic Imaging Section
Department of Radiology
The University of Chicago Medicine
Chicago, IL

Brett W. Carter, MD
Thoracic Radiology
Associate Professor of Radiology
Director of Thoracic CT, Co-Director of Thoracic MRI
The University of Texas MD Anderson Cancer Center
Houston, Texas

Kristopher W. Cummings, MD
Assistant Professor of Radiology
Cardiothoracic Imaging
Mayo Clinic Arizona
Scottsdale, Arizona

Travis S. Henry, MD
Assistant Professor of Clinical Radiology
Cardiac and Pulmonary Imaging Section
Department of Radiology & Biomedical Imaging
University of California, San Francisco
San Francisco, California

Cylen Javidan-Nejad, MD
Associate Professor of Radiology
Fellowship Director
Cardiothoracic Imaging Section
Mallinckrodt Institute of Radiology
Washington University in St. Louis
St. Louis, Missouri

Clinton E. Jokerst, MD
Assistant Professor of Radiology
Cardiothoracic Imaging
Mayo Clinic Arizona
Scottsdale, Arizona

Brent P. Little, MD
Assistant Professor
Division of Cardiothoracic Imaging
Department of Radiology and Imaging Sciences
Emory University School of Medicine
Atlanta, Georgia

Felipe Martínez, MD
Staff Radiologist
Imaging Institute
Cleveland Clinic Florida
Weston, Florida

Bethany Milliron, MD
Radiology Resident
Department of Radiology and Imaging Sciences
Emory University
Atlanta, Georgia

Diana Palacio, MD
Associate Professor
Department of Medical Imaging
The University of Arizona College of Medicine
Tucson, Arizona

Nadeem Parkar, MD
Assistant Professor of Radiology and Internal Medicine
Chief, Cardiac and Thoracic Imaging
Department of Radiology
St. Louis University
St. Louis, Missouri

Constantine Raptis, MD
Associate Professor of Radiology
Co-Director Emergency Radiology
Cardiothoracic Imaging Section
Mallinckrodt Institute of Radiology
Washington University in St. Louis
St. Louis, Missouri

Tyler H. Ternes, MD
Cardiothoracic Radiology
Wichita Radiological Group
Wesley Medical Center
University of Kansas School of Medicine–Wichita
Wichita, Kansas

Aalok Turakhia, MD
Radiologist
Bay Imaging Consultants
Walnut Creek, California

Christopher M. Walker, MD
Thoracic Radiology
St. Luke's Hospital of Kansas City
University of Missouri
Kansas City, Missouri

Section I

Introduction to Chest Radiology

CHAPTER 1

Introduction to Chest Radiology

Melissa L. Rosado-de-Christenson

Introduction

Chest imaging is an integral part of the evaluation of patients who present with thoracic complaints. Chest radiography is usually performed in the initial evaluation of patients with cough, dyspnea, or chest pain. However, it is also frequently performed in asymptomatic individuals undergoing a routine physical exam, a hospital admission, and preoperative assessment, despite its documented low yield for the detection of occult disease in surgical candidates. In addition, a large number of chest radiographs are obtained on hospital inpatients. The latter are frequently performed using portable technique and are often repeated daily.

Chest computed tomography (CT) is also frequently performed, with a marked recent increase in utilization for the evaluation of cardiovascular diseases, particularly by cardiologists. There has also been a modest increase in the utilization of chest CT for noncardiovascular indications. Thoracic magnetic resonance imaging (MRI) outside of cardiovascular indications is not as frequently performed and is reserved mostly for problem solving and further evaluation of abnormalities detected on chest radiography or CT.

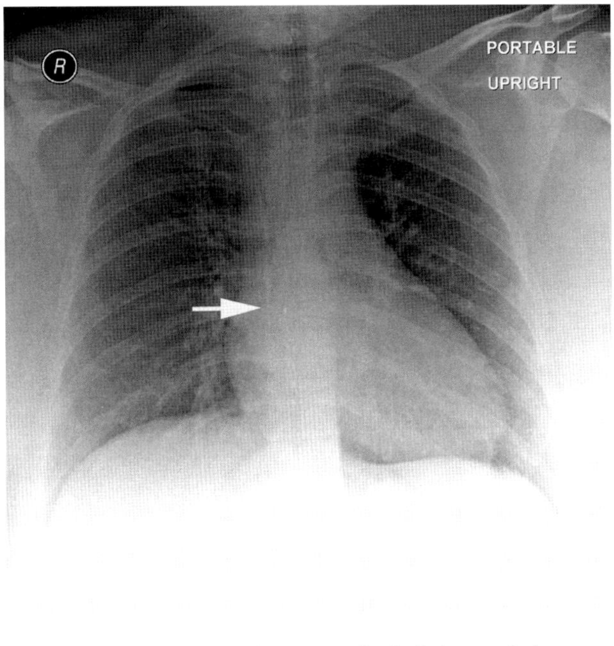

Figure 1.1. Radiography of obese patients. Anteroposterior portable chest radiograph shows a peripherally inserted central catheter (PICC) with tip near the superior cavoatrial junction (arrow). Although radiographic technique and patient positioning are optimal, the PICC tip is difficult to visualize in this large patient.

The Role of the Radiologist

Image Quality

Radiologists should partner with radiologic technologists to continuously assess and improve image quality and ensure optimal technique. Radiologic technologists and quality assurance personnel will benefit from education and guidance regarding issues related to patient positioning and technique. The radiologist must also strive to control radiation exposure to all patients, particularly children, young patients, and pregnant women. Radiographic imaging of obese patients is increasingly performed and presents additional challenges (Fig. 1.1).

Patient Identity

The radiologist should carefully investigate all cases in which the image in question and the comparison image do not appear to belong to the same individual. This problem may be encountered in busy practices and particularly in patients undergoing portable chest radiography. In these cases, imaging features of degenerative osseous changes, prior trauma or surgery, and intrathoracic calcifications can be used to establish that the images indeed belong to the same individual. In patients without the previously mentioned distinguishing features, comparison of the transverse processes of the T1 vertebra, the adjacent posteromedial first ribs, the spinous processes, and the scapular wings has been shown to be very useful in establishing that the radiographs belong to the same subject (Fig. 1.2).

Right Versus Left

Radiologists must always pay attention to right and left markers to determine whether the technologist accurately placed them. Unidentified errors may adversely impact the performance of invasive procedures. Because most patients have the heart and gastric bubble on the left, this is not often an issue on chest radiography. However, the

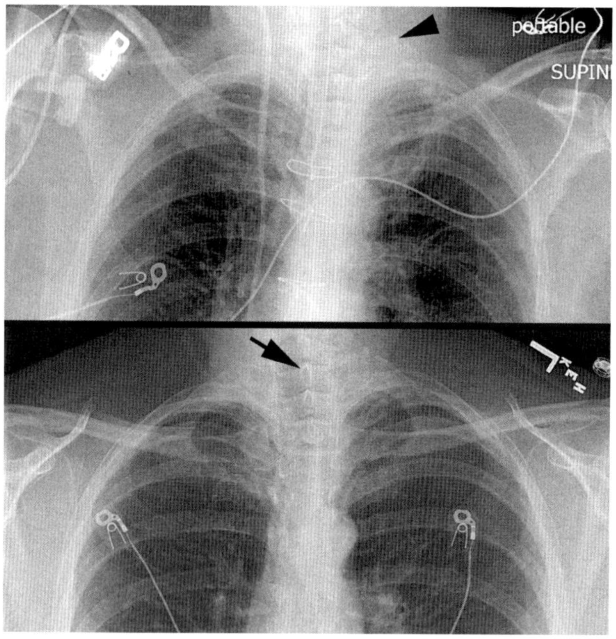

Figure 1.2. Patient identification. Composite image with portable (top) and preoperative (bottom) posteroanterior (PA) chest radiographs shows identical morphologic features of T1 and its spinous (arrow) and transverse (arrowhead) processes, documenting that the images belong to the same patient despite new surgical changes.

radiologist should investigate new cases of aberrant situs to exclude a marker placement error (Fig. 1.3). Although rare, similar mislabeling errors may occur in chest CT, particularly when prone imaging is used, and can usually be solved by reviewing the raw data.

Viewing Conditions

Chest radiographic interpretation requires optimal viewing conditions. Reading rooms should be assessed for noise and lighting levels as well as ambient temperature. Viewing monitors must be clean and must provide appropriate illumination to optimize image viewing and identification of subtle findings.

Imaging Interpretation

Chest imaging remains one of the most challenging areas of diagnostic radiology. Evaluation of the thorax often begins with chest radiography, one of the most difficult studies to interpret given the broad range of structures imaged and the superimposition of complex tissues of air, water, fat, and bone density together with various radiopaque medical devices. In addition, important abnormalities such as early lung cancer may be subtle and easily missed. Thus, radiographic interpretation requires a thorough knowledge of normal imaging anatomy.

Although chest CT is somewhat easier to interpret, accurate assessment is time-consuming and requires a systematic evaluation of the airways, lungs, pleura, mediastinum, and chest wall skeletal structures and soft tissues. In addition, chest imaging with CT often includes portions of the upper abdomen that must also be thoroughly assessed. Given the large number of structures imaged, assessment is typically accomplished in a variety of planes using window and level settings that optimize visualization of various organs. Contrast-enhanced studies require additional scrutiny of contrast-filled cardiovascular structures. Chest

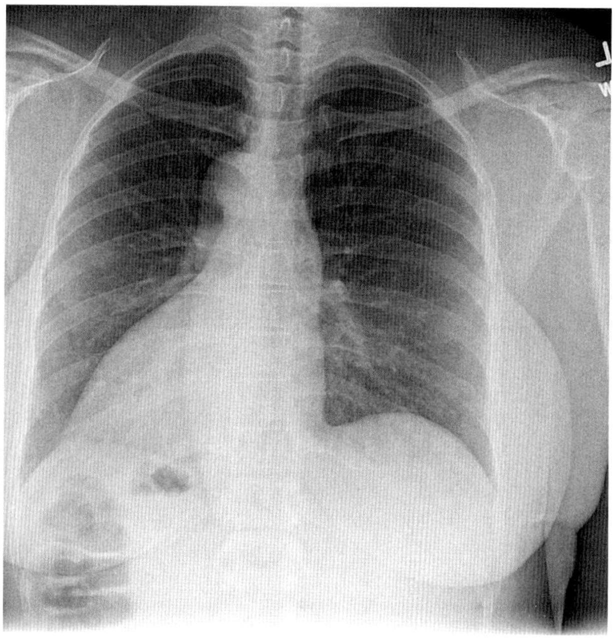

Figure 1.3. Right and left markers. PA chest radiograph of a patient with situs inversus shows a correctly placed left marker that allows the radiologist to suggest the diagnosis despite the unusual appearance of the mediastinal and upper abdominal structures.

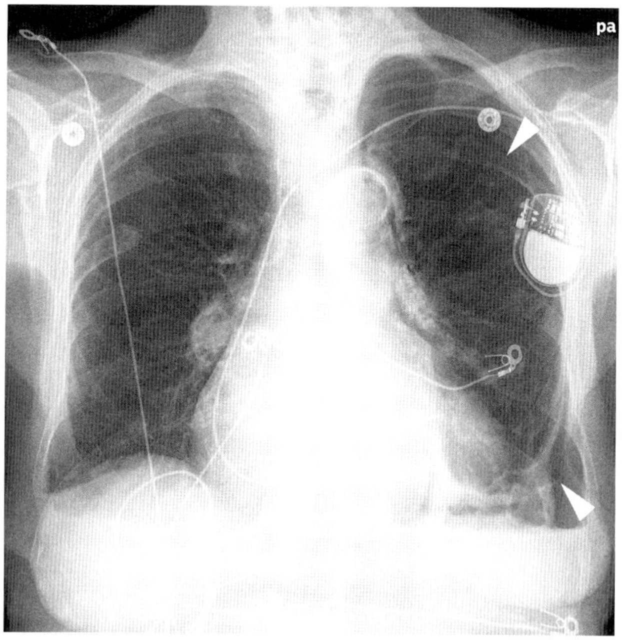

Figure 1.4. Critical findings. PA chest radiograph of a patient status post placement of a left pectoral single-chamber transvenous pacer shows a new left hydropneumothorax (arrowheads), a complication of the procedure. Such critical findings should be promptly communicated to the clinical team.

MRI presents additional challenges because specific imaging sequences and protocols must be employed to optimize evaluation of the structures of interest. Regardless of imaging modality, comparison to prior studies is critical for detecting subtle new findings.

Radiologic Report

The radiologic report should document the imaging study performed, the date of the study, demographic information, clinical indications, a description of the imaging findings, and a clear and unambiguous impression. Abnormal and pertinent incidental findings should be included. Radiologists should carefully review reports for typographical errors. Management recommendations should be included when appropriate. It is generally agreed that structured reporting provides a consistent report format with standardized headings that is advantageous to both radiologists and referring physicians.

Critical Findings

The radiologist should communicate urgent and unexpected findings to the referring physician or a member of the clinical team to expedite appropriate patient management. Such communications should be documented on the report, including the name of the person receiving the communication, the date, and the time (Fig. 1.4).

The Visible Radiologist

Because imaging is such an integral part of clinical diagnosis, radiologists need to partner with clinicians in order to play a greater role in clinical decision-making. There is a current effort to bring the radiologist out of the reading room and render him or her more visible to both consultants and patients. Radiologists have much to contribute to patient care via interdisciplinary medical conferences during which management decisions are made. Patients have increasing access to their medical records, including radiologic reports, and may have questions regarding their content and language. Radiologists should strive to embrace their role as valuable members of the health care team and enhance communication with clinicians, administrators, and patients.

Suggested Reading

American College of Radiology. *ACR Practice Guideline for Communication of Diagnostic Imaging Findings, Revised 2010 (Resolution 11)*. Reston, VA: American College of Radiology; 2010.

Bhalla M, Noble ER, McLean FM, Norris DM, Hicklin OM, Henschke C. Radiographic features useful for establishing patient identity for improperly labeled portable chest radiographs. *J Thorac Imaging*. 1994;9:35–40.

Boland GW. Visibility of radiologists: Helping to secure your future. *AJM Am J Roentgenol*. 2009;192:1373–1374.

Weiss DL, Langlotz CP. Structured reporting: Patient care enhancement or productivity nightmare? *Radiology*. 2008;249:739–747.

CHAPTER 2

Imaging Modalities

Melissa L. Rosado-de-Christenson

Introduction

Various imaging modalities are used to evaluate the thorax. The initial imaging evaluation of patients with thoracic complaints is usually performed with chest radiography. Chest radiographic abnormalities are often further assessed with chest computed tomography (CT), which allows more accurate lesion localization and characterization. Magnetic resonance imaging (MRI) is frequently used in the assessment of cardiovascular abnormalities, and it may be used to evaluate selected cases of mediastinal and chest wall lesions. Positron emission tomography (PET) and PET/CT are routinely employed for staging and restaging patients with malignancy. Ultrasound is used in the assessment of patients with pleural effusion, and it is increasingly employed at the bedside to diagnose pneumothorax. Fluoroscopy is usually performed to evaluate diaphragmatic function. Ventilation–perfusion scintigraphy is used to diagnose pulmonary thromboembolic disease. Skeletal scintigraphy is helpful in the evaluation of osseous lesions identified on radiography or CT and may be used to assess the malignant potential of such lesions. Specialized scintigraphy studies may be used to evaluate glandular abnormalities and specific neoplasms.

Chest Radiography

Posteroanterior (PA) chest radiography (Fig. 2.1a) is optimally performed at full inspiration with the patient in the upright position and the anterior chest placed against the image receptor. The term *PA* refers to the direction of the x-ray beam as it traverses the patient. The scapulae are moved laterally (and away from the lungs) by placing the dorsal wrists against the hips and rotating the shoulders anteriorly. The source–image distance (SID) is 72 in. The beam should be collimated to include the lateral skin surfaces, C7 superiorly and the upper abdomen 3 in. below the costophrenic angles inferiorly. The spinous process of T3 should be equidistant to the medial clavicles, the medial scapulae

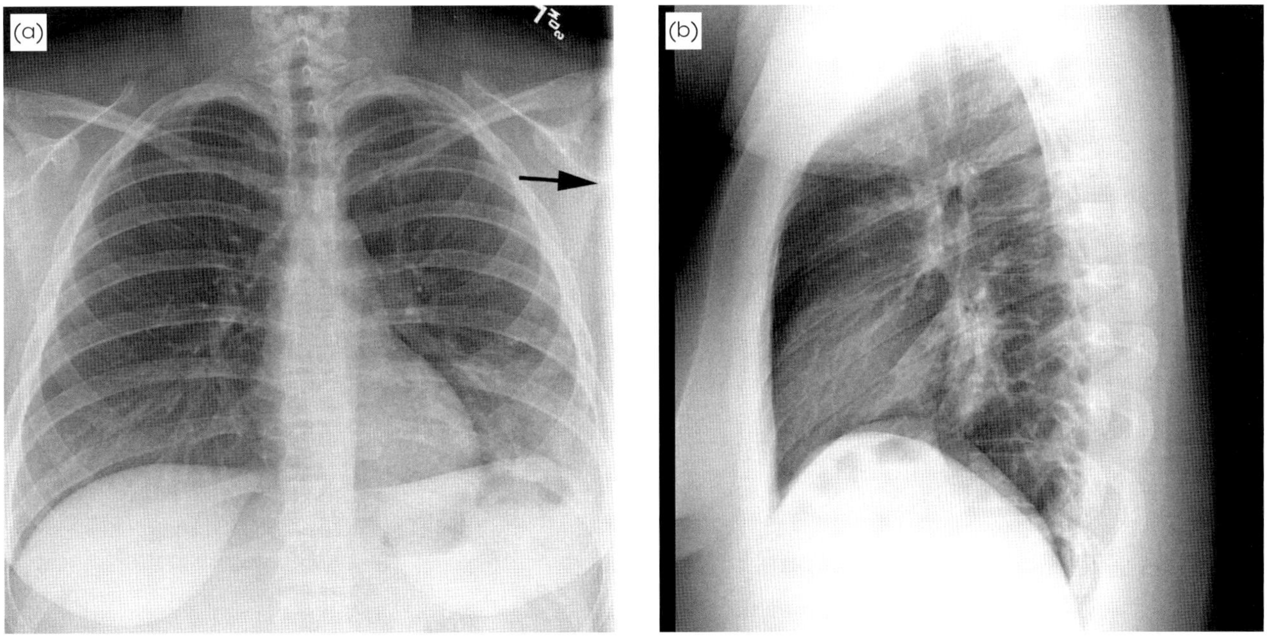

Figure 2.1. PA and lateral chest radiography. (a) PA chest radiograph of a patient with left lower lobe pneumonia shows consolidation in the left base. Patient positioning is not optimal because the left scapula partially overlies the lung. Collimation (arrow) is also not optimal because the left lateral skin surface is excluded. (b) Lateral chest radiograph of the same patient confirms the lower lobe location of the abnormality situated posterior to the major fissure. Patient positioning is not optimal because the soft tissues of the upper extremities overlie the anterior lung apices.

should not be superimposed on the lungs, and the larynx and costophrenic sulci should be visible. Adequate inspiration usually results in displacement of the domes of the hemidiaphragms below the posterior ninth ribs. The posterior basal lung and its pulmonary vessels should be visible through the soft tissue structures of the upper abdomen. Thoracic vertebrae and pulmonary vessels should be visible through the cardiomediastinal silhouette. Entrance skin exposure should not exceed 0.3 mGy, high kilovoltage technique (120–150 kVp) should be used, and scatter should be reduced with a grid. High kilovoltage radiographs allow greater penetration of the mediastinum and osseous structures. The shorter exposure time allows pulmonary structures to appear sharper.

Lateral chest radiography (Fig. 2.1b) is optimally performed with the patient in an upright nonrotated position with the left chest against the image receptor (left lateral chest radiograph). The arms should be raised above the head to avoid superimposition over the thorax.

Anteroposterior (AP) chest radiography (Figs. 2.2 and 2.3) is often performed on infants and critically ill, debilitated, and traumatized patients. AP chest radiography may be performed in the supine, semi-upright, or sitting positions with the patient's back against the image receptor. The x-ray beam traverses the patient in an anteroposterior direction. The clavicles usually follow a horizontal course, and the scapulae are often superimposed on the lateral aspects of the upper lungs. AP chest radiographs are typically exposed with a SID of 40 in. This shorter SID results in magnification of structures. Because high kilovoltage techniques cannot be used, there is less penetration of dense structures and increased exposure times with resultant decreased sharpness of visualized pulmonary structures.

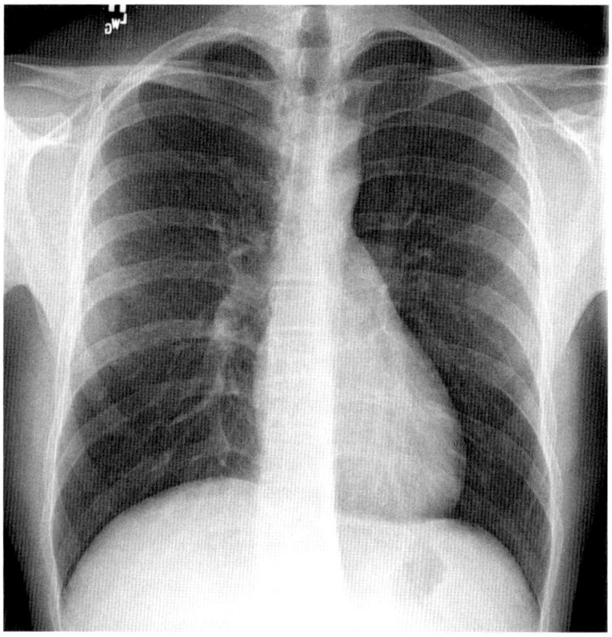

Figure 2.2. Portable chest radiography. Normal AP chest radiograph of a relatively healthy patient shows horizontal orientation of the medial clavicles and the bilateral scapulae overlying the lateral aspects of the lungs. Imaging should be reserved for symptomatic patients, and patients should be imaged with PA and lateral chest radiography whenever possible.

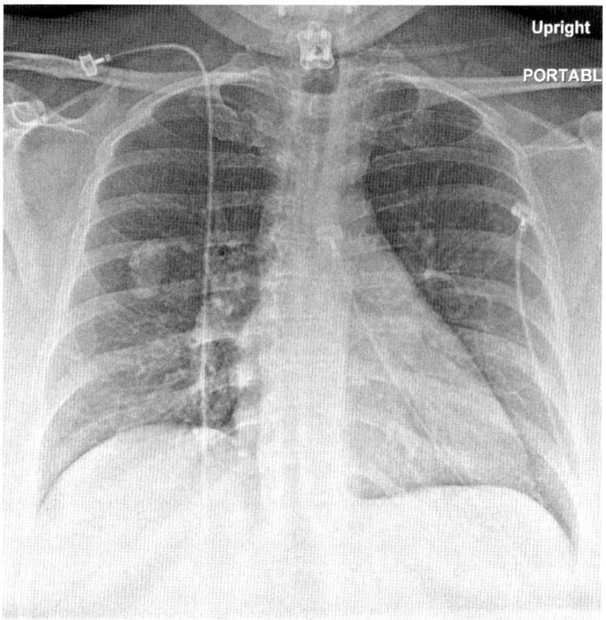

Figure 2.3. Portable chest radiography. AP portable chest radiograph of a patient who presented with cough shows a large right mid lung zone calcified granuloma. Note the horizontal orientation of the medial clavicles and superimposition of the scapulae over the lateral aspects of the lungs. The lordotic projection is not intentional but frequently seen on AP radiography.

Apical lordotic chest radiography is achieved by cranial angulation of the x-ray beam and results in the clavicles projecting above the lung apices in order to visualize apical abnormalities. In fact, many AP portable chest radiographs exhibit features of the lordotic radiographic projection.

Decubitus chest radiography (Fig. 2.4) may be used to assess pleural effusion or pneumothorax and to exclude aspirated foreign bodies in infants and young children. The patient is imaged on his or her side using AP or PA technique and a horizontal x-ray beam. Visualization of the recumbent side is facilitated by "raising" the patient from the table using a foam mat.

Fluoroscopy

Fluoroscopy allows evaluation of diaphragmatic motion during respiration. The patient is asked to sniff or breathe in rapidly through the nose (sniff test) to elicit paradoxical hemidiaphragmatic motion in cases of paralysis (abnormal cephalad movement of the paralyzed hemidiaphragm and caudal movement of the normal hemidiaphragm).

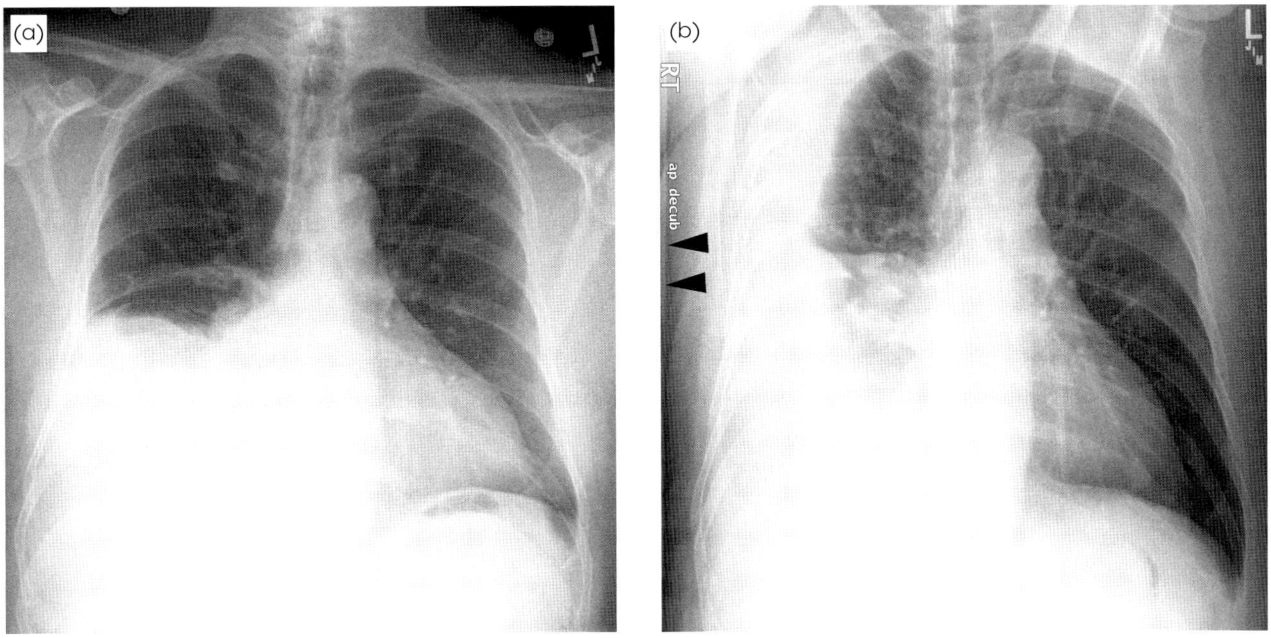

Figure 2.4. Decubitus chest radiography. (a) PA chest radiograph of a patient with dyspnea shows a large right pleural effusion that manifests as right basilar opacity with a superior convexity that mimics the hemidiaphragm. (b) Right lateral decubitus chest radiograph of the same patient confirms a large free right pleural effusion layering in the dependent right pleural space. Visualization of the right lateral pleural surface and right chest wall is achieved by placing the patient on a foam mat (arrowheads).

Chest CT

Chest CT is often used to evaluate radiographic abnormalities and to assess the vascular structures of the chest. CT cross-sectional imaging allows a systematic assessment of the lungs, airways, pleura, mediastinal structures, and chest wall. Additional multiplanar images, minimum and maximum intensity projections, and surface shaded display images may help further evaluate or optimally demonstrate specific findings.

Unenhanced chest CT is usually sufficient for the assessment of the lung, airways, and mediastinal lymph nodes. Evaluation of pulmonary nodules is enhanced with thin-section images to detect calcification and to determine attenuation characteristics including ground-glass attenuation and cavitation.

Contrast-enhanced chest CT is used to evaluate the heart, blood vessels, thymus, and hilar lymph nodes. It is particularly helpful in staging and restaging malignancy. CT angiography is used extensively in the evaluation of pulmonary thromboembolic disease, acute aortic syndrome, and traumatic vascular injury (Fig. 2. 5).

High-resolution chest CT (HRCT) is used to evaluate diffuse infiltrative pulmonary processes (Fig. 2.6). It is characterized by thin (1–2 mm) collimation of images and a high spatial frequency (preferably bone) algorithm. Expiratory HRCT allows identification of air-trapping in patients with small airways disease. Prone imaging allows distinction between dependent atelectasis (which resolves in the prone position) and subtle posterior subpleural interstitial lung disease (Fig. 2.6).

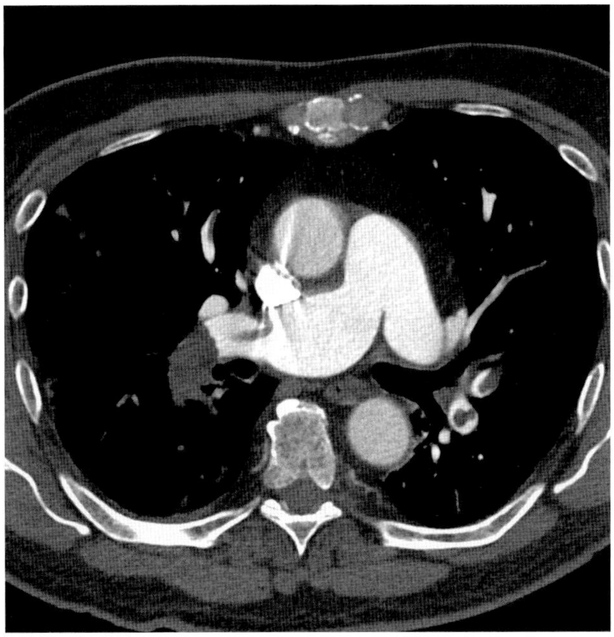

Figure 2.5. Chest CT: CT pulmonary angiography. Contrast-enhanced CT pulmonary angiogram shows enlargement of the pulmonary arteries and extensive pulmonary thromboemboli. Contrast-enhanced chest CT is optimal for vascular imaging.

Chest MRI

Chest MRI is often used to further assess specific abnormalities, including chest wall involvement by neoplasms (including Pancoast tumors) and vascular involvement by mediastinal malignancies (superior vena cava obstruction

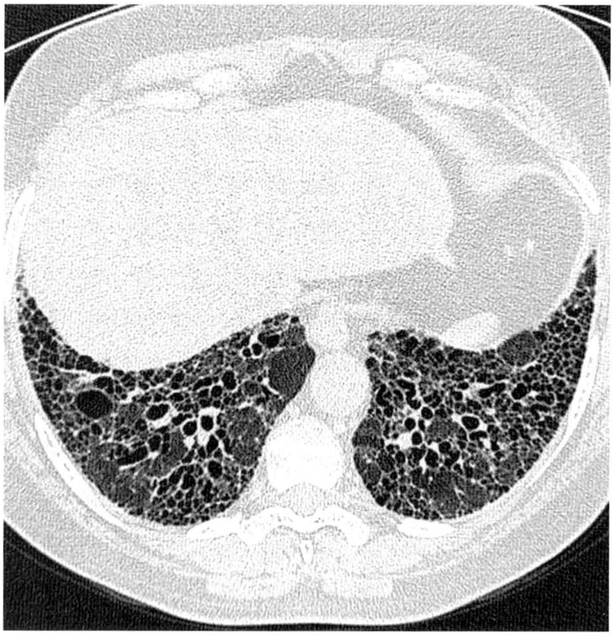

Figure 2.6. Chest CT: high-resolution CT. Unenhanced HRCT of a patient with usual interstitial pneumonia (UIP) and chronic dyspnea shows basilar honeycombing and traction bronchiectasis. The patient was imaged in the prone position to minimize posterior-dependent atelectasis. HRCT is the imaging modality of choice for evaluating diffuse infiltrative lung disease.

and vascular invasion). MRI is particularly useful in the evaluation of the thymus for distinction between hyperplasia and neoplasia based on signal drop on in-phase and out-of-phase imaging (Fig. 2.7). Thymic MRI is also helpful in distinguishing solid from cystic thymic lesions. MRI angiography is routinely used in some centers for the evaluation of aortic pathology and pulmonary thromboembolic disease.

FDG PET/CT

PET imaging is frequently employed for oncologic imaging. It relies on the intravenous administration of fluorodeoxyglucose (2-deoxy-2[^{18}F]-fluoro-D-glucose) or FDG, and images show the rate of glucose metabolism in the body. Combined PET/CT imaging allows fusion of FDG PET with corresponding CT images to anatomically localize metabolic abnormalities. FDG PET/CT allows identification of areas of avid glucose metabolism characteristic of metabolically active malignant neoplasms (Fig. 2.8). However, indolent malignant neoplasms may show little metabolic activity, and benign infectious or inflammatory conditions may be intensely FDG-avid, producing false-negative and false-positive findings, respectively.

Scintigraphy

Ventilation–perfusion (V/Q) scintigraphy is used for the evaluation of pulmonary thromboembolism. Although most patients with suspected pulmonary thromboembolism are usually imaged with CT pulmonary angiography, V/Q scintigraphy remains a valuable imaging modality, particularly when taking into account clinical probability, D-dimer assay, and findings on chest radiography. The lower radiation dose to the chest makes this test ideally suited for the evaluation of young patients, especially young women and pregnant women.

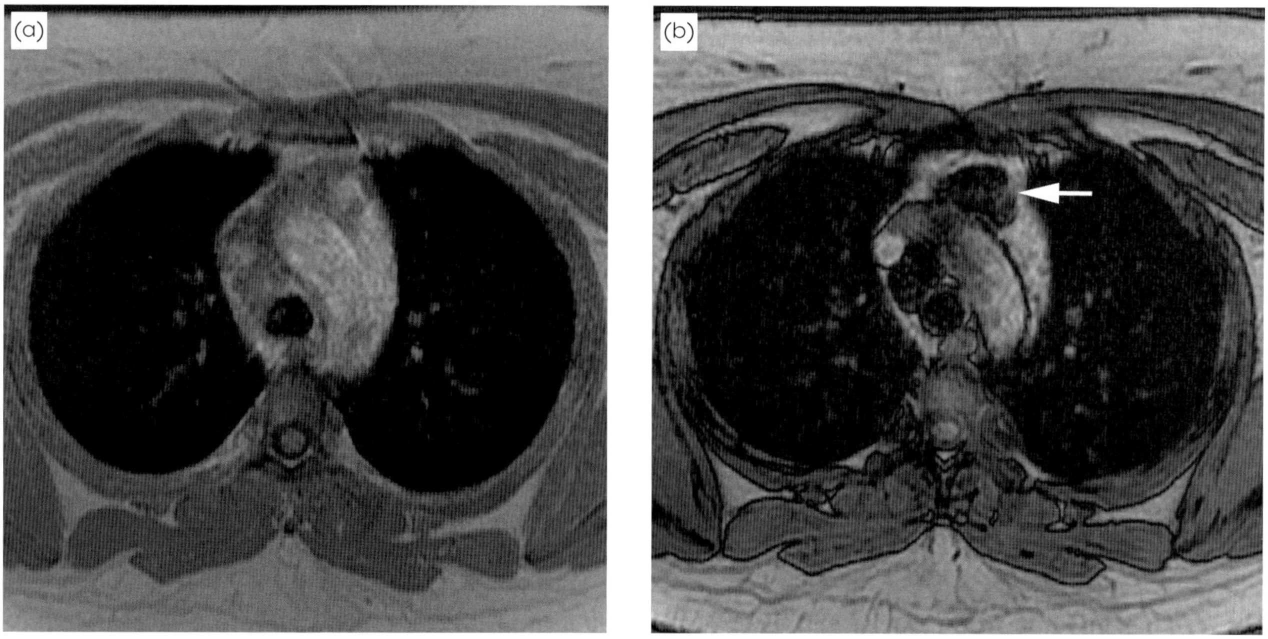

Figure 2.7. Chest MRI: chemical shift thymic imaging. In-phase (a) and opposed-phase (b) gradient-echo T1-weighted MR images show decrease in the signal intensity of the thymus (arrow) consistent with the diagnosis of thymic hyperplasia.

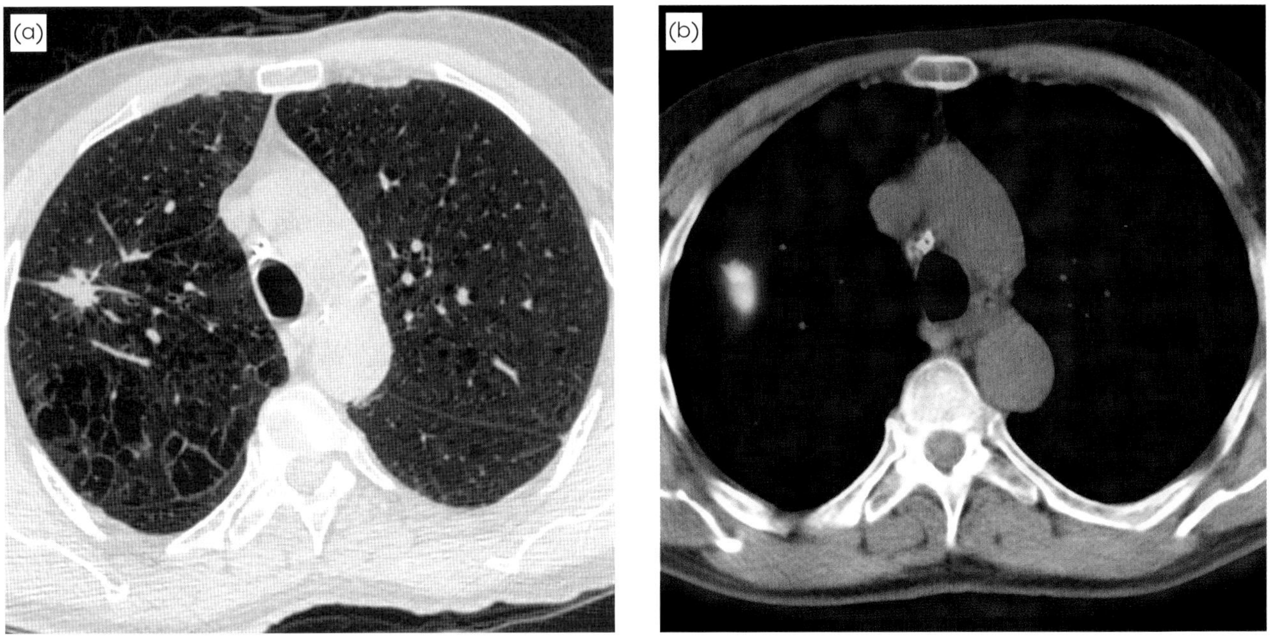

Figure 2.8. FDG PET/CT. (a) Unenhanced chest CT shows a primary squamous cell carcinoma manifesting as a spiculated right upper lobe nodule with a pleural tag on a background of centrilobular and paraseptal emphysema. (b) PET/CT of the same patient shows intense FDG uptake in the nodule consistent with malignancy.

Iodine nuclear scintigraphy is used for the evaluation of the thyroid gland and particularly ectopic thyroid tissue. Parathyroid radionuclide imaging (sestamibi) is used for identifying hyperfunctioning parathyroid tissue. Somatostatin receptor scintigraphy with ^{111}In-octreotide is useful in the evaluation of carcinoid tumors.

Ultrasound

Thoracic ultrasound is useful in the assessment of the abnormal pleural space, specifically for the detection and characterization of pleural effusions. Thoracic ultrasound is also routinely employed for image-guided fluid drainage and lesion biopsy. Thyroid ultrasound is widely utilized for the assessment of thyroid lesions and for image-guided biopsy of suspicious thyroid abnormalities.

Comment

Recent advances in chest CT including the introduction of multidetector CT, optimized scanning protocols, and image reformations have greatly facilitated the expeditious noninvasive diagnosis of thoracic abnormalities. However, the ease of performance and wide availability of CT imaging has brought about an increased utilization of CT with a resultant increase in the radiation dose received by the population imaged. The radiologist should play an active role and work closely with radiation technologists and physicists toward dose reduction from medical imaging through optimization of CT protocols. Radiologists should also strive to open avenues of communication with clinicians and other health care providers and educate them regarding the optimal imaging study for the specific clinical indication.

Suggested Reading

Hansell DM, Lynch DA, McAdams HP, Bankier AA, eds. Technical considerations. In: *Imaging of Diseases of the Chest*, 5th ed. Philadelphia: Mosby; 2010:1–37.

Inaoka T, Takahashi K, Mineta M, et al. Thymic hyperplasia and thymus gland tumors: Differentiation with chemical shift MR imaging. *Radiology*. 2007;243:869–876.

Kuyumcu S, Adalet I, Sanli Y, Turkmen C, Ozkan ZG, Yilmazbayhan D. Somatostatin receptor scintigraphy with ^{111}In-octreotide in pulmonary carcinoid tumors correlated with pathological and 18 FDG PET/CT findings. *Ann Nucl Med*. 2012;26:689–697.

Moss IC, Klok FA, Kroft LJ, de Roos A, Huisman MV. Imaging tests in the diagnosis of pulmonary embolism. *Semin Respir Crit Care Med*. 2012;33:138–143.

Smith-Bindman R, Miglioretti DL, Johnson E, et al. Use of diagnostic imaging studies and associated radiation exposure for patients enrolled in large integrated healthcare systems, 1996–2010. *JAMA*. 2012;307:2400–2409.

CHAPTER 3

Overview of Normal Thoracic Imaging Anatomy

Melissa L. Rosado-de-Christenson

Definition

The word "anatomy" derives from the Greek *anatemnŏ*, which means to "cut open" and refers to the scientific study of the body. Although basic knowledge of anatomy is principally based on dissection studies, medical imaging provides the opportunity to study anatomy in vivo. Because disease processes alter the normal anatomy and physiology of various organs, there has been recent significant growth in the use of medical imaging for the initial evaluation of suspected disease. Radiographic anatomy is complex given the superimposition of numerous structures and organs of various anatomic densities and the fact a radiograph is a two-dimensional image of a three-dimensional body region. Orthogonal imaging (imaging at 90° angles) is crucial for the radiographic localization of structures in three dimensions. Computed tomography (CT) and magnetic resonance imaging (MRI) allow visualization and identification of structures in the *x*, *y*, and *z* axes and precise localization of abnormalities as they relate to adjacent structures. Knowledge of normal imaging anatomy allows the radiologist to readily recognize and assess anatomic variants and abnormalities, even when subtle.

Thoracic Anatomy

Thoracic imaging allows visualization and evaluation of the lungs, airways, pulmonary vessels, hila, pleura, mediastinum, and the osseous and soft tissue structures of the chest wall.

Lungs

The lungs are mostly composed of air-filled alveoli and the intervening pulmonary interstitium. The normal interstitium is not visible on radiography, and its visualization should suggest interstitial lung disease. The interstitium is also typically invisible on CT, but the location of interlobular septa may be inferred based on visualization of peripheral pulmonary veins (which course in the interlobular septa). The interlobar fissures divide the lungs into lobes, are often visible on radiography, and are consistently visualized on chest CT.

Airways

Radiography allows identification of the central airways: trachea, mainstem bronchi, and some lobar and segmental bronchi. Normal bronchi in the mid to peripheral lungs are not visible on radiography. Chest CT provides optimal visualization of bronchi, which are paired with corresponding pulmonary artery branches. CT demonstrates great variation in airway branching patterns. Normal bronchioles are not usually visible on CT.

Pulmonary Vessels

Central pulmonary arteries and veins are readily visualized on radiography. Distinction between arteries and veins can be made on cross-sectional imaging based on vessel course and location with respect to adjacent airways.

Systemic Vessels

The aorta gives rise to the great vessels of the head and upper body as well as intercostal and bronchial arteries. The bilateral brachiocephalic veins anastomose to form the superior vena cava, which also receives venous tributaries from the azygos and hemiazygos venous systems. The aorta, left subclavian artery, and superior and inferior vena cava interfaces are visible on radiography and all systemic vessels are well visualized on CT and MRI.

Hila

The hilum is the point of connection between the medial lung and the adjacent mediastinum. Bronchi and vessels course between lung and mediastinum through the hilum. The hilum contains pulmonary arteries, pulmonary veins, central airways, lymph nodes, and intervening fat. However, the radiographic hilar opacity is predominantly composed of pulmonary arteries and superior pulmonary veins. The hila should always be evaluated for their position with respect to each other because abnormal hilar displacement is a sign of volume loss. Contrast-enhanced chest CT and chest MRI allow visualization and characterization of the vascular, airway, and lymph node components of the hila.

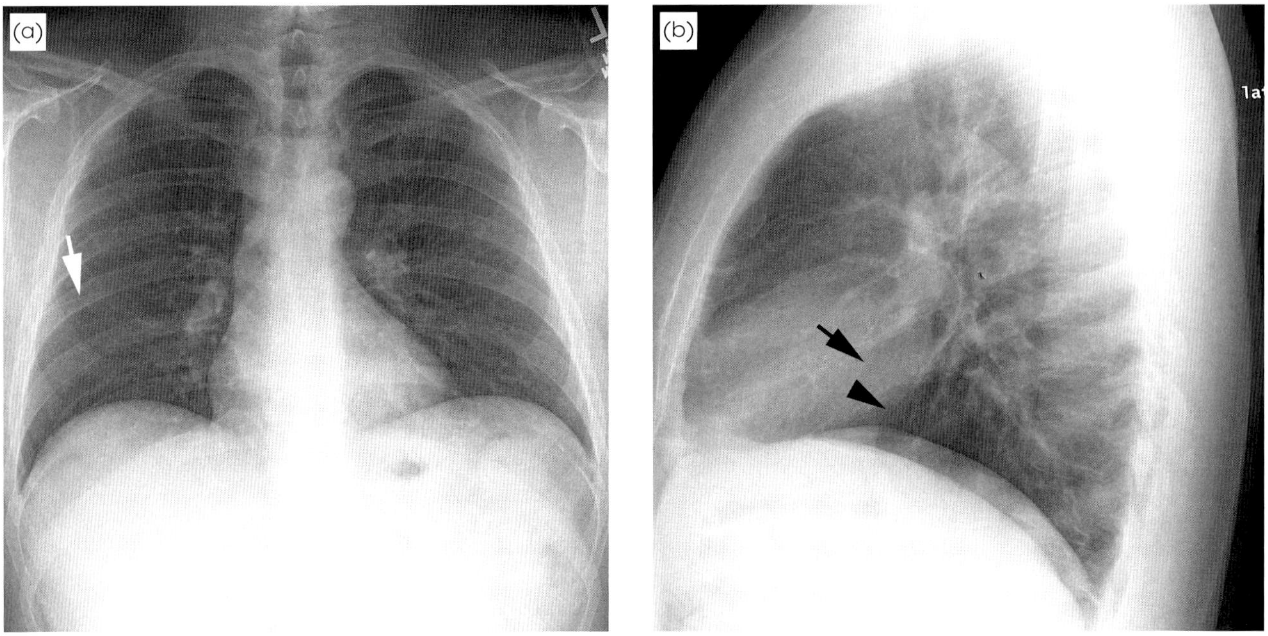

Figure 3.1. Lung lobes and interlobar fissures. (a) Normal posteroanterior (PA) chest radiograph shows partial visualization of the minor fissure (arrow) located between the right upper and middle lobes. (b) Lateral chest radiograph of the same patient shows partial visualization of the right (arrow) and left (arrowhead) major fissures located between the lower lobes posteriorly and the upper and middle lobes anteriorly. The normal interlobar fissures may be subtle on radiography.

Mediastinum

The mediastinum is the space between the lungs and pleural spaces, extends from the thoracic inlet to the diaphragm, and is bound anteriorly by the chest wall and posteriorly by the vertebral bodies. The paravertebral areas are not part of the mediastinum proper but form part of the radiographic posterior mediastinum in the Felson classification of mediastinal compartments. The mediastinum contains the heart, pericardium, thymus, trachea, esophagus, great arteries and veins, thoracic duct, nerves, lymph nodes, and fat.

Pleura

The pleura is a continuous surface epithelium consisting of visceral and parietal components according to the thoracic structures it lines. The visceral pleura lines the lungs (including the fissures) and the parietal pleura lines the nonpulmonary surfaces, including the chest wall, diaphragm, and mediastinum. The apposition of these pleural surfaces forms a potential space called the pleural space.

Chest Wall

The chest wall is composed of skeletal (vertebrae, ribs, and sternum) and soft tissue (skin, muscle, fat, nerves, lymphatics, blood vessels, and endothoracic fascia) structures.

Thoracic Imaging Anatomy

Chest radiography allows assessment of structures in all thoracic anatomic regions. Cross-sectional imaging with CT and MRI provides excellent visualization and characterization of structures in all anatomic areas.

Lungs and Pleura

- The right lung has three lobes: upper, middle, and lower.
- The left lung has two lobes: upper and lower.
- Each lung lobe is supplied by lobar, segmental, and subsegmental bronchi and accompanying vascular structures.
- Each lobe is lined by visceral pleura; interlobar fissures are composed of two apposed visceral pleural layers and are often incomplete. Radiographic visualization of interlobar fissures allows identification of pulmonary lobes.
- The normal pleura may be visible at the interlobar fissures. The minor fissure courses horizontally from the hilum on frontal radiography and is located anteriorly on lateral radiographs. It manifests as an ovoid lucency devoid of vasculature on axial CT. The major fissures are optimally visualized on lateral chest radiography and are visible as thin soft tissue lines on axial CT (Figs. 3.1 and 3.2).
- Accessory fissures include azygos (Fig. 3.3), superior accessory (Fig. 3.2), inferior accessory, and left minor.
- The right upper lobe abuts the upper mediastinum and is located above the minor fissure and anterior to the major fissure. The middle lobe abuts the right cardiac border and is located between the minor fissure and the inferior aspect of the major fissure. The right lower lobe abuts the mediastinum and paravertebral region and is posterior to the major fissure.

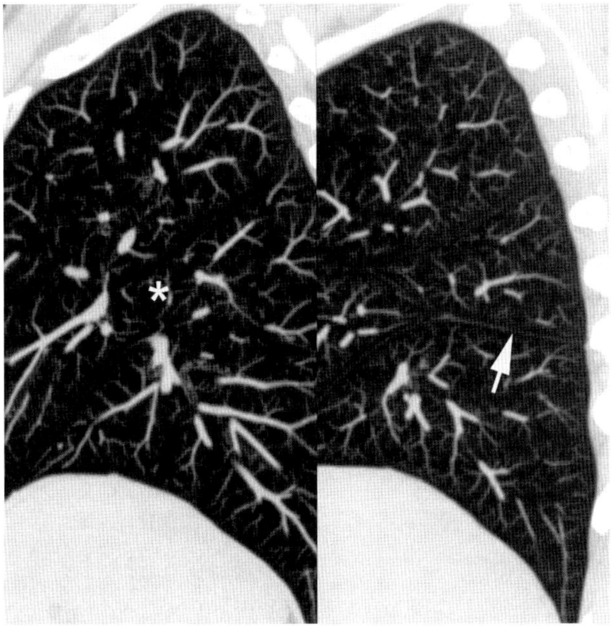

Figure 3.2. Interlobar and accessory fissures. Composite image with sagittal chest CT shows an incomplete major fissure with a "bridge" of lung (asterisk) connecting the upper and lower lobes. The superior accessory fissure (arrow) separates the lower lobe superior segment from the basilar segments.

- The left upper lobe abuts the mediastinum and is located anterior to the major fissure. The lingular segments abut the left cardiac border. The left lower lobe abuts the mediastinum and paravertebral region and is located posterior to the major fissure.

Airways

- The trachea courses vertically and slightly to the right of midline.
- The right mainstem bronchus gives rise to upper, middle, and lower lobe bronchi. The bronchus intermedius is immediately below the origin of the right upper lobe bronchus and gives rise to the middle and right lower lobe bronchi (Figs. 3.4 and 3.5).
- The left mainstem bronchus gives rise to upper and lower lobe bronchi (Figs. 3.4 and 3.5).
- The right upper lobe bronchus is eparterial and arises above the right pulmonary artery; the left upper lobe bronchus is hyparterial and arises below the left pulmonary artery (Fig. 3.6).
- Right upper lobe bronchus branches: Apical, anterior, and posterior segmental bronchi.
- Middle lobe bronchus branches: Medial and lateral segmental bronchi.
- Right lower lobe bronchus branches: Superior, medial basilar, anterior basilar, lateral basilar, and posterior basilar segmental bronchi.
- Left upper lobe bronchus branches: Apicoposterior, anterior, superior lingular, and inferior lingular segmental bronchi.
- Left lower lobe bronchus branches: Superior, anteromedial basilar, lateral basilar, and posterior basilar segmental bronchi.
- Bronchial branching is highly variable.

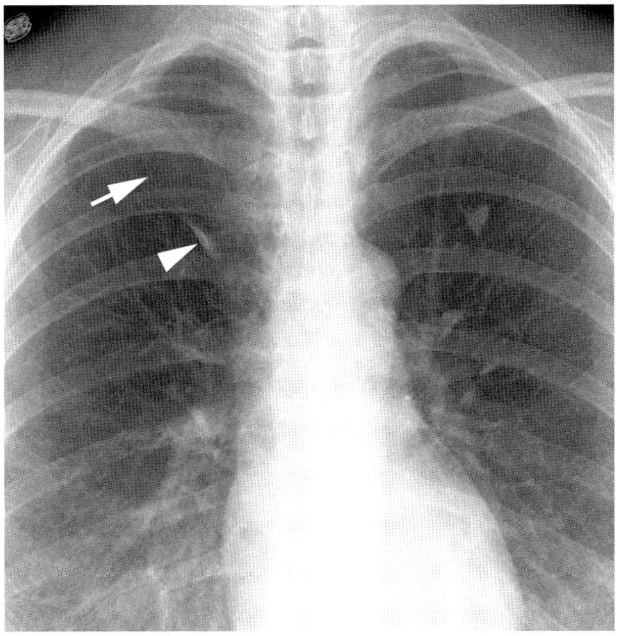

Figure 3.3. Accessory azygos fissure. Coned-down PA chest radiograph shows an accessory azygos fissure that manifests as a right upper lobe thin arcuate line (arrow) that terminates in the tear-shaped azygos arch (arrowhead). Note the absence of the azygos arch at the right tracheobronchial angle.

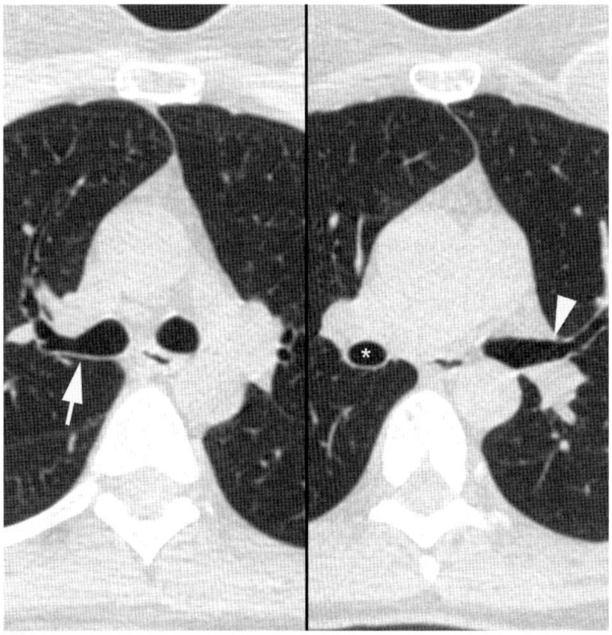

Figure 3.4. Central bronchi. Composite image with unenhanced chest CT shows the right (arrow) and left (arrowhead) upper lobe bronchi. The bronchus intermedius (asterisk) is the continuation of the right tracheobronchial tree below the orifice of the right upper lobe bronchus.

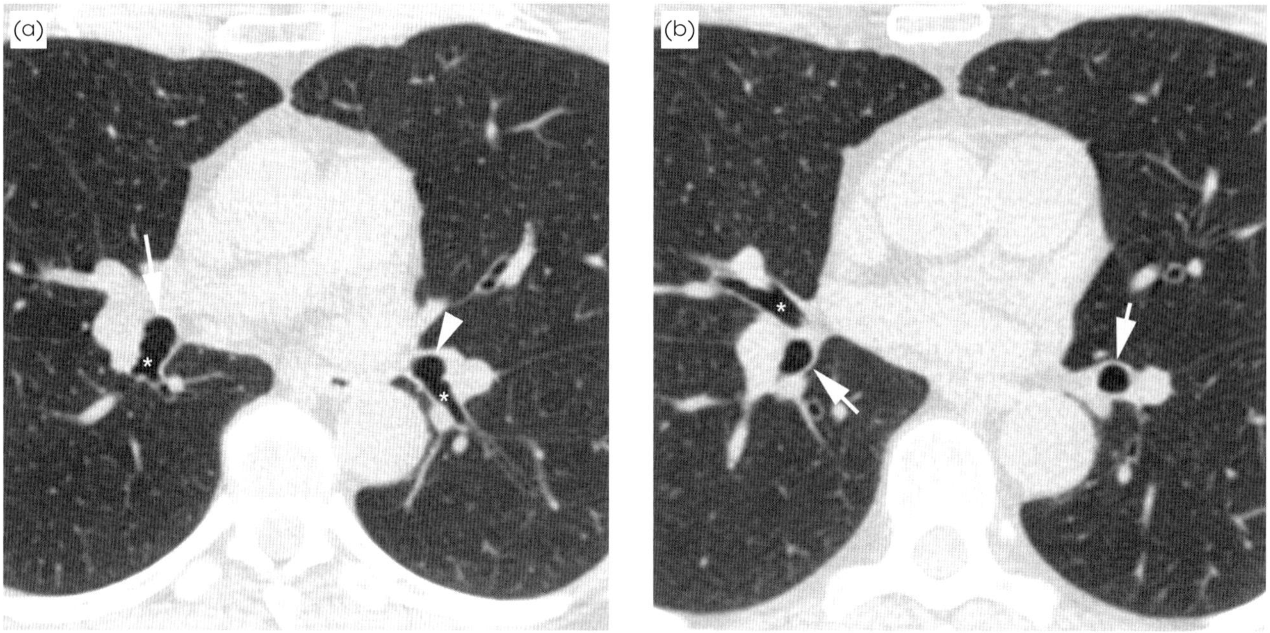

Figure 3.5. Central bronchi. (a) Unenhanced chest CT shows the right (arrow) and left (arrowhead) lower lobe bronchi giving rise to corresponding superior segmental bronchi (asterisks). (b) Unenhanced chest CT shows the middle lobe bronchus (asterisk) and the bilateral lower lobe truncus basalis bronchi (arrows) above the origins of the basilar segmental lower lobe bronchi.

Pulmonary Vessels

- See Fig. 3.7.
- The pulmonary trunk arises from the right ventricular outflow tract and gives rise to right and left pulmonary arteries. It contributes to the radiographic left mediastinal border caudal to the aortopulmonary window and cephalad to the left atrial appendage. It is anterior and to the left of the ascending aorta on cross-sectional imaging and normally measures up to 28.6 mm transversely at the level of the bifurcation.
- The pulmonary arteries supply each lung and branch along their corresponding bronchi.
- The interlobar pulmonary arteries course inferiorly from the hila.
- The pulmonary artery branches are generally located medial to the corresponding airways in the upper lobes and lateral to the corresponding airways in the lower lobes.
- The pulmonary veins follow a relatively horizontal course toward the left atrium and are generally located lateral to the airways in the upper lobes and medial to the airways in the lower lobes.
- Pulmonary vessel size tapers toward the lung periphery.

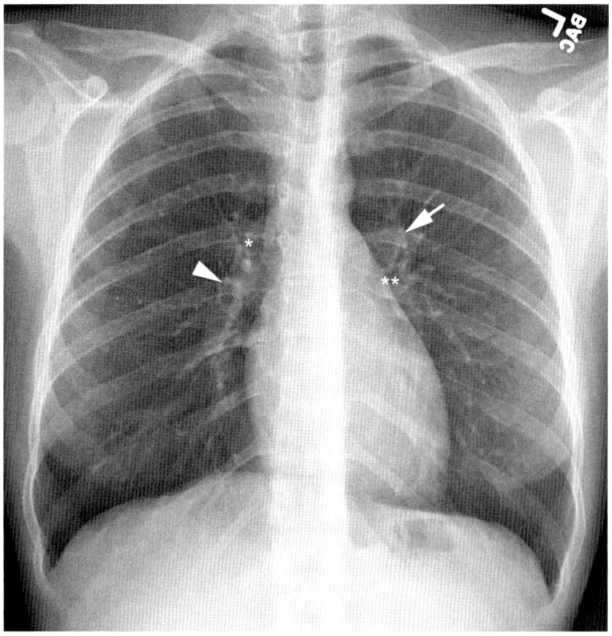

Figure 3.6. Upper lobe bronchial morphology. PA chest radiograph shows normal tracheobronchial morphology. The right upper lobe bronchus (asterisk) is eparterial and arises above the ipsilateral pulmonary artery (arrowhead). The left upper lobe bronchus (double asterisk) is hyparterial and arises below the ipsilateral pulmonary artery (arrow).

Systemic Vessels

- See Fig. 3.7.
- The thoracic aorta arises from the left ventricular outflow tract and consists of the ascending thoracic aorta, the aortic arch, and the descending aorta. The ascending aorta is located posterior and to the right of the pulmonary trunk. Most patients have a left aortic arch. The aortic arch gives rise to the brachiocephalic, left common carotid, and left subclavian arteries. The descending aorta is usually located to the left of midline.

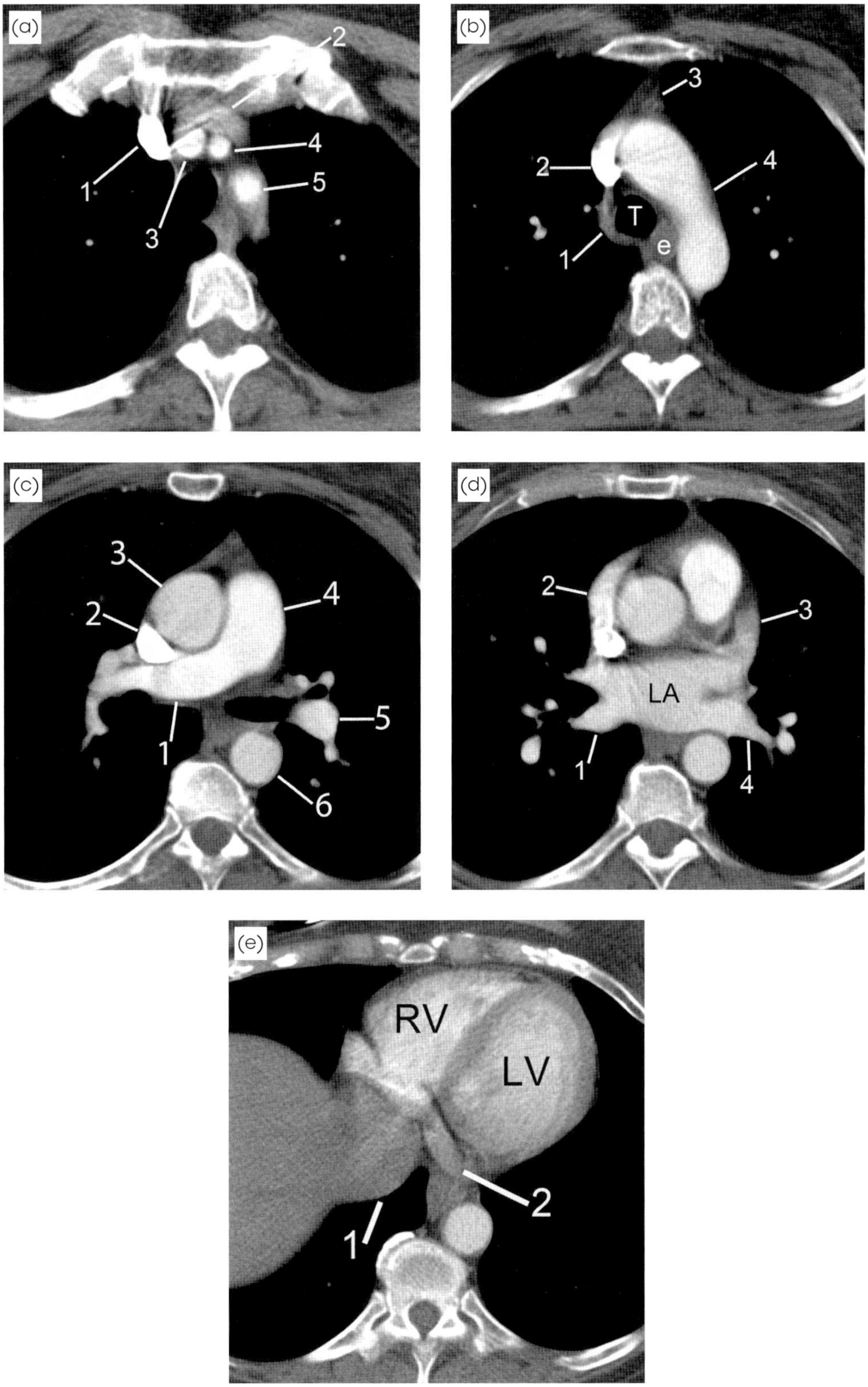

Figure 3.7. Thoracic vessels and other structures on axial contrast-enhanced chest CT. (a) Right (1) and left (2) brachiocephalic veins and the brachiocephalic (3), left common carotid (4), and left subclavian (5) arteries. (b) Azygos arch (1), superior vena cava (2), thymus (3), and aortic arch (4). e, esophagus; T, trachea. (c) Right pulmonary artery (1), superior vena cava (2), ascending aorta (3), pulmonary trunk (4), left interlobar pulmonary artery (5), and descending aorta (6). (d) Right inferior pulmonary vein (1), right atrial appendage (2), left atrial appendage (3), and left inferior pulmonary vein (4). LA, left atrium. (e) Inferior vena cava (1) and coronary sinus (2). LV, left ventricle; RV, right ventricle.

- The inferior vena cava drains into the lower right atrium.
- The superior vena cava is formed by the anastomosis of the right and left brachiocephalic veins and drains into the upper right atrium.
- The azygos and hemiazygos veins drain into the posterior wall of the inferior vena cava via the azygos arch, which is located at the right tracheobronchial angle.
- The azygos vein ascends on the right adjacent to the right anterior aspect of the lower and midthoracic vertebral bodies.
- The hemiazygos vein ascends on the left adjacent to the left anterior aspect of the lower and midthoracic vertebral bodies and crosses the midline to drain into the azygos vein.

Hila

- See Fig. 3.8.
- The right hilum is lower than the left on frontal radiography in 97% of cases, and it is at the same level as the left in 3% of cases (Fig. 3.6).
- On lateral radiography, the right hilum is anterior and inferior to the distal trachea, and the left hilum is posterior and inferior. The right hilar density is composed of pulmonary arteries and veins and is called the right hilar vascular opacity; the left hilar density is mostly composed of the left pulmonary artery.
- On lateral radiography, the right upper lobe bronchus is located cephalad to the left. The right upper lobe bronchus is visible in 45% of normal radiographs, whereas the left upper lobe bronchus (left mainstem–left upper lobe bronchus continuum) is visible in 75%.
- The posterior walls of the right mainstem bronchus and bronchus intermedius form the intermediate stem line, which measures less than 4 mm in thickness.

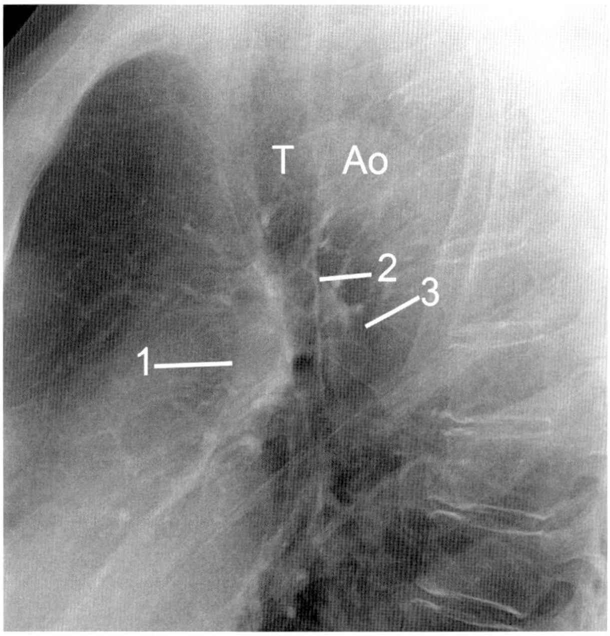

Figure 3.8. Hila on lateral radiography. Right hilar vascular opacity (1), intermediate stem line (2), and left interlobar pulmonary artery (3). Ao, aortic arch; T, trachea.

Mediastinum

- See Fig. 3.9.
- Frontal chest radiography: Right mediastinal contours from cephalad to caudad include the superior vena cava interface and the right atrium. Left mediastinal contours from cephalad to caudad include the left subclavian artery interface, the aortic arch, the aortopulmonary window, the pulmonary trunk, the left atrial appendage, and the left ventricle.

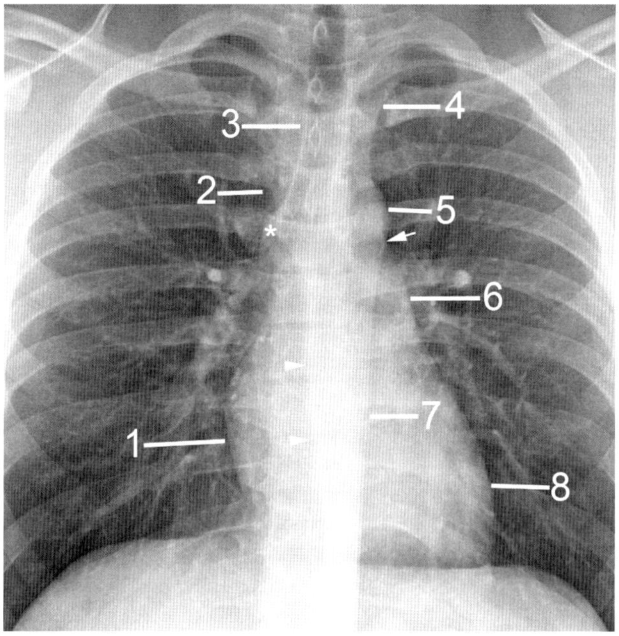

Figure 3.9. Mediastinal interfaces on radiography. Right atrium (1), superior vena cava interface (2), right paratracheal stripe (3), left subclavian artery interface (4), aortic arch (5), pulmonary trunk (6), left paraaortic interface (7), and left ventricle (8). Azygoesophageal recess (arrowheads), azygos arch (asterisk), and aortopulmonary window (arrow).

- Lateral chest radiography: Anterior mediastinal contours from cephalad to caudad include pulmonary trunk and right ventricle. Posterior mediastinal contours include thoracic aorta, left atrium, left ventricle, and inferior vena cava.
- Mediastinal lines: The anterior junction line represents the points of contact of the upper lobes (and pleural surfaces) anterior to the mediastinum. The posterior junction line represents the points of contact of the upper lobes (and pleural surfaces) posterior to the mediastinum (Fig. 3.10).

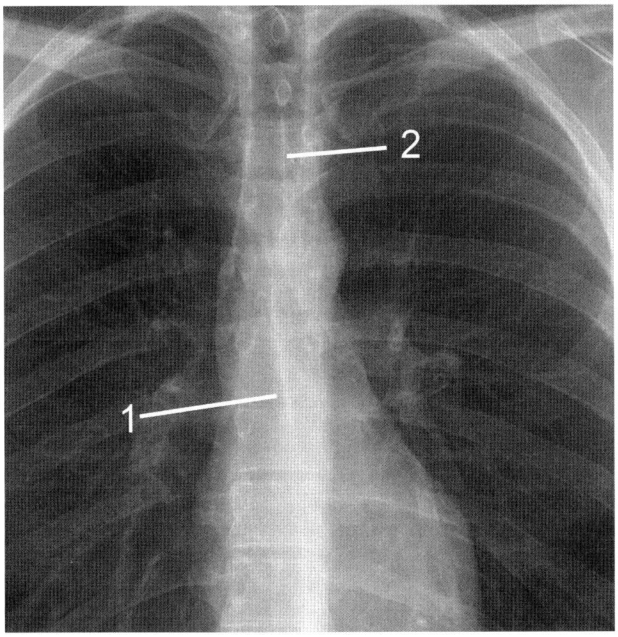

Figure 3.10. Mediastinal lines on radiography. Anterior junction line (1) and posterior junction line (2).

- Mediastinal stripes: The right and left paratracheal stripes result from contact of aerated lung with the lateral tracheal walls and surrounding mesenchymal tissues and extend from the thoracic inlet to the azygos arch on the right and to the aortic arch on the left (Fig. 3.9). The paravertebral stripes result from contact of aerated lung with the thoracic vertebrae and their surrounding mesenchymal tissues. The posterior tracheal stripe or tracheoesophageal stripe results from contact between the aerated right upper lobe and the posterior tracheal wall and its surrounding mesenchymal tissues.
- Mediastinal interfaces: The azygoesophageal recess results from contact of aerated right lower lobe with the adjacent mediastinum near the azygos vein and the esophagus (hence the name). The left para-aortic interface results from contact of aerated left lower lobe with the descending thoracic aorta (Fig. 3.9).

Chest Wall

Osseous Structures

- Shoulders: Humeri, scapulae, and clavicles with glenohumeral, acromioclavicular, and sternoclavicular joints.
- Sternum: Manubrium sternum superiorly and sternal body inferiorly; xiphoid process articulates with inferior sternal body.
- Clavicles: Connect sternum to scapulae.
- Scapulae: Paired triangular flat bones.
- Ribs: Twelve pairs—ribs 1–7 articulate with sternum via costal cartilages, ribs 8–10 articulate with costal cartilage of rib 7, and ribs 11 and 12 do not articulate with sternum or rib costal cartilages.
- Rib costal cartilages: May calcify and be visible on radiography; male pattern of calcification tubular, and female pattern of calcification peripheral tram track-like.
- Spine: Twelve thoracic vertebral bodies and their intervertebral disk spaces.

Soft Tissues

- Muscles: Include pectoral, intercostal, and back muscles.
- Vessels: Internal thoracic (formerly internal mammary) arteries and veins, intercostal arteries and veins, lymphatics.
- Nerves: Intercostal nerves, brachial plexi, paravertebral sympathetic ganglia and nerves.
- Skin and subcutaneous tissues: Breast, subcutaneous fat.

Anatomic Regions

- Thoracic inlet: Opening that allows communication between the neck and upper intrathoracic region; bound by T1 posteriorly, clavicles laterally, and superior aspect of manubrium sternum anteriorly.
- Thoracic outlet: Opening between inferior thorax and abdomen; bound by T12 posteriorly, 12th ribs and inferior-most costal cartilages laterally, and xiphoid process anteriorly.
- Supraclavicular region: Soft tissues above the bilateral clavicles and below the adjacent neck.
- Axillae: Pyramidal space between upper lateral chest and adjacent proximal upper extremities.
- Breast and pectoral region: Located in anterior superior chest wall and visible as increased soft tissue density depending on size.
- Nipples may manifest as nodular opacities overlying the anterior chest and should not be confused with pulmonary nodules.

Suggested Reading

Federle MP, Rosado-de-Christenson ML, Raman SP, et al. *Imaging Anatomy: Chest, Abdomen, Pelvis*. Second Edition. Philadelphia, PA: Elsevier; 2017.

CHAPTER 4

The Radiology Report

Gerald F. Abbott

The radiology report is a vital document in patient care that must communicate the results of imaging studies to the health care team in a clear, accurate, and timely manner. It represents a distillation of the radiologist's medical knowledge, experience, and medical judgment. The ability of radiologists to effectively communicate their observations and form a summary impression of their findings is largely the basis on which they are judged by their clinical colleagues. The report also serves as a means for communication to the patient. In addition, when medicolegal situations arise, the report is often a key document that may provide the basis on which legal judgment may be made as to whether a standard of care was met. The report may also be used for billing purposes, accreditation requirements, quality improvement, research, and teaching purposes.

The key elements of a radiology report are (1) administrative information, (2) patient identification, (3) clinical history and indications for the examination, (4) imaging technique, (5) comparison with prior studies, (6) observations/imaging findings, (7) summary or impression, and (8) signature.

As shown in Box 4.1, *administrative information* includes the name of the imaging facility, identifies the referring provider, and indicates the date and time of service. *Patient identification* includes such basic demographic information as the patient's name, date of birth, identifying medical record number, and a number specific to that particular episode of care (e.g., imaging study accession number). The *clinical history and indications* section briefly describes the patient's medical history, lists any risk factors or known allergies, and indicates the reason for the examination. The *imaging technique* section indicates what study was done, including the specific examination protocol and type and amount of any contrast material used or medication administered. Any adverse reaction to intravenous contrast administration must also be documented in the report. The *comparison with prior studies* section indicates the date, time, and type of previous studies that have been reviewed and compared with the current study, if applicable. The *observations/imaging findings* section of the report describes the abnormalities detected by the radiologist and whether those findings are new or have progressed or improved. Comparison with prior studies may also reveal that previously demonstrated abnormalities have resolved.

Box 4.1 Components of the Radiology Report

The radiology report should include the following components, as recommended by the Radiology Reporting Committee of the Radiological Society of North America:

- Administrative information: Imaging facility, referring provider, date and time of service
- Patient identification: Name, identifier (e.g., medical record number, Social Security number), date of birth, sex
- Clinical history: Medical history, risk factors, allergies, reason for examination, including medical necessity
- Imaging technique: Time of image acquisition, imaging device, image acquisition parameters, patient positioning, interventions, contrast materials and other medications administered, radiation dose
- Comparison: Date and type of previous examinations reviewed, if applicable
- Observations/imaging findings: Narrative description or itemization of findings, including measurements, image annotations, and identification of key images
- Summary or impression: Key observations, inferences, and conclusions, including any recommendations
- Signature: The date and time of electronic signature for each responsible provider, including attestation statement for physicians supervising trainees, if applicable

The findings section may also include pertinent negatives with regard to the clinical setting and question at hand (e.g., "No pulmonary emboli are demonstrated"). The *summary or impression* section provides a brief summary of findings and a short list of the most likely possibilities that take into consideration the patient's clinical history. The most pertinent findings should be listed at the top of the *impression* section in decreasing order of importance. The *signature* section indicates the date and time of electronic signature for each responsible provider, including any necessary attestation statement for physicians supervising trainees, if applicable.

The previously discussed scheme of organization is an essential element of "structured reporting," a communication technique endorsed by the American College of Radiology (ACR) and recommended by the ACR Intersociety Conference—an annual gathering of 50 member organizations representing the leading subspecialty societies in diagnostic imaging. Another key element of structured reporting is consistent organization or "itemized reporting." In thoracic imaging reports, for example, imaging findings are typically organized as separate paragraphs with headings such as (1) tubes and lines, (2) lungs and airways, (3) pleura, (4) heart and mediastinum, (5) bones, and (6) soft tissues. This format is preferred by clinicians because information pertaining to specific organ systems can be retrieved more easily than in a free-form narrative report format.

In some practices, this structure is amplified by utilization of templates, with text in place describing normal findings. The interpreting radiologist may then use that default text when normal findings are observed or may modify or replace it to indicate specific abnormalities in each of the previously mentioned anatomic sections of the report.

Surveys have shown that referring clinicians value accuracy in radiology reports above all other factors, but they also cite clarity, completeness, and timeliness of reporting as very important features. Clarity requires the use of plain English instead of radiology jargon or obscure abbreviations. Brevity is achieved by constructing concise, clear sentences that avoid rambling descriptions and redundant phrases. For instance, reporting that "No pulmonary nodules are demonstrated" is preferred to "Review of the scan at lung windows shows no evidence of pulmonary nodules." The pertinence of findings is also important, particularly when composing a summary of findings or impression. Findings should be listed in the *impression* section in the order of their importance, with the most important finding listed first and the least important listed last.

According to the Physician Insurers Association of America, communication errors are one of the top five reasons radiologists are sued for medical malpractice. The ACR stresses the importance of communicating important findings to the referring physician by direct communication that is clearly documented in the report of that examination. Direct communication is defined in the current version of the ACR's guideline as communication accomplished in person or by telephone, usually as doctor-to-doctor communication. In some circumstances of urgency or unusual complexity, delivery and receipt of a report may be handled through surrogates (e.g., nurse, ordering physician's call partner, or another representative of the ordering physician). The ACR does caution, however, that any failure on the part of the surrogate would likely be attributed to the radiologist.

Documentation of such communications creates a history of what has been communicated for the purpose of substantiating facts and events. In the event of litigation, such documentation serves as strong evidence that a radiologist acted reasonably.

In some circumstances, a preliminary or "draft" report may be issued as a verbal or written communication, typically when limited or incomplete clinical information is available and there is a need for immediate management of a patient. By its very nature, such a report may not contain all reportable findings. The key feature of a preliminary report is that it is time sensitive—made for the purpose of providing information necessary for prompt medical management of a patient. Preliminary reports should be clearly labeled as such in order to alert clinicians that additional information may be available at a later time and also to avoid confusion with the subsequent final report. The ACR guidelines recommend that all verbal preliminary reports be reduced to written form as soon as possible and that such authentication be done by the physician who interpreted the study.

Ideally, the radiology report will adhere to a consistent and structured framework of organization and display its content in a clear, concise, and readable format; also, critical findings will be communicated to the referring physician and health care team in a timely and effective manner. By adhering to the basic elements defined in the ACR's *Practice Guideline for Communication*, radiologists will maintain their role as highly valued and effective members of the health care team.

Suggested Reading

American College of Radiology. *ACR Practice Guideline for Communication of Diagnostic Imaging Findings*. Reston, VA: American College of Radiology; 2005.

Berlin L. Malpractice issues in radiology: Radiology reports. *AJR Am J Roentgenol*. 1997;169:943–946.

Dunnick NR, Langlotz CP. The radiology report of the future: A summary of the 2007 Intersociety Conference. *J Am Coll Radiol*. 2008;5(5):626–629.

Kahn CE, Langlotz CP, Burnside ES, et al. Towards best practices in radiology reporting. *Radiology*. 2009;252(3):852–856.

Kushner DC, Lucey LL; American College of Radiology. Diagnostic radiology reporting and communication: The ACR guideline. *J Am Coll Radiol*. 2005;2(1):15–21.

Reiner BI, Knight N, Siegel EL. Radiology reporting, past, present, and future: The radiologist's perspective. *J Am Coll Radiol*. 2007;4(5):313–319.

Sistrom CL, Langlotz CP. A framework for improving radiology reporting. *J Am Coll Radiol*. 2005;2(2):159–167.

Weiss DL, Langlotz CP. Structured reporting: Patient care enhancement or productivity nightmare? *Radiology*. 2008; 249(3):739–747.

CHAPTER 5

Basic Signs in Chest Radiology: Silhouette, Hilar Overlay, and Hilar Convergence Signs

Gerald F. Abbott

Definition

An imaging "sign" is a combination of findings considered "classic" for a specific observation—one that narrows the differential diagnosis to a more precise list of considerations. Just as traffic signs enable motorists to proceed more accurately, imaging signs often lead the radiologist to a more precise diagnostic conclusion. Familiarity with imaging signs facilitates rapid recognition of complex imaging patterns that often suggest a specific diagnosis or narrow the diagnostic possibilities to be considered. The imaging signs discussed in this chapter pertain to chest radiography and computed tomography (CT) and are among the most common that occur in thoracic imaging.

Silhouette Sign

The silhouette sign, described by Felson in 1950, was one of the first imaging signs described in chest radiography. It enabled radiologists to localize intrathoracic lesions on posteroanterior (PA) chest radiographs by applying the principle that when two objects of the same radiographic density come into contact with each other, the edge or margin between them disappears (i.e., is "silhouetted"). For example, the margins of the heart, aorta, and hemidiaphragms are normally visible when in apposition with normal aerated lung parenchyma, but their margins are obscured when the alveolar air in adjacent lung parenchyma is replaced by water density material (e.g., exudate of pneumonia, pulmonary hemorrhage, pulmonary edema, or aspiration) or by the presence of a mass.

The location of the silhouette sign within the chest helps to localize the detected abnormality to a specific portion of the lung. The following are classic locations of the silhouette sign on the PA or anteroposterior (AP) chest radiograph: (1) The right superior mediastinum (e.g., superior vena cava, paratracheal stripe, and superior aspect of right hilum) may be silhouetted by a process that opacifies the right upper lobe; (2) the right heart border may be obscured ("silhouetted") by an airspace filling process involving the middle lobe or, less commonly, the medial aspect of the right lower lobe; (3) the aortic arch may be obscured by opacification of the apicoposterior segment of the left upper lobe; (4) the left heart border may be obscured by opacification of the lingular segment of the left upper lobe; and (5) either hemidiaphragm may be obscured by opacity within the basilar segments of the ipsilateral lower lobe (Fig. 5.1) or by an ipsilateral pleural effusion. Note that either hemidiaphragm may remain visible (not silhouetted) when opacification of the ipsilateral lower lobe is posterior to the dome of that hemidiaphragm. Left lower lobe opacity may also obscure (silhouette) the lateral margin of the descending aorta (Fig. 5.1).

On the lateral chest radiograph, the posterior margin of the heart or posterior left hemidiaphragm may be obscured by a left lower lobe process (sometimes mimicked

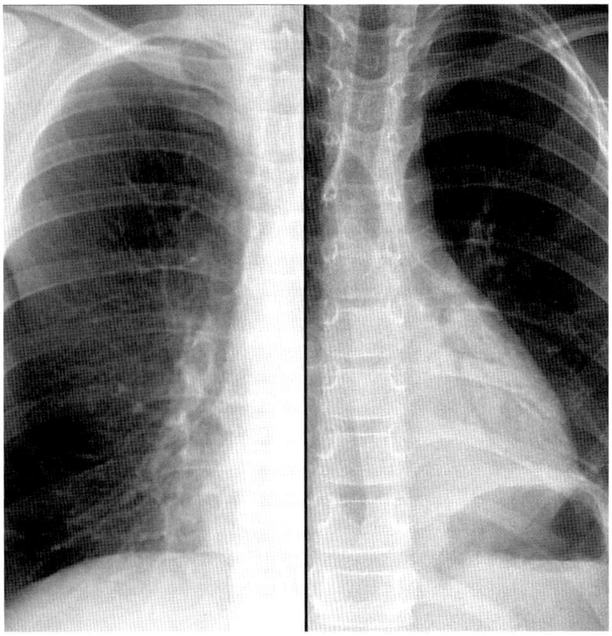

Figure 5.1. Silhouette sign. Coned-down PA chest radiographs show middle lobe atelectasis that obscures (silhouettes) the right heart border (left) and left lower lobe pneumonia that silhouettes the left hemidiaphragm and lower thoracic aorta (right). Air bronchograms are apparent in the left lower lobe (right) due to consolidation.

by a hiatal hernia), the anterior right hemidiaphragm may be silhouetted by a right middle lobe process, and the posterior right hemidiaphragm may be obscured by opacification of the right lower lobe.

The silhouette sign is most commonly a manifestation of pneumonia, atelectasis, or pleural effusion, but it may also be produced by a mass involving the lung, mediastinum, pleura, or chest wall. Further evaluation by CT may be a useful next step, but comparison with prior imaging studies is sometimes revealing.

Air Bronchogram

The air bronchogram sign refers to visualization of air-filled bronchi in a background of opacified lung parenchyma, classically seen in consolidation of lung parenchyma (Fig. 5.1). A variety of alveolar-filling disease processes may produce the air bronchogram sign, and differential diagnostic considerations include pneumonia (infectious, aspiration, or lipoid), alveolar pulmonary edema, alveolar pulmonary hemorrhage, or cicatrization (fibrosis) that may be related to radiation therapy or advanced interstitial lung disease (e.g., sarcoidosis, usual interstitial pneumonia, and nonspecific interstitial pneumonia), and neoplasm (lymphoma and mucinous adenocarcinoma). Visualization of the air bronchogram sign implies patency of proximal bronchi supplying that region of lung.

On chest radiography, air bronchograms manifest within areas of dense lung parenchyma as tapering, tubular lucencies that may branch. On CT, air bronchograms may be more clearly visualized as air-filled tapering bronchi, surrounded by dense lung parenchyma that may be consolidated or atelectatic.

In a febrile patient, air bronchograms are suggestive of pneumonia. Follow-up chest radiography is recommended in 6–8 weeks to document resolution of the findings and exclude an underlying malignancy. In some instances of lung consolidation, air bronchograms may not be visible. For example, pulmonary infarction may result in consolidation without air bronchograms when blood fills airways in the affected area of lung parenchyma; and mucus or pus may fill the airways in a segment of lung affected by pneumonia.

Deep Sulcus Sign

Radiologists should be aware that 30% of pneumothoraces are detected on supine chest radiography. The deep sulcus sign indicates pneumothorax—typically in a supine patient—and refers to the asymmetric appearance of lucency (air) within the lateral costophrenic angle, extending more inferiorly (i.e., appearing deeper in extent) than the normal contralateral costophrenic angle (Fig. 5.2). Its appearance is based on the caudal extent of the parietal pleura (costal and diaphragmatic surfaces), which is normally in close apposition within the lateral costophrenic sulcus and not visible on normal chest radiographs. When a pneumothorax occurs in a supine individual, air rises to

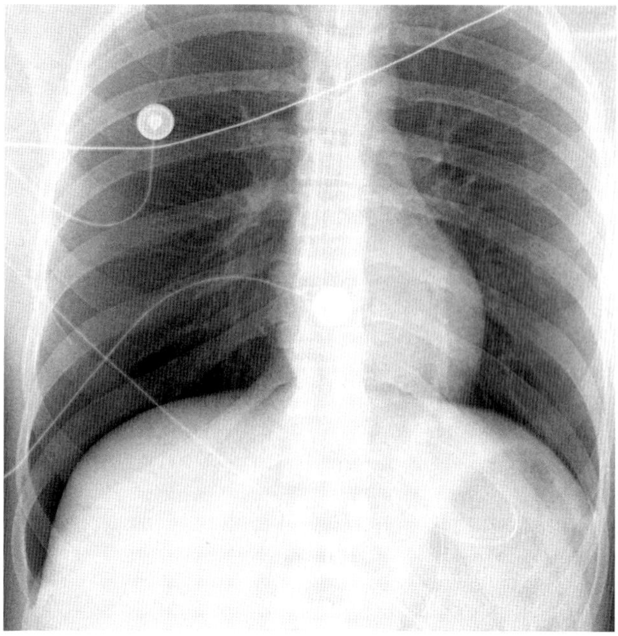

Figure 5.2. Deep sulcus sign. AP supine chest radiograph of a patient with a right pneumothorax shows abnormal lucency in the right lower hemithorax that extends into the right costophrenic sulcus, forming the "deep sulcus sign" of pneumothorax that may occur in supine patients.

the least dependent part of the involved hemithorax—along the costophrenic interface—and manifests as abnormal lucency within the involved costophrenic sulcus on supine chest radiography. The lucency may extend across the anterior surface of the ipsilateral hemidiaphragm from the costophrenic sulcus to the hypochondrium. The ipsilateral hemidiaphragm may also be depressed when an element of tension is present. A thin pleural line along the inferolateral aspect of the ipsilateral lung may sometimes be visualized within the area of lucency, confirming the presence of pneumothorax. Air may also outline the undersurface of the ipsilateral lung and/or the surface of the hemidiaphragm, mediastinal fat, and the adjacent heart border.

The deep sulcus sign is most useful in patients in intensive care units and those being evaluated following trauma. It is also helpful in patients with pleural adhesions that may alter the normal configuration of a pneumothorax.

Incomplete Border Sign

The incomplete border sign refers to the border characteristics of an abnormal finding on chest radiography—one that manifests with a combination of well-defined and ill-defined borders (i.e., incomplete) (Fig. 5.3). The sign implies that the lesion (e.g., mass) is in an extrapulmonary location—typically pleural or chest wall in origin. The incomplete borders may be manifest on both orthogonal (PA and lateral) views and appear discrepant when compared. CT reveals the contours of the pleural, chest wall, or cutaneous lesion—often demonstrating obtusely angled interfaces between the edges of the mass and the adjacent pleural surface (Fig. 5.3).

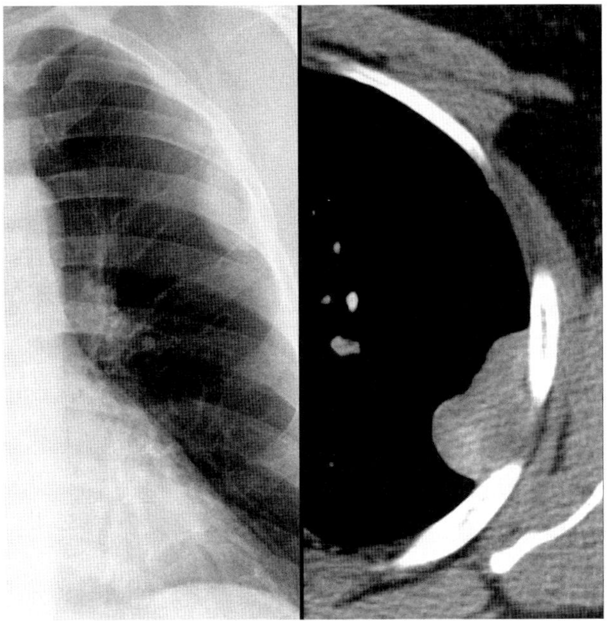

Figure 5.3. Incomplete border sign. Coned-down PA chest radiograph (left) and chest CT (right) show a pleural metastasis from malignant melanoma. The mass exhibits incomplete borders on chest radiography (left) and both obtuse and acutely angled interfaces with the adjacent pleural surface on chest CT (right).

The obtuse angles at such interfaces lack the tangential relationship between the bulk of the mass and the x-ray beam, producing incomplete borders on the chest radiograph.

The most common pleural abnormalities that may manifest with the incomplete border sign are loculated pleural effusion (focal or multifocal), pleural plaques, metastasis, solitary (localized) fibrous tumor, and mesothelioma. Chest wall lesions to consider include lipoma, metastasis, plasmacytoma, primary osseous malignancy, nipples, and skin nodules.

Hilar Convergence Sign

The hilar convergence sign may be used to resolve a potential imaging challenge: An enlarged main pulmonary artery may simulate a hilar mass; conversely, a hilar mass may be mistaken for an enlarged main pulmonary artery.

On chest radiography, if pulmonary vascular structures converge to and merge with the margins of a mass-like hilar opacity, that "mass" is likely the main pulmonary artery (Fig. 5.4, left). Conversely, if the vascular structures appear to course through such an opacity—or do not converge to it—the opacity is likely a hilar or mediastinal mass (Fig. 5.4, right).

Hilum Overlay Sign

The hilum overlay sign refers to another potential imaging challenge: Cardiomegaly may mimic an anterior mediastinal mass; conversely, an anterior mediastinal mass may mimic cardiomegaly. Visualization of normal hilar vascular structures through a mass-like opacity implies that the opacity arises in the anterior mediastinum (Fig. 5.5).

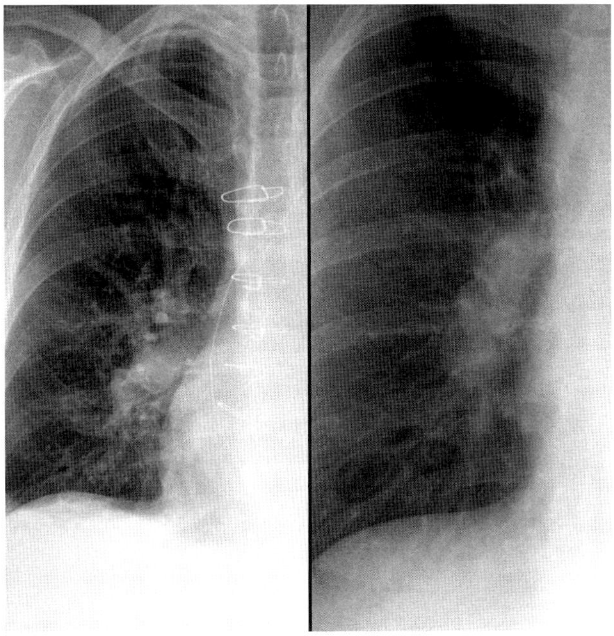

Figure 5.4. Hilar convergence sign. Coned-down PA chest radiographs demonstrate vascular structures converging to the right hilum in a patient with pulmonary hypertension (left) and vascular structures projecting through—not converging into—a hilar mass (right).

S Sign of Golden

In 1925, Dr. Ross Golden described a useful radiographic sign indicating right upper lobe atelectasis caused by a right hilar mass. The "S sign of Golden" refers to an S-shaped sharp interface formed by the combined contours of the minor fissure (bowed upward and concave) and the outer margin of a

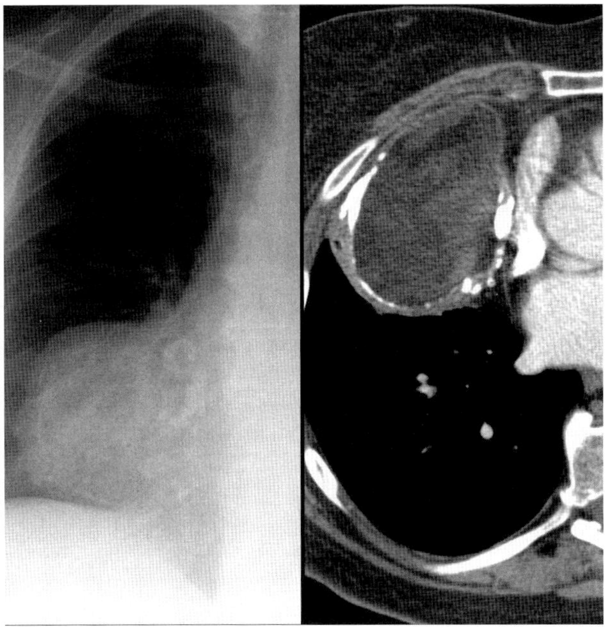

Figure 5.5. Hilum overlay sign. Coned-down PA chest radiograph (left) shows right hilar/perihilar vessels projecting through an anterior mediastinal mass. Chest CT (right) shows an anterior mediastinal teratoma.

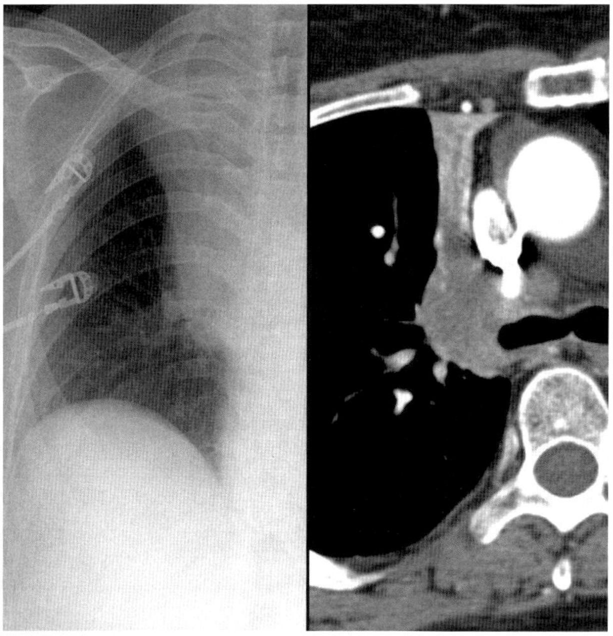

Figure 5.6. S sign of Golden. Coned-down PA chest radiograph (left) demonstrates the S sign of Golden—an S-shaped sharp interface formed by the combined contours of the minor fissure (bowed upward and concave) and the convex outer border of a central hilar mass. Chest CT (right) shows a right hilar mass with convex borders that occludes the right upper lobe bronchus, with resultant atelectasis of the right upper lobe. The outer border of the atelectatic upper lobe, formed by the displaced minor fissure, is slightly concave.

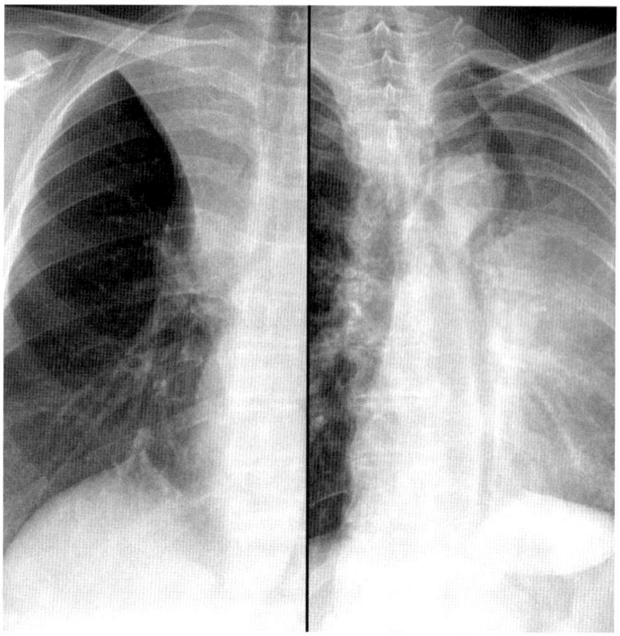

Figure 5.7. Juxtaphrenic peak sign and luftsichel sign. Coned-down PA chest radiographs demonstrate a triangular-shaped opacity projecting superiorly along the right hemidiaphragm of a patient with right upper lobe atelectasis resulting from a central obstructing lung cancer (left). A patient with left upper lobe atelectasis caused by lung cancer demonstrates the luftsichel sign—a sickle-shaped lucency along the left mediastinal border at the level of the aortic arch (right). The lucency results from hyperinflation of the superior segment of the left lower lobe.

central hilar mass (convex) (Fig. 5.6). The resultant S-shaped interface, coursing from the hilum to the periphery, is a radiographic "sign" suggesting the presence of a central, obstructing lung cancer. Although originally described in association with right upper lobe atelectasis, the "S sign" may occur at other sites of lobar atelectasis caused by central tumors.

Juxtaphrenic Peak Sign

The juxtaphrenic peak sign may occur in atelectasis of either upper lobe or following upper lobe resection, and it is less often seen in cases of middle lobe atelectasis. The sign consists of a triangular-shaped opacity projecting superiorly along the ipsilateral hemidiaphragm, with its apex ("peak") pointed upward (Fig. 5.7, left). In the early years of chest radiography, this finding was referred to as "tenting" due to its tent-like shape. Reports in the literature have associated some instances of this sign as related to the presence of an inferior accessory fissure—a vertical fissure that separates the medial basilar segment of a lower lobe from the other basilar segments.

Luftsichel Sign

The luftsichel sign is sometimes detected in patients with moderate to marked left upper lobe atelectasis. *Luftsichel* is a German word meaning "air sickle," referring to a sickle-shaped lucency that may occur along the left mediastinal border in some cases of left upper lobe atelectasis (Fig. 5.7, right). The lucency is produced by a portion of the superior segment of the left lower lobe that hyperinflates in a compensatory manner in the presence of left upper lobe atelectasis. It may then insinuate itself between the mediastinum and the collapsed upper lobe, producing a sickle-shaped lucency as it extends along the aortic knob and adjacent mediastinal border. It should not be mistaken for a pneumothorax or pneumomediastinum. The luftsichel sign does not always occur with left upper lobe atelectasis; it has been reported in some cases of right upper lobe atelectasis.

Cervicothoracic Sign

The cervicothoracic sign, described by Felson in 1968, helps to distinguish between anterior and posterior mediastinal lesions on the PA chest radiograph. It is based on the knowledge of anatomic boundaries—that the anatomic extent of the anterior mediastinum ends at the level of the clavicles, whereas the boundary of the posterior mediastinum extends above the level of the clavicles. Therefore, any mass that disappears at the clavicles is likely anterior and may be silhouetted by the soft tissues of the neck (Fig. 5.8, left); whereas any mass sharply outlined in the thoracic apex is likely posterior and located within the chest (Fig. 5.8, right).

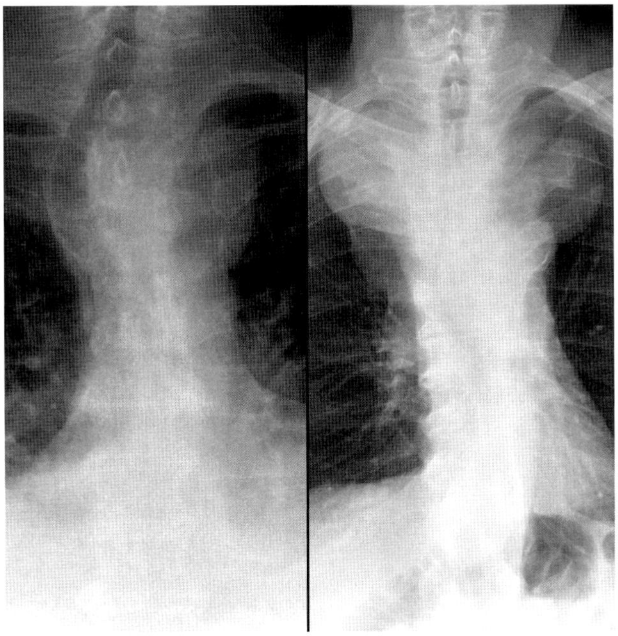

Figure 5.8. Cervicothoracic sign. Coned-down PA chest radiographs demonstrate a thyroid goiter in the anterior mediastinum that does not extend above the level of the clavicles (left) and a mediastinal liposarcoma that remains well-defined within the apical region, indicating its extension into the posterior aspect of the upper thorax (right).

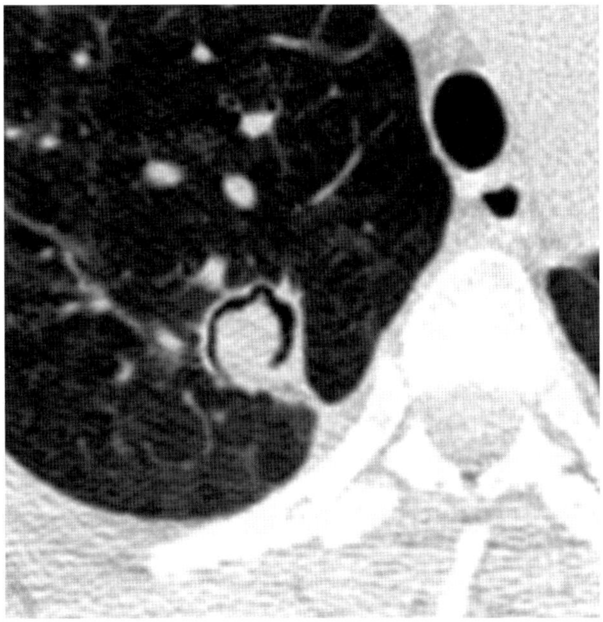

Figure 5.9. Air crescent sign. Chest CT demonstrates circumferential cavitation forming a crescentic collection of air around a nodular lesion within an area of consolidation in the right upper lobe. In a neutropenic patient, this sign is highly suggestive of invasive aspergillosis and typically manifests with the return of neutrophil function, suggesting a favorable prognosis.

Air Crescent Sign

In cases of angioinvasive aspergillosis, the chest radiograph and CT may demonstrate the air crescent sign. Typically seen as the patient's immune system is recovering (typically 2 weeks after the onset of infection), a crescent-shaped collection of air forms around a nodular opacity that represents retracted, infarcted lung associated with crescentic or circumferential cavitation (Fig. 5.9). The air crescent sign is seen in approximately 50% of patients with angioinvasive aspergillosis, particularly when the initial lesion manifested as consolidation or a mass. The parenchymal cavitation that forms the air crescent sign typically occurs 2 weeks after detection of an initial radiographic abnormality and coincides with the return of neutrophil function, suggesting a favorable prognosis. Although not specific for invasive aspergillosis, the sign is highly characteristic in the proper clinical setting. It may also be seen in cavitating tumors, tuberculosis, intracavitary hemorrhage, and vasculitis (e.g., Wegener granulomatosis).

In a different clinical setting, a variant of the air crescent sign may occur that manifests as a crescent-shaped collection of air along the margins of a mycetoma (fungal ball) and is referred to as the Monod sign. Mycetomas occur in immunocompetent hosts with preexisting structural lung disease, typically associated with tuberculosis, infection, or sarcoidosis.

Halo Sign

The halo sign refers to a "halo" of ground-glass opacity surrounding one or more pulmonary nodules (Fig. 5.10). In a neutropenic patient with fever, the halo sign almost always indicates infection by angioinvasive aspergillosis. The halo correlates with the presence of hemorrhage, surrounding a central nodular area of septic infarction. The

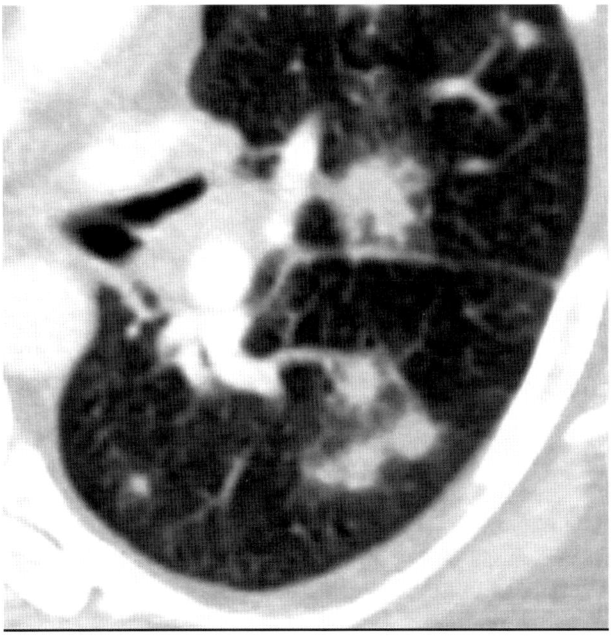

Figure 5.10. Halo sign. Chest CT shows multiple nodules in the left lung, each with a surrounding "halo" of ground-glass opacity. In a neutropenic patient with fever, the halo sign almost always indicates infection by angioinvasive aspergillosis and correlates with the presence of hemorrhage surrounding a central nodular area of septic infarction.

halo sign may also be seen in other infections (mucormycosis, candida, herpes simplex virus, and cytomegalovirus), Wegener granulomatosis, hemorrhagic metastasis, and Kaposi sarcoma.

Suggested Reading

Federle MP, Rosado de Christenson ML, Woodward PJ, Abbott GF, et al. Hila. In: *Diagnostic and Surgical Imaging Anatomy: Chest, Abdomen, Pelvis*. Salt Lake City, UT: Amirsys; 2006.

Felson B. More chest roentgen signs and how to teach them: Annual oration in memory of L. Henry Garland, M.D., 1903–1966. *Radiology*. 1968;90:429–441.

Felson B, Felson H. Localization of intrathoracic lesions by means of the postero-anterior roentgenogram; The silhouette sign. *Radiology*. 1950;55:363–374.

Kuhlman JE, Fishman EK, Siegelman SS. Invasive pulmonary aspergillosis in acute leukemia: Characteristic findings on CT, the CT halo sign, and the role of CT in early diagnosis. *Radiology*. 1985;157:611–614.

McAdams HP, Rosado-de-Christenson ML, Templeton PA, Lesar M, Moran CA. Thoracic mycoses from opportunistic fungi: Radiologic–pathologic correlation. *RadioGraphics*. 1995;15:271–286.

Mintzer RA, Sakowicz BA, Blonder JA. Lobar collapse: Usual and unusual forms. *Chest*. 1988;94:615–620.

Pugatch RD. Differentiation of pleural and pulmonary lesions using computed tomography. *J Comput Assist Tomogr*. 1978: 2:601–606.

Rossi SE, Erasmus JJ, McAdams HP, Donnelly LF. Thoracic manifestations of neurofibromatosis—I. *AJR Am J Roentgenol*. 1999; 173:1631–1638.

Woodring JH, Reed JC. Radiographic manifestations of lobar atelectasis. *J Thorac Imaging*. 1996;11:109–144.

Section II

Bedside Radiography

Medical Devices

CHAPTER 6

Introduction to Portable Chest Radiography: Support Devices

Melissa L. Rosado-de-Christenson

Introduction

Portable or bedside chest radiographs are frequently obtained in hospitalized patients. These studies are particularly useful in critically ill and unstable patients who cannot be safely transported to the radiology department for conventional radiography. Portable radiography is also used for imaging debilitated and bed-ridden patients who may not be critically ill. In addition, portable chest radiographs are frequently obtained in the emergency department for the initial imaging of traumatized patients and for imaging patients with acute cardiothoracic conditions who are deemed unstable or critically ill. Typically, only a frontal anteroposterior (AP) chest radiograph is obtained with the patient in the supine, semi-upright, or upright position. Portable chest radiographs should not be obtained to increase patient throughput and are not considered an appropriate substitute for posteroanterior (PA) and lateral chest radiographs. In fact, the latter should be obtained whenever the patient's clinical condition permits.

Portable Chest Radiography

Portable chest radiographs are AP radiographs. The term "AP" refers to the direction of the x-ray beam as it traverses the patient from anterior to posterior. The image receptor is placed behind the patient. The source-to-image receptor distance is usually 40 in. (as opposed to 72 in. in PA chest radiography). As a result, there is magnification of normal anteriorly located structures, particularly the heart. Because the kilovoltage (kVp) is lower (because portable units are unable to deliver high kVp), exposure times are longer, resulting in increased image blur. In addition, pulmonary structures including lung nodules appear less sharp and may be poorly visualized.

Characteristics of AP Chest Radiography

- Lordotic projection is common.
- Clavicles are horizontally oriented.
- Scapulae often project over the lateral upper lung zones.
- The heart and mediastinum are often magnified.

Approach to Portable Chest Radiographs

Because portable chest radiographs are typically reserved for critically ill patients, external monitoring devices will frequently project over the areas of interest and must be distinguished from internally placed medical devices (Fig. 6.1). As a general rule, one must account for every radiopaque object, structure, or device identified on any radiograph in order to exclude an unsuspected foreign body. This is particularly important in the case of portable chest radiographs because they are interpreted without the benefit of orthogonal or lateral radiographs that allow localization of a structure or object in three dimensions and distinction of internal versus external objects or structures.

The radiologist needs to identify and assess each medical device and determine whether or not it is appropriately positioned (Fig. 6.2). A systematic assessment of the lungs, airways, pleura, mediastinum, skeleton, and soft tissues follows. Patients in the intensive care unit (ICU) may undergo chest radiography frequently and sometimes on a daily basis. It is important for the radiologist to systematically assess each radiograph and compare the positions of medical devices and the various radiographic abnormalities on each subsequent examination. Unsuspected new findings should be promptly communicated to the clinical team (Fig. 6.2), particularly when such findings require immediate intervention, in which case direct verbal communication is the standard of care.

Important Findings on Portable Chest Radiographs

Medical Devices

Typical medical devices seen frequently on portable chest radiographs include endotracheal tubes, enteric tubes, and vascular catheters. Various cardiac conduction devices are also frequently encountered on both portable and non-portable chest radiographs, including cardiac pacemakers, implantable cardioverter defibrillators, vagus nerve stimulators, and spinal cord stimulators. Implantable loop recorders are used for long term monitoring of patients with arrhythmias. Ventricular assist devices now serve

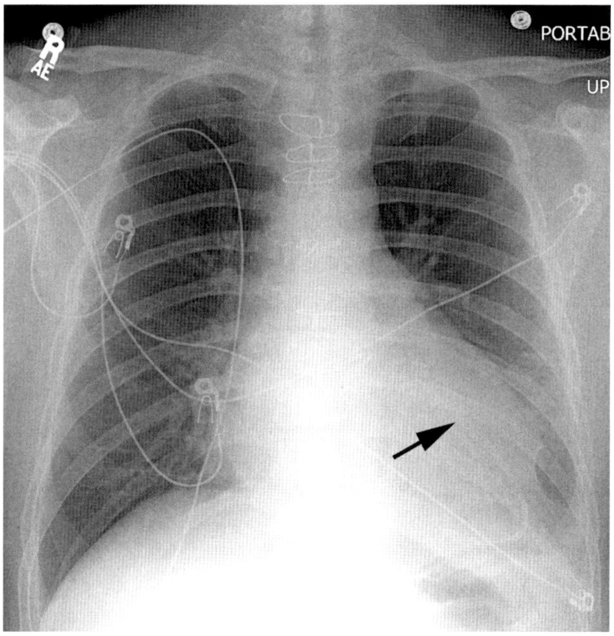

Figure 6.1. Extraneous monitoring devices. AP portable chest radiograph shows characteristic findings of lordotic projection, horizontally oriented clavicles, and superimposition of the scapulae over the lungs. External monitoring devices project over the thorax. Note the pericardial drainage catheter (arrow) for treatment of pericardial tamponade.

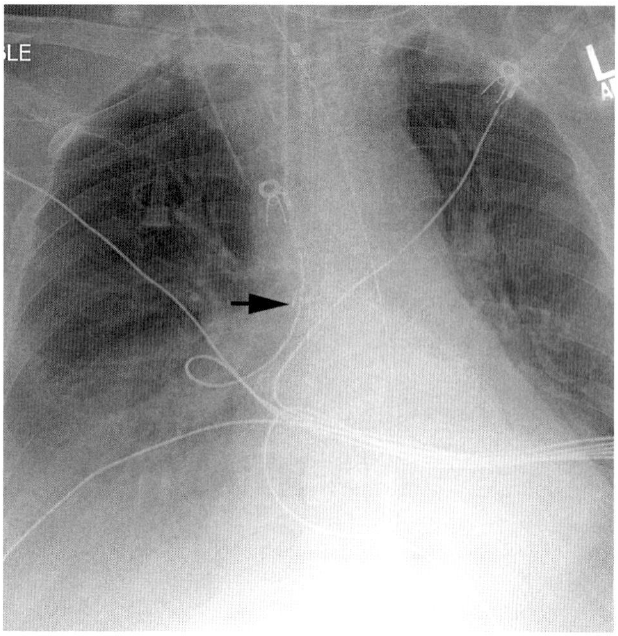

Figure 6.2. Support devices. AP chest radiograph shows a right internal jugular central venous catheter, an endotracheal tube, an enteric tube, and several overlying external monitoring devices. Note the malpositioned temperature probe with tip (arrow) in the right mainstem bronchus.

as destination therapy (or permanent alternative to heart transplantation) for patients with severe chronic heart failure. However, these devices may also be used as a bridge to recovery or transplantation.

Various drainage tubes and catheters may also be used in the hospital setting, particularly for drainage of air or fluid collections in the pleura, pericardium, and mediastinum.

The radiologist should assess the position of all visible medical devices and document any significant changes. Device malposition should be immediately communicated to the clinical team and the communication should be documented on the radiology report. Radiologists may need to research the appearance and function of emerging medical devices in the interest of accurate image interpretation. When an unusual medical device is encountered, consultation with the electronic medical record usually helps in its identification and determination of proper placement (Figs. 6.3 and 6.4).

Frequency of Imaging

Although it is common practice to perform routine daily portable chest radiographs in patients in the ICU, the American College of Radiology Appropriateness Criteria® state that such practices are not indicated. The following are indications for performing chest radiography in the ICU setting:

- Initial placement of endotracheal and enteric tubes, vascular catheters, or any other life-support device
- Change in the patient's clinical condition

General Assessment

Once medical devices have been evaluated, the radiologist must evaluate the rest of the thorax. This includes determination of lung volume; identification of airspace and/or interstitial opacities; and assessment of the pulmonary vasculature, the mediastinum, and the pleural spaces—the latter for identification of pleural effusion and/or pneumothorax. The chest wall should also be evaluated for acute fractures and soft tissue abnormalities, particularly in the setting of trauma. In rare cases, the exact position of a support device cannot be determined with certainty on portable chest radiography. In these instances, additional imaging with PA and lateral chest radiographs or advanced imaging with CT will be required.

Key Points

- Portable chest radiographs are used for imaging critically ill and bed-ridden patients who are not able to undergo PA and lateral chest radiography.
- Routine portable chest radiography of patients in the ICU is not recommended. Such radiographs should be obtained on initial placement of medical devices and for specific clinical indications.
- All radiopaque objects seen on radiography must be identified and assessed.
- Portable chest radiographs are often compromised by extraneous devices superimposed on the areas of interest.

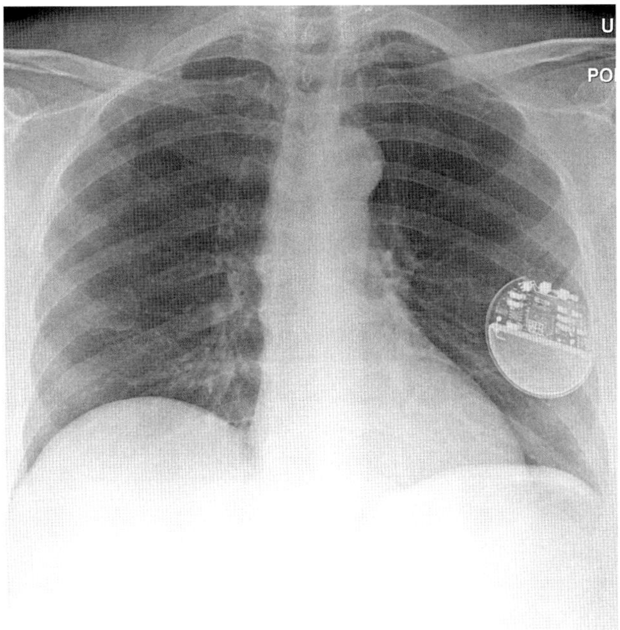

Figure 6.3. Vagus nerve stimulator. AP chest radiograph shows a vagus nerve stimulator with a left pectoral generator and leads coursing into the left neck. Vagus nerve stimulation may be used to treat seizures and depression. Correlation with the electronic medical record allows accurate identification of unusual medical devices.

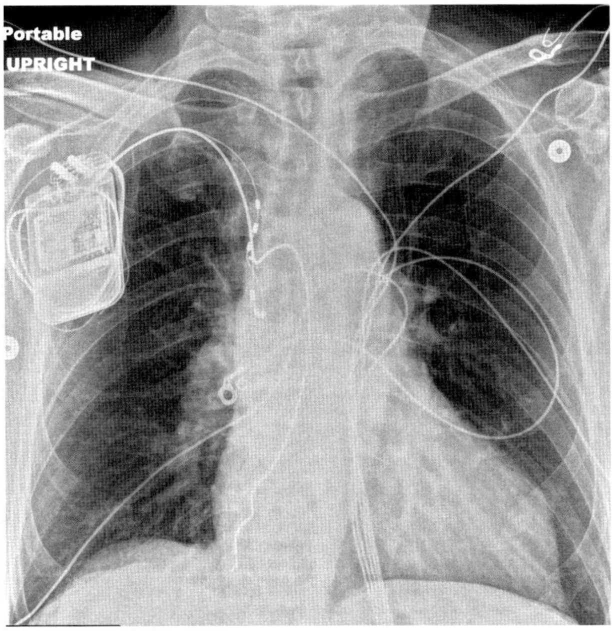

Figure 6.4. Transvenous phrenic nerve stimulator. AP chest radiograph shows a transvenous phrenic nerve stimulator consisting of a pulse generator, a stimulation lead coiled in the superior vena cava (near the phrenic nerve), and a sensing lead coursing into the azygos vein and terminating near the right hemidiaphragm. This device is used for management of central sleep apnea. Correlation with the electronic medical record and research allow accurate identification and assessment of emerging medical devices.

- All medical devices should be assessed for appropriate positioning and potential complications of placement.
- In some cases, patients evaluated with portable chest radiography will require further imaging with lateral chest radiography or more advanced imaging with chest CT.

Suggested Reading

Amorosa JK, Bramwit MP, Mohammed TH, et al. ACR Appropriateness Criteria® routine chest radiographs in intensive care unit patients. *J Am Coll Radiol.* 2013;10:170–174.

Oba Y, Zaza T. Abandoning daily routine chest radiography in the intensive care unit: Meta-analysis. *Radiology.* 2010;255:386–395.

CHAPTER 7

Endotracheal and Enteric Tubes

Tyler H. Ternes

Definition

An endotracheal tube (ETT) is a catheter placed in the trachea to protect the airway and provide adequate gas exchange (Fig. 7.1). An enteric tube is a thin, flexible, hollow catheter used for enteric suctioning or administration of drugs and/or nutrition (Fig. 7.2).

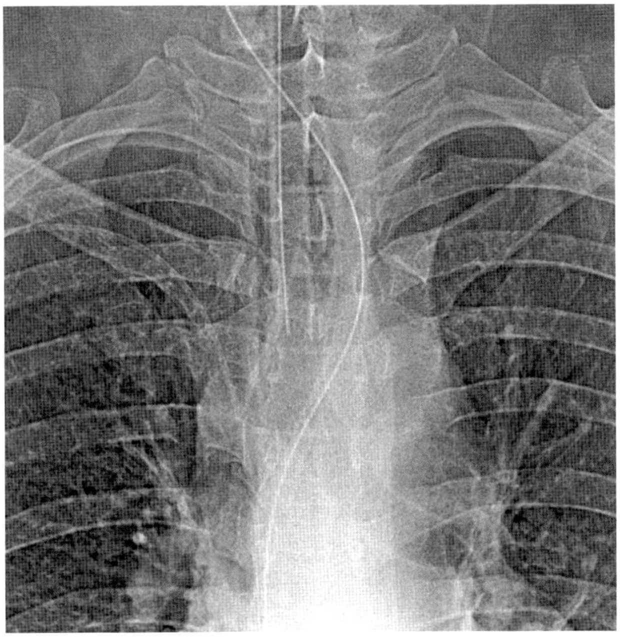

Figure 7.1. Appropriately positioned ETT. Portable chest radiograph shows an appropriately positioned ETT. The ETT tip should be approximately 3–7 cm above the carina. Note that the enteric tube follows an undulating course along the length of the esophagus, a common finding.

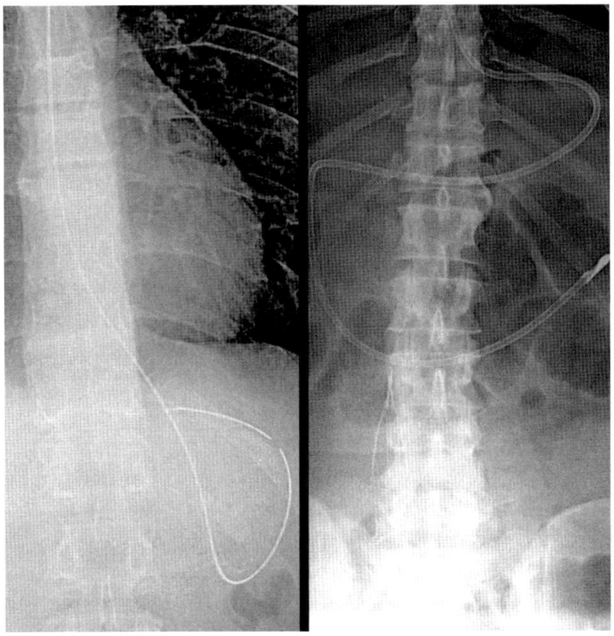

Figure 7.2. Appropriately positioned enteric tubes. Composite image with chest radiographs from 2 different patients. An enteric tube (left) has its sideport and tip well below the gastroesophageal junction. A feeding tube (right) shows the tip near the duodenal-jejunal junction (ligament of Treitz).

Clinical Features

An ETT is placed orally or nasally to maintain airway patency and to provide mechanical ventilation for patients undergoing surgery and for those with respiratory failure (Fig. 7.3). Most ETTs have an inflatable cuff used to prevent air leakage. A malpositioned ETT may extend too far inferiorly into the right mainstem bronchus or bronchus intermedius, resulting in poor left lung and/or right upper lobe ventilation (Fig. 7.4). A malpositioned ETT may also be placed too high, with resultant inadvertent extubation or vocal cord injury. Esophageal intubation may occur, resulting in absent pulmonary ventilation and gaseous distention of the stomach. Overinflation of the ETT balloon cuff may rarely lead to tracheal injury or stenosis. Tracheal rupture complicating intubation is rare. Tracheostomy tubes are used for patients who require long-term intubation. They are placed via a surgical stoma created in the anterior trachea, with the tip ideally halfway between the stoma and the carina. Tracheostomy tubes uncommonly lead to stenosis at the stoma site.

Enteric tubes may be orogastric or nasogastric and are typically used for gastric decompression and drug administration. The ideal tube tip position is in the stomach so that the tube sideport is beyond the gastroesophageal junction. Smaller caliber enteric tubes are often used for feeding and to administer drugs. Usually, these are placed nasally and advanced past the pylorus to decrease the risk of reflux and/or aspiration. Malpositioned enteric tubes may be incompletely advanced into the stomach or may

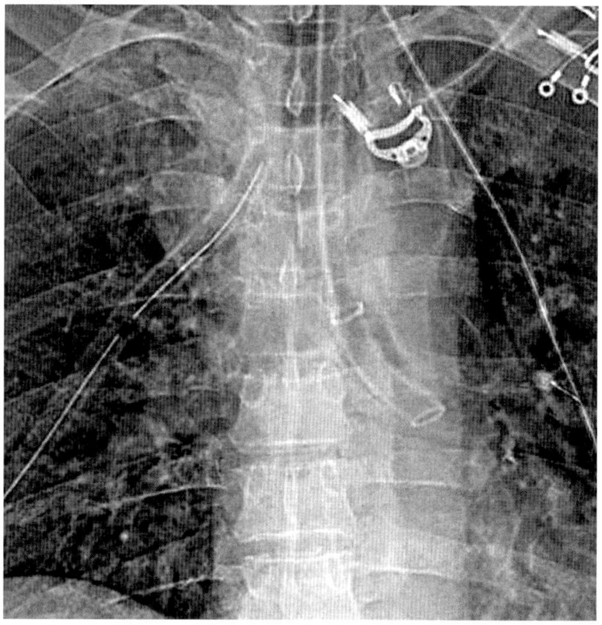

Figure 7.3. Appropriately positioned ETT. Portable chest radiograph shows an ETT extending into the left mainstem bronchus. During surgery, the left lung was selectively intubated and ventilated while surgery was performed on the decompressed right lung.

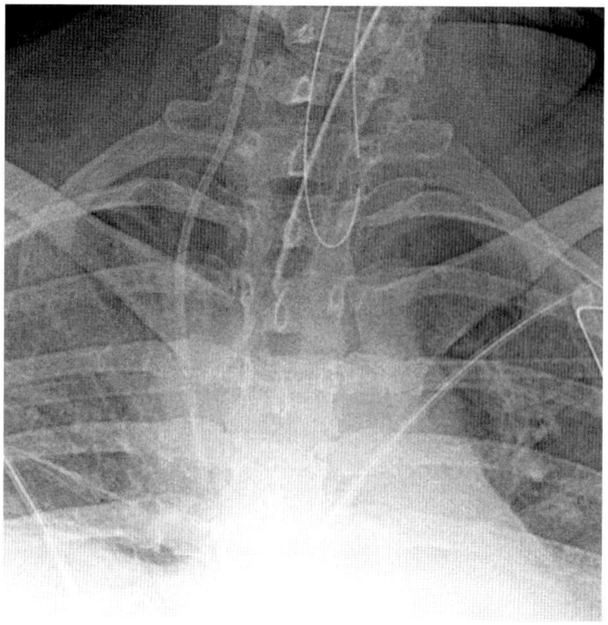

Figure 7.5. Malpositioned enteric tube. Portable chest radiograph shows an ETT with the tip projecting just above the medial clavicles. The enteric tube is coiled in the upper esophagus and ascends superiorly beyond the field of view. Repositioning of the tubes is required, and this finding should be verbally communicated to the clinical team.

exhibit hypopharyngeal or esophageal coiling (Fig. 7.5). Inadvertent placement of an enteric tube into the airway, lung, or pleural space may occur and may result in aspiration, pneumonia, lung injury, hemothorax, empyema, and pneumothorax (Fig. 7.6). Esophageal and gastric perforation have also been reported (Fig. 7.7).

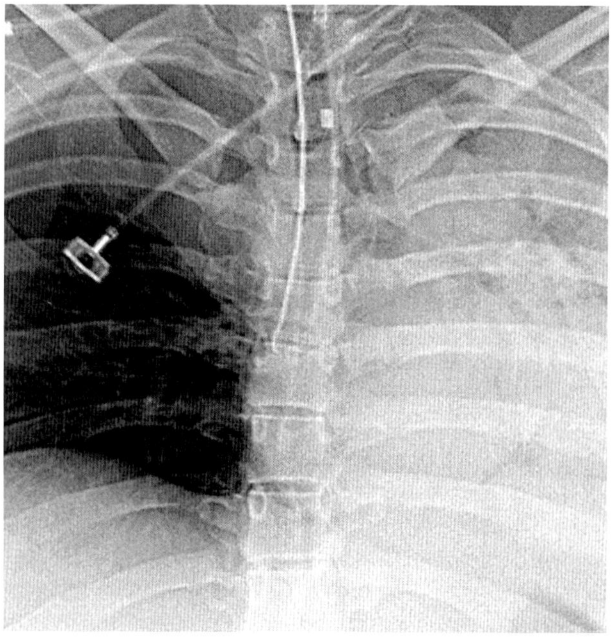

Figure 7.4. Malpositioned ETT. Portable chest radiograph shows a malpositioned ETT with tip in the bronchus intermedius and resultant left lung and right upper lobe atelectasis.

Anatomy and Physiology

Ideally, the ETT tip resides 5 cm above the carina. Confident evaluation of ETT placement requires an understanding of the normal airway anatomy. The tracheal carina

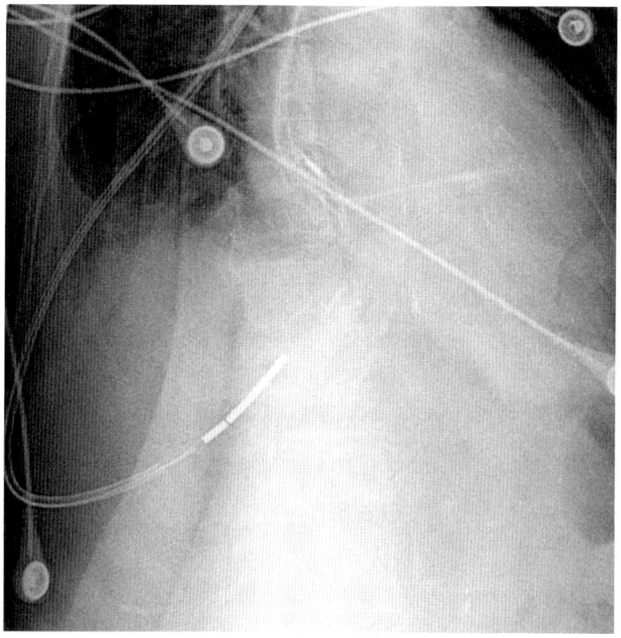

Figure 7.6. Malpositioned feeding tube. Portable radiograph of the lower chest/upper abdomen of an obtunded patient shows a feeding tube inadvertently placed into the right mainstem bronchus and advanced into the right pleural space. A deep sulcus sign relates to a right pneumothorax resulting from pulmonary perforation.

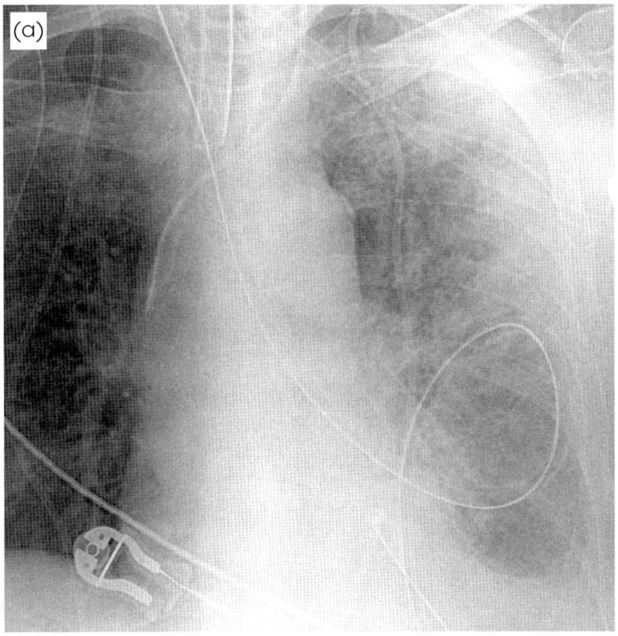

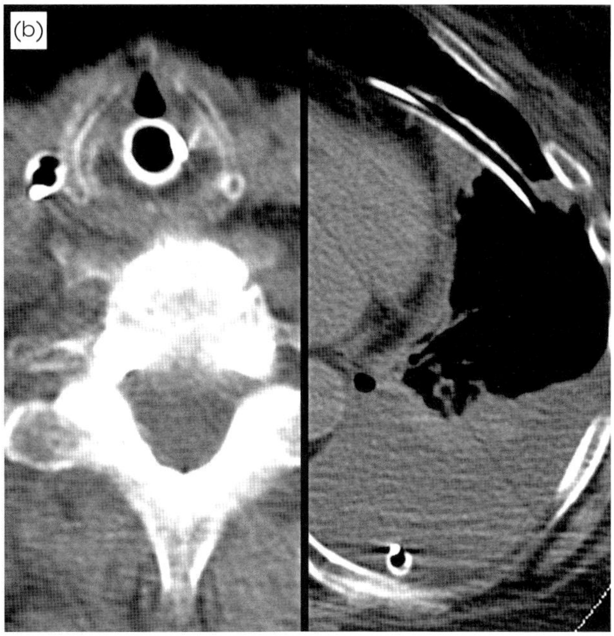

Figure 7.7. (a) Malpositioned enteric tube. Portable chest radiograph obtained after placement of multiple support devices shows an appropriately positioned ETT. However, the enteric tube takes an unexpected course, projecting over the left hemithorax. (b) Composite image of an unenhanced chest CT of the same patient shows the proximal aspect of the enteric tube located lateral to the right thyroid cartilage (left) due to pharyngeal perforation during placement. The distal aspect of the enteric tube (right) courses into the left pleural space.

is typically at the T5 to T7 level. ETT tip excursion corresponds to head position. With cervical flexion, the ETT tip may descend up to 2 cm. With cervical extension, the ETT tip may ascend up to 2 cm. Evaluation of enteric tubes also requires knowledge of normal and variant anatomy. Enteric tubes should be advanced well below the diaphragm, unless a large hiatal hernia is present. For feeding purposes, a vertical descent of the abdominal portion of the enteric tube to the right of midline is considered consistent with transpyloric placement.

How to Approach the Image

Portable chest radiographs are typically obtained following ETT and enteric tube placement to confirm appropriate positioning. Radiographic interpretation requires assessment of these and all other medical support devices. Comparison to prior studies is crucial for identification of interval device malpositioning. Any malpositioned device should be immediately reported to the clinical team. If radiographic findings are equivocal, repeat radiography should be performed with oblique or lateral radiographs as needed. CT may be required in complex cases.

What Not to Miss

Endotracheal and Tracheostomy Tubes

- Exclude esophageal intubation.
- Exclude tip position that is too high or too low.
- Exclude pneumomediastinum and/or pneumothorax.
- Ensure that balloon cuff is not overinflated.

Enteric Tubes

- Document tip position and exclude intraluminal coiling.
- Exclude airway intubation or other extraesophageal enteric tube position.
- Exclude pneumomediastinum and/or pneumothorax.
- Confirm feeding tube placement into duodenum.

Differential Diagnosis

Overlying Support and Monitoring Devices

Many patients imaged at the bedside commonly have external cardiac leads and defibrillator patches. These typically do not follow the same course as internal devices.

External Portion of Enteric Tube

- External portion may project over the thorax but can usually be determined to be external to the patient.
- Enteric tube positioned in large hiatal hernia or neoesophagus.
- External portion may simulate endobronchial position of enteric tube. Comparison with prior studies is beneficial.

Dual-Lumen ETT

- May be misinterpreted as unintentional bronchial intubation.

Imaging Findings

Endotracheal Tube Appropriate Position

- See Fig. 7.1.
- Most have a vertical radiopaque thin line for easier identification.
- Ideal tip position is 5 cm above carina (3–7 cm).
- Balloon cuff should not exceed tracheal diameter.

Endotracheal Tube Malposition

- See Fig. 7.4.
- Too high: ETT tip should be at least 3 cm below vocal cords to prevent injury; ETT tip may not be visible.
- Too low: ETT tip typically cannulates right main bronchus. May result in left lung atelectasis and potentially right upper lobe atelectasis if placed into bronchus intermedius.
- Balloon cuff overinflation: ETT cuff should fill the trachea but should not expand the tracheal walls (Fig. 7.8).
- Esophageal intubation: ETT lateral to tracheal air column; gaseous distention of the stomach.
- Tracheal injury: Suspect in cases of unexplained subcutaneous air, pneumomediastinum, or pneumothorax following intubation.

Enteric Tube Appropriate Position

- See Fig. 7.2.
- Majority of nasogastric (suction) tubes have a vertical radiopaque line that helps identify tube course and position.
- Feeding tubes are of smaller caliber and often have a stiff segmental metallic density tip.
- Enteric tube should parallel the course of the esophagus.
- Enteric tube tip should be well below gastric cardia (in the gastric antrum), with sideport below the gastroesophageal junction.
- Feeding tube tip is ideally in the second to fourth portion of the duodenum or the C loop. Confirmation of anatomic position can be achieved with contrast injection.

Enteric Tube Malposition

- See Figs. 7.5–7.7.
- Tube coiling in the hypopharynx or esophagus.
- Tube tip and/or sideport above gastroesophageal junction.
- Tube descending along the course of the airway.

Clinical Issues

Endotracheal Tube

- ETTs are used for patients with respiratory failure or for airway protection. Assessment and documentation of proper ETT position is crucial to ensure adequate ventilation. Malpositioned ETTs may manifest with persistent hypoxia or respiratory failure.
- A malpositioned ETT often results in varying degrees of atelectasis. The degree of volume loss is often heightened in ventilated patients because inspired

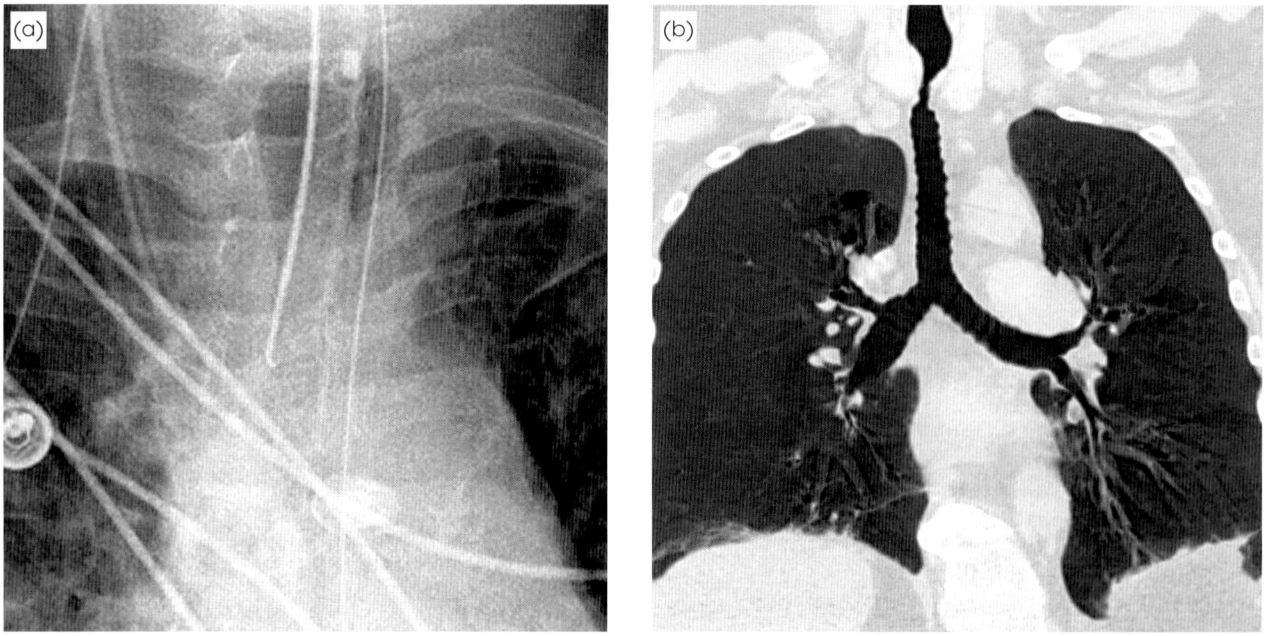

Figure 7.8. (a) Overinflated ETT balloon cuff. Coned-down portable chest radiograph shows an appropriately positioned ETT tip. However, there is greater than expected distention of the endotracheal tube balloon cuff, depicted as the lucency surrounding the tube. (b) Coronal minimum intensity projection unenhanced chest CT of the same patient obtained several weeks later shows focal tracheal stenosis near the thoracic inlet. Prolonged ETT balloon cuff overdistention may result in subsequent acquired airway stenosis.

oxygen concentrations may approach 100%, resulting in more rapid air shift and atelectasis.

- An ETT balloon cuff positioned too high may lead to vocal cord injury. Persistent balloon cuff overinflation within the trachea may result in tracheal stenosis.
- Ventilated patients may develop barotrauma wherein high peak pressures lead to alveolar rupture that may manifest as interstitial emphysema, pneumomediastinum, or pneumothorax.
- A dual-lumen ETT allows asymmetric lung ventilation for surgical procedures and accommodates differences in lung compliance. It also allows bronchopulmonary lavage while avoiding transbronchial contamination.
- Tracheostomy tubes are preferred for long-term mechanical ventilation.

Enteric Tubes

- Enteric tubes are used for suctioning or feeding. Improper placement is not uncommon, and it should be excluded with radiographic assessment.
- Inappropriate enteric tube placement in the airway, lung, or pleural space could result in devastating consequences, including aspiration, lung injury, and pneumothorax.
- An enteric tube that is not properly advanced may contribute to reflux and aspiration.

Key Points

- Confirmation of appropriate positioning of endotracheal and enteric tubes as well as other medical support devices is essential.
- ETTs should ideally be positioned 5 cm above the carina.
- Ideal position of an enteric tube tip is in the gastric antrum.
- Feeding tube tips should reside in the second to fourth portion of the duodenum.

Suggested Reading

Godoy MC, Leitman BS, de Groot PM, Vlahos I, Naidich DP. Chest radiography in the ICU: Part 1. Evaluation of airway, enteric, and pleural tubes. *AJR Am J Roentgenol.* 2012 Mar; 198(3):563–571.

Hunter TB, Taljanovic MS, Tsau PH, Berger WG, Standen JR. Medical devices of the chest. *RadioGraphics.* 2004 Nov–Dec; 24(6):1725–1746.

CHAPTER 8

Vascular Catheters

Tyler H. Ternes

Definition

Vascular catheters are medical devices used to gain access to the circulatory system in patients requiring medications, dialysis, resuscitative fluids, or hemodynamic monitoring.

Clinical Features

Central venous catheters are typically placed via a large-caliber vein (internal jugular, subclavian, and femoral). Vascular catheters are often placed at the bedside using anatomic landmarks for guidance, although there is increasing utilization of ultrasound guidance. Many of these catheters are for short-term use. For long-term vascular access, a small-caliber peripherally inserted central catheter (PICC) can be placed via an antecubital vein (Fig. 8.1). Subcutaneous ports and dialysis catheters are also used for long-term access (Fig. 8.2). They are placed surgically and are used in patients who require chemotherapy and multiple blood samplings. Imaging assessment of these catheters is important to exclude malpositioning (Figs. 8.3–8.6).

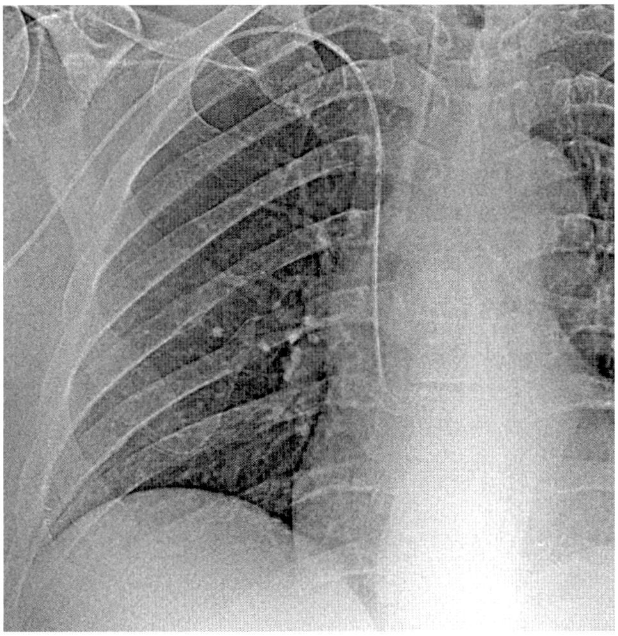

Figure 8.1. Portable chest radiograph of a 63-year-old man with osteomyelitis requiring a long course of intravenous antibiotics shows a right PICC with the tip in the distal superior vena cava near the desired location of the superior cavoatrial junction.

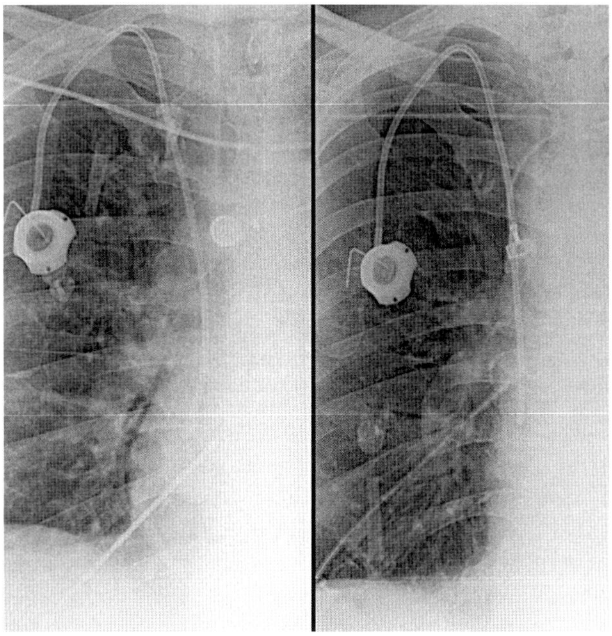

Figure 8.2. Composite image with posteroanterior (PA) chest radiographs of a 72-year-old man with lung cancer obtained on the same day. The apparent position of the catheter tip changes, seemingly in the right atrium on expiration (left) and at the superior cavoatrial junction on inspiration (right).

Hemodialysis catheters typically have a large caliber to accommodate large volumes and flow rates, and they often have multiple lumens (Fig. 8.7).

Pulmonary artery catheters (PACs) are predominantly used in critically ill and postoperative patients (Fig. 8.8). PACs are diagnostic and monitoring tools, but they are not effective for therapeutic purposes. They are often used in the intensive care unit to differentiate between various types of shock. Like other venous catheters, PACs are placed via large central veins, but they are advanced into the pulmonary artery. The catheter has a distal balloon that can be inflated in the pulmonary arterial tree and allows measurement of central venous, intracardiac, pulmonary arterial, and pulmonary capillary wedge pressures. Note that the utilization of PACs is controversial, and their use has generally decreased. Several studies have shown no change in mortality or length of hospital stay with the use of PACs.

An intra-aortic balloon pump (IABP) is a counterpulsation device consisting of a long inflatable balloon mounted on a catheter (Fig. 8.9). As the name implies, the catheter

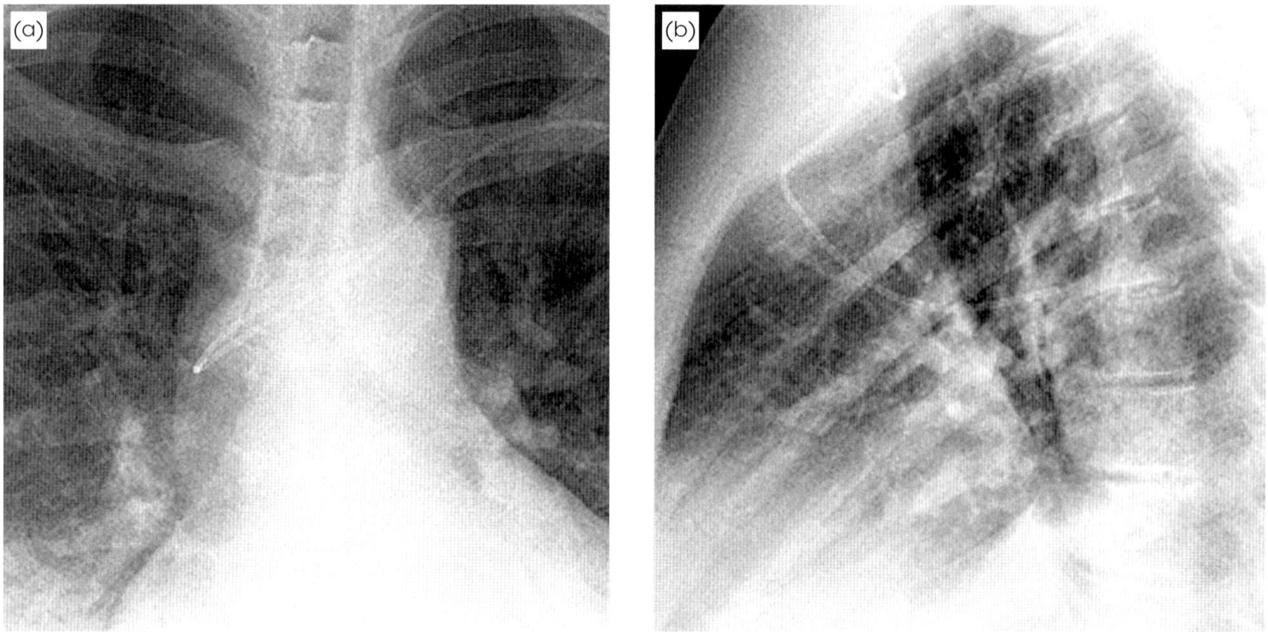

Figure 8.3. (a) PA chest radiograph shows an abnormal position of the distal aspect of a left PICC, with the tip appearing to coil above the right tracheobronchial angle, in the expected region of the azygos arch. (b) Lateral chest radiograph of the same patient shows that the PICC courses posteriorly, confirming its location within the azygos arch. The catheter malposition warrants notification to the clinical team and recommendation for repositioning.

is placed in the aorta and is used to monitor patients with critically compromised heart function. The balloon portion of the IABP is located in the descending thoracic and upper abdominal aorta and should be placed above the origins of the celiac, mesenteric, and renal arteries. Its purpose is to assist patients with hemodynamic shock by increasing coronary flow during diastole and decreasing left ventricular afterload during systole.

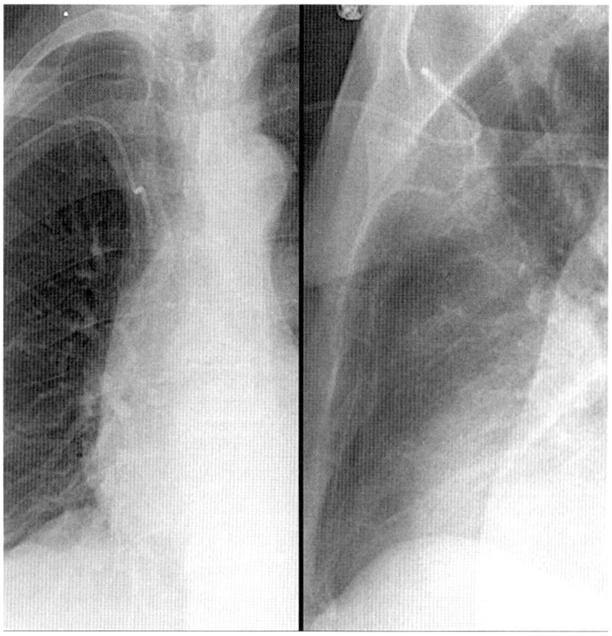

Figure 8.4. Composite image with PA and lateral chest radiographs shows a right PICC with an abnormal distal course (left). The lateral chest radiograph (right) shows that the catheter courses anteriorly and caudally, consistent with insertion into the right internal thoracic/mammary vein.

Anatomy and Physiology

The majority of central venous catheters are placed via subclavian or internal jugular vein approach. The ideal tip position is within the superior vena cava, near the superior cavoatrial junction. This rule applies for central venous catheters, PICCs, subcutaneous ports, and dialysis catheters. If the tip is too high, there is an increased risk of vessel injury or reflux of potentially toxic intravenously administered drugs. If the tip is too low (in the right atrium), cardiac arrhythmia could potentially be induced. Variation in inspiratory depth may change the apparent tip position, with decreased inspiration resulting in a more inferior position of the catheter tip. Pulmonary artery catheter tip position is preferably in the left or right pulmonary arteries and not extending beyond 2 cm from the hilum. The balloon tip should always be deflated except when actively measuring pressures.

An IABP is typically placed via the femoral artery and then positioned to terminate in the descending thoracic aorta, with the tip distal to the left subclavian artery. The balloon component is typically 25 cm in length. IABPs may also be surgically placed via the subclavian artery, typically the right.

How to Approach the Image

The American College of Radiology Appropriateness Criteria® for Routine Chest Radiographs in Intensive Care

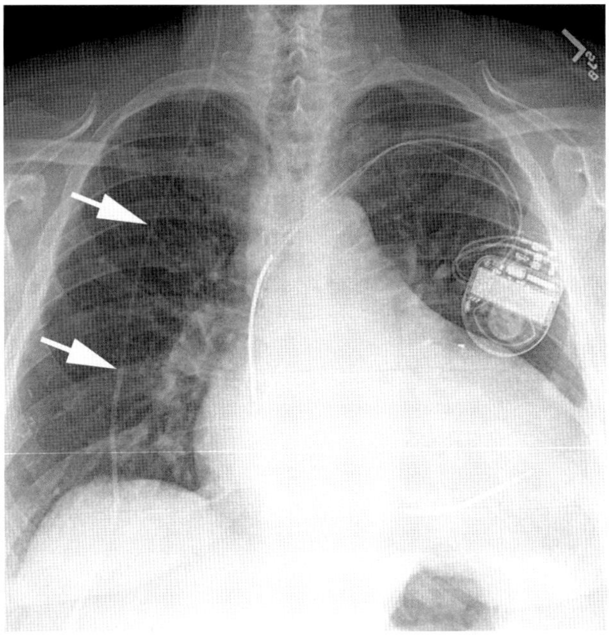

Figure 8.5. Portable chest radiograph shows a malpositioned right internal jugular vein catheter coursing superiorly into the neck. The external aspect of the catheter (arrows) projects over the right hemithorax and mimics ventriculoperitoneal shunt tubing given its course.

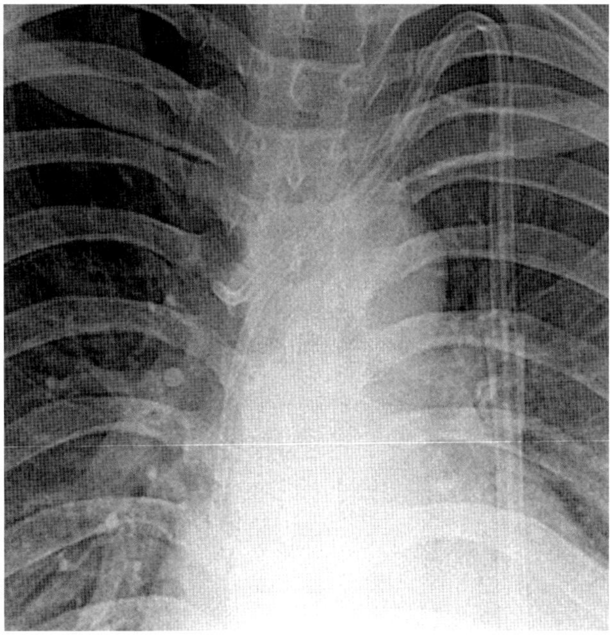

Figure 8.7. Frontal chest radiograph of a 64-year-old man with a left internal jugular vein dual-lumen catheter for hemodialysis. One of the catheter tips is appropriately positioned near the superior cavoatrial junction, but the other catheter tip shows an abnormal course into the azygos arch.

Unit Patients recommend chest radiographic evaluation following placement of central venous catheters and upon an appropriate clinical indication. To not overlook a malpositioned medical device, it is imperative to know the type and number of support devices that the patient is reported to have. Because this information is rarely available on the requisition, the radiologist must account for each radiopaque device seen on radiography. Comparison to prior studies is also required. A malpositioned device should be immediately reported to the clinical team to avoid

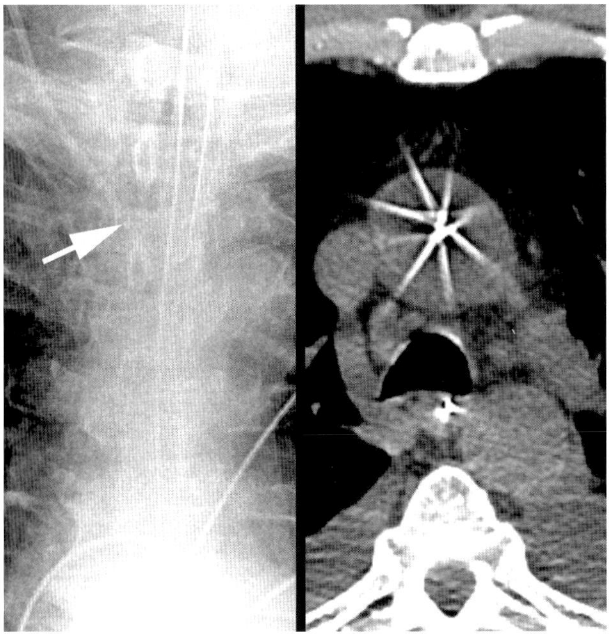

Figure 8.6. Composite image with portable chest radiograph and unenhanced chest CT shows an abnormal course (arrow) of a presumed right internal jugular central venous catheter (left) secondary to inadvertent right carotid artery puncture. CT (right) documents catheter placement in the ascending aorta.

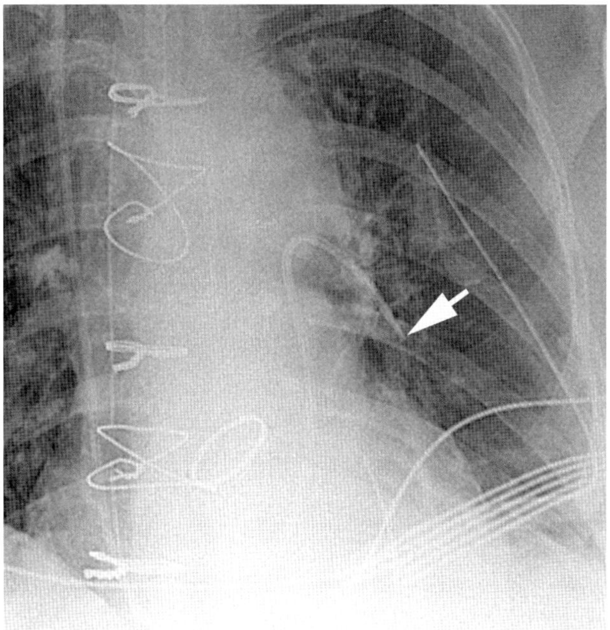

Figure 8.8. AP chest radiograph obtained following aortic valve replacement shows a pulmonary artery catheter with tip (arrow) in the left interlobar pulmonary artery. The catheter tip is in an acceptable position, within 2 cm of the hilum.

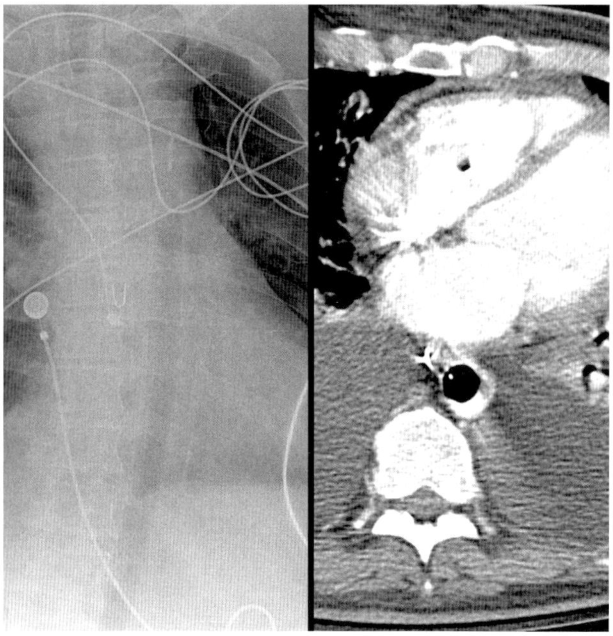

Figure 8.9. Composite image with portable chest radiograph and contrast-enhanced chest CT shows the tubular air-filled IABP balloon along the descending aorta and the radiopaque marker (IABP tip) projecting just below the aortic arch. Chest CT (right) shows the air-filled intra-aortic balloon.

complications. In difficult cases, such as in situations with multiple or overlapping devices and in cases with superimposed extraneous radiopaque equipment, the radiologist may request repeat examinations. These may be performed in oblique or lateral projections to further assess medical device location and tip position.

What Not to Miss

In addition to analyzing the appropriate position of each medical device, radiologists must carefully scrutinize the image for detection of other complications, including catheter fracture, pneumothorax, and mediastinal hemorrhage.

Differential Diagnosis

Several factors may complicate image interpretation:

Overlying Equipment or Extraneous Devices

Several types of external monitoring equipment may be misinterpreted as a malpositioned catheter. These are often recognized by their course on radiography as external to the patient.

Variant Anatomy

Variant vascular anatomy such as persistent left superior vena cava may result in the misdiagnosis of a malpositioned vascular catheter. Correlation with orthogonal or cross-sectional imaging may be helpful in complicated cases.

Imaging Findings

Knowledge of normal radiographic anatomy is crucial for accurate interpretation. The right first anterior intercostal space corresponds to the approximate location of the junction of the brachiocephalic veins to form the superior vena cava. The inferior aspect of the bronchus intermedius is the approximate location of the superior cavoatrial junction. The proximal descending aorta is located below the transverse aortic arch. The radiologist must be able to identify the following complications of catheter placement.

Malposition

- See Figs. 8.3–8.6.
- Abnormal catheter course into the azygos, internal jugular, internal mammary, or superior intercostal veins; central catheter tip in the right atrium or ventricle; pulmonary artery catheter in a peripheral vessel branch; IABP extending above the aortic arch or positioned too low.
- Catheter kinking or looping.
- Placement into an anomalous vessel or through a septal defect.

Catheter Fracture

- Catheter "pinch off" between the first rib and clavicle.

Vascular Injury

- Catheter may perforate a vessel and course into the pleural space, producing a new apical cap or a new pleural effusion (hemothorax or infusothorax).
- Catheter may perforate a vessel and course into the mediastinum or pericardium, producing mediastinal widening from hemorrhage or new enlargement of the cardiopericardial silhouette secondary to hemopericardium.

Unintentional Arterial Puncture

- Aberrant catheter course medial to that of the normal superior vena cava, often projecting over the aortic arch.

Unintentional Lung Puncture

- Pneumothorax; may exhibit deep sulcus sign due to supine patient position.

Clinical Issues

- Pneumothorax is the second most common acute complication of vascular catheter placement and should be excluded on every post-procedure radiograph.
- Vascular injury may produce life-threatening hemothorax, hemopericardium, or mediastinal hemorrhage.

- Catheter infection is a potential complication, most frequently due to *Staphylococcus* species.
- Catheter thrombosis may cause soft tissue swelling, as well as pulmonary embolism.
- Pulmonary artery catheters extending into a peripheral vessel branch may result in pulmonary infarction or pseudoaneurysm formation.
- IABP balloon extending above the aortic arch may obstruct the great vessels; IABP balloon positioned too low may occlude mesenteric and renal arteries.
- A fibrin sheath may form around a long-term indwelling catheter and manifests as a catheter that can be flushed but through which blood cannot be aspirated. Injection of tissue plasminogen activator through the catheter may prove therapeutic.

Key Points

- The radiologist must assess all vascular catheters for appropriate positioning and to exclude complications.
- When findings are equivocal or confusing, the radiologist should not hesitate to recommend additional imaging.
- The most common complication of vascular catheter placement is malposition.
- Identification of catheter malposition must be verbally communicated to the clinical team and documented on the radiologic report.

Suggested Reading

Godoy MC, Leitman BS, de Groot PM, Vlahos I, Naidich DP. Chest radiography in the ICU: Part 2. Evaluation of cardiovascular lines and other devices. *AJR Am J Roentgenol.* 2012 Mar;198(3):572–581.

Hunter TB, Taljanovic MS, Tsau PH, Berger WG, Standen JR. Medical devices of the chest. *RadioGraphics.* 2004 Nov–Dec;24(6):1725–1746.

Rajaram SS, Desai NK, Kalra A, et al. Pulmonary artery catheters for adult patients in intensive care. *Cochrane Database Syst Rev.* 2013 Feb 28;2:CD003408.

CHAPTER 9

Cardiac Conduction Devices

Tyler H. Ternes

Definition

Cardiac pacemakers and implantable cardioverter defibrillators (IDCs) are electronic devices used for management of cardiac conduction abnormalities and designed for permanent use (Figs. 9.1 and 9.2). An ICD differs from a pacemaker in its ability to defibrillate the heart via the discharge of a single high-voltage impulse. These permanent conduction devices consist of a pulse generator and electrical leads.

The generator houses the battery, which has a 5- to 10-year life span. Computer hardware and software are also components of the generator and allow monitoring and correction of arrhythmias, as well as event recording. The information stored in the generator can be sent electronically via the Internet for further evaluation. The central portion of the lead is the conductor wire. The leads are attached to the generator with connector pins. The conductor wires are insulated in silicone or polyurethane. The leads are implanted in the heart by active or passive fixation. Active fixation involves a helical tip screwed into the myocardium. Passive fixation involves radiolucent tines that are "passively" caught within trabeculae along the inner lining of the heart.

Clinical Features

Cardiac conduction devices may be used for temporary or permanent pacing. Epicardial leads are placed for temporary use in the event that immediate pacing is needed (e.g., during heart surgery) and may be removed prior to discharge. Pacemakers are used for management of sinoatrial (SA) and atrioventricular (AV) nodal abnormalities. ICDs are particularly useful for treatment of rapid ventricular arrhythmias.

Anatomy and Physiology

The precise purpose of a permanent conduction device can only be determined through a process called interrogation, wherein manufacturer-specific equipment communicates

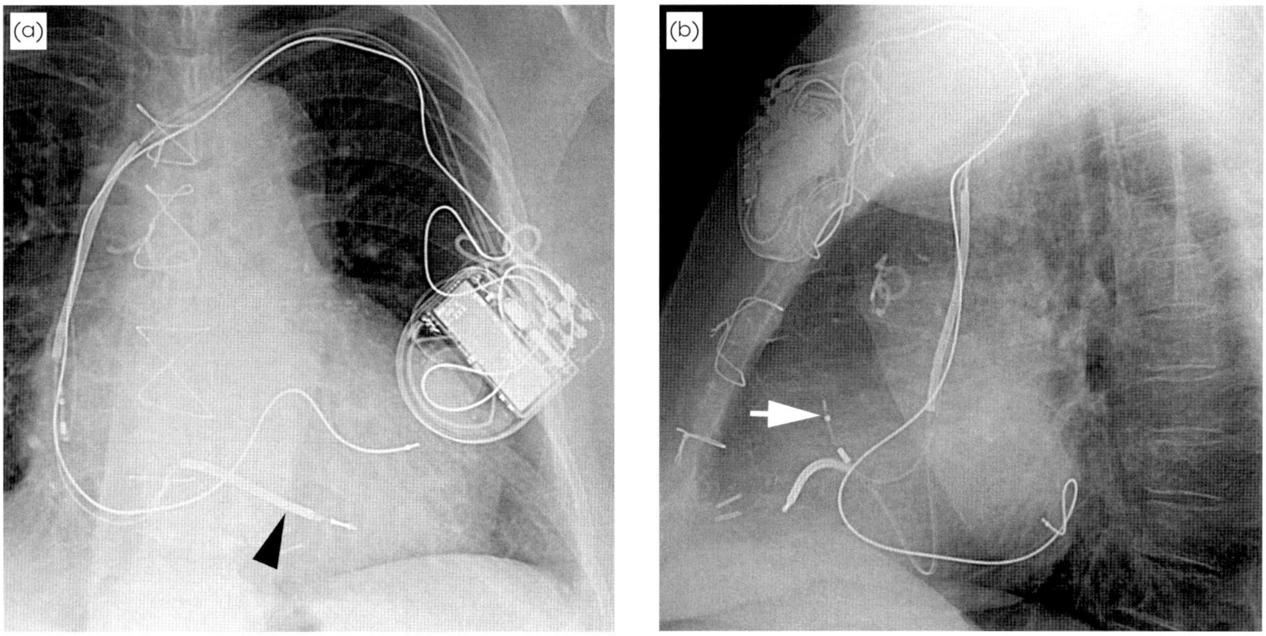

Figure 9.1. Expected appearance of cardiac conduction device. Posteroanterior (PA) (a) and lateral (b) chest radiographs show a left pectoral transvenous, dual-chamber biventricular ICD/pacemaker. The generator is in the left anterior chest wall, and the leads attach to it by connector pins. The thick "shock coils" (arrowhead) of the right ventricular lead indicate that this is an ICD. The right atrial appendage lead tip (arrow) is J-shaped on the lateral radiograph. The right ventricular lead tip is in the right ventricular apex. The third lead is positioned along the posterior heart border via the coronary sinus.

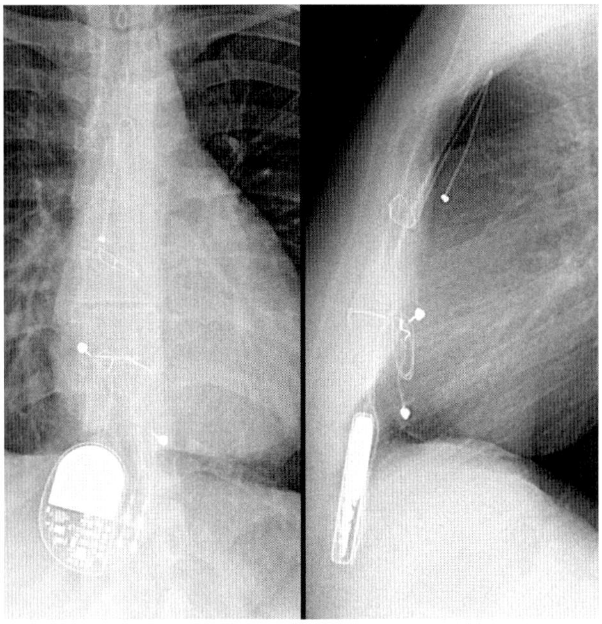

Figure 9.2. Composite image with PA and lateral chest radiographs of a young woman with congenital heart disease shows epicardial wires placed via the subxyphoid approach. Navigation of pacemaker wires may be difficult in children with complex congenital heart disease and variant anatomy, and these patients may require epicardial placement. Patients with abnormal or occluded veins may also require epicardial placement.

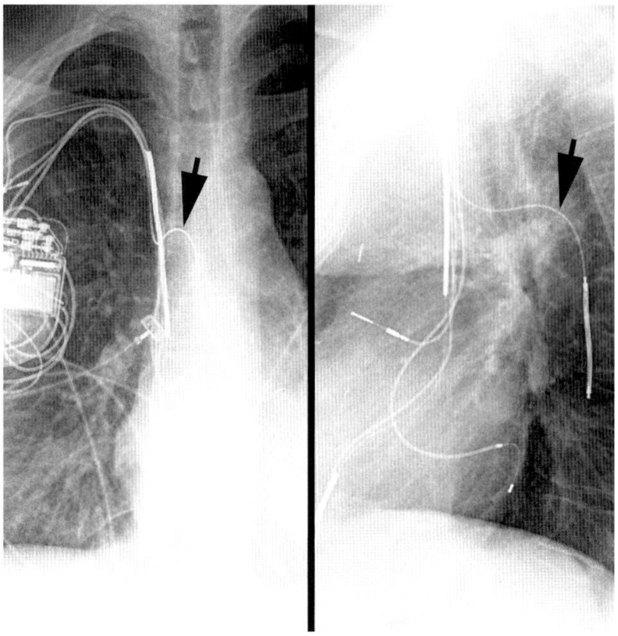

Figure 9.3. Composite image with PA and lateral chest radiographs of a patient with ventricular arrhythmias shows an unexpected course of one of the leads positioned in the azygos vein (arrows). Any lead placement in an unusual position should be communicated to the referring clinician.

directly with the device. However, the general purpose of the device may be inferred from its radiographic appearance. The leads of permanent conduction devices are typically placed via transvenous approach and vary in number from one to three. The generator is positioned subcutaneously in the anterior chest wall, with leads traversing the subclavian and brachiocephalic veins, and the superior vena cava. Single-chamber pacers are typically placed with the lead in the right ventricular apex and are usually employed to manage SA node disease in patients with preserved AV node function. Conversely, dual-chamber pacers are used to treat patients with AV block and have leads in the right atrial appendage and right ventricular apex. Biventricular pacing may be used in patients with cardiomyopathy and interventricular dysynchrony to provide coordinated contraction of the ventricles and thereby improve cardiac function. This has also been termed resynchronization therapy. The additional left ventricular stimulation is usually achieved via a lead placed into the coronary sinus and terminating in a branch vein positioned over the left ventricular surface. An ICD lead is typically placed in the right ventricle to sense and defibrillate a ventricular tachyarrhythmia. Frequently, pacemakers and ICDs are merged into a single device, in which there are pacer leads in the right atrium and coronary sinus, respectively, in addition to a combined pacer/ICD lead in the right ventricle.

How to Approach the Image

Interpretation of chest radiographs must include a thorough assessment of all medical support devices. It is common practice to begin radiographic assessment with a description of the medical devices for two reasons. First, the devices may be overlooked, and important findings such as unexpected lead positions could be missed (Figs. 9.3 and 9.4). Second, the types of support devices may provide clues to the patient's underlying condition.

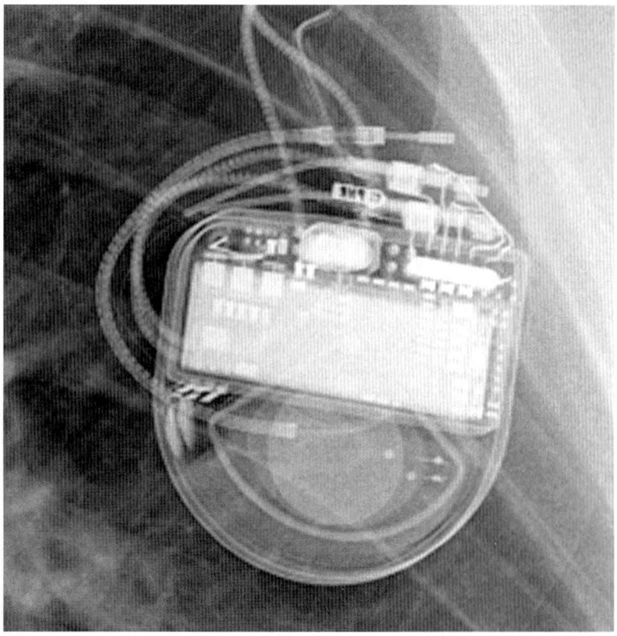

Figure 9.4. Disconnected lead. Coned-down PA chest radiograph of a patient with a prior pacemaker revision shows that one of the leads is disconnected from the generator. In this case, the lead was intentionally abandoned, but in patients with pacemaker malfunction, the cause may a disconnected lead.

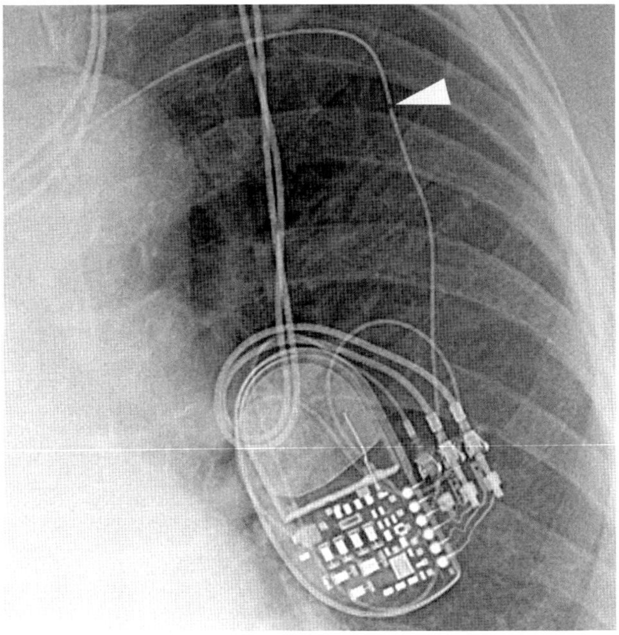

Figure 9.5. Fractured lead. PA chest radiograph of a patient with pacemaker malfunction shows that one of the pacer leads is fractured (arrowhead); this required additional lead placement. The finding of fractured pacer leads should be promptly communicated to the referring physician.

The generator should not change in position or configuration on serial radiographs in the absence of intervention. The connector pins should be assessed to ensure they are engaged at the port sites. The wires should also be evaluated for kinks or fractures (Fig. 9.5). Wire malposition (or interval change in position) should be excluded in every case. The atrial lead should show a characteristic upward and anterior curve into the right atrial appendage that is J-shaped on lateral radiography. A right ventricular lead should ideally be positioned in the right ventricular apex, just to the left of the spine on a frontal radiograph and along the anterior/inferior aspect of the cardiac silhouette on a lateral radiograph. Other positions (e.g., the right ventricular outflow tract) are preferred by cardiologists in certain cases. Left ventricular pacer leads in tributary veins of the coronary sinus often appear as a lead coursing toward the left heart border on the frontal radiograph and coursing along the posterior heart border on the lateral radiograph. The presence of thick shock coils indicates that the device is an ICD. Most manufacturers place a company logo near the generator to aid programmers in determining which device to use for detection.

The chest radiograph must be assessed for potential complications immediately after placement of a cardiac conduction device.

What Not to Miss

Immediately Following Placement of a Pacemaker or ICD

- New pleural effusion or apical cap should raise concern for hemothorax secondary to vascular injury.
- Pneumothorax should be excluded on every radiograph, given the potential for lung puncture during placement.
- Interval enlargement of the cardiopericardial silhouette should suggest hemopericardium from rare myocardial perforation and should prompt urgent evaluation (Fig. 9.6).
- Lead malposition.

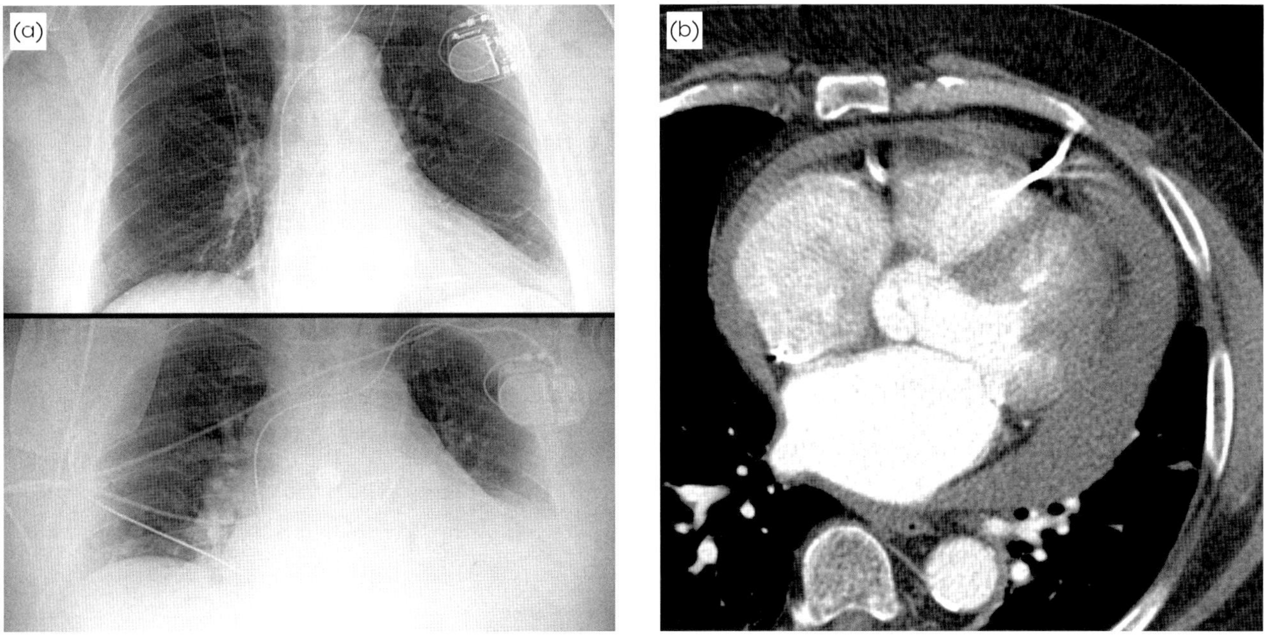

Figure 9.6. (a) Composite image with anteroposterior (AP) chest radiographs obtained immediately after pacemaker placement (top) and several hours later (bottom) shows interval widening of the cardiac silhouette and vascular pedicle concerning for hemopericardium or mediastinal hemorrhage. (b) Contrast-enhanced chest CT of the same patient shows myocardial perforation into the pericardium by the right ventricular pacer lead. Typically, ventricular perforation is of little consequence, but in this patient there was an associated moderate hemopericardium.

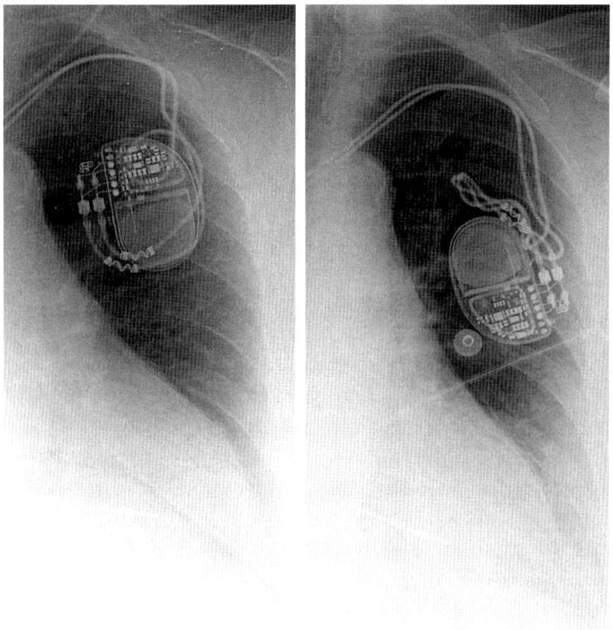

Figure 9.7. Composite image with AP chest radiographs obtained at baseline (left) and 8 months later (right) shows a new orientation of the pulse generator (right) and an abnormal configuration of the pacer wires that exhibit a twisted appearance, consistent with Twiddler's syndrome.

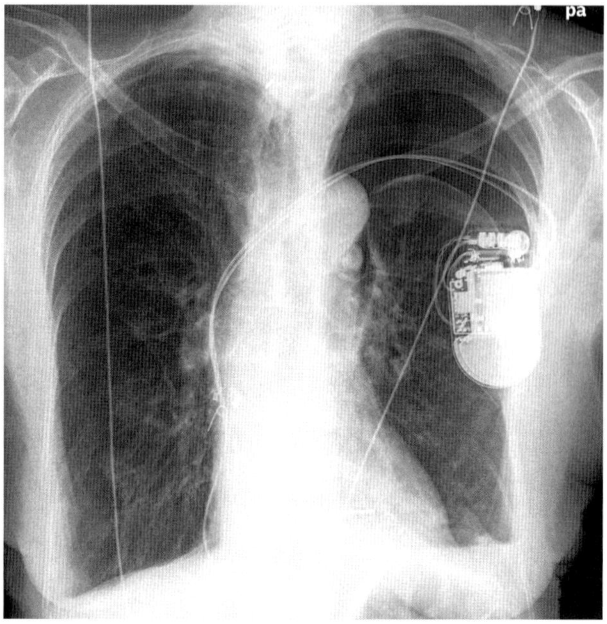

Figure 9.8. PA chest radiograph obtained immediately following left transvenous pacemaker/ICD placement shows a large left pneumothorax. Pneumothorax is one the the most common acute complications of placement of cardiac conduction devices.

Serial Radiographs in Patients with Pacemakers or ICDs

- Twiddler's syndrome: Manipulation of the generator by the patient manifesting as a change in its position or orientation with potential changes in lead position or lead fracture (Fig. 9.7).
- Lead fracture that typically occurs due to pinch-off near the clavicle (Fig. 9.5).
- Infection that may manifest as persistent gas surrounding generator or persistent gas, fluid, and inflammation in the subcutaneous tissues surrounding the generator on computed tomography (CT).
- Dislodged or "backed-out" connector pin at the port site in the generator that may produce pacer/ICD malfunction (Fig. 9.4).

Differential Diagnosis

Abandoned Leads

- The number of active leads should equal the number of ports. An abandoned lead may mimic an unintentionally disconnected lead. However, if all the connector ports are occupied, the disconnected lead was likely intentionally abandoned (replaced) due to malfunction.
- Abandoned lead fragments in the absence of a generator and in association with sternal wires typically indicate prior heart transplantation.

Deep Brain and Vagus Nerve Stimulators

- Deep brain stimulator: Used in patients with neurodegenerative disorders such as Parkinson's disease; may mimic a pacemaker generator, but leads extend superiorly beyond the field of view.
- Vagus nerve stimulator: Used for epilepsy treatment; may mimic cardiac conduction devices, but the wire terminates in the cervical region near the vagus nerve.

Imaging Findings

Pacemaker

Cardiac conduction devices usually consist of a generator that houses the battery and connector ports. Pins should be engaged with their respective ports. Pacer wires extend into the heart.

- Single-chamber pacemaker: Lead in right ventricular apex.
- Dual-chamber pacemaker: Leads in right atrium and right ventricle.
- Single-chamber biventricular pacemaker: Leads in right ventricle and coronary sinus.
- Dual-chamber biventricular pacemaker: Leads in right atrium, right ventricle, and coronary sinus.

ICD

- Identified by the thick shock coils on at least one of the leads, typically the right ventricular lead.

Clinical Issues

- The typical life span of the battery is 5–10 years.
- The majority of pacing abnormalities require assessment with a process called interrogation.
- Myocardial perforations are classified as gross (symptomatic) versus microperforation (asymptomatic). Given the relatively low pressures in the right ventricle, perforations are frequently asymptomatic. A symptomatic patient with new cardiac enlargement should be assessed with contrast-enhanced CT. The rate of perforation is estimated at 1–10%. A perforating right ventricular lead typically maintains normal function (Fig. 9.6).

Key Points

- Pacemakers are complex devices used for a variety of cardiac conduction abnormalities. Lead placement depends on the underlying cardiac pathology.
- ICDs are used for ventricular tachyarrhythmias, and they deliver a high voltage for defibrillation. They are identified on radiography by the presence of thick shock coils.
- Radiologists must assess complications following pacemaker and ICD placement, including pneumothorax, hemothorax, and hemopericardium acutely and Twiddler's syndrome, lead fracture, and lead malposition chronically (Figs. 9.6, 9.7, and 9.8).

Suggested Reading

Aguilera AL, Volokhina YV, Fisher KL. Radiography of cardiac conduction devices: A comprehensive review. *RadioGraphics.* 2011;31(6):1669–1682.

Costelloe CM, Murphy WA Jr, Gladish GW, Rozner MA. Radiography of pacemakers and implantable cardioverter defibrillators. *AJR Am J Roentgenol.* 2012;199(6): 1252–1258.

CHAPTER 10

Thoracostomy Tubes and Mediastinal Drains

Tyler H. Ternes

Definition

Chest or thoracostomy tube is a broad term used to describe any type of hollow catheter used for draining the pleural space. When intentionally placed in the mediastinum, the term mediastinal drain is preferred.

Clinical Features

One of the main uses of thoracostomy tubes is treatment of large or symptomatic pneumothorax. The larger the pneumothorax, the higher the probability that chest tube placement will be required. Another common use of thoracostomy tubes is drainage of pleural fluid, including infected pleural fluid collections (empyema) and hemothorax. These processes require chest tube placement due to poor resorption and clearance of purulent or hemorrhagic pleural fluid.

Chest tube sizes range from 6F to 40F and include large surgically placed chest tubes and small-caliber pigtail catheters. Typically, a larger caliber tube is placed for traumatic pneumothorax and viscous pleural fluid. Small-caliber catheters (≤14F) can often be placed with Seldinger technique using a coaxial needle and guidewire. Large-bore catheters (>16F) are often placed via blunt dissection into the pleural space.

Mediastinal drainage can also be performed with many different catheter sizes. It is most commonly performed following cardiac surgery. The drain may be positioned in various locations, including the pericardial space. Mediastinal drainage helps prevent pericardial tamponade and reduces the risk of subsequent pericarditis.

Anatomy and Physiology

The goal of thoracostomy tube placement is to position the tube in the pleural space, between the visceral and parietal pleural surfaces. Large-caliber tubes usually enter the pleural space at the midaxillary line. Small-caliber (pigtail) tubes may be placed via the second intercostal space at the midclavicular line.

A chest tube used for pneumothorax evacuation is positioned with the tip directed toward the apical pleural space following an anterior superior course due to the nondependent location of pleural air (Fig. 10.1). Conversely, a chest tube placed for evacuation of pleural fluid is ideally positioned at the basilar pleural space following a posterior inferior course due to the dependent location of pleural fluid (Fig. 10.2). In some cases, the chest tube is specifically directed toward areas of loculated pleural fluid or air. During placement, the tube should ideally be advanced along the superior margin of the adjacent rib to avoid injury to the intercostal vessels that course just along the inferior rib margin.

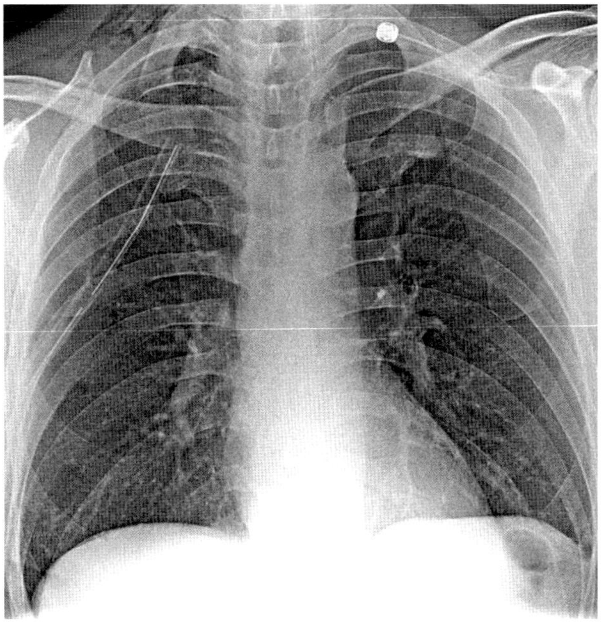

Figure 10.1. Appropriately positioned chest tube. Portable chest radiograph of a 39-year-old man after chest tube placement for spontaneous right pneumothorax shows that the tube courses toward the right apex with the sideport projecting over the right hemithorax.

How to Approach the Image

A crucial element of radiographic interpretation of hospitalized patients involves evaluation of all medical support devices. This includes assessment of chest tube position. A thoracostomy tube is usually placed into the pleural space with the tip directed apically for pneumothorax evacuation and toward the base for pleural fluid evacuation. Chest

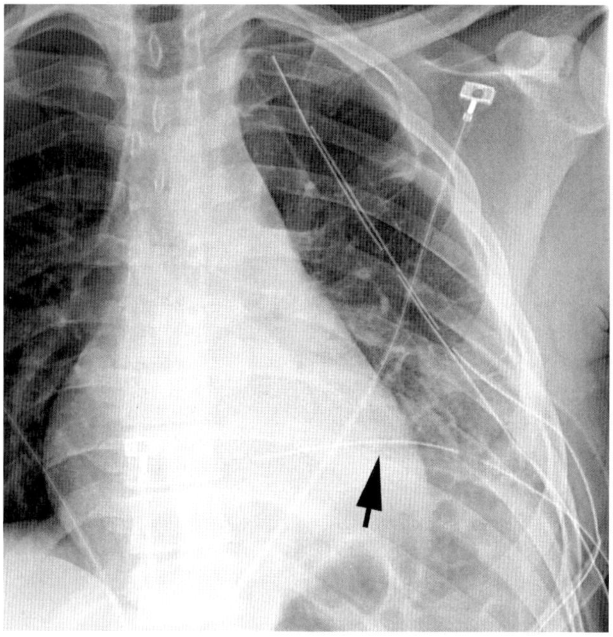

Figure 10.2. Appropriately positioned chest tube. Portable chest radiograph of a 51-year-old man with chest tube placement after video-assisted thoracoscopy for evacuation of left empyema shows one tube directed toward the base (arrow) for evacuation of residual pleural fluid and two tubes directed apically for evacuation of pneumothorax.

tubes typically have a longitudinal radiopaque line with a small focal interruption indicating the site of the tube sideport. One should ensure that the sideport is also located within the pleural space for optimal function. Mediastinal drain position is variable (Fig. 10.3).

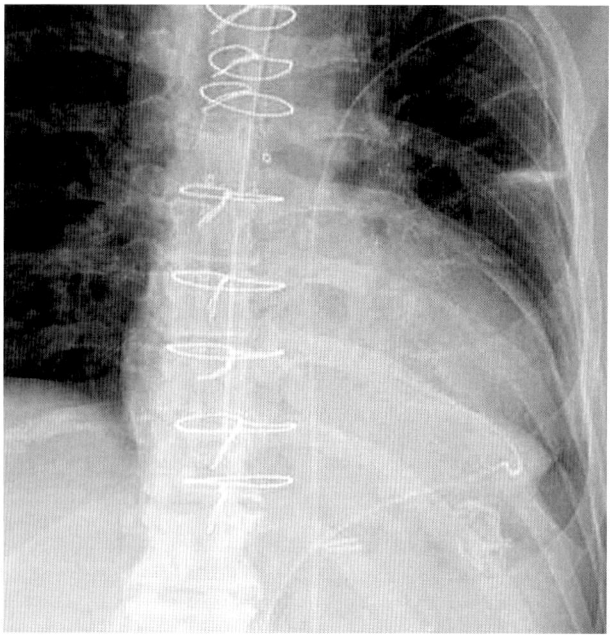

Figure 10.3. Appropriately positioned mediastinal drains. Anteroposterior (AP) chest radiograph of a patient status post coronary artery bypass graft surgery shows midline and left basilar mediastinal drains.

What Not to Miss

Chest Tube

- Nonresolving pneumothorax or pleural effusion suggesting chest tube malfunction.
- Chest tube or sideport located in chest wall soft tissues (Fig. 10.4).
- Intrafissural chest tube placement (Fig. 10.5).
- Intraparenchymal chest tube placement (Figs. 10.6 and 10.7).
- Chest tube kinking.
- Inadvertent mediastinal or abdominal chest tube placement (Fig. 10.8).

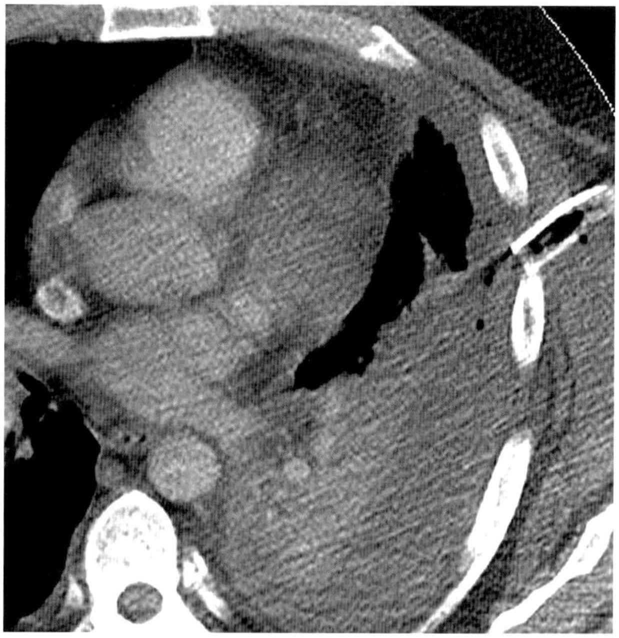

Figure 10.4. Malpositioned chest tube. Axial contrast-enhanced chest CT of a patient with empyema and poor chest tube drainage shows retraction of the chest tube tip (and sideport) into the left chest wall outside the pleural space, which precluded adequate empyema drainage.

Mediastinal Drain

- Progressive mediastinal widening indicates worsening mediastinal hemorrhage or poorly functioning mediastinal drain.

Differential Diagnosis

Overlying Extraneous Equipment

- External portions of tubes, particularly enteric tubes, may mimic an aberrant course of a chest tube.

Chest Tube in Profile

- May mimic a focal kink or malpositioning; absence of kinking may be confirmed with oblique or lateral radiography.

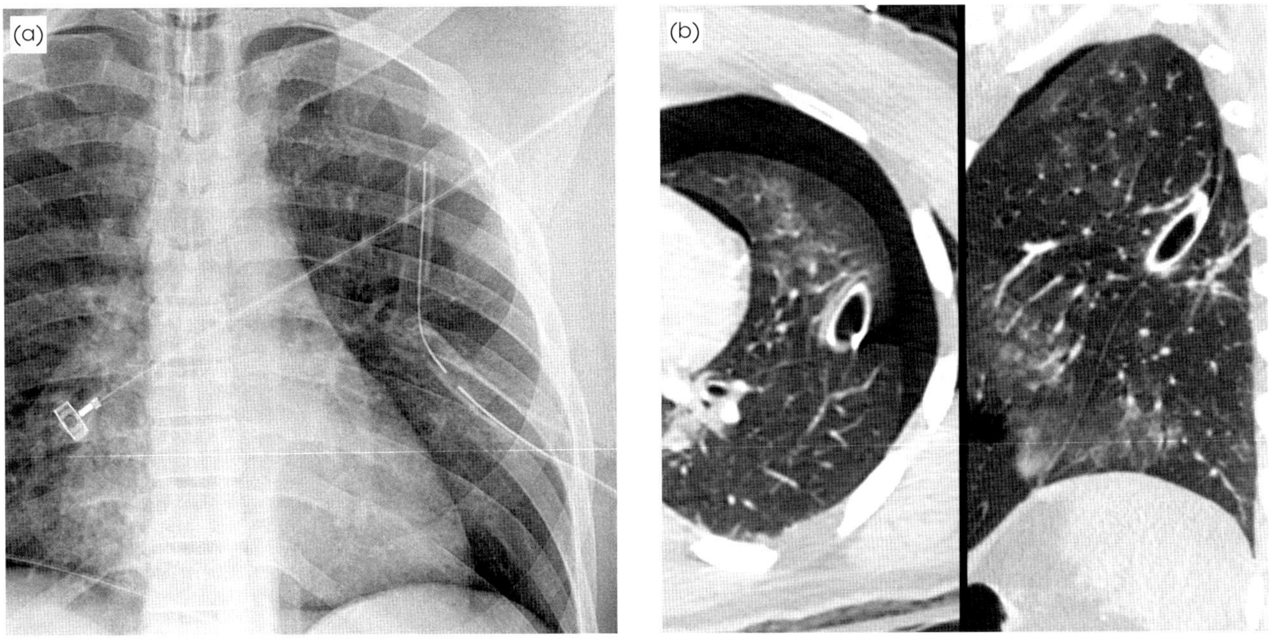

Figures 10.5. Malpositioned chest tube. (a) AP chest radiograph of a 32-year-old man involved in a motor vehicle collision shows a left chest tube oriented toward the apex with a somewhat vertical distal course. (b) Composite image with contrast-enhanced chest CT of the same patient shows a left pneumothorax and a chest tube located within the left major fissure (left), confirmed on the sagittal reformatted image (right). Reformatted images may be useful for accurate assessment of chest tube location.

Bullous Emphysema

- May mimic pneumothorax.
- Bullae are identified by visualization of thin bulla walls.

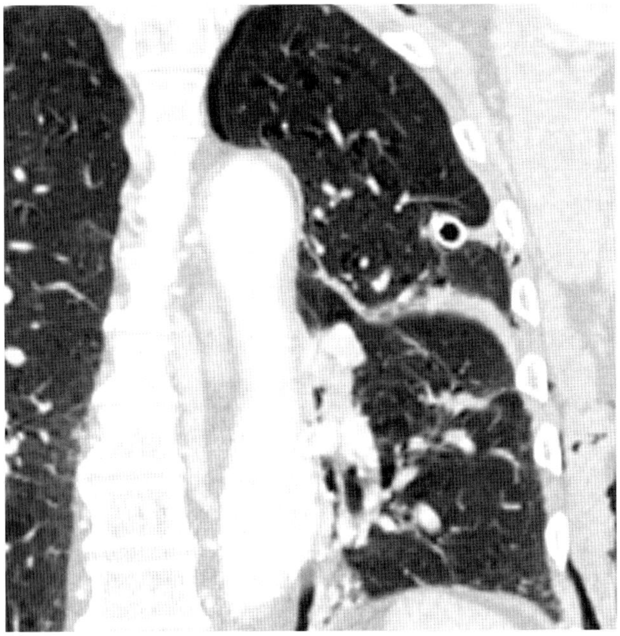

Figure 10.6. Malpositioned chest tube. Coronal contrast-enhanced chest CT shows a left chest tube indenting the left upper lobe and completely surrounded by lung parenchyma.

Imaging Findings

Chest Tube

- Large-bore chest tubes manifest as parallel thin linear opacities with a thin metallic density line along the course of the tube.
- Small-bore chest tubes typically do not exhibit a metallic density line.
- A small focal interruption in the chest tube's metallic line indicates the sideport location.
- Ideally, both the tube tip and the sideport should be within the pleural space and project within the thoracic cavity.
- Chest tube course should be directed toward the posterior base for pleural fluid drainage and toward the anterior apex for pneumothorax evacuation.
- A focal or acute angulation along the chest tube course suggests a kink and the need for potential repositioning.
- Computed tomography (CT) may demonstrate soft tissue attenuation within the chest tube lumen due to debris or hemorrhage that may produce obstruction.
- Multiplanar reformatted CT images may allow identification of intrafissural or intraparenchymal chest tube malpositioning.

Mediastinal Drain

- Devices of various sizes manifesting with parallel radiopaque lines projecting over the mediastinum. May exhibit a longitudinal metallic density line.

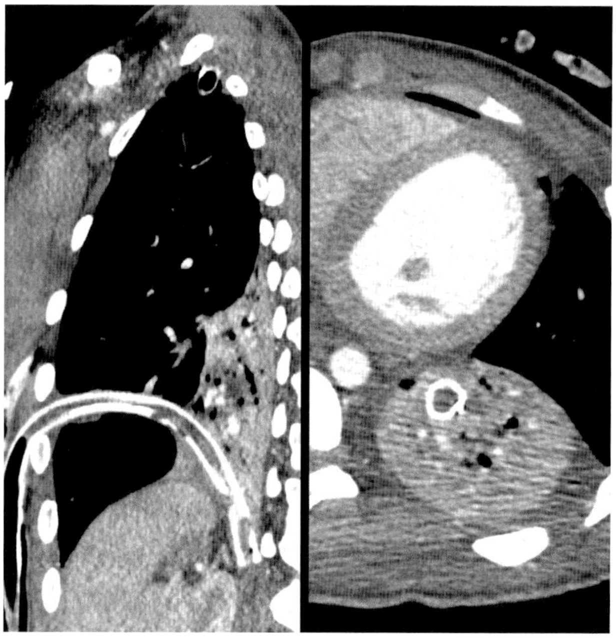

Figure 10.7. Malpositioned chest tube. Composite image with contrast-enhanced chest CT shows an anterior-to-posterior chest tube course inconsistent with the expected location of the pleural space (left). The axial image (right) confirms intraparenchymal chest tube placement. High density in the chest tube lumen is consistent with hemorrhage.

- Often placed via subxyphoid approach.
- Tube tip directed at surgeon's discretion.
- Focal angulation suggests kink and potential need for repositioning.

Clinical Issues

- Appropriate thoracostomy tube size is debatable. Recently, there has been a trend toward using smaller tube sizes (≤14 Fr) because many authors suggest that small-bore tubes are more easily placed, are adequate for drainage of most pleural collections, and result in less patient discomfort. However, some pleural abnormalities, such as recurrent pneumothorax (particularly in mechanically ventilated patients), may require large-bore tubes.
- Silastic drains are preferred by some surgeons for drainage of the mediastinum and/or pleural space after cardiothoracic surgery. Advantages include smaller size (19 Fr) and increased flexibility compared to typical large-bore plastic chest tubes. These factors may contribute to increased patient comfort and mobility. These tubes are fluted throughout their length to increase fluid drainage. However, their use is not widespread, partially due to concern for obstruction by large clots.
- The method of chest tube placement is at the discretion of the physician. Small-bore catheters are most commonly placed with the Seldinger technique, wherein the pleural space is accessed with a coaxial needle and guidewire and the tube is advanced over the wire. Alternatively, a trocar technique (direct puncture) can be used, but only in selected cases due to the danger of injuring the adjacent lung. Large-bore tubes are positioned via blunt dissection involving a skin incision and dissection of the subcutaneous

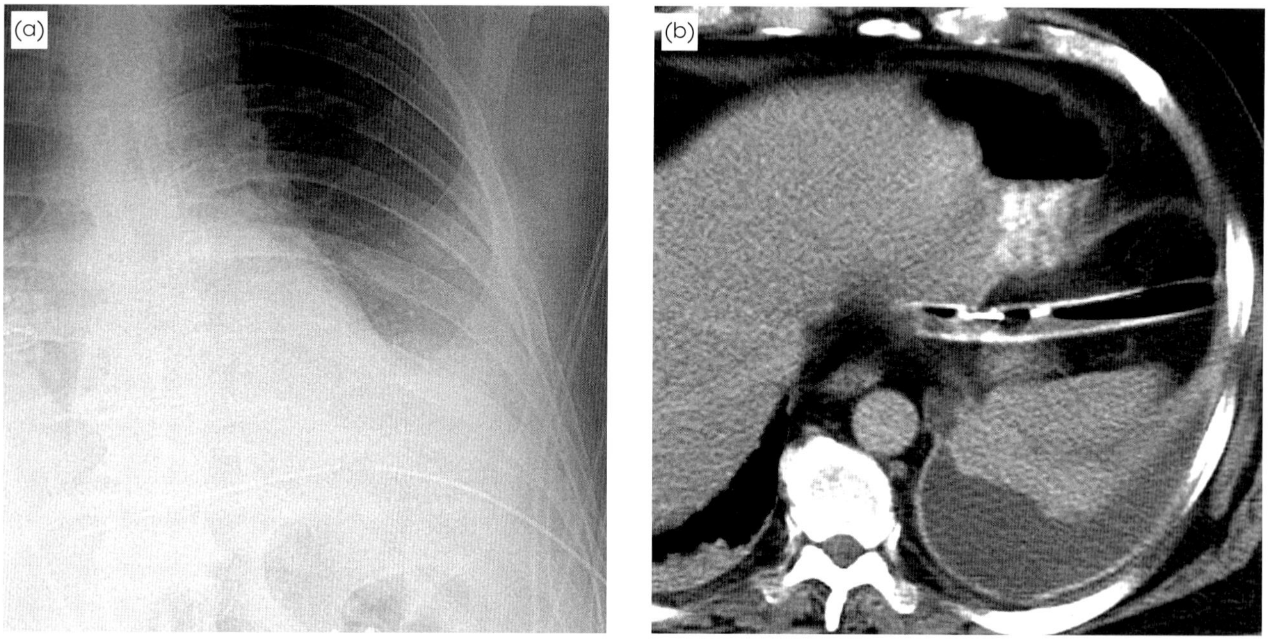

Figure 10.8. Malpositioned chest tube. (a) AP chest radiograph of a patient with suspected left empyema shows a left basilar chest tube that crosses the midline and exhibits a lower than expected position. (b) Contrast-enhanced chest CT of the same patient shows chest tube placement below the diaphragm within the abdomen and also the tube tip abutting the liver. The finding of any malpositioned medical device should be immediately communicated to the the clinical team.

space and intercostal muscles. This technique also allows digital palpation of the pleural space.
- A chest tube should not be placed into a bulla.

Key Points

- Chest tubes and mediastinal drains are used to evacuate the pleural space and mediastinum, respectively.
- Anteroapical chest tube placement is recommended for pneumothorax evacuation. Inferoposterior chest tube placement is recommended for pleural effusion drainage.
- Chest tubes may be straight or pigtail-shaped. Small-bore catheters (≤14 Fr) have been increasingly advocated due to increased patient comfort.
- Like every other medical device, chest tubes and mediastinal drains should be assessed on each radiograph. Nonresolving pneumothorax or pleural effusion should prompt evaluation for a potential cause of poor chest tube function, including kinking or malposition outside the pleural space, within the fissure, or in the lung parenchyma.

Suggested Reading

Godoy MC, Leitman BS, de Groot PM, Vlahos I, Naidich DP. Chest radiography in the ICU: Part 1. Evaluation of airway, enteric, and pleural tubes. *AJR Am J Roentgenol.* 2012 Mar;198(3):563–571.

Hunter TB, Taljanovic MS, Tsau PH, Berger WG, Standen JR. Medical devices of the chest. *RadioGraphics.* 2004 Nov–Dec;24(6):1725–1746.

Mahmood K, Wahidi MM. Straightening out chest tubes: What size, what type, and when. *Clin Chest Med.* 2013 Mar;34 (1):63–71.

Section III

Bedside Radiography

Common Abnormalities

CHAPTER 11

Common Abnormalities on Portable Chest Radiography

Brent P. Little

Introduction

The chest radiograph is the most commonly performed radiographic examination, and bedside radiography plays an important role in assessing acute cardiopulmonary disease in the inpatient setting, particularly within intensive care units. Radiologists must be aware of the range of abnormalities that manifest on bedside chest radiography in order to optimize patient care.

Technique

Portable radiographs may be challenging to interpret. The typical bedside chest radiographic examination is obtained as a single anteroposterior (AP) view with the detector panel placed under or behind the patient. The resulting AP radiograph magnifies the heart, great vessels, and hila. Lack of a lateral radiograph limits evaluation of the posterior lower lobes, which are partially obscured by the cardiac silhouette and hemidiaphragms. Although portable radiographs are often obtained with the head of the bed elevated, supine positioning is routinely used for many critical ill and intubated patients—causing pleural fluid to layer posteriorly and pneumothoraces to collect anteroinferiorly within the costophrenic sulci.

Approach to Common Findings at Bedside Radiography

Assessment of Technique

Recognition of the limitations of portable radiographic technique is critical. AP radiographs obtained with patient rotation and the beam oblique to the anterior chest may cause a normal mediastinum to appear widened. Hypoinflation may cause crowding of bronchovascular structures at the lung bases, which may be confused with atelectasis or pneumonia, or hide true pathology. Underexposed radiographs may obscure portions of the mediastinum, whereas overexposed radiographs may create artifactual pulmonary hyperlucency.

Time Course of the Disease

Certain conditions, such as aspiration pneumonitis, pulmonary edema, and lobar atelectasis, develop and resolve rapidly, whereas pneumonia and acute respiratory distress syndrome (ARDS) have a less fluctuating course. Comparison studies may enable discrimination of acute abnormalities from chronic lung diseases such as pulmonary fibrosis or scarring from prior infection.

Common Findings on Bedside Chest Radiography

Many common pulmonary diseases in the inpatient setting manifest as abnormal increased opacity of the lung. Several patterns should be recognized:

- Airspace (alveolar) opacity: Filling of alveoli and distal (respiratory) bronchioles with fluid, pus, blood, or cells of any type causes abnormal attenuation of the x-ray beam and ranges from patchy, hazy opacity to dense "consolidation" (obscuring underlying bronchovascular structures). Airspace opacities are common in pneumonia (Fig. 11.1), aspiration (Fig. 11.2), alveolar edema, and, less frequently, pulmonary hemorrhage.
- Interstitial opacities: The axial interstitium and lymphatics course along the bronchovascular bundles. Thickening of these structures manifests as linear or nodular opacities, "peribronchial cuffing," and/or hilar indistinctness. The peripheral interstitium courses along the subpleural lung and interlobular septa and, when thickened with fluid or cells, manifests as septal or Kerley B lines in the lung periphery. Interstitial pulmonary edema and infection with an interstitial component are common causes of interstitial opacities in the inpatient setting.
- Atelectasis: Atelectasis (from the Greek for "incomplete expansion") is partial or complete lung collapse. In contrast to other airspace opacities, atelectasis is associated with volume loss instead of airspace filling. Lobar or total lung atelectasis can be recognized by displacement of the interlobar fissures and hila or shift of the mediastinum toward the side of the

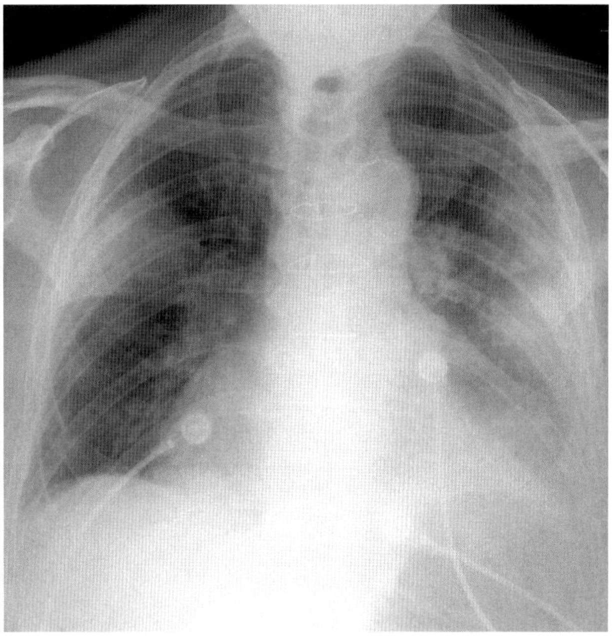

Figure 11.1. Pneumonia. Portable AP chest radiograph shows consolidation in the right upper lobe and patchy airspace opacities in the left upper and lower lobes. Sputum culture grew *Streptococcus pneumoniae*.

atelectasis, as well as increased opacity of the involved lung. Subsegmental atelectasis can be linear or band-like on both chest radiography and CT.

- Pleural fluid: Blunting of the costophrenic angles or a meniscoid opacity at the lung periphery are reliable signs of pleural fluid. When the patient is supine, pleural fluid may layer posteriorly, causing a gradient of diminishing opacity on chest radiography extending cranially from the lung bases. Pleural fluid can also cause dense basilar opacity that at times is difficult to distinguish from airspace opacity.
- Pneumothorax: Patients being evaluated with portable chest radiography may be susceptible to development of pneumothorax as a result of barotrauma related to mechanical ventilation, underlying lung disease (e.g., ARDS and emphysema) (Fig 11.3), or thoracic interventions. It is important to recognize radiographic mimics of pneumothorax, most often skin folds (Fig. 11.4).

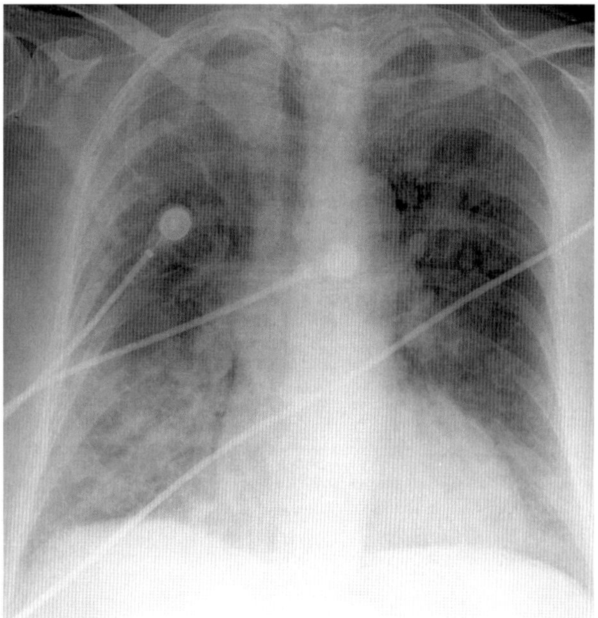

Figure 11.2. Aspiration. Portable mildly rotated AP chest radiograph shows multifocal airspace opacities in both upper and lower lobes that were new imaging findings compared to a prior radiograph obtained 8 hours earlier.

Differential Diagnosis

Once an abnormality is detected and described, a differential diagnosis is formulated based on the clinical history and radiographic findings. In the inpatient, the following common diseases should be considered:

- Pneumonia: Community-acquired and health care-associated pneumonias are common and usually manifest with patchy airspace opacity and/or consolidation. Interstitial opacities commonly occur in viral and atypical pneumonias.
- Aspiration: Aspiration is common in traumatized patients, the neurologically impaired, and patients with impaired swallowing mechanisms or tracheostomies. Aspiration is characterized by dependent, bronchocentric airspace opacities and/or consolidation

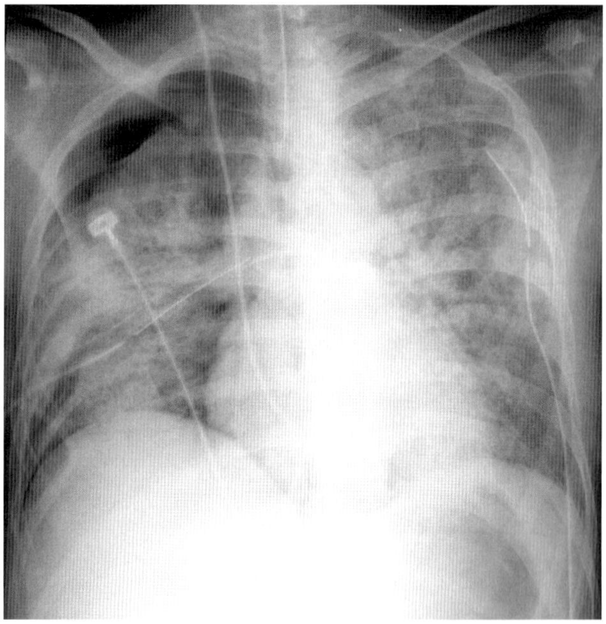

Figure 11.3. Pneumothorax (ARDS). Portable AP chest radiograph shows an endotracheal tube, bilateral chest tubes, and a right apical pneumothorax manifesting as abnormal lucency in the outer aspect of the right upper hemithorax. Both lungs are opacified by diffuse airspace and interstitial opacities—manifestations of diffuse alveolar damage (DAD). Clinically, the patient fulfilled criteria for the diagnosis of ARDS.

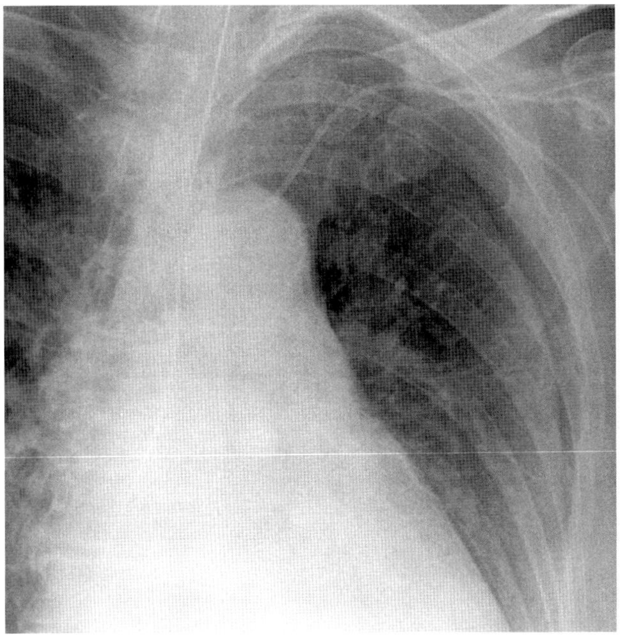

Figure 11.4. Skin fold mimicking pneumothorax. Coned-down portable AP chest radiograph shows a well-defined interface in the left upper and mid hemithorax that parallels the outer aspect of the lung and mimics a pneumothorax. Lung markings extend beyond the interface, and there is no abnormal lucency in the lung periphery, a characteristic finding in pneumothorax.

with centrilobular nodules and tree-in-bud opacities. The findings are often bilateral but asymmetric.

- Pulmonary edema: Interstitial opacities occur in the early stages (interstitial edema). Airspace opacities, often perihilar and relatively symmetric, occur in alveolar edema.
- ARDS: ARDS is persistent severe hypoxemia due to a variety of pulmonary and systemic causes. In the early stages, bilateral hazy airspace or interstitial opacities are common. In later phases, superimposed bibasilar consolidation may be seen.
- Atelectasis: Lobar or total lung atelectasis is usually due to mucous plugging or aspiration when detected in inpatients. Volume loss in the involved lung and mediastinal shift to the side of collapse are the rule.
- Pleural effusions or hemothorax: Pleural effusions are common in inpatients, especially those with heart failure or recovering from surgery. A rapidly developing pleural collection after surgery or trauma suggests hemothorax (or, less commonly, chylothorax).

Conclusion

Several acute pulmonary diseases are common in the inpatient setting. Appreciation of the clinical presentations and common imaging findings of these diseases is essential in interpreting bedside chest radiography.

Suggested Reading

Khan A, Hamdan AJ, AL-Ghanem S, Alaa G. Reading chest radiographs in the critically ill: Part II. Radiography of lung pathologies common in the ICU patient. *Ann Thorac Med.* 2009;4(3):149–157.

Rubinowitz AN, Siegel MD, Tocino I. Thoracic imaging in the ICU. *Crit Care Clin.* 2007;23(3):539–557.

CHAPTER 12

Pulmonary Venous Hypertension and Edema

Brent P. Little and Travis S. Henry

Definition

Pulmonary edema is defined as abnormal pulmonary extravascular fluid accumulation. It is commonly characterized as "cardiogenic" or "noncardiogenic." In cardiogenic edema, impaired cardiac function leads to elevated left atrial and pulmonary venous hydrostatic pressures with resultant fluid accumulation in the lungs. Noncardiogenic pulmonary edema is caused by increased capillary permeability that occurs in lung injury (e.g., acute respiratory distress syndrome (ARDS)), hypoalbuminemia, or fluid volume overload.

Clinical Features

Pulmonary edema is a common finding at inpatient bedside radiography. However, because radiographic findings can overlap with other diseases such as increased capillary permeability edema (ARDS), diffuse pneumonia, pulmonary hemorrhage, and other conditions, accurate diagnosis relies heavily on correlation with clinical findings. Cardiogenic edema with systolic dysfunction can be detected at echocardiography as a decreased left ventricular ejection fraction, but diastolic dysfunction can also be a source of edema despite a normal ejection fraction. Elevated brain natriuretic peptide (BNP) levels may also be a clue to the underlying cause of the edema.

Pulmonary capillary wedge pressure is the gold standard for diagnosing congestive heart failure, allowing characterization as mild, moderate, or severe. Normal wedge pressure is less than12 mm Hg. Mild congestive failure correlates with a pulmonary capillary wedge pressure of 12–19 mm Hg; on upright radiographs, upper lobe vessels are distended and referred to as "pulmonary venous redistribution" or "cephalization." Moderate congestive failure (20–25 mm Hg) results in interstitial pulmonary edema, with thickening of the interlobular septa on chest radiographs (Kerley B lines) and CT. Severe failure (>25 mm Hg) correlates with pulmonary alveolar edema, which manifests as airspace opacity on radiographs and CT.

Anatomy and Physiology

Fluid is dynamically filtered across the endothelium of the pulmonary capillaries and resorbed by pulmonary lymphatics. A balance in hydrostatic and oncotic pressures maintains equilibrium, and a disturbance in either force can result in abnormal fluid accumulation (edema):

- Cardiogenic (hydrostatic) edema: Intravascular hydrostatic pressure is too high, driving fluid into the lungs. This is usually caused by increased venous pressure (e.g., left heart failure).
- Noncardiogenic (permeability) edema: Imbalance of oncotic pressures. Low protein states (e.g., liver or renal failure) result in decreased intravascular oncotic pressure, whereas alveolar damage can increase permeability of the endothelium, causing proteins to leak into the interstitium with resultant increased extravascular oncotic pressure. Either process causes a net outward movement of fluid. Pulmonary edema occurs when the resulting increase in outward fluid filtration overwhelms the lung's capacity for lymphatic drainage.

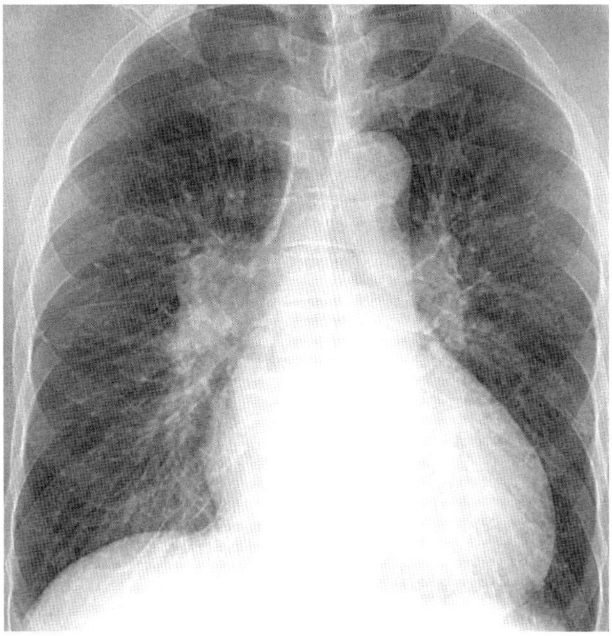

Figure 12.1. Pulmonary venous hypertension. Posteroanterior (PA) chest radiograph (upright patient) shows cardiomegaly and upper lobe vessels equal in caliber or larger than vessels at the lung bases, a radiographic sign of pulmonary venous hypertension in an upright patient. Normally, a gravitational gradient is present, with a 1:3 size ratio of upper zone to lower zone vessels.

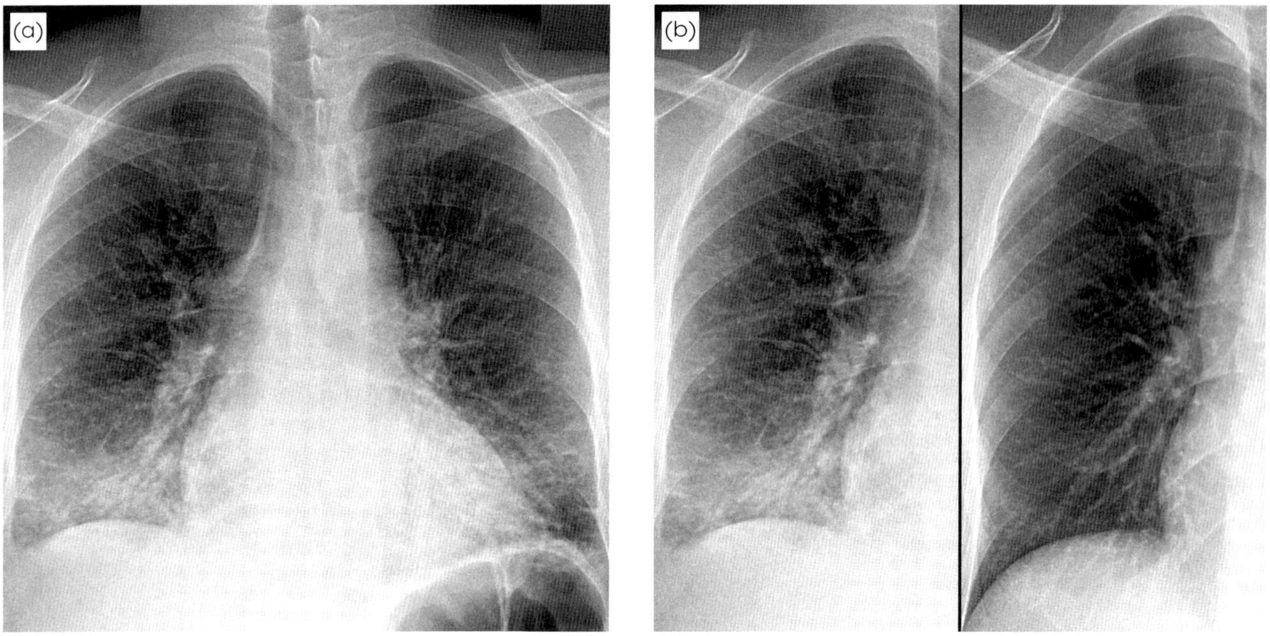

Figure 12.2. Interstitial pulmonary edema. (a) PA chest radiograph of a renal transplant patient shows findings of interstitial edema with bilateral peripheral Kerley B lines, mild thickening of the minor fissure, and pulmonary venous redistribution ("cephalization"). Mild cardiomegaly, small bilateral pleural effusions, and engorgement of the azygous arch are all ancillary findings of pulmonary edema. (b) Composite of coned-down PA views of the right lung show Kerley B lines at the lung periphery (left) and blurring of pulmonary vascular structure; a subsequent radiograph (right) shows resolution of the septal thickening and pleural effusions, with persistent cephalization remaining.

How to Approach the Image

What Is the Time Course of the Abnormality?

Comparison with prior radiographs is extremely useful. Rapid onset, rapid fluctuation, and/or rapid resolution of opacities suggest pulmonary edema (especially cardiogenic edema). Permeability edema may persist in the setting of ARDS, but in general, chronic abnormalities point to other etiologies.

What Is the Radiographic Technique?

Portable chest radiography can complicate the diagnosis of pulmonary edema. Supine positioning may cause distension of upper lobe vessels in the absence of pulmonary venous hypertension, and layering pleural effusions may mimic pulmonary edema (see Fig. 12.2). Moreover, anteroposterior (AP) technique can magnify the cardiac silhouette and vessels. Low lung volumes or hypoinflated lungs may also mimic pulmonary venous hypertension.

Are There Ancillary Findings of Cardiogenic Edema or Volume Overload?

Dilation of the superior vena cava and azygous vein suggests volume overload and may widen the vascular pedicle. Cardiomegaly is often seen in cardiogenic edema. Pleural effusions are commonly seen with volume overload or cardiogenic edema but are not as common in ARDS. Thickening of the fissures and peribronchial cuffing are other helpful clues signaling the presence of interstitial pulmonary edema.

What Not to Miss

Several acute and chronic lung diseases may resemble pulmonary edema on imaging studies. Clinical information and the time course of findings should be considered to avoid misinterpretation. In the acute setting, pulmonary hemorrhage and diffuse pneumonia may manifest with bilateral perihilar consolidation and interstitial thickening. In the chronic setting, fibrosing interstitial lung disease may manifest with progressive basilar reticular opacities.

Typical characteristics of pulmonary edema include the following:

- Rapid onset and rapidly changing appearance on chest radiography
- Ancillary findings of cardiomegaly and pleural effusions (in cardiogenic edema)
- Typically more symmetric than other causes of airspace and interstitial opacity

Differential Diagnosis

Other Causes of Increased Vascularity

- Shunt vascularity: A left-to-right shunt such as an atrial septal defect or patent ductus arteriosus causes increased pulmonary arterial flow. Pulmonary arteries are enlarged centrally and taper in the lung periphery. However, shunt vascularity should not result in airspace or interstitial edema.

- "Cephalization" on supine radiographs: True pulmonary venous redistribution to the upper lungs ("cephalization") is a reliable finding only on upright radiographs. In the supine position, the normal gravitational gradient of blood distribution is lost, and upper lobe vessels appear as large as lower lobe vessels.

Other Causes of Interstitial Thickening

- Pneumonia: Pneumonias with interstitial components (e.g., viral, *Pneumocystis* pneumonia) may mimic interstitial edema, manifesting with haziness of the hila, indistinctness of pulmonary vessels, and Kerley A and B lines. Airspace opacities may also be present, mimicking alveolar edema.
- Interstitial lung disease: Diffuse lung diseases with interstitial components such as pulmonary fibrosis and sarcoidosis can cause interstitial thickening that may mimic interstitial edema. Persistently reduced lung volumes and coarse, irregular septal lines are imaging clues to underlying pulmonary fibrosis or other interstitial lung diseases.
- Lymphangitic carcinomatosis: May manifest as chronic smooth and/or nodular septal thickening. The findings may be focal or diffuse and, when smooth, may mimic pulmonary edema.

Other Causes of Bilateral Airspace Opacities

- Other diffuse airspace diseases: Common conditions such as pneumonia, diffuse alveolar damage, pulmonary hemorrhage, and aspiration pneumonitis and less common diseases such as hypersensitivity pneumonitis, multifocal primary pulmonary adenocarcinoma, and alveolar proteinosis may cause bilateral airspace opacities.
- Layering pleural effusions: On supine radiographs, free-flowing effusions layer posteriorly, and the resulting increased opacity of the hemithorax can be confused with edema. Layering pleural effusions cause a gradient of decreasing opacity extending cranially from the base, and sharp vessel contours are seen through the hazy increased opacity of the affected hemithorax.

Imaging Findings

Pulmonary Venous Hypertension

- Distended upper lobe pulmonary vessels: In the upright position, lower lobe vessels are normally two or three times larger than upper lobe vessels due to the gravitational gradient. In pulmonary venous hypertension (Fig. 12.1), excess fluid within the lower lungs causes a larger amount of pulmonary venous flow to the upper lobes, increasing the diameter of the upper lobe vessels to an equal or larger size compared to the lower zone vessels—a finding called "pulmonary venous vascular redistribution" or "cephalization."
- Increased vascularity: In the supine patient, the normal craniocaudal blood distribution gradient is disrupted even in the absence of pulmonary venous hypertension. However, an overall impression of increased pulmonary vascularity is often present in patients with congestive heart failure, even on supine chest radiography.

Interstitial Edema

- Smooth septal thickening: Excess fluid within the septa that border the secondary pulmonary lobule manifests as "septal thickening" on CT and as peripheral Kerley B lines on chest radiography (Fig. 12.2b).
- Fissural thickening: Excess fluid within the septa at the periphery of the secondary pulmonary lobule causes "septal thickening" manifesting as "Kerley B" lines at the periphery of the lung on chest radiographs. Subpleural interstitial edema manifests as transient thickening of the interlobar fissures that disappears with resolution of the edema (Figs. 12.2a and 12.2b).
- Peribronchial "cuffing": Edema may cause thickening of the peribronchovascular interstitium surrounding bronchial walls and is usually accompanied by interlobular septal thickening—a finding that distinguishes edema from true bronchial wall thickening (Figs. 12.3a and 12.3b).
- Vascular indistinctness: Perihilar haze from interstitial edema causes indistinctness of vessel borders, often best seen in the perihilar region and especially along the borders of the right interlobar pulmonary artery (Figs. 12.2a and 12.3b).
- Hilar fullness and indistinctness: Hilar vessels appear engorged and indistinct. Individual hilar structures become difficult to distinguish.

Alveolar Edema

- Airspace opacities: Alveolar fluid results in hazy airspace opacities (ground glass on CT) and consolidation. The opacities are often bilateral and perihilar, and at times they may manifest as a "batwing" pattern (Fig. 12.4). Findings of interstitial edema often coexist.
- Rapid interval change: When not part of a capillary leak syndrome, the airspace opacities of pulmonary edema can change rapidly (often within hours), and a shifting distribution may be seen on serial chest radiographs.
- Asymmetric pulmonary edema: Common causes of asymmetric pulmonary edema (Fig. 12.5) include patient positioning (continuously lying on one side in bed), regional sparing due to underlying emphysema or oligemia, mitral regurgitation with increased hydrostatic pressures transmitted to the right lung (usually after papillary muscle rupture from myocardial infarction), and re-expansion pulmonary edema after drainage of pleural effusion or pneumothorax (Fig. 12.6).

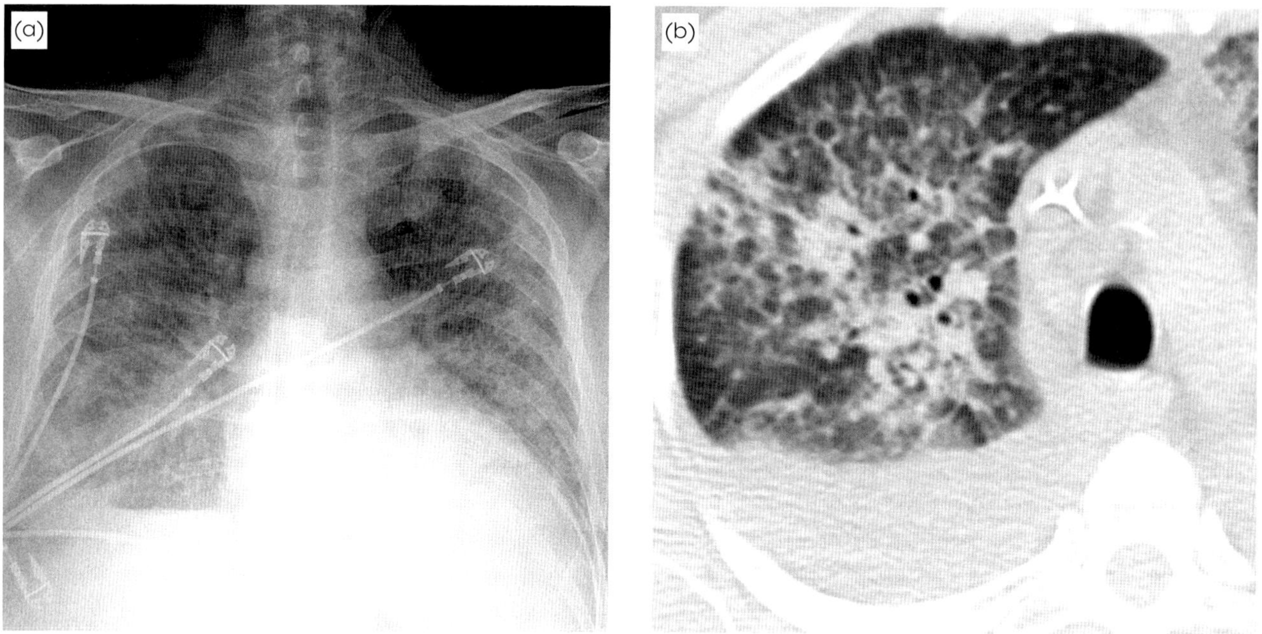

Figure 12.3. Alveolar pulmonary edema. (a) PA chest radiograph of a 64-year-old man with aortic stenosis and shortness of breath shows diffuse bilateral airspace and interstitial opacities. The pulmonary vasculature and hila are indistinct, and peribronchial cuffing is demonstrated in the right suprahilar region. The azygous arch and superior vena cava are dilated, evidence of elevated intravascular volume. (b) Axial CT of the right lung shows findings that were bilateral and symmetric, with ground-glass opacities and patchy consolidation with a central predominance, consistent with interstitial and alveolar pulmonary edema. Bilateral moderate-sized pleural effusions are present.

Ancillary Findings in Patients with Edema

- Cardiomegaly, pleural effusions, and dilatation of the central veins can be seen in congestive heart failure and volume overload; however, these findings occur less frequently in patients with ARDS and diffuse pneumonia.

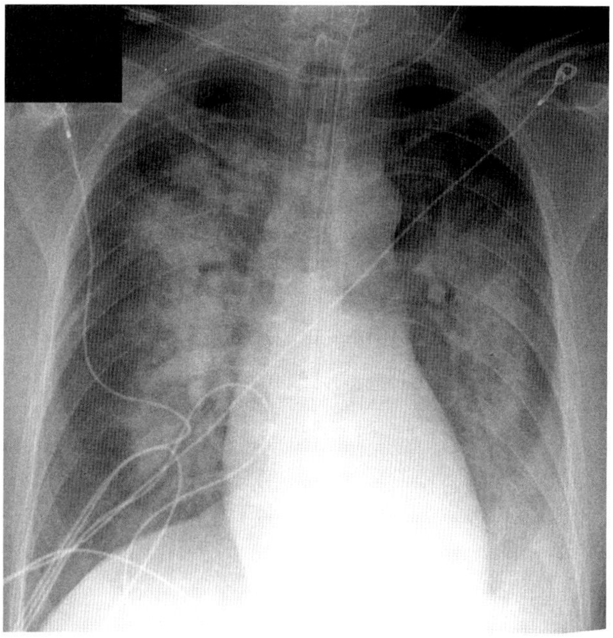

Figure 12.4. Pulmonary edema, "batwing" pattern. AP chest radiograph of a 55-year-old man with severe mitral regurgitation and pulmonary edema demonstrates dense bilateral perihilar opacities (batwing pattern) that appeared rapidly and cleared promptly following diuresis. Mild asymmetry of radiograph findings, as in this case, is common in patients with pulmonary edema.

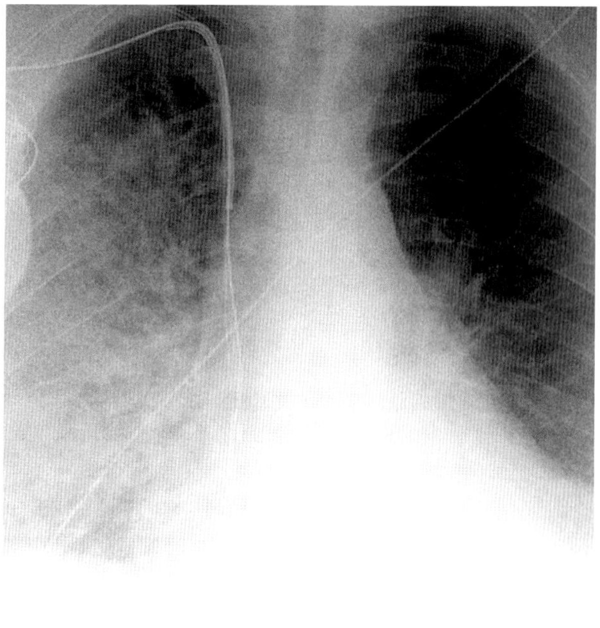

Figure 12.5. Asymmetric pulmonary edema. AP chest radiograph of a 64-year-old man with congestive heart failure demonstrates asymmetric pulmonary edema, with airspace and interstitial opacities in the right lung but minimal findings in the left perihilar region. Causes of asymmetric pulmonary edema include patients lying on one side in bed, underlying emphysema, and mitral regurgitation.

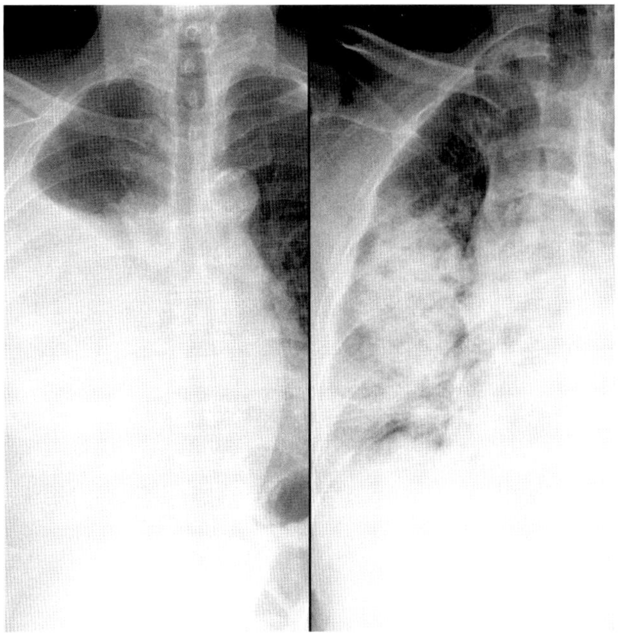

Figure 12.6. Re-expansion pulmonary edema. Composite image of PA chest radiographs of a 70-year-old woman before (left) and soon after (right) drainage of a large pleural effusion shows re-expansion pulmonary edema (right) manifesting as patchy dense consolidation in the right mid-lung that mimics pneumonia or aspiration.

Clinical Issues

- BNP is produced by cardiac myocytes. Serum levels are elevated in cardiogenic edema and can be used to support a suspected diagnosis of pulmonary edema at imaging. Although BNP can also be elevated in a variety of lung diseases, low BNP levels suggest a diagnosis other than cardiogenic pulmonary edema.
- Pulmonary edema is often diagnosed and monitored through noninvasive means (including BNP monitoring, clinical assessment, and imaging studies) rather than pulmonary artery catheterization. A large randomized trial published in 2005 (the ESCAPE trial) found no significant difference in outcomes between patients monitored with pulmonary artery catheters and those managed with noninvasive monitoring.
- Treatment of cardiogenic edema usually involves medical therapy (inotropic agents and preload/afterload reduction) and ventilation support to improve oxygenation. Supportive devices such as intra-aortic balloon pumps can be used to stabilize patients with severe heart failure.

Key Points

- Cardiogenic edema can be characterized in three phases—pulmonary venous hypertension, interstitial edema, and alveolar edema—each with different radiographic findings.
- Radiographic and clinical findings must be correlated to achieve an accurate diagnosis of pulmonary edema because other causes of interstitial and airspace opacities can have overlapping appearances.

Suggested Reading

Asrani A, Kaewlai R, Digumarthy, et al. Urgent findings on portable chest radiography: What the radiologist should know—Review. *AJR Am J Roentgenol.* 2011;196(6 Suppl.):S45–S61.

Binanay C, Califf RM, Hasselblad V, et al. Evaluation study of congestive heart failure and pulmonary artery catheterization effectiveness: The ESCAPE trial. *JAMA.* 2005; 294(13):1625–1633.

Gluecker T, Capasso P, Schnyder P, et al. Clinical and radiologic features of pulmonary edema. *RadioGraphics.* 1999; 19(6):1507–1531.

Khan A, Hamdan AJ, Al-Ghanem S, Alaa G. Reading chest radiographs in the critically ill: Part II. Radiography of lung pathologies common in the ICU patient. *Ann Thorac Med.* 2009;4(3):149–157.

Murray JF. Pulmonary edema: Pathophysiology and diagnosis. *Int J Tuberculosis Lung Dis.* 2011;15(2):155–160.

Rubinowitz AN, Siegel MD, Tocino I. Thoracic imaging in the ICU. *Crit Care Clin.* 2007;23(3):539–573.

CHAPTER 13

Atelectasis, Pneumonia, and Aspiration

Brent P. Little and Travis S. Henry

Definition

Atelectasis and pneumonia are commonly encountered in the inpatient setting, particularly in intensive care units, when patients are intubated and seriously ill and often subject to a variety of comorbidities. The two entities are often confused because they have overlapping imaging appearances and may coexist. Atelectasis represents incomplete expansion of the lung parenchyma, with associated loss of volume, whereas pneumonia is an infection of the parenchyma and not typically associated with volume loss. Recognition of the characteristic imaging findings of these diseases allows a confident diagnosis to be made in many cases and a helpful differential diagnosis to be offered in others.

Clinical Features

Atelectasis

Atelectasis is a very common imaging finding in the inpatient setting, especially in postoperative patients, for whom the incidence has been estimated to be as high as 90%. Common etiologies include subsegmental atelectasis due to hypoinflation; passive (relaxation) atelectasis due to compression from adjacent pleural effusion; and obstructive atelectasis from mucous plugging, aspiration, or foreign bodies. Affected patients may be asymptomatic if the atelectasis is mild, but the sudden onset of hypoxemia and respiratory distress may accompany more severe forms of atelectasis (i.e., lobar or whole lung), and chest radiographs may change as rapidly as the patient's symptoms. In such cases, tube suctioning over an existing endotracheal/tracheostomy tube, chest respiratory therapy, or bronchoscopic retrieval of a mucous plug may improve symptoms. Historically, atelectasis has been purported to cause early postoperative fever, but that notion has been challenged by recent analyses suggesting that the presence of atelectasis is unrelated to fever.

Pneumonia

Hospitalized patients are at increased risk of pneumonia due to exposure to virulent organisms in the inpatient setting and/or prolonged intubation. Whereas gram-positive organisms are common causative agents in community-acquired pneumonia, gram-negative organisms such as *Klebsiella* are important causes of health care-associated pneumonia. In immunosuppressed patients, certain pathogens, such as fungi (e.g., aspergillus and mucormycosis), pneumocystis, and viruses (e.g., cytomegalovirus), are important considerations. Tuberculosis is yet another pathogen that is still relevant and must not be forgotten, particularly in today's world of widespread global travel.

More than 1 million patients are hospitalized annually for pneumonia in the United States. The most common complications resulting in admission include a necrotizing or cavitary pneumonia (especially bacterial or fungal etiologies) and/or empyema. Less common complications, such as empyema with bronchopleural fistula, may cause persistent pneumothorax and result in significant morbidity/mortality.

Aspiration

An aspiration pneumonitis can occur hours after the inhalation of gastric contents and is more common in neurologically impaired patients, patients with tumors or previous surgeries that impair the normal swallowing mechanism, and victims of severe trauma. A chemical pneumonitis may resolve in a matter of hours or days, but it can evolve into aspiration pneumonia. Poor dentition is a particular risk factor for development of aspiration pneumonia, usually due to gram-negative organisms.

Anatomy and Physiology

Atelectasis occurs when the negative pressure within the pleural space is insufficient to maintain complete expansion of the alveolar walls; alveolar collapse ensues, with loss of volume in the involved lung. Decreased respiratory effort or bronchial obstruction can cause atelectasis, and passive atelectasis may occur adjacent to a pleural effusion or pneumothorax.

Pneumonia is an infection of the lung involving the pulmonary parenchyma and occasionally the airways. Infection may spread via the airways, via tiny connections between terminal bronchioles and adjacent alveoli (canals of Lambert), and through interalveolar openings (pores of Kohn), with these factors combining to allow spread of infection within pulmonary lobes.

How to Approach the Image

Evaluate the Time Course

- Lobar collapse due to a mucous plug occurs rapidly and may promptly resolve following treatment (Fig. 13.1a).
- Aspiration pneumonitis may develop within hours.
- Pneumonia usually has an indolent course, and imaging findings may lag behind the resolution of clinical symptoms but typically resolve within 6–8 weeks.

Look for Asymmetry/Volume Loss

- Shift of the mediastinum toward a parenchymal opacity suggests ipsilateral lobar or total lung atelectasis (Fig. 13.1b).
- Hilar or fissural displacement, or new upward displacement of a hemidiaphragm, are additional indirect signs of atelectasis.
- Increased opacity in a hemithorax without evidence of significant volume loss suggests another process (e.g., pneumonia and pleural effusion or mass).

Localize the Abnormality

- The "silhouette sign" refers to obscuration of adjacent structures by a parenchymal process, with specific points of obscuration indicating which pulmonary lobe or lobes are likely to be involved by consolidation or atelectasis (Figs. 13.1a and 13.2a).

Assess the Distribution and Morphology

- A homogeneous opacity with one or more sharply defined borders (fissural boundary) suggests lobar atelectasis (Fig. 13.2b). Look for displacement of the involved fissure(s) and crowding of underlying bronchovascular structures—both of which are direct signs of atelectasis.
- Patchy, nodular, or mass-like opacities may be manifestations of pneumonia on chest radiography and CT.
- A dependent and/or bronchocentric distribution of findings suggests aspiration.
- Rapidly developing central consolidation can be seen in edema, typically bilateral and fairly symmetric, but asymmetric pulmonary edema may also occur.
- Peripheral wedge-shaped consolidation in an acute clinical setting suggests lung infarction; chronic peripheral consolidation can be seen in organizing pneumonia or eosinophilic pneumonia.

Use the Clinical History

- Does the patient have fever or leukocytosis to suggest pneumonia?
- Does the patient have a history of heart failure or clinical signs of volume overload?
- Are acute symptoms mild or absent, suggesting a more sinister pathology such as an obstructing cancer?

What Not to Miss

Inspect serial chest radiographs carefully because new parenchymal opacity may indicate pneumonia, aspiration, or atelectasis.

Lobar collapse due to a mucous plug occurs rapidly.

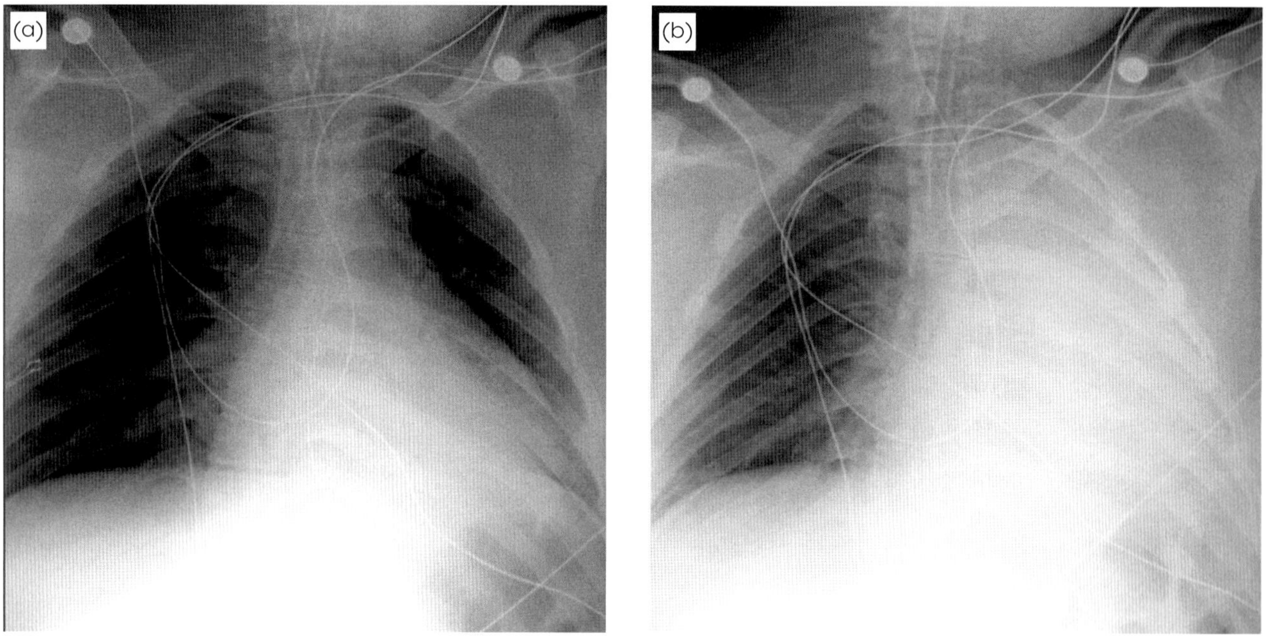

Figure 13.1. Atelectasis. (a) Anteroposterior (AP) chest radiograph of a 25-year-old woman with progressive atelectasis of the left lung due to mucous plugging shows dense retrocardiac opacity in the left lower lobe that obscures (silhouettes) the aortic margin and left hemidiaphragm. (b) Chest radiograph obtained 4 hours later shows complete atelectasis of the left lung with diffuse opacification of the left hemithorax and shift of the mediastinal structures to the left.

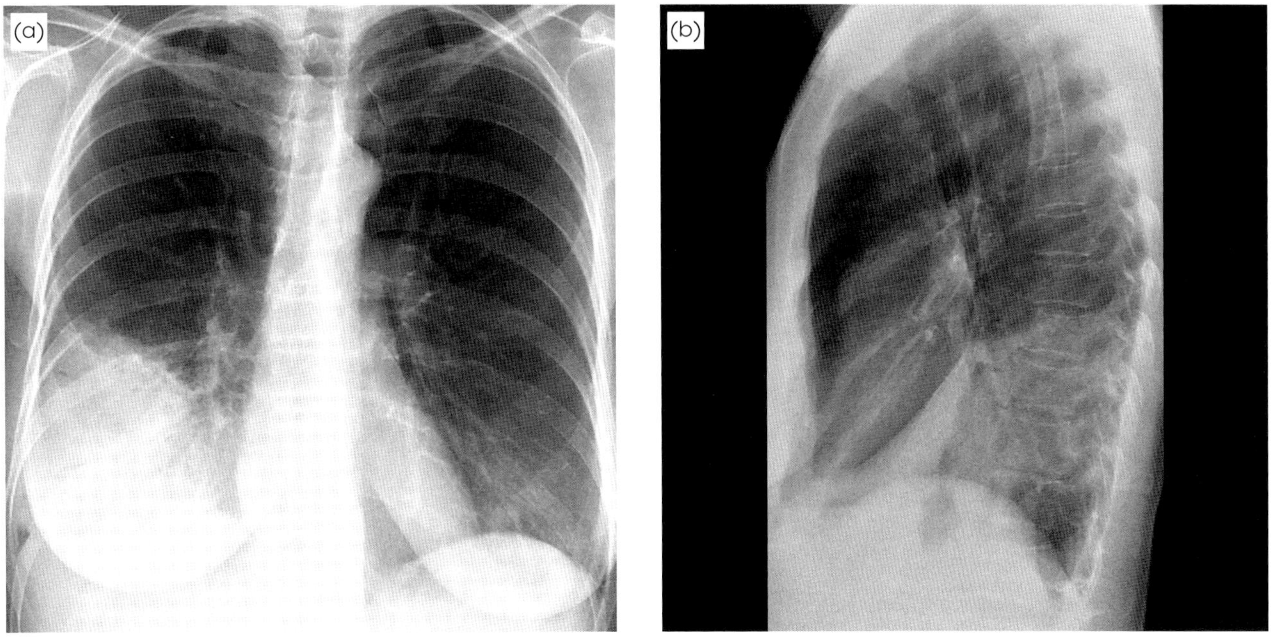

Figure 13.2. Right lower lobe pneumonia. (a) PA chest radiograph shows confluent airspace opacity in the right lower lobe that contains faint air bronchograms and obscures the right hemidiaphragm. In contradistinction to atelectasis, there is no shift of the mediastinal structures. (b) Lateral chest radiograph of the same patient shows dense consolidation, faint air bronchograms, and a sharp interface along the anterior aspect of the consolidation representing the lower portion of the right major fissure and localizing the pneumonia to the right lower lobe. The consolidation also obscures most of the right hemidiaphragm.

Differential Diagnosis

Acute Causes of Consolidation

Pulmonary Hemorrhage

- Patchy or diffuse ground-glass opacity and/or consolidation (Fig 13.3).

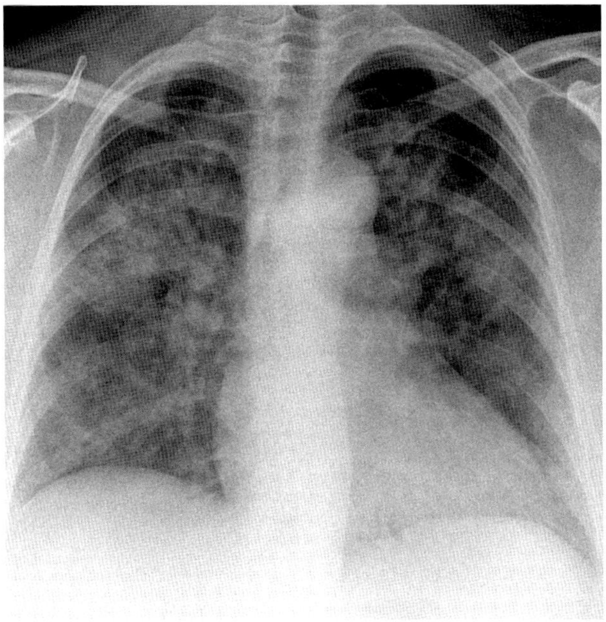

Figure 13.3. Diffuse pulmonary hemorrhage. PA chest radiograph of a 38-year-old man with systemic lupus erythematosus and hemoptysis shows bilateral patchy consolidation that resembles pneumonia.

- May be due to various etiologies, including vasculitis, drug reaction, and other causes, or may be idiopathic.
- May have a rapid or subacute onset.
- Usually resolves more slowly than pulmonary edema.

Pulmonary Infarction

- Peripheral wedge-shaped consolidation; may form a "Hampton's hump" on chest radiography.
- Large infarcts may mimic segmental or lobar pneumonia.
- A small ipsilateral pleural effusion is a common associated finding.

Pulmonary Edema

- Often bilateral and symmetric, perihilar.
- Rapid onset and/or change suggests the diagnosis.
- Common ancillary findings include dilated superior vena cava/azygous vein, bilateral pleural effusions, or interstitial (septal and interlobar fissural) thickening.

Subacute/Chronic Consolidation

Organizing Pneumonia

- Patients present with dyspnea, cough, and fever over several weeks, with symptoms similar to those of pneumonia (Fig 13.4).
- A pattern of peripheral consolidation developing over days to months is common.
- The "atoll sign" (or "reverse halo" sign) may occur (a peripheral rim of consolidation with central ground-glass opacity)—may offer a clue to the diagnosis.
- Transbronchial or open lung biopsy may confirm diagnosis.

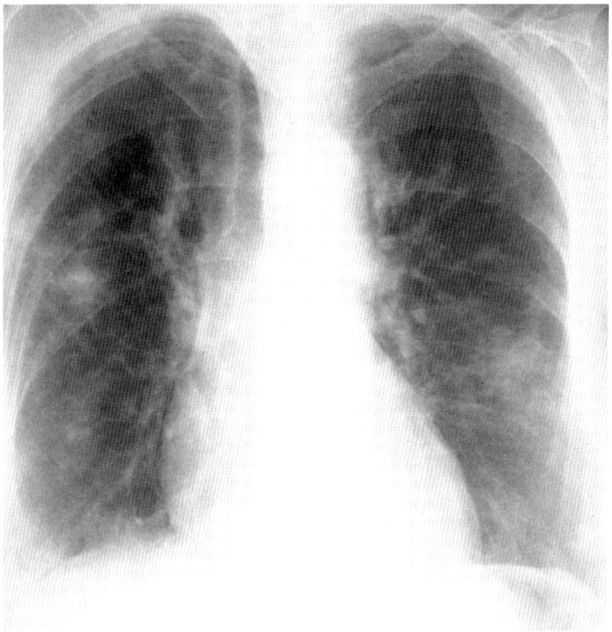

Figure 13.4. Organizing pneumonia. PA chest radiograph of a 52-year-old man with dry cough demonstrates bilateral patchy areas of consolidation that were peripheral and peribronchovascular in distribution on chest CT (not shown).

Eosinophilic Pneumonia

- Peripheral ground-glass opacity or consolidation is common.
- A "fleeting" pattern of consolidation may occur, with patchy consolidation that may change or migrate over the course of days or weeks.
- Peripheral and/or tissue eosinophilia detected concurrent with consolidation.

Malignancy Mimicking Pneumonia

- A central lung tumor may cause post-obstructive pneumonia.
- Follow-up radiographs are often recommended in 6–8 weeks to document resolution of the pneumonia.
- Primary adenocarcinoma of the lung and certain types of metastatic adenocarcinoma may manifest as consolidation.

Granulomatous Inflammatory Diseases

- Sarcoidosis and pneumoconiosis may manifest with consolidation that is bilateral, usually symmetric and bronchocentric, and upper lobe predominant.
- Perilymphatic nodules clustered along bronchovascular structures, fissures, and interlobular septa are imaging clues.
- Polyangitis with granulomatosis (formerly Wegener granulomatosis) may manifest as nodules, mass-like consolidations, or even lobar consolidation—often due to hemorrhage.

Imaging Findings

Atelectasis

On radiographs and CT, volume loss is the key to the diagnosis; on contrast-enhanced CT, atelectatic lung will enhance more than consolidation due to pneumonia.

- Subsegmental atelectasis: Usually band-like or linear/discoid opacities. Less commonly, subsegmental atelectasis may exhibit a patchy appearance similar to pneumonia.
- Passive/relaxation atelectasis: In the supine patient, relatively homogeneous basilar opacities with a gradient decreasing in opacity from lung base to apex may represent posteriorly layering pleural effusions with passive atelectasis in the adjacent lung.
- Obstructive atelectasis: Volume loss and displacement of fissures and hila, usually rapid in onset and resolution and often involving an entire lobe or lung. In the hospitalized patient, mucous plugging and/or aspiration are common causes of atelectasis (Fig. 13.1b).
- Lobar atelectasis: Volume loss forming a triangular/fan-shaped homogeneous opacity with sharp margins obscuring adjacent structures. Lower lobe collapse is very common in inpatients, typically forming a triangular-shaped opacity and causing obscuration of the adjacent hemidiaphragm and mediastinal shift to the ipsilateral side (Fig. 13.1a).
- Total lung atelectasis may occur with obstruction at the level of the main bronchus. Lobar or multilobar loss of volume may precede total lung atelectasis. Total lung atelectasis causes complete opacification of a hemithorax, and it usually causes mediastinal shift to the same side as the collapse (Fig. 13.1b).
- Cicatricial atelectasis: Caused by fibrosing lung disease or prior infection, especially tuberculosis. Linear or nodular scarring and a chronic time course are easily recognized upon comparison with prior studies.

Pneumonia

Pneumonia may manifest on imaging studies in a bronchopneumonia (lobular) or lobar/multilobar pattern, or it may manifest with diffuse interstitial findings.

- Lobar/multilobar pneumonia: May manifest as consolidation of one or more lobes. Air bronchograms may occur because the infectious exudate is centered in and opacifies the involved alveoli, which surround air-filled bronchi (Fig. 13.2a).
- Bronchopneumonia: Infection is centered in the bronchiolar epithelium; it may involve multiple lobes

and manifest as centrilobular nodules or consolidation; usually seen with bacterial pathogens or tuberculosis; air bronchograms are typically absent.

- Interstitial pneumonia: Imaging reflects an inflammatory process involving the pulmonary interstitium, usually secondary to viral pathogens or *Pneumocystis jirovecii*. Common findings include ground-glass opacity or consolidation, septal thickening, bronchial wall thickening, and centrilobular nodules. Pleural effusions are usually absent (especially in patients with *Pneumocystis* pneumonia).

Complications of Pneumonia

- Necrosis/cavitation and abscess formation: Occur in aggressive bacterial, fungal, or mycobacterial pneumonias or septic emboli. Look for cystic lucencies or air fluid levels. On CT, early necrosis may manifest as foci of low attenuation within consolidated lung (Fig. 13.5).
- Parapneumonic effusion and empyema: Parapneumonic effusion (either transudative or exudative) that usually layers. Empyema may develop and is characterized by a loculated effusion and thickening of visceral and parietal pleura (split pleura sign). Air within a pleural fluid collection is most often due to communication with a bronchus (bronchopleural fistula) and less often due to recent intervention.

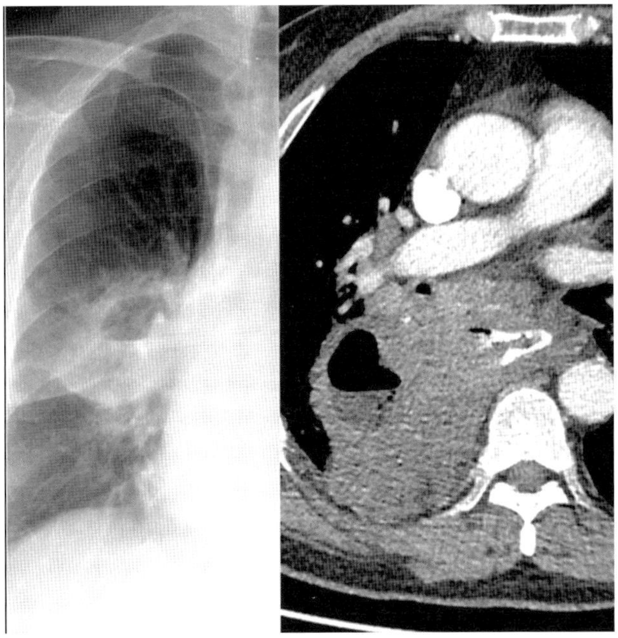

Figure 13.5. Lung abscess. Composite image of PA chest radiograph (left) and contrast-enhanced chest CT (right) of a 62-year-old man with esophageal cancer, pneumonia, and a lung abscess shows a thick-walled cavitary mass with an air–fluid level in the right lower lobe. Extensive adjacent consolidation is demonstrated on the CT, contiguous with esophageal thickening by tumor. In this clinical setting, pneumonia may have resulted from aspiration or from an esophageal–airway fistula.

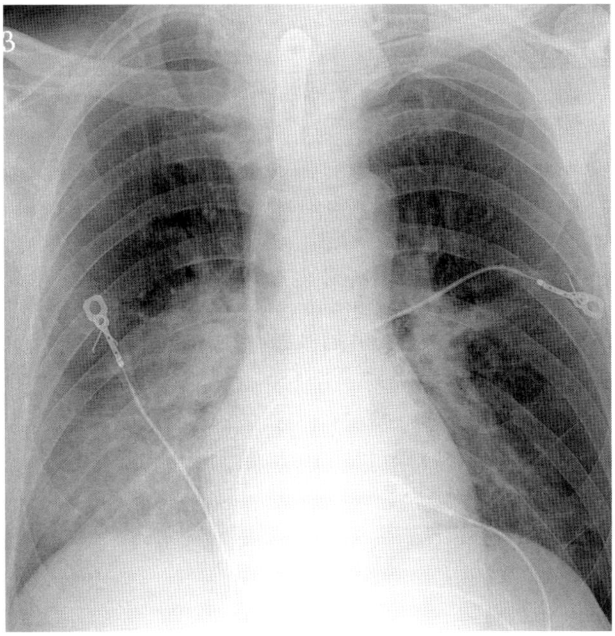

Figure 13.6. Aspiration pneumonia. AP chest radiograph of a 46-year-old man shows bilateral lower lung consolidation that developed acutely following a witnessed aspiration event.

Aspiration

- Radiographic abnormalities develop rapidly after an aspiration event (Fig. 13.6).
- Distribution may be unilateral or bilateral, usually dependent (most often posterior segments of upper lobes and superior and posterior basal segments of lower lobes) with a bronchocentric distribution.
- Findings may range from small centrilobular nodules and tree-in-bud opacities to frank consolidation.
- Massive aspiration may manifest as extensive bilateral airspace opacity; may be difficult to distinguish from edema.

Clinical Issues

- Chest radiographs may change rapidly in patients affected by aspiration or the more severe forms of atelectasis (i.e., lobar or whole lung), and patients' symptoms typically change just as rapidly—frequently developing hypoxemia and respiratory distress.
- Whereas atelectasis in the inpatient setting is a common finding, outpatients who present with lobar atelectasis should be suspected to have an obstructing tumor until proven otherwise (except for patients with cystic fibrosis or asthma).

Key Points

- Volume loss and parenchymal enhancement on CT are key findings that differentiate atelectasis from other causes of consolidation.
- Clues to lobar or total lung atelectasis include volume loss, mediastinal shift, fissural and hilar displacement, and a homogeneous opacity with straight borders obscuring adjacent structures (e.g., hemidiaphragm or heart border).
- Pneumonia may manifest with many different patterns—often nonspecific for a given organism; however, the pattern may help to narrow the differential diagnostic considerations.
- Aspiration most commonly manifests with dependent centrilobular nodules and/or consolidation.

Suggested Reading

Asrani A, Kaewlai R, Digumarthy S, et al. Urgent findings on portable chest radiography: What the radiologist should know—Review. *AJR Am J Roentgenol.* 2011;196(6 Suppl.):S45–S61.

Godoy MCB, Leitman BS, de Groot PM, Vlahos I, Naidich DP. Chest radiography in the ICU: Part 2. Evaluation of cardiovascular lines and other devices. *AJR Am J Roentgenol.* 2012;198(3):572–581.

Khan A, Hamdan AJ, Al-Ghanem S, Alaa G. Reading chest radiographs in the critically ill: Part II. Radiography of lung pathologies common in the ICU patient. *Ann Thorac Med.* 2009;4(3):149–157.

Rubinowitz AN, Siegel MD, Tocino I. Thoracic imaging in the ICU. *Crit Care Clin.* 2007;23(3):539–573.

CHAPTER 14

Acute Respiratory Distress Syndrome

Brent P. Little and Travis S. Henry

Definition

Acute respiratory distress syndrome (ARDS) is a clinical diagnosis of severe hypoxemia due to diffuse lung injury and permeability edema in the setting of normal cardiac function.

Clinical Features

Causes of ARDS may be divided into primary pulmonary and extrapulmonary/systemic etiologies. Pneumonia, aspiration, inhalational lung injury, and local chest trauma are important pulmonary causes. Sepsis, pancreatitis, transfusion-related lung injury, drug reactions, and severe multiorgan trauma are important extrapulmonary causes. A typical clinical presentation is dyspnea and tachypnea progressing during the first 1–3 days after the inciting event, eventually requiring mechanical ventilation. Progressive hypoxemia despite increasing concentrations of supplemental oxygen suggests progression of a primary lung disease (e.g., pneumonia) to ARDS.

The American–European Consensus Conference (AECC) criteria (1994) and the newer Berlin criteria (2011) have been used as clinical guidelines for diagnosing ARDS. Both define ARDS as acute-onset respiratory failure with bilateral pulmonary opacities on chest radiography or CT. However, the AECC criteria utilize a wedge pressure of less than 18 mm Hg, whereas the Berlin criteria replace assessment of wedge pressure with echocardiographic evaluation of ventricular function and recognize that cardiogenic edema can coexist with ARDS. In addition, the AECC definition of PaO_2/FiO_2 of less than 200 mm Hg is divided into three categories: mild (>200 mm Hg), moderate (100–200 mm Hg), and severe (<100 mm Hg).

ARDS has a high mortality rate, with outcomes correlating with the Berlin classification (27% mortality for mild, 32% for moderate, and 45% for severe ARDS). In addition to progressive respiratory failure, complications of ARDS include pneumothorax, pneumomediastinum, and subcutaneous gas due to barotrauma during the organizing and fibrotic phases.

Because high ventilatory pressures are associated with accelerated lung remodeling and lung damage in ARDS, the mainstay of therapy is a protective lung ventilation protocol used in the Acute Respiratory Distress Syndrome Network trial (2000), known as the "ARDS Net" protocol. A lower tidal volume of 4–6 ml/kg patient body weight and controlled 25–30 cm H_2O plateau pressure led to a mortality reduction from 40% to 31%.

Anatomy and Physiology

In ARDS, lung injury incites abnormal capillary permeability and development of diffuse interstitial and alveolar edema in the setting of a normal pulmonary wedge pressure. The acute, *exudative phase* is characterized by leakage of high-protein-content edema and neutrophils across capillary walls into the pulmonary interstitium and alveoli, with an associated decrease in lung compliance. In the later *organizing phase*, type II pneumocytes and hyaline membranes proliferate, leading to early fibrosis. During this phase, the hypoxemia characteristic of ARDS is partially due to persistent alveolar collapse in the setting of diminished lung surfactant production by damaged endothelium. A gravitational gradient of edematous, partially atelectatic lung tends to develop, correlating with the appearance of dependent atelectasis and consolidation on chest radiography and CT. A third phase, characterized by fibrosis and possible recovery, may follow if the patient survives the acute lung injury.

The pathologic hallmark of ARDS is diffuse alveolar damage, characterized by edema, interstitial inflammation, and hyaline membranes in the acute setting and by type II pneumocyte hyperplasia and loose organizing fibrosis in the organizing phase. These findings may reverse in the recovery phase, or the alveolar damage may progress to fibrosis and "honeycombing"—small cystic spaces with fibrous walls.

How to Approach the Image

- What is the time course of abnormalities? The findings of ARDS tend to remain stable over several days or weeks in the organizing phase, in contrast to the evolving changes that occur with many other causes of diffuse airspace opacities.
- What is the distribution of airspace opacities? Hazy bilateral airspace opacities in ARDS tend to be diffuse or at times peripheral in distribution

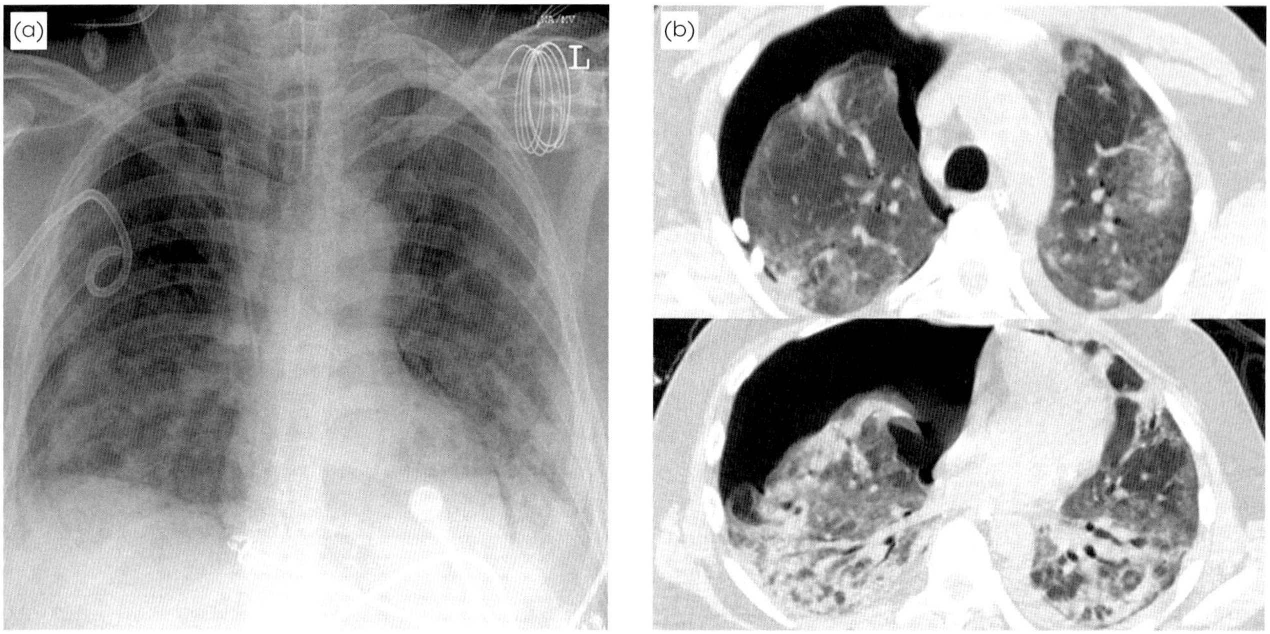

Figure 14.1. ARDS and H1N1 viral pneumonia. (a) Anteroposterior (AP) chest radiograph of a 52-year-old man with ARDS and H1N1 viral pneumonia shows diffuse bilateral patchy and hazy airspace and interstitial opacities. Lucency at the right apex represents a right pneumothorax, a known complication of ARDS. (b) Composite image of contrast-enhanced chest CT shows bilateral symmetric ground-glass opacity and patchy consolidation in the lower lobes, a right pneumothorax, and trace pneumomediastinum.

(Figs. 14.1 and 14.2) rather than central/perihilar, as in pulmonary edema.

- Are there complications of ARDS? The decreased compliance of the lungs in the organizing phase of ARDS calls for a high index of suspicion for complications of barotrauma, such as pneumothorax (Fig. 14.1) and pneumomediastinum (Fig. 14.3). Chronic pulmonary fibrosis in ARDS may have an anterior predominance—an uncommon distribution for other fibrosing lung diseases.

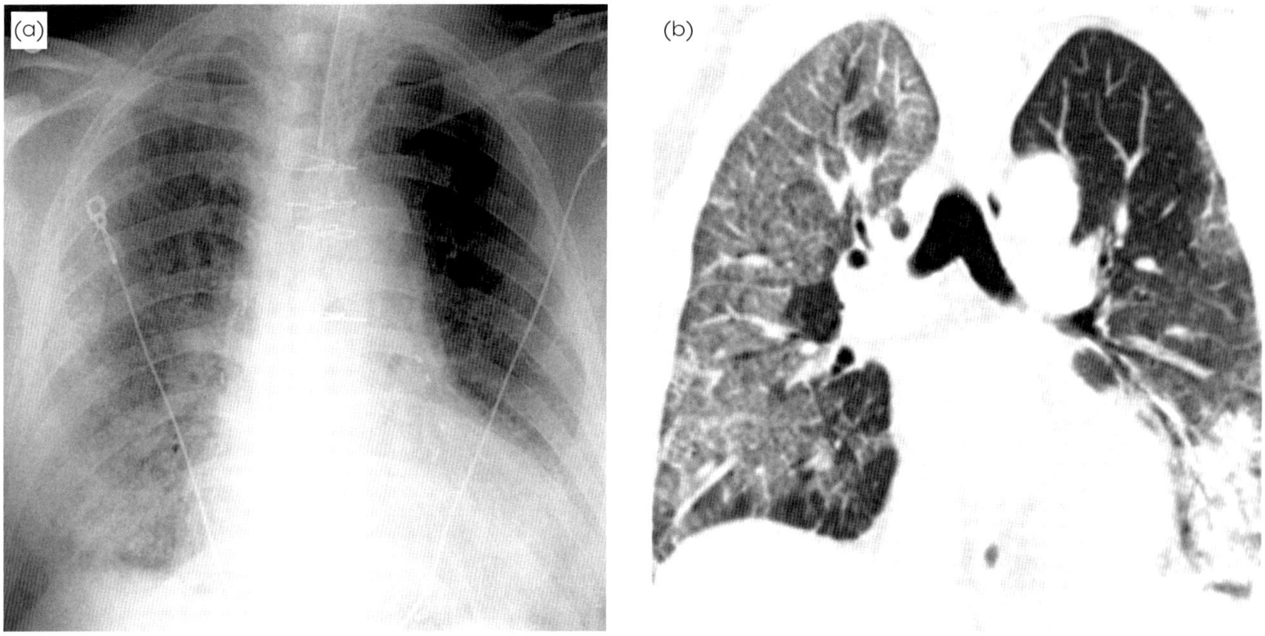

Figure 14.2. ARDS following coronary artery bypass surgery. (a) AP chest radiograph of a 66-year-old man with pneumonia and ARDS shows bilateral hazy airspace opacity. Consolidation in the left lower lobe and lingula obscure the left heart border. (b) Coronal CT shows asymmetric bilateral ground-glass opacity with interlobular septal thickening ("crazy paving pattern") and consolidation in the left lower lung. Intrapulmonary causes of acute respiratory syndrome produce an asymmetric pattern of airspace opacity more often than do extrapulmonary causes.

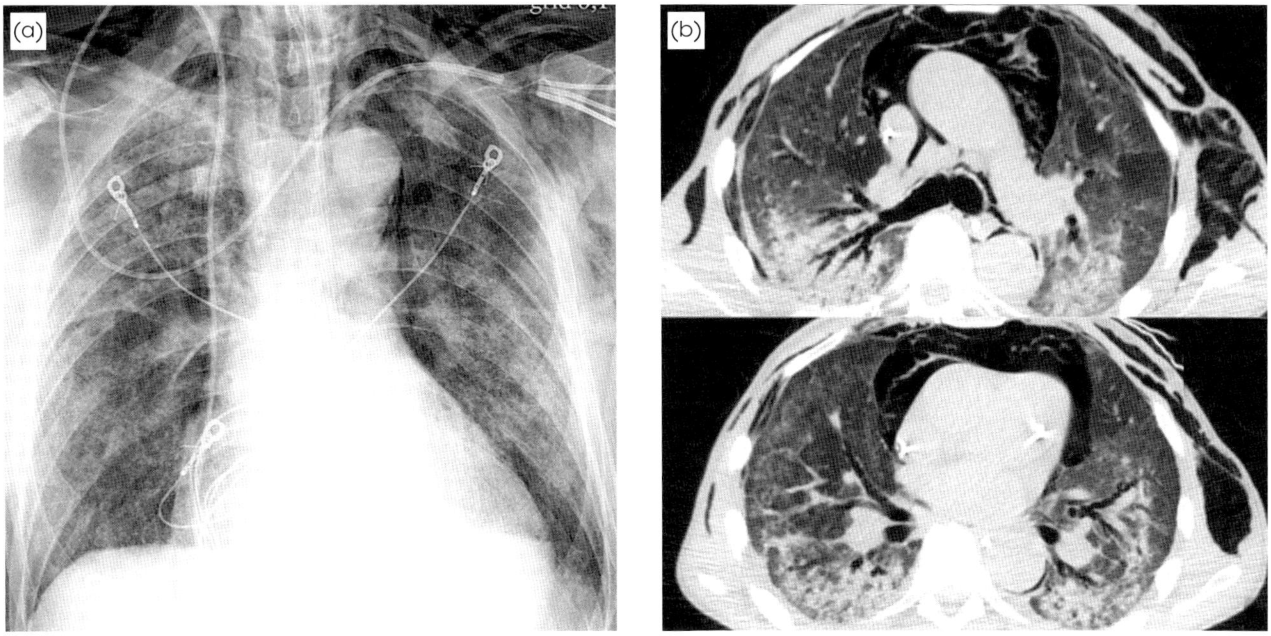

Figure 14.3. ARDS. (a) AP chest radiograph of a 78-year-old man with ARDS shows bilateral hazy airspace opacity, a diffuse fine reticular pattern, and subcutaneous emphysema in the lower neck and upper chest wall. Curvilinear lucency along the left mediastinal border represents pneumomediastinum that extends into the neck. (b) Composite image of chest CT images shows bilateral ground-glass opacity and consolidation in the posterior-dependent aspect of the upper and lower lobes, with pneumomediastinum and subcutaneous emphysema. Areas of varicoid bronchiectasis are demonstrated in both lungs, a finding associated with the organizing phase of ARDS.

What Not to Miss

Look for imaging findings of ARDS in patients with progressive dyspnea and tachypnea who require mechanical ventilation.

Pneumothorax may occur in patients with ARDS due to barotrauma, with minimal loss of volume of the ipsilateral lung due to its increased density and decreased compliance (Fig. 14.1).

Differential Diagnosis

- Pulmonary edema: Especially in its early phase, ARDS may have an appearance indistinguishable from pulmonary edema on chest radiographs, with bilateral interstitial thickening and airspace opacities. The opacities in ARDS are more constant than those of edema, maintaining a similar daily distribution and extent. Ancillary findings of congestive heart failure (dilated central veins, pleural effusions, and cardiomegaly) are often absent.
- Diffuse pneumonia or aspiration: A diffuse distribution of hazy airspace opacities and a basilar and dependent distribution of consolidation are suggestive of ARDS. However, ARDS may have an appearance indistinguishable from certain viral or atypical pneumonias, including pneumocystis pneumonia. In addition, because pneumonia, aspiration, and other primary lung processes are potential causes of ARDS, those conditions may coexist.
- Pulmonary hemorrhage: Alveolar hemorrhage may manifest with bilateral hazy airspace opacities with interstitial thickening and consolidation. Hemoptysis may be a clue to the diagnosis, as well as positive immunologic markers in the setting of vasculitis.
- Diffuse pulmonary adenocarcinoma: Comparison with prior radiographs will show a slow, progressive course. Clinical course will be similarly chronic.

Imaging Findings

Exudative, Early Phase

- Onset 24–72 hours after inciting event.
- Hazy bilateral airspace opacities with either a diffuse or somewhat peripheral predominance (Fig. 14.1a) (rather than the characteristic central/perihilar distribution of cardiogenic edema).
- Interstitial thickening.
- Findings change slowly (over days or weeks) rather than the rapid change typical of hemorrhage or edema (over several hours).
- Asymmetric lung disease (e.g., pneumonia) can lead to asymmetric imaging findings of ARDS (Fig. 14.2a).

Organizing, Intermediate Phase

- Hazy bilateral airspace opacities persist.
- Consolidation may develop in a basilar and dependent gradient distribution.

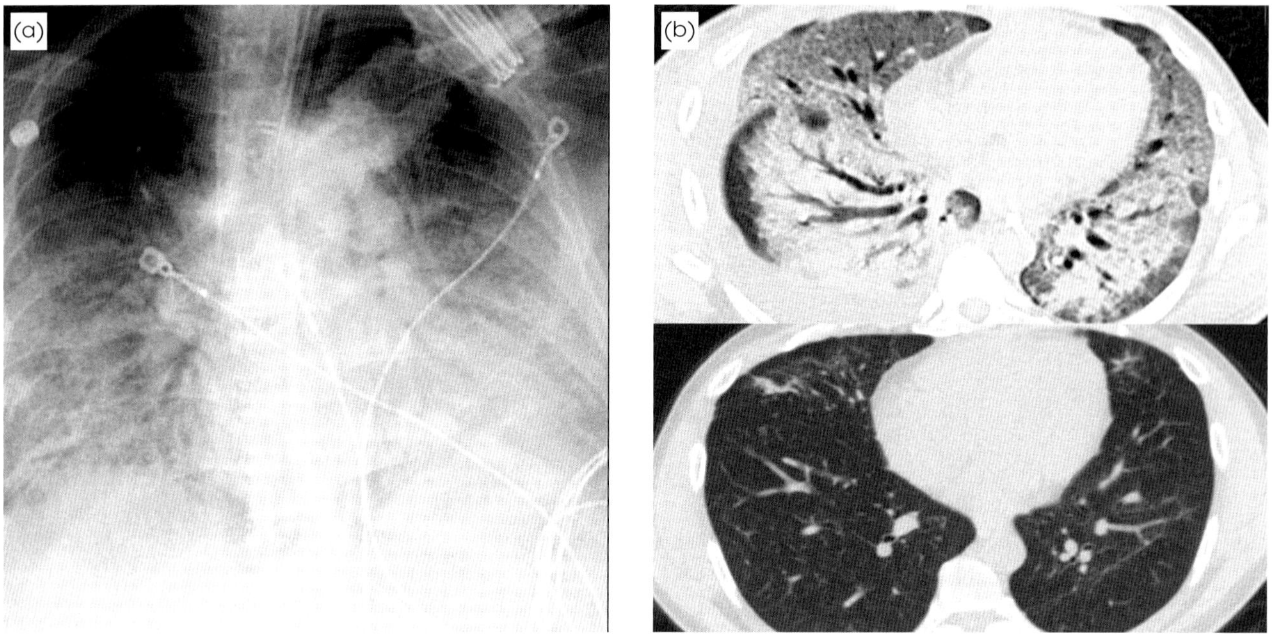

Figure 14.4. ARDS and cytomegalovirus pneumonia. (a) AP chest radiograph of a 45-year-old man with ARDS due to cytomegalovirus pneumonia shows diffuse bilateral hazy airspace opacity with patchy areas of consolidation and air bronchograms in the lower lobes. (b) Composite image of chest CT shows diffuse bilateral ground-glass opacity and posterior consolidation and bronchiectasis in the right lower lobe (top) that almost completely resolved in chest CT obtained 10 months later (bottom). Minimal volume loss and scarring is demonstrated in the anterior aspect of the middle lobe and lingula. This pattern of anterior areas of fibrosis is common in survivors of ARDS.

- Bronchial dilatation, often irregular/varicose, may develop rapidly over the course of days to weeks; this finding is more easily detected on CT than radiography (Fig. 14.4).
- Barotrauma and decreased lung compliance may lead to pneumothorax and/or pneumomediastinum.

Recovery or Fibrotic Phase

- Some degree of architectural distortion is usually apparent on imaging studies.
- In some cases, the lungs may return to a normal appearance.
- Fibrosis in an anterior distribution with associated areas of bronchiectasis is a common finding due to barotrauma; the typical dependent consolidation may limit injury to those portions of lung.
- Severe fibrosis may occur, and it may require lung transplantation.

Clinical Issues

- ARDS carries a high morbidity and mortality rate, with mortality as high as 50%.
- Measurement of pulmonary wedge pressure may help differentiate ARDS from cardiogenic pulmonary edema; however, the two can coexist, and an elevated wedge pressure does not exclude ARDS.
- Adequate ventilation using a low tidal volume and reduced plateau pressures is paramount in preventing damage to the lung from barotrauma.
- Acute interstitial pneumonia is a clinical syndrome of idiopathic ARDS, associated with severe shortness of breath, cough, and other symptoms that develop over several days in a previously healthy patient. Diffuse airspace opacities are characteristic imaging findings, and the histology of diffuse alveolar damage is identical to that seen in ARDS.

Key Points

- ARDS is a clinical diagnosis of diffuse lung injury leading to severe hypoxemia despite high inspired oxygen concentrations.
- Histologically, ARDS manifests as diffuse alveolar damage.
- Intrapulmonary causes of ARDS include pneumonia, inhalational injuries, aspiration, and chest trauma.
- Extrapulmonary or systemic causes include sepsis, multiorgan failure, transfusion reaction, pancreatitis, and drug toxicity.
- The early exudative phase occurs within 72 hours of the precipitating cause, and it usually manifests with diffuse bilateral airspace opacities.
- The organizing phase occurs later, with a dependent gradient of consolidation worse in the posterior lower lungs; bronchial dilatation may develop rapidly.
- In survivors, the lung may return to a relatively normal state or may develop fibrosis. Fibrosis is often more severe in the anterior portions of the lungs due to the protective effect of the typically posterior-dependent consolidation and atelectasis of ARDS.

Suggested Reading

Caironi P, Carlesso E, Gattinoni L. Radiological imaging in acute lung injury and acute respiratory distress syndrome. *Semin Respir Crit Care Med.* 2006;27(4):404–415.

Desai SR. Acute respiratory distress syndrome: Imaging of the injured lung. *Clin Radiol.* 2002;57(1):8–17.

Fanelli V, Vlachou A, Ghannadian S, Simonetti U, Slutsky AS, Zhang H. Acute respiratory distress syndrome: New definition, current and future therapeutic options. *J Thorac Dis.* 2013; 5(3):326–334.

Ferguson ND, Fan E, Camporota L, Antonell M, Anzueto A, Beale R, et al. The Berlin definition of ARDS: An expanded rationale, justification, and supplementary material. *Intensive Care Med.* 2012;38(10):1573–1582.

Section IV

Volume Loss

CHAPTER 15

Volume Loss

Christopher M. Walker

Introduction

The term *atelectasis* refers to loss of volume in the lung. It is one of the most frequently encountered imaging findings on chest radiography and CT, but it may be misinterpreted as other diseases causing lung opacification (e.g., pneumonia and aspiration) (Fig. 15.1). It is important for radiologists to understand the various mechanisms of volume loss and know the direct and indirect imaging signs of atelectasis in order to optimize patient care.

Types of Atelectasis

There are four types of atelectasis: resorption, relaxation, adhesive, and cicatricial.

Resorption atelectasis is the most common form of volume loss and occurs with obstruction of small or large airways by a nodule or mass, a foreign body, or mucus. With small or large airway obstruction, alveolar air is absorbed by circulating pulmonary blood but is not replaced with inspired air, leading to progressive reduction in alveolar volume. In patients breathing room air, an obstructed portion of lung may become completely atelectatic in 24 hours. In intubated patients breathing a high concentration of inspired oxygen, complete resorption and atelectasis may occur within 1 hour. Rapid air absorption may also occur when an endobronchial mass acts as a ball valve.

Resorption atelectasis is common in patients following major surgery when small bronchioles are obstructed by mucus from impaired mucociliary transport. Air bronchograms may be present when mucus obstructs small peripheral airways (Fig. 15.1) but are absent when a mass or mucus obstructs a central airway. As air is absorbed from the lung, intrapleural pressure decreases, causing fluid and blood to be drawn into the collapsed lung. Thus, atelectatic lung weighs more than expanded lung of the same volume. Occasionally, a large amount of fluid and blood is drawn into the obstructed portion of lung and results in little or no volume loss (i.e., drowned lung).

Relaxation or passive atelectasis occurs when pneumothorax, pleural effusion, or a mass allows the lung to "relax" and lose volume (Fig. 15.2). Compressive atelectasis, used

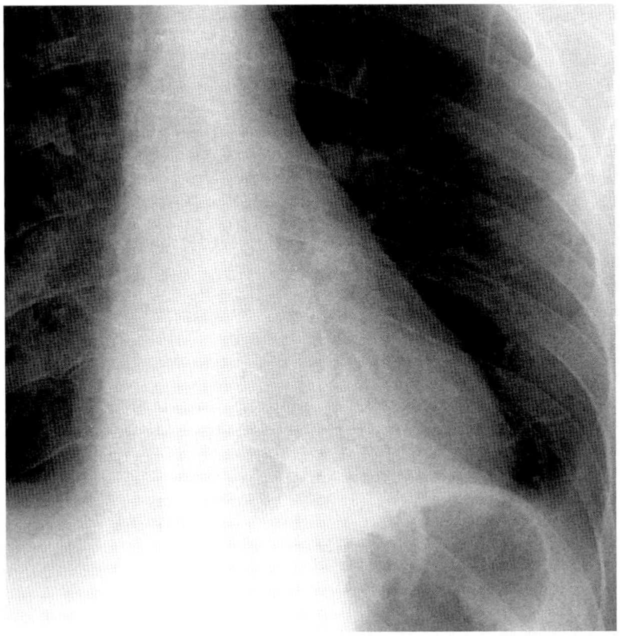

Figure 15.1. Signs of volume loss. Coned-down posteroanterior (PA) chest radiograph shows a triangular-shaped retrocardiac opacity representing left lower lobe atelectasis following aspiration. Air bronchograms within the opacity indicate patency of the proximal airways. The atelectatic lung obscures the adjacent left hemidiaphragm.

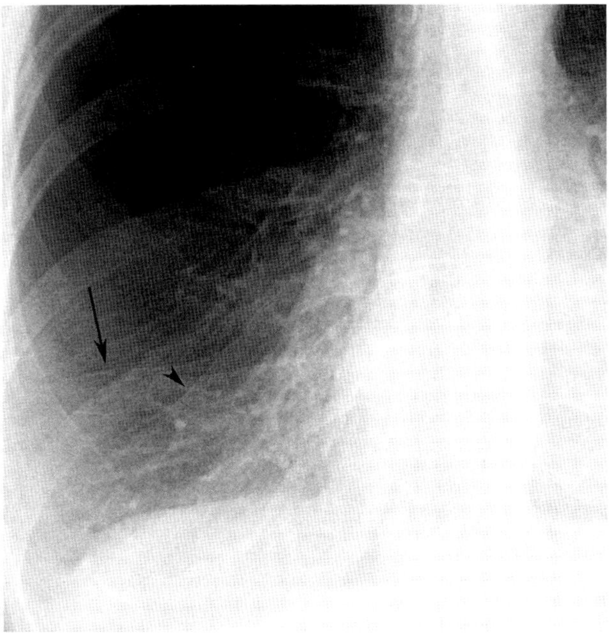

Figure 15.2. Relaxation (compressive) atelectasis from a giant bulla. Coned-down PA chest radiograph shows abnormal lucency in the right mid-lung from a giant bulla that produces relaxation atelectasis of the middle and right lower lobes characterized by bronchovascular crowding and displacement of the minor (arrow) and major (arrowhead) fissures—two direct signs of atelectasis. The right hilum is displaced inferomedially, an indirect sign of atelectasis.

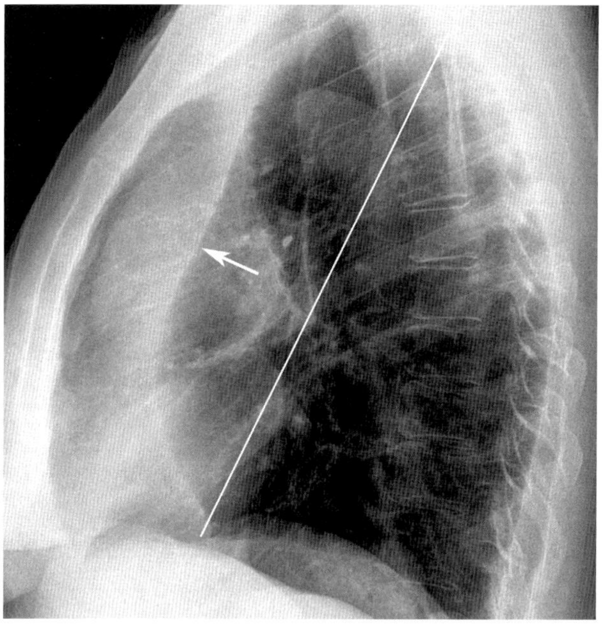

Figure 15.3. Fissural displacement in left upper lobe atelectasis. Lateral chest radiograph shows marked anterior displacement of the left major fissure from its normal position (white line) to lie parallel to the anterior chest wall as a sharp interface (arrow) that separates the dense atelectatic left upper lobe anteriorly from the aerated left lower lobe, which exhibits compensatory hyperinflation.

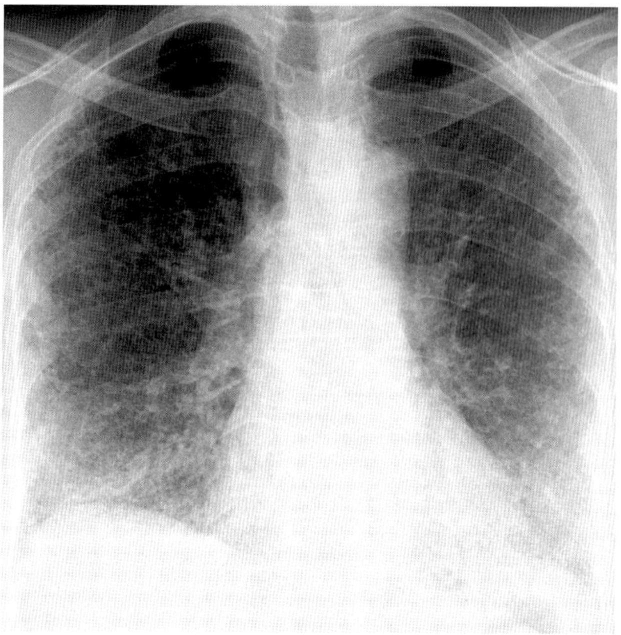

Figure 15.4. Diffuse cicatricial atelectasis from idiopathic pulmonary fibrosis. PA chest radiograph shows bilateral low lung volumes from pulmonary fibrosis manifesting as diffuse bilateral, predominantly basilar reticular opacities.

interchangeably with relaxation atelectasis by many radiologists, implies lung atelectasis beyond its normal resting state. When lung collapses, pulmonary blood flow decreases. Because the density of lung is dependent not only on the number of alveoli but also on the pulmonary vasculature, the density of the collapsed lung may not increase until the atelectasis is severe (Fig. 15.3).

Adhesive atelectasis occurs with surfactant deficiency. Surfactant is produced by type II pneumocytes and helps prevent alveolar collapse during exhalation. Adhesive atelectasis is most frequently encountered in premature infants who suffer from the infant respiratory distress syndrome related to surfactant deficiency. Adult causes of adhesive atelectasis include smoke inhalation, acute respiratory distress syndrome, cardiac surgery, pulmonary embolism, acute radiation pneumonitis, and pneumonia.

Cicatricial atelectasis refers to volume loss associated with pulmonary fibrosis and may be focal or diffuse (e.g., idiopathic pulmonary fibrosis) (Fig. 15.4). Signs of fibrosis (e.g., reticulation, bronchiectasis or bronchiolectasis, architectural distortion, and honeycombing) usually accompany this type of atelectasis.

Direct Imaging Signs of Atelectasis

The two direct signs of atelectasis are displacement of interlobar fissures and crowding of bronchovascular structures (Figs. 15.2 and 15.3).

- Fissural displacement may be the only direct sign of volume loss on chest radiography. The minor (horizontal) fissure is usually visible on frontal and lateral chest radiographs, and portions of both major (oblique) fissures are typically visible on lateral radiographs. Fissures are displaced toward the atelectatic lobe or lobes (Figs. 15.2 and 15.3). The various imaging patterns of lobar atelectasis are discussed in subsequent chapters.
- Crowding of bronchovascular structures is easiest to detect on CT and is a helpful sign of volume loss when fissural displacement is not readily appreciated. Crowded bronchovascular structures may also be seen on chest radiography when an atelectatic lobe contains residual air (Fig. 15.2).

Indirect Imaging Signs of Atelectasis

The indirect imaging signs of atelectasis include increased lung opacity (Figs. 15.1–15.3), mediastinal shift, hilar displacement, diaphragmatic elevation, compensatory lung hyperinflation, and the shifting granuloma sign. The indirect signs are most helpful in diagnosing volume loss when seen in combination.

- Lung opacity increases in areas of atelectasis, and involved segments, lobes, or an entire lung may become progressively more opaque as the degree of atelectasis increases.
- In most patients, the right hemidiaphragm is higher or at the same level as the left hemidiaphragm. With

volume loss—especially involving the lower lobes—the ipsilateral hemidiaphragm may shift upward (Figs. 15.1 and 15.4). Comparison with prior chest radiographs is often helpful in recognizing elevation of a hemidiaphragm.

- Left hilar structures are positioned more superiorly than right hilar structures in most patients. Lower lobe atelectasis may cause downward displacement and vertical reorientation of the ipsilateral hilar structures (Fig. 15.2), whereas upper lobe atelectasis causes outward rotation and elevation of the associated hilum.
- The trachea, heart, and mediastinal structures may shift to the side of volume loss. This sign is most helpful in distinguishing whole lung atelectasis from a large pleural effusion. Whole lung atelectasis is usually accompanied by ipsilateral mediastinal shift, whereas a large pleural effusion displaces the mediastinum to the contralateral side. In some cases, these two conditions may coexist and mediastinal shift may be minimal.
- In segmental or lobar atelectasis, the remainder of the affected lung may expand (compensatory hyperinflation) and exhibit decreased density and splaying of bronchovascular structures on radiography and CT.
- Approximation of the ribs may occur in lobar atelectasis. This finding is always seen in association with other signs of volume loss and should not be used in isolation as a sign of atelectasis.
- The shifting granuloma sign refers to movement of a known parenchymal lesion (e.g., calcified granuloma) from its previous position and usually indicates atelectasis within the same or an adjacent lobe.

Suggested Reading

Woodring JH, Reed JC. Types and mechanisms of pulmonary atelectasis. *J Thorac Imaging*. 1996;11:92–108.

CHAPTER 16

Atelectasis: Opaque Hemithorax

Christopher M. Walker

Definition

An opaque hemithorax results from unilateral absence of aerated lung parenchyma that results in homogeneous water density of the affected hemithorax without visualization of pulmonary markings. It often indicates serious underlying disease that may be pleural (effusion or neoplasm) or pulmonary in origin (pneumonia, pneumonectomy, mass, or complete lung atelectasis) or a combination of those entities.

Clinical Features

Patients affected by sudden collapse of an entire lung are generally symptomatic with dyspnea, hypoxia, or cough. However, if the atelectasis develops slowly, patients may have minimal or no symptoms. Centrally obstructing lesions may result in symptoms of cough, wheezing, dyspnea, and, in some cases, hemoptysis. Patients with severe unilateral pneumonia will typically present with signs and symptoms of infection. Patients with pneumonectomy are generally asymptomatic in the absence of tumor recurrence.

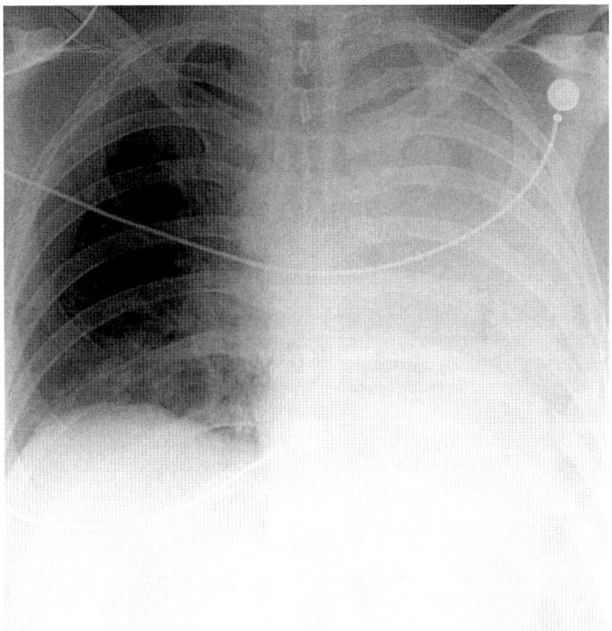

Figure 16.1. "Drowned lung" from mucous plugging. Anteroposterior (AP) chest radiograph of a patient with sudden hypoxia shows an opaque left hemithorax without mediastinal shift. A prior chest radiograph obtained 8 hours earlier was normal. "Drowned lung" was diagnosed based on rapid onset and trace pleural fluid on bedside ultrasound.

Anatomy and Physiology

Total lung atelectasis is usually caused by lung cancer obstructing the right or left main stem bronchus, but it can also be the result of foreign body aspiration, mucus plugging, contralateral intubation of a mainstem bronchus, or bronchial stricture. In the setting of mainstem bronchus obstruction, alveolar air is resorbed by circulating pulmonary blood but not replaced with inspired air, leading to progressive reduction of alveolar volume. Complete resorption of room air takes 24 hours, but resorption occurs more rapidly if a patient is breathing higher concentrations of oxygen. As air is absorbed, intrapleural pressure decreases and fluid and blood are drawn into the collapsed lung. Occasionally, a large amount of fluid and blood may be drawn into the collapsed lung with little or no loss of volume, resulting in a so-called "drowned lung" (Fig. 16.1).

How to Approach the Image

When an opaque hemithorax is encountered on chest radiography, the volume of the opaque hemithorax must be compared to that of the contralateral side for signs of mediastinal shift, such as tracheal displacement or displacement of the cardiomediastinal silhouette (Fig. 16.2). Complete lung atelectasis, lung hypoplasia/aplasia, and pneumonectomy (Figs. 16.3 and 16.4) cause a decreased volume in the affected hemithorax, ipsilateral mediastinal shift, elevation of the ipsilateral hemidiaphragm, and narrowing of the rib interspaces. Conversely, pleural effusion and a large intrathoracic mass cause increased volume in the affected hemithorax, contralateral mediastinal shift (Figs. 16.5 and 16.6), inferior displacement of the ipsilateral hemidiaphragm, and widening of the rib interspaces. The position of the hemidiaphragm is indirectly inferred by evaluation of abdominal gas-containing structures, such as the adjacent stomach or colon, or by assessment of the inferior aspect of the liver. Occasionally, opaque hemithorax occurs without appreciable mediastinal shift, typically

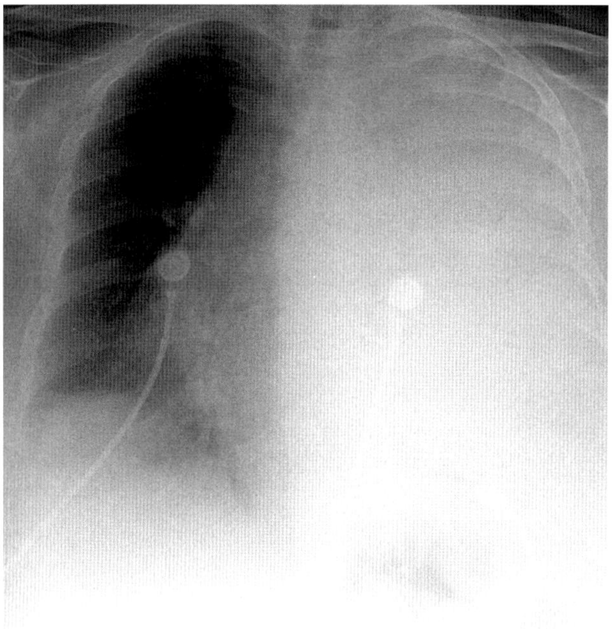

Figure 16.2. Hemothorax from trauma. AP chest radiograph of a patient with hemothorax from blunt chest trauma shows an opaque left hemithorax and contralateral tracheal and mediastinal shift. The inferomedial displacement of the gastric bubble is consistent with inferior displacement of the left hemidiaphragm.

when atelectasis and pleural effusion coexist or in the setting of acute lung collapse with drowned lung (Fig. 16.1). In all cases, contrast-enhanced chest CT is very useful in evaluating these findings.

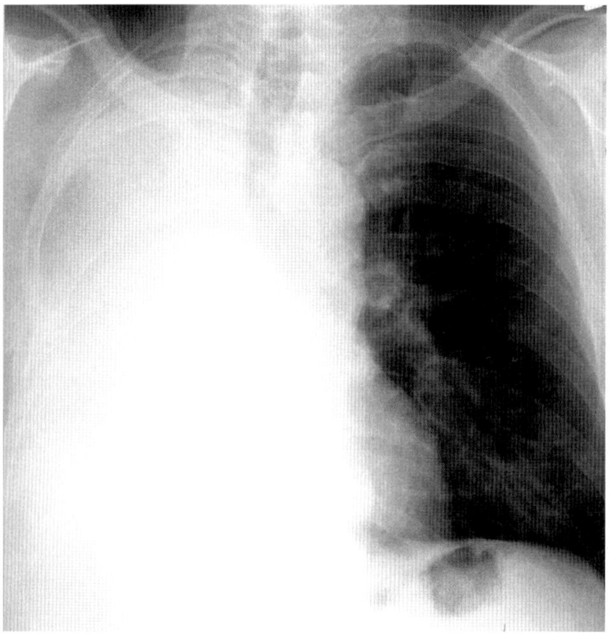

Figure 16.3. Pneumonectomy. PA chest radiograph of a patient who had a right pneumonectomy shows an opaque right hemithorax and ipsilateral shift of the trachea and mediastinum. Note surgical absence of the posterior fifth rib.

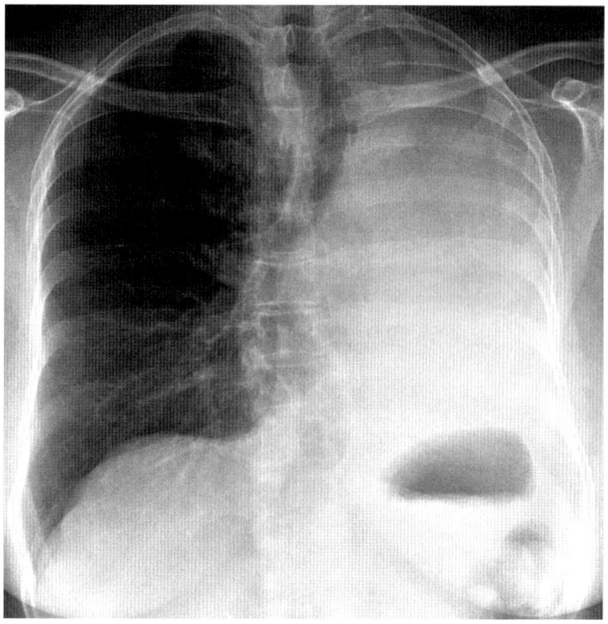

Figure 16.4. Centrally obstructing lung cancer. PA chest radiograph shows an opaque left hemithorax, ipsilateral tracheal and mediastinal shift, and upward displacement of the gastric bubble consistent with elevation of the left hemidiaphragm. There is compensatory hyperinflation of the right lung rotates across the midline.

What Not to Miss

- Total collapse of the lung is generally a marker of a serious condition.
- Outpatients with opaque hemithorax typically have a centrally obstructing, often advanced lung cancer, and a careful radiographic analysis for secondary signs of malignancy including lymphadenopathy, pulmonary nodules, and skeletal metastases must be performed. Further evaluation with contrast-enhanced CT and bronchoscopy is usually warranted.
- Inpatients with complete lung atelectasis often have a centrally obstructing mucous plug or mainstem bronchus intubation.

Differential Diagnosis

- Pleural effusion
  - Hemothorax (Fig. 16.2)
  - Empyema
  - Malignant pleural effusion
  - Chylothorax from trauma or conditions such as lymphangioleiomyomatosis (Fig. 16.5)
- Tumor
- Pneumonia: Uncommon cause of opaque hemithorax; affected patients symptomatic with fever, cough, and sputum production
- Pneumonectomy (Fig. 16.3): History of prior surgery
- Pulmonary agenesis or hypoplasia

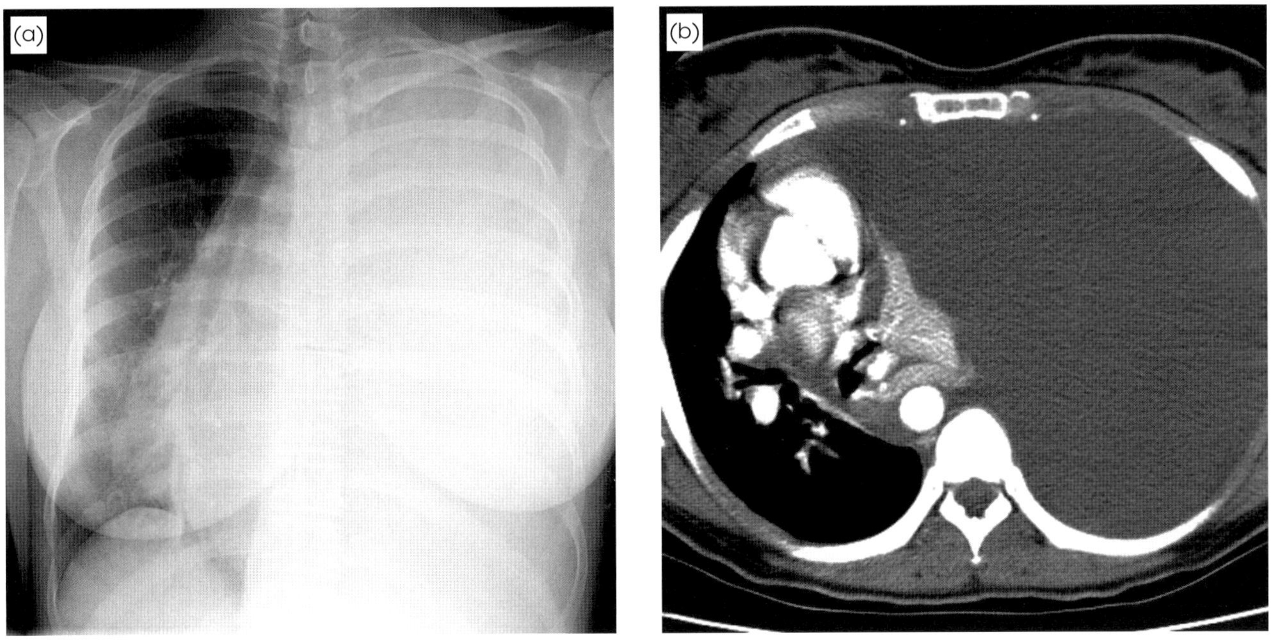

Figure 16.5. Large left chylous effusion. (a) PA chest radiograph of a patient with lymphangioleiomyomatosis shows an opaque left hemithorax, contralateral mediastinal and tracheal shift, and widened left rib interspaces. (b) Contrast-enhanced chest CT of the same patient shows a large left chylous pleural effusion causing contralateral mediastinal shift and total atelectasis of the left lung. Chylous effusion cannot be differentiated from other pleural effusions based on CT Hounsfield units.

Imaging Findings

Atelectasis

Radiography

- Tracheal shift toward opaque hemithorax
- Mediastinal shift toward opaque hemithorax (Fig. 16.4); absence of shift in drowned lung (Fig. 16.1)
- Mediastinal rotation to the affected side occurs more commonly in chronic collapse and manifests as increased retrosternal lucency on the lateral chest radiograph.
- Elevated hemidiaphragm and narrowed rib interspaces
- Compensatory hyperinflation of unaffected lung
- Associated findings of lymphadenopathy, pleural effusion, and skeletal metastases in advanced centrally obstructing lung cancer

CT

- Assessment of central airways for endoluminal neoplasm or mucus plug
- Contrast-enhanced studies for differentiation of atelectatic lung from underlying mass

Pleural Effusion

Radiography

- Contralateral mediastinal shift and ipsilateral hemidiaphragm depression in large pleural effusions (Figs. 16.2 and 16.5). The differential diagnosis for unilateral large pleural effusion includes the following:
  - Malignant pleural effusion
  - Hemothorax
  - Chylothorax
  - Empyema

CT

- Differentiation of higher attenuation or enhancing atelectatic lung from lower attenuation surrounding pleural fluid (Fig. 16.5b)
- Assessment of pleural fluid for the following:
  - Associated pleural thickening or masses in malignant effusion
  - Gas in patients with empyema
  - High-attenuation pleural fluid or hematocrit effect (high-attenuation fluid–fluid levels) in hemothorax

Ultrasound

- Helps confirm pleural effusion
- Facilitates therapeutic and diagnostic thoracentesis

Tumor

- A large pleural or parenchymal tumor may increase the volume of the hemithorax, leading to contralateral mediastinal shift and hemidiaphragm depression (Fig. 16.6).
- Assessment with contrast-enhanced CT allows visualization of parenchymal or pleural mass and differentiation from uninvolved lung parenchyma and pleural fluid.

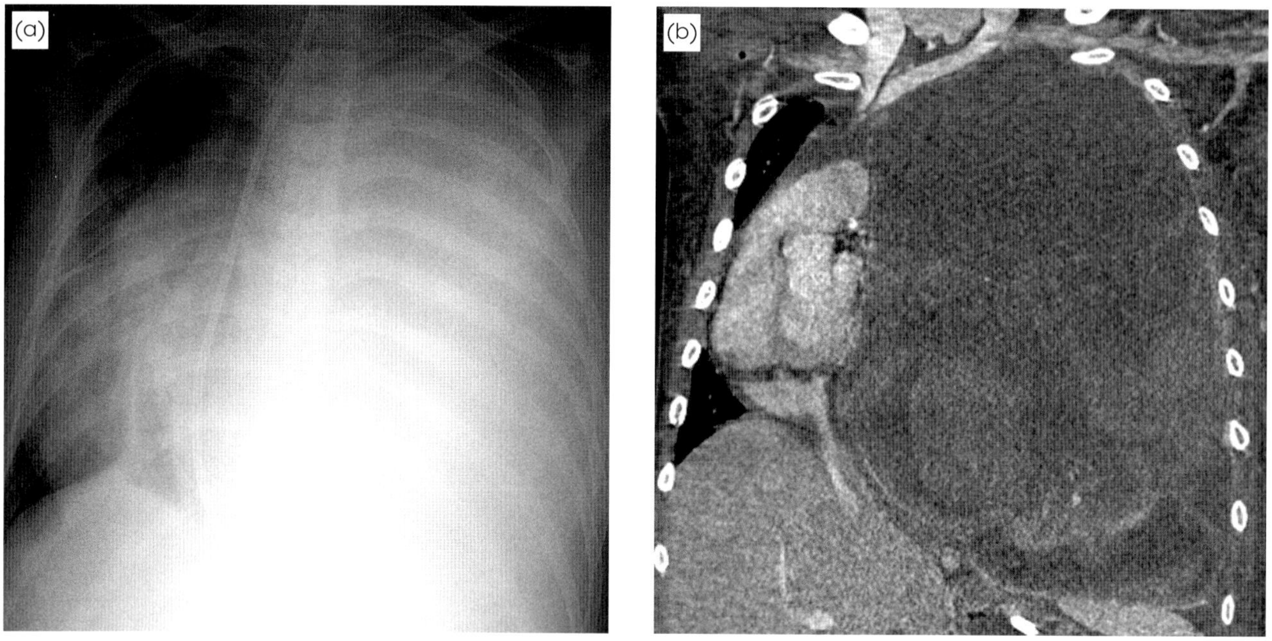

Figure 16.6. Metastatic mediastinal sarcoma. (a) AP chest radiograph of a patient with metastatic sarcoma shows an opaque left hemithorax with contralateral mediastinal and tracheal shift suggesting a large pleural effusion and/or a large mass. (b) Coronal contrast-enhanced chest CT of the same patient shows a large heterogeneously enhancing mass in the left hemithorax with associated large left pleural effusion that produces contralateral mediastinal shift and inversion of the ipsilateral hemidiaphragm.

Pneumonectomy

- Following lung resection, the pneumonectomy space is initially air-filled and gradually fills with fluid during the following 2 weeks.
- Progressive volume loss and shift of the mediastinum toward the pneumonectomy space (Fig. 16.3).
- Imaging signs of thoracotomy including surgical clips or staples and partial rib resection (usually the posterior fifth or sixth rib).
- Progressive shift of contralateral lung across anterior mediastinum with increased retrosternal lucency on the lateral chest radiograph.

Pneumonia

- The presence of aerated or consolidated lung within opaque hemithorax should suggest pulmonary infection but does not exclude underlying malignancy.
- Little or no volume loss with absence of tracheal or cardiomediastinal shift.

Clinical Issues

- Acute opaque hemithorax in an inpatient should suggest mucus plugging and should be communicated to the clinical staff for prompt relief of the obstruction.
- Opaque hemithorax in an outpatient typically requires further evaluation with CT, ultrasound, and/or bronchoscopy for exclusion of underlying centrally obstructing tumor.
- Treatment of whole lung atelectasis is generally directed at the underlying cause. A large pleural effusion is generally treated with therapeutic thoracentesis; mucus plugging may be managed with aggressive suctioning, chest physiotherapy, or bronchoscopy.
- Whole lung atelectasis from an obstructing cancer may require surgery, radiation therapy, and/or chemotherapy.

Key Points

- Unilateral opaque hemithorax often signifies a serious condition. The direction of mediastinal shift helps in the formulation of a short differential diagnosis.
- Consider complete lung collapse if there is a small hemithorax with ipsilateral mediastinal shift and hemidiaphragm elevation (Fig. 16.4).
- Consider a large pleural effusion or mass if there is contralateral mediastinal shift with hemidiaphragm depression (Figs. 16.2, 16.5, and 16.6).
- The differential diagnosis for a large, unilateral pleural effusion includes trauma with hemothorax, infection with empyema, malignancy with a malignant pleural effusion, or chyle with chylothorax.
- Collapsed lung is differentiated from pleural fluid on CT by looking at its density and greater degree of contrast enhancement. Collapsed lung is slightly denser than pleural fluid on noncontrast CT (Fig. 16.5b).

Suggested Reading

Woodring JH, Reed JC. Radiographic manifestations of lobar atelectasis. *J Thorac Imaging*. 1996;11:109–144.
Woodring JH, Reed JC. Types and mechanisms of pulmonary atelectasis. *J Thorac Imaging*. 1996;11:92–108.

CHAPTER 17

Upper and Middle Lobe Atelectasis

Christopher M. Walker

Definition

Upper and middle lobe atelectasis represents partial (segmental or subsegmental) or complete volume loss of the affected lobe. It is a common chest radiographic finding in postsurgical patients but may be a manifestation of lung cancer when detected in outpatients.

Clinical Features

Symptoms associated with upper and middle lobe atelectasis vary depending on its cause and the degree of lung collapse. Patients may be asymptomatic or present with vague complaints, and the radiologist may be the first to suggest the diagnosis. Patients may be asymptomatic if atelectasis develops slowly. However, if atelectasis develops suddenly, patients may present with respiratory compromise. Patients with underlying lung cancer as the cause of atelectasis may present with hemoptysis, cough, or dyspnea. Patients with a causative mucus plug or aspirated foreign body often present with the sudden onset of dyspnea and hypoxia.

Anatomy and Physiology

Knowledge of normal hilar vascular structures and mediastinal contours and interfaces is essential for making the diagnosis of lobar atelectasis, which generally follows specific patterns:

- The right upper lobe (RUL) collapses medially, superiorly, and anteriorly and maintains its contiguity with the hilum and peripheral lung.
- The middle lobe collapses medially, inferiorly, and superiorly.
- The left upper lobe (LUL) collapses anteriorly and superiorly.

How to Approach the Image

The first step is identifying an abnormal opacity and differentiating atelectasis from consolidation by looking for direct and indirect signs of volume loss. The second step in the imaging diagnosis of upper or middle lobe atelectasis is identifying displaced hilar vascular structures. The third step is identifying distorted mediastinal contours and obscured mediastinal interfaces (silhouette sign). The fourth step requires inspection of the lateral chest radiograph to confirm abnormalities seen on the posteroanterior (PA) chest radiograph. As a final step, search for the cause of lobar atelectasis, focusing on central structures in particular, and look for any associated findings. Contrast-enhanced CT is helpful in most cases to evaluate for central obstructing neoplasm.

What Not to Miss

Lobar atelectasis is often the initial imaging manifestation of lung cancer.

- Inspect every chest radiograph for direct and indirect signs of volume loss, including displaced hilar vascular structures and obscured mediastinal interfaces.
- Once lobar atelectasis is identified, search for associated abnormalities (e.g., lymphadenopathy and skeletal metastases).
- All adult outpatients with lobar atelectasis should be further evaluated with contrast-enhanced chest CT.

Differential Diagnosis

Atelectasis must be differentiated from consolidation that is usually caused by pneumonia, aspiration, or hemorrhage. The easiest clues to diagnosing atelectasis are to search for the direct and indirect signs of volume loss. The differential diagnosis for lobar atelectasis is influenced by the patient's age, clinical presentation, and location at the time of imaging.

Adult Inpatient

- Mucus plugging with poor mucociliary function
- Malpositioned endotracheal tube with selective right (or left) mainstem bronchial intubation

Adult Outpatient (>40 Years of Age)

- Endobronchial obstructing tumor (lung cancer or endobronchial metastasis)
- Extrinsic bronchial obstruction (mediastinal mass or lymphadenopathy)

Adult Outpatient (<40 Years of Age)

- Endobronchial obstructing mass (carcinoid, hamartoma, and foreign body; less likely lung cancer)
- Extrinsic bronchial obstruction (mediastinal mass or lymphadenopathy)
- Bronchial stenosis (bronchomalacia and postinfectious stricture)

Child

- Foreign body aspiration

Imaging Findings

Right Upper Lobe Atelectasis

Radiography

- The minor fissure rotates superomedially in a clockwise direction and is higher laterally because its medial aspect is anchored at the hilum. The fissure is visible as a sharp interface between the opacified right upper lobe and aerated middle lobe.
- The *S sign of Golden* (Fig. 17.1) was initially described on chest radiography and indicated right upper lobe atelectasis due to a central obstructing hilar mass. The sign refers to an S-shaped interface formed by the concave elevated minor fissure and the contiguous medially located convex contour of the hilar mass.
- Other indirect signs may be seen including rightward tracheal shift, right hemidiaphragm elevation, hyperexpansion of the middle and right lower lobes, and a juxtaphrenic peak.
- On the lateral chest radiograph, the superior aspect of the major fissure is displaced anteriorly and the minor fissure superiorly. The collapsed RUL assumes a triangular shape anchored at the hilum with the base at the lung apex—called the "mediastinal wedge" by some authors.
- The truncus anterior (i.e., RUL pulmonary artery) and right superior pulmonary vein (RSPV) are displaced upward and inward toward the mediastinum. With complete atelectasis, these structures obscure the upper right mediastinal border and are not visualized. The interlobar pulmonary artery rotates superiorly and laterally, and the normal hilar angle formed by the RSPV and interlobar pulmonary artery is lost.

CT

- Upward displacement of minor fissure and anterior displacement of superior aspect of major fissure.
- Crowding of bronchovascular structures within atelectatic lung.
- A hilar mass may be differentiated from atelectatic lung on CT by noting their differences in attenuation following contrast administration. Atelectatic lung typically enhances more than an adjacent hilar mass, but the tumor margin may be poorly defined (Fig. 17.1b).

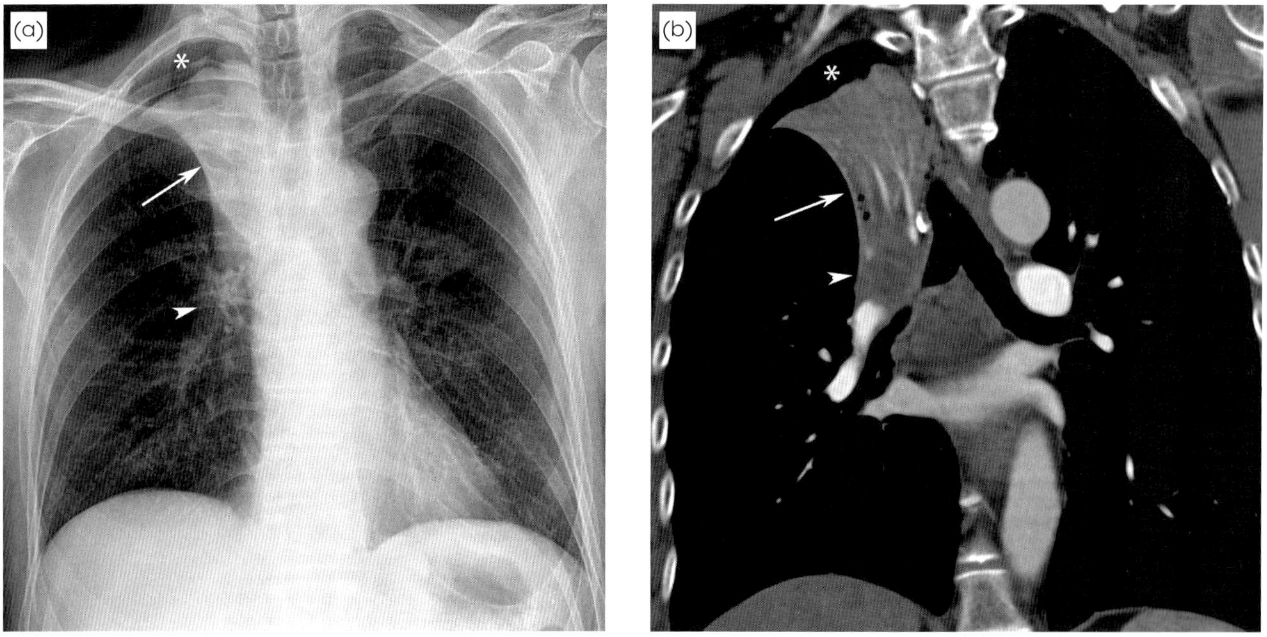

Figures 17.1. Right upper lobe atelectasis (lung cancer). (a) PA chest radiograph shows upward and medial displacement of the minor fissure forming a sharp, concave interface (arrow) and the convex border of a right hilar mass (arrowhead)—the two contours combining to produce the S sign of Golden. Right apical pneumothorax (asterisk) resulted from an abrupt drop in intrapleural pressure from sudden lobar collapse (pneumothorax ex vacuo). (b) Coronal contrast-enhanced CT of the same patient shows right upper lobe atelectasis, the displaced minor fissure (arrow), a right hilar mass (arrowhead), and adjacent subcarinal lymphadenopathy. The hilar mass is differentiated from the atelectatic lobe by its relative hypoattenuation.

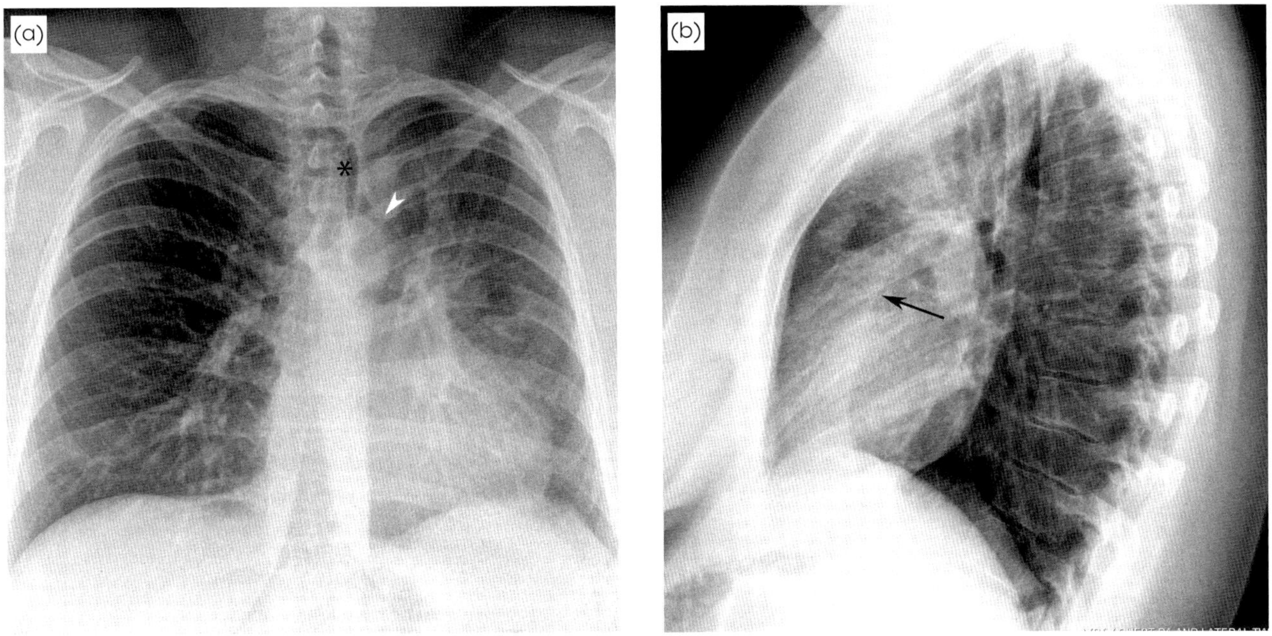

Figures 17.2. Left upper lobe atelectasis (lung cancer). (a) PA chest radiograph shows hazy left lung opacity that obscures the left heart border, left tracheal (asterisk) shift, and an elevated left hemidiaphragm. A sickle-shaped lucency (arrowhead) outlines the aortic arch (Luftsichel sign) and is produced by the hyperinflated left lower lobe superior segment located between the aorta and the collapsed upper lobe. (b) Lateral chest radiograph of the same patient shows anterior displacement and mild bowing of the left major fissure (arrow) forming a sharp interface between the atelectatic upper lobe and the hyperinflated lower lobe.

Left Upper Lobe Atelectasis

Radiography

- The left upper mediastinum and left heart border are obscured, and there is a veil-like opacity on the PA view.
- With further collapse, the lobe loses volume and is less apparent on the frontal radiograph. Portions of the left mediastinum and heart may remain visible. The left main bronchus assumes a horizontal course or is angled upward.
- The hyperinflated superior segment of the left lower lobe occasionally outlines the transverse aortic arch forming a crescentic (sickle-shaped) collection of air on the frontal radiograph termed the *Luftsichel sign* (German for "air crescent") (Figs. 17.2a and 17.3).
- There are often indirect signs of volume loss, including leftward mediastinal shift, elevation of the left hemidiaphragm, and a juxtaphrenic peak.
- The left upper lobe pulmonary artery and the left superior pulmonary vein move up and in toward the mediastinum and may be obscured in severe atelectasis. The interlobar pulmonary artery supplying the left lower lobe rotates superiorly and laterally.
- The lateral chest radiograph shows the left major fissure as an arcuate edge displaced anteriorly.

CT

- Anterior displacement of major fissure (Fig. 17.4)
- Crowding of bronchovascular structures within atelectatic lung
- Obstructing lesion usually better appreciated on contrast CT as hypodense mass in contrast to densely enhancing atelectatic lung

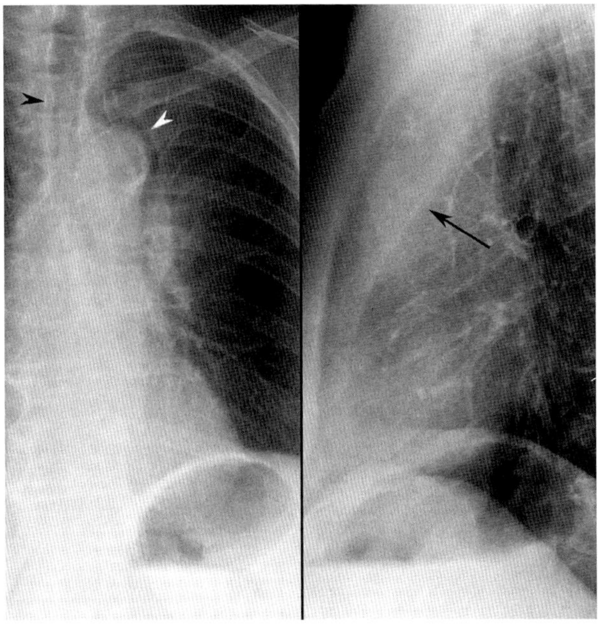

Figures 17.3. Left upper lobe atelectasis (lung cancer). Composite image with PA (left) and lateral (right) chest radiographs shows hazy opacity along the left heart border, horizontal orientation of the left mainstem bronchus, elevation of the left hemidiaphragm, and mild tracheal deviation to the left (black arrowhead). The Luftsichel sign manifests as a sickle-shaped lucency adjacent to the aortic arch (white arrowhead). Note anterior displacement of the left major fissure (arrow), a direct imaging sign of atelectasis.

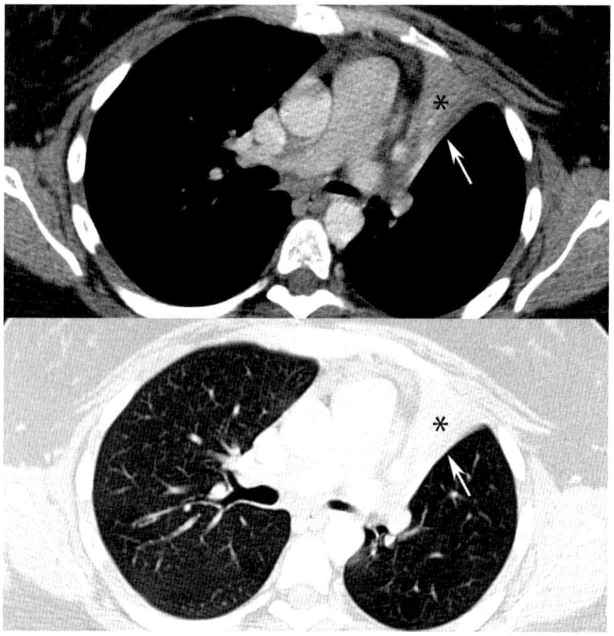

Figure 17.4. Chronic left upper lobe atelectasis (airway stricture). Composite image with chest CT in soft tissue (top) and lung (bottom) window shows left upper lobe atelectasis (asterisks) with leftward mediastinal shift and displacement of the left major fissure (arrows).

Middle Lobe Atelectasis

Radiography

- On the PA chest radiograph, the atelectatic middle lobe obscures all or part of the right heart border unless the medial segment is not involved (Fig. 17.5).
- The right hemidiaphragm remains visible because the aerated right lower lobe abuts its surface.
- On the lateral chest radiograph, the minor fissure moves inferiorly and the inferior part of the right major fissure moves superiorly, approximating to form a triangular opacity that is usually apparent.
- A collapsed middle lobe may be differentiated from pleural fluid in the major fissure by inspecting its margins. Fluid in the major fissure typically has biconvex margins, whereas middle lobe atelectasis has biconcave or flat margins. In most cases, the minor fissure can also be seen as separate from the pleural fluid opacity.
- Indirect signs of volume loss (i.e., mediastinal or hilar displacement) are usually not apparent due to the small volume of the middle lobe.

CT

- Minor fissure moves inferiorly and the inferior part of the right major fissure moves superiorly, approximating to form a triangular opacity.
- Right middle lobe syndrome is chronic or recurrent middle lobe atelectasis caused by extrinsic compression or obstruction of the central or peripheral airways. It occurs in patients with complete major and minor fissures that limit collateral air drift between lobes and hampers the ability to clear secretions. Associated bronchiectasis is a common imaging finding.

Combined Right Upper and Middle Lobe Atelectasis

- Rare; resembles complete LUL atelectasis
- Usually caused by lung cancer

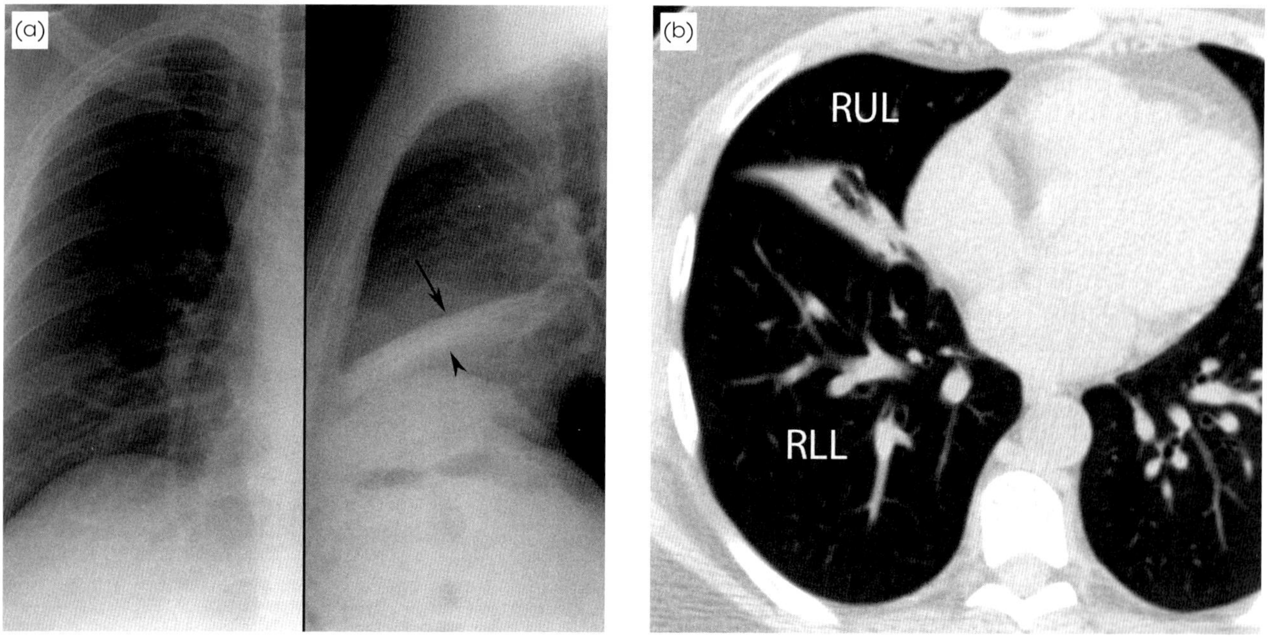

Figure 17.5. Chronic middle lobe atelectasis (middle lobe syndrome). (a) Composite image with PA (left) and lateral (right) chest radiographs shows subtle obscuration of the right heart border (left), inferior displacement of the minor fissure (right, arrow), and elevation of the lower aspect of the right major fissure (arrowhead) indicating middle lobe atelectasis. (b) Unenhanced chest CT shows the triangular-shaped atelectatic middle lobe that contains bronchiectatic airways and is interposed between the upper lobe anteriorly (RUL) and the lower lobe posteriorly (RLL).

Clinical Issues

Treatment of lobar atelectasis is directed at the underlying cause:

- Proximal mucus plugging is managed by suctioning and bronchoscopy.
- Suspected foreign body aspiration is managed with bronchoscopy.
- Distal mucus plugging with proximal air bronchograms may be managed with chest physiotherapy.
- Suspected obstructing tumor should have staging examinations (e.g., PET/CT, mediastinoscopy, and bronchoscopy) and biopsy to determine the appropriate therapy.

Key Points

- Lobar atelectasis in an adult outpatient is lung cancer until proven otherwise, and CT should be performed for further evaluation.
- CT features of malignant bronchial obstruction include irregular narrowing or occlusion of the airway and a central mass causing a convex bulge in the proximal aspect of the collapsed lobe (Fig. 17.1b).
- A hilar mass may be differentiated from atelectatic lung on CT by noting their differences in attenuation following contrast administration. Atelectatic lung typically enhances more than an adjacent hilar mass, but the tumor margin may be poorly defined (Fig. 17.1b).
- Lobar atelectasis that develops in an inpatient is generally from mucus plugging or a malpositioned endotracheal tube. The absence of air bronchograms suggests proximal airway obstruction, and affected patients may benefit from bronchoscopy and aggressive suctioning.
- Total lobar atelectasis may be difficult to appreciate on chest radiography and may simulate a loculated pleural effusion or mediastinal mass. Identifying displaced hilar structures or other signs of volume loss may facilitate the diagnosis (Fig. 17.1a).

Suggested Reading

Molina PL, Hiken JN, Glazer HS. Imaging evaluation of obstructive atelectasis. *J Thorac Imaging*. 1996;11:176–186.

Woodring JH, Reed JC. Radiographic manifestations of lobar atelectasis. *J Thorac Imaging*. 1996;11:109–144.

CHAPTER 18

Lower Lobe Atelectasis

Christopher M. Walker

Definition

Lower lobe atelectasis refers to volume loss in the right or left lower lobe. Atelectasis may be partial (segmental or subsegmental) or complete. The former commonly affects patients who have undergone surgery, and it may be indistinguishable from aspiration or pneumonia on portable chest radiographs. Lower lobe atelectasis is frequently overlooked because the increased density of the atelectatic lobe often overlies the heart and mediastinum on frontal radiography and the spine on lateral radiography (Figs. 18.1–18.4).

Clinical Features

Symptoms associated with lower lobe atelectasis vary depending on the cause and the degree of lung atelectasis. Patients with lung cancer and lobar atelectasis may be asymptomatic or may present with hemoptysis, cough, or dyspnea. Patients with a mucus plug or foreign body aspiration often have sudden onset of dyspnea and hypoxia.

Anatomy and Physiology

The lower lobes collapse posteromedially and inferiorly along the ipsilateral paravertebral region because they are anchored by the inferior pulmonary ligament.

Partial or complete left lower lobe atelectasis is common following open-heart surgery and is seen in up to 90% of patients undergoing such surgical procedures, but it is usually of no clinical significance. Some theories regarding the pathogenesis of lower lobe atelectasis in these cases include hypothermic damage to the left phrenic nerve, left main bronchus kinking, and direct trauma to the left lower lobe during surgery.

A centrally obstructing mass or aspirated foreign body may cause complete resorption atelectasis as described in Chapter 15 (Fig. 18.3). Subsegmental, partial. or complete lobar atelectasis may also occur in asthmatics.

How to Approach the Image

The first step in the imaging diagnosis of lower lobe atelectasis is identifying retrocardiac or lower lobe opacities and differentiating atelectasis from consolidation. Atelectasis typically causes inferior displacement and obscuration of hilar vascular structures. The second step relies on the recognition of direct and indirect signs of volume loss, including ipsilateral mediastinal shift, hemidiaphragm elevation, and displacement of the fissures. The third step uses the lateral radiograph to confirm the lower lobe atelectasis suspected on the frontal radiograph. Finally, search for the cause of lobar atelectasis and any associated findings such as lymphadenopathy, obstructing endoluminal airway lesion, or bony metastases.

What Not to Miss

Lobar atelectasis is often the initial presentation of lung cancer. When assessing a chest radiograph, make sure you see the para-aortic interfaces, paravertebral regions, and the hemidiaphragm contours in their entirety. All adult outpatients presenting with lobar atelectasis should be further evaluated with contrast-enhanced computed tomography (CT).

Partial or complete left lower lobe atelectasis is common following open-heart surgery and should not be misdiagnosed as pneumonia or aspiration.

Differential Diagnosis

Differential diagnosis of lobar atelectasis is highly influenced by the age of the patient, clinical presentation, and patient location at time of imaging (inpatient vs. outpatient). As in the case of upper lobe atelectasis, many outpatients presenting with lower lobe atelectasis have an endobronchial obstructing neoplasm such as lung cancer, endobronchial metastasis, carcinoid, or foreign body aspiration. The majority of inpatients with lobar atelectasis have mucus plugging or a malpositioned endotracheal tube causing the atelectasis. There are several other conditions that may be mistaken for partial or complete lower lobe atelectasis. Identification of these conditions is often accomplished with radiography, but in some cases CT may be required.

Pleural Effusion

- No inferior hilar displacement.
- Interlobar pulmonary artery remains visible.

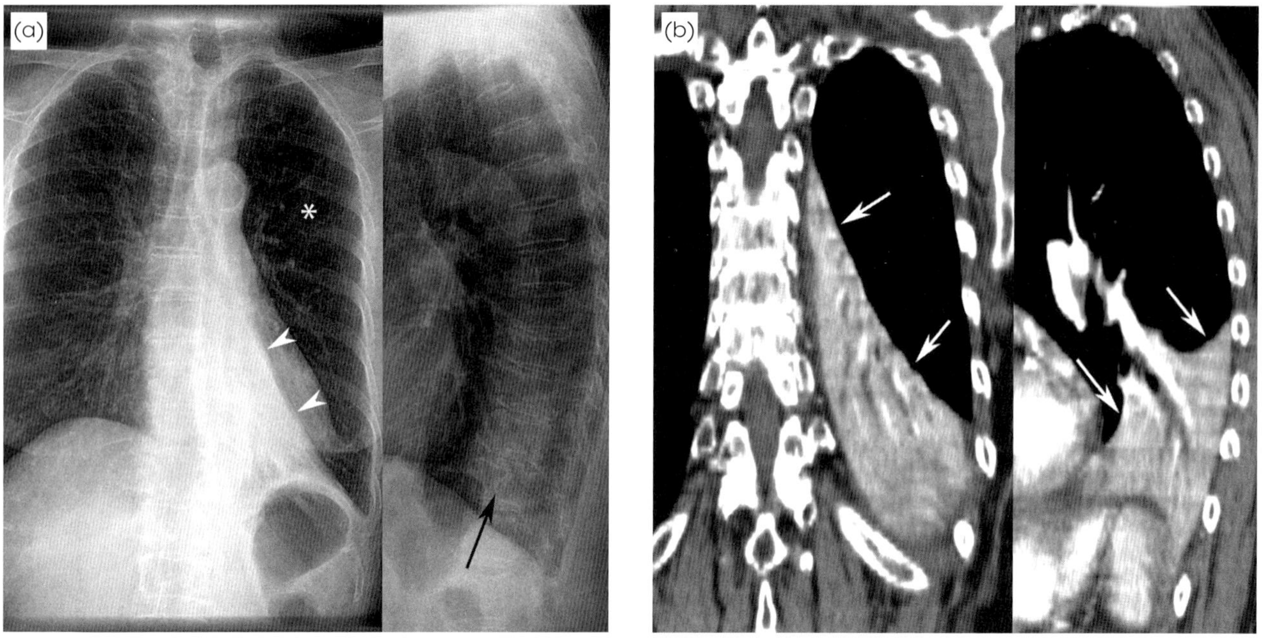

Figure 18.1. Chronic left lower lobe atelectasis. (a) Composite image with posteroanterior (PA) (left) and lateral (right) radiographs shows LLL atelectasis manifesting as a retrocardiac triangular opacity. The major fissure (arrowheads) migrates medially and posteriorly. The atelectatic lobe obscures the medial and posterior hemidiaphragm (arrow). Left upper lobe (asterisk) hyperlucency is due to compensatory hyperinflation. (b) Composite image with coronal (left) and sagittal (right) contrast-enhanced chest CT of the same patient shows posteromedial and inferior LLL atelectasis, major fissure (arrows) retraction toward the LLL, and crowded mucus-filled airways.

- Pleural fluid opacity is higher laterally with a meniscus sign, whereas opacity from lower lobe atelectasis is higher medially.

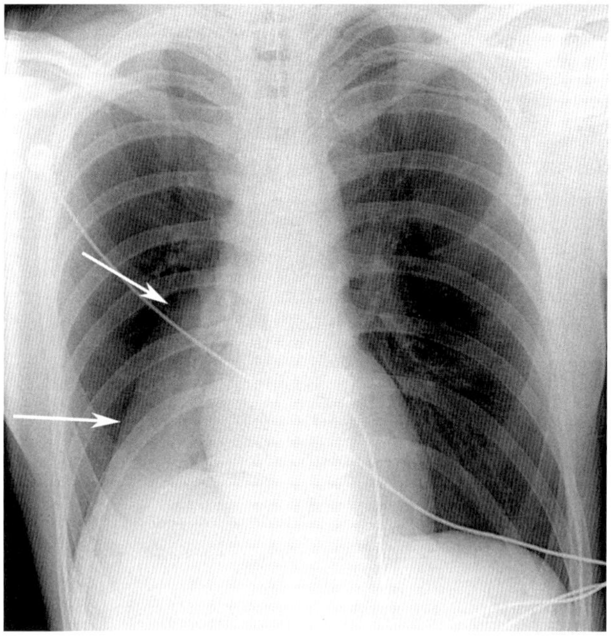

Figure 18.2. Right lower lobe atelectasis (mucus plugging). PA chest radiograph shows right lung volume loss, slight right shift of the heart, and increased right lower hemithorax opacity with a well-defined outer border (arrows) that represents the major fissure. There is obscuration of the right hemidiaphragm and the interlobar pulmonary artery, but the right heart border remains visible due to the normally aerated middle lobe.

Aspiration

- The lower lobes are a common location for aspiration (superior segments in the supine position and basal segments when upright).
- Aspiration may cause distal atelectasis, minimal volume loss, or no volume loss.
- On CT, aspiration causes gravity-dependent consolidation, centrilobular nodules, and tree-in-bud opacities.
- Patients may be asymptomatic, and approximately 50% of normal adults have minor episodes of aspiration during sleep that manifest as small tree-in-bud opacities on CT.
- Aspiration occurs in patients with impaired swallowing (stroke, drug or alcohol intoxication, head and neck cancers, esophageal dysmotility, etc.).
- Aspiration frequently appears and disappears suddenly within hours.
- Aspiration may progress to pneumonia or abscess formation.

Pneumonia

- The best differentiating feature is clinical history suggestive of pneumonia (i.e., fever, cough, and sputum production) in association with lower lobe opacity.
- Pneumonia generally causes little or no volume loss and may even expand the lobe.
- Pneumonia may occur in atelectatic lung and is best differentiated on contrast-enhanced CT. Pneumonia is often hypoenhancing, whereas atelectatic lung is hyperenhancing.

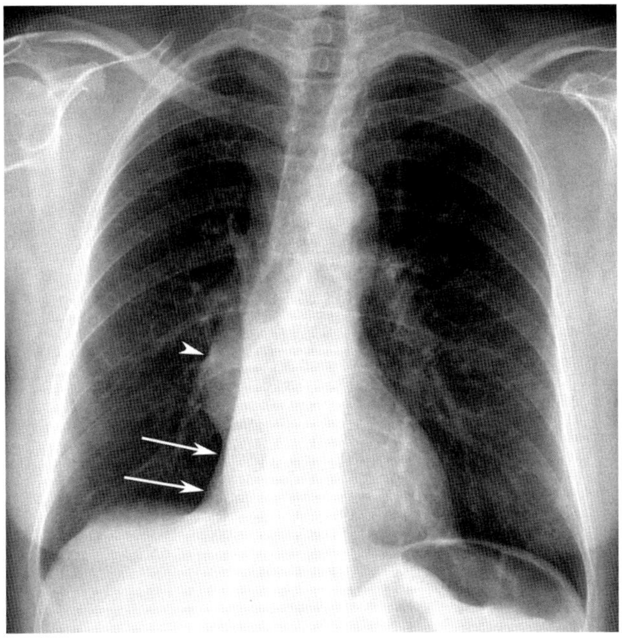

Figure 18.3. Complete right lower lobe atelectasis (carcinoid tumor). PA chest radiograph shows complete right lower lobe atelectasis due to a large right hilar mass (arrowhead). The collapsed lobe has a narrow triangular shape adjacent to the mediastinum outlined by the major fissure laterally (arrows). There is compensatory hyperinflation of the middle and upper lobes, and the right heart border remains visible due to the aerated middle lobe.

Imaging Findings

Left Lower Lobe Atelectasis

Radiography

- Early atelectatic lobe exhibits a superolateral curvilinear, convex margin on frontal radiography and may project beyond left heart border.
- Lateral radiography shows posterior displacement of the major fissure.
- Descending thoracic aorta and ipsilateral paravertebral stripe are obscured, but the left heart border remains visible outlined by aerated lingula of the left upper lobe.
- Left mainstem bronchus is inferiorly and medially displaced.
- Left interlobar pulmonary artery is eventually obscured as it abuts collapsed lower lobe.
- Left upper lobe pulmonary artery and left superior pulmonary vein are displaced inferolaterally resulting in a small hilum
- Initially, left lower lobe (LLL) atelectasis may obscure the entire left hemidiaphragm. With further atelectasis, the hemidiaphragm paradoxically becomes more visible as the hyperinflated left upper lobe fills the space previously occupied by the LLL.
- Elevation of the left hemidiaphragm with ipsilateral mediastinal shift.

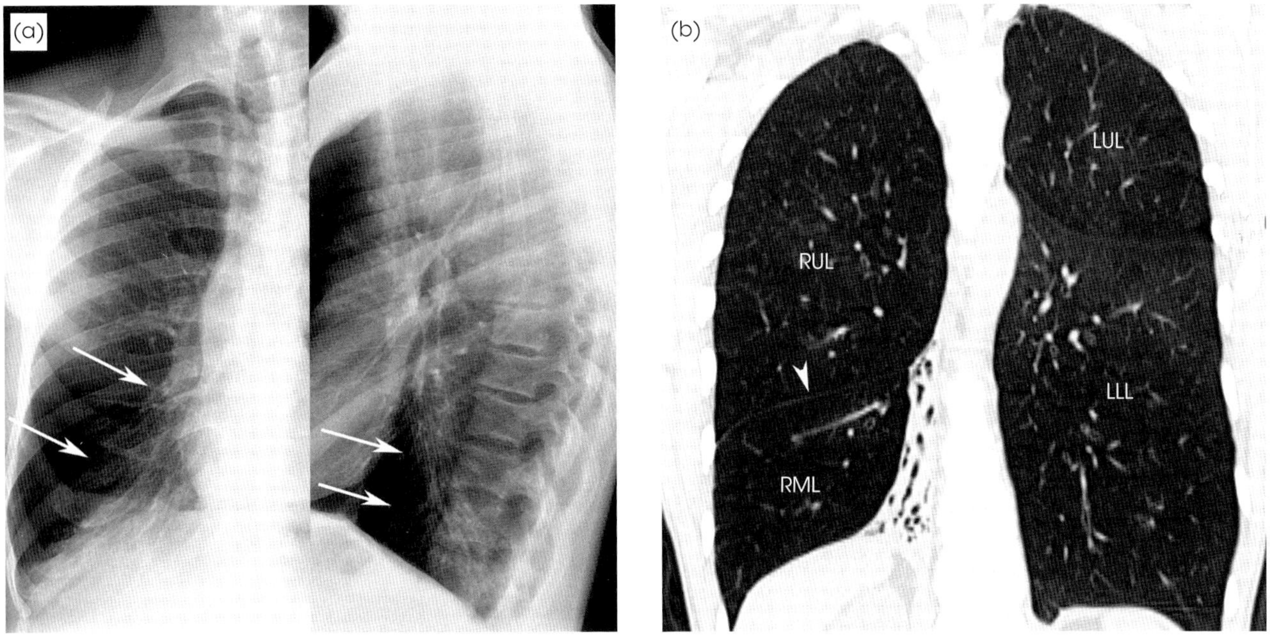

Figure 18.4. Chronic right lower lobe atelectasis (constrictive bronchiolitis). (a) Composite image with PA (left) and lateral (right) chest radiographs shows RLL atelectasis and visualization of the displaced major fissure (arrows) on the PA and lateral radiographs. Note crowded bronchovascular structures within the atelectatic RLL. (b) Coronal unenhanced chest CT shows severe RLL atelectasis extending along the right paravertebral region and bounded laterally by the major fissure. Note the inferiorly displaced minor fissure (arrowhead) and that the middle lobe (RML) now abuts the majority of the right hemidiaphragm. Diffuse mosaic attenuation reflects constrictive bronchiolitis. LLL, left lower lobe; LUL, left upper lobe; RUL, right upper lobe.

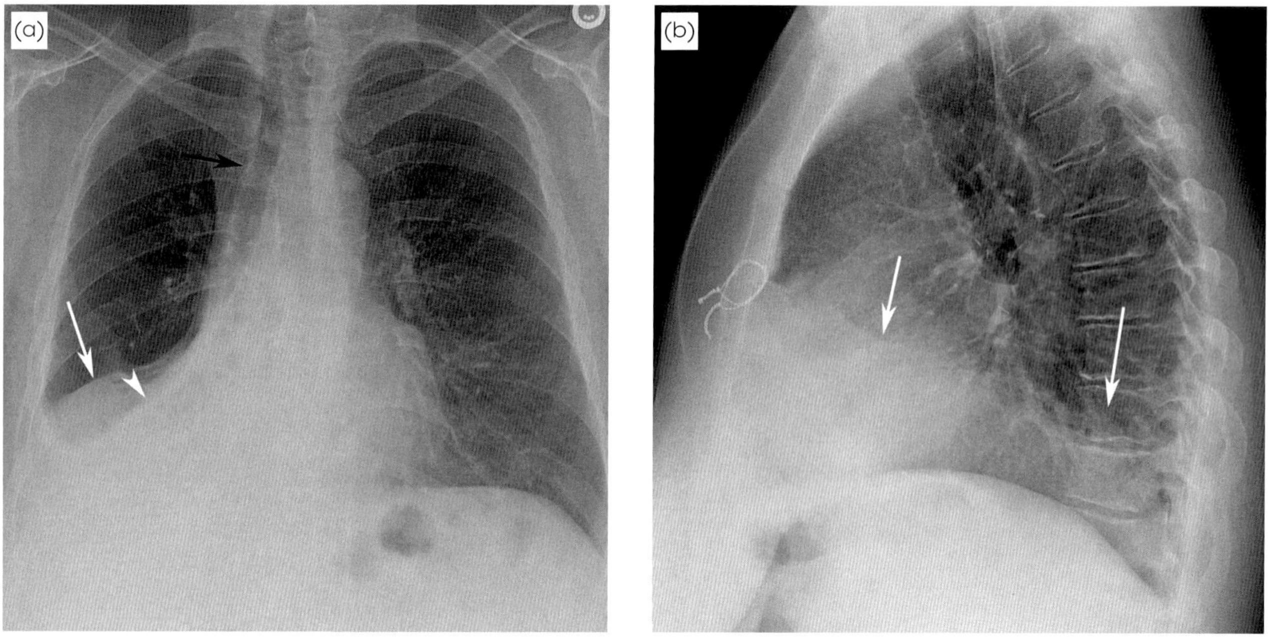

Figure 18.5. Combined middle and right lower lobe atelectasis. (a) PA chest radiograph shows right lower lobe atelectasis with inferior minor fissure (white arrow), medial major fissure (arrowhead) displacement, and rightward tracheal (black arrow) shift. Note hyperlucent right upper lobe from compensatory hyperinflation. (b) Lateral chest radiograph shows a band of opacity over the lower lung extending from anterior to posterior (arrows). CT (not shown) revealed a right hilar lung cancer encasing the bronchus intermedius and right pulmonary artery.

- *Top of the knob sign* represents obscuration of the superomedial aspect of aortic arch (knob) as mediastinal structures shift to the left.
- *Flat waist sign* represents flattening of the left heart border and mediastinum from posterior rotation and leftward shift of the heart.
- *Nordenström sign* represents linear atelectasis in the lingula due to vertical reorientation and kinking of lingular bronchi.

CT

- Direct visualization of displaced fissures and crowding of bronchovascular structures.
- Direct visualization of cause of atelectasis (e.g., mucus-filled bronchi, foreign body, or obstructing endoluminal neoplasm).
- Atelectatic lung is hyperenhancing on contrast-enhanced CT, whereas tumor is typically hypoenhancing.

Right Lower Lobe Atelectasis
Radiography

- Right lower lobe (RLL) atelectasis is virtually identical to LLL atelectasis.
- The first sign is posterior displacement of the major fissure on lateral radiography.
- Minor fissure may be inferiorly displaced on frontal radiography.
- Early atelectatic lobe has superolateral curvilinear, convex margin on frontal radiograph, and right heart border remains visible, being outlined by aerated middle lobe.
- Right hilum and right mainstem bronchus are inferomedially displaced, and bronchus intermedius is more vertically oriented.
- Right interlobar artery is obscured by the collapsed RLL.
- Right upper lobe pulmonary artery and right superior pulmonary vein are inferiorly and laterally displaced.
- Initially, RLL atelectasis may obscure the entire right hemidiaphragm. With further atelectasis, the right hemidiaphragm paradoxically becomes more visible as the hyperinflated right middle lobe and eventually the right upper lobe contact the hemidiaphragm and fill the space previously occupied by the RLL.
- Elevation of the right hemidiaphragm with ipsilateral mediastinal shift.
- *Upper triangle sign* represents visualization of the anterior junction line and shift of the upper mediastinal structures to the right due to volume loss that resembles a triangle. The apex of the triangle points toward the hilum.
- *Gatling gun sign* represents visualization of aerated clustered end-on bronchi within the collapsed right lower lobe that resembles the appearance of a machine gun.

CT

- Direct visualization of displaced fissures and crowding of bronchovascular structures.
- Direct visualization of the cause of atelectasis (e.g., mucus-filled bronchi, foreign body, or obstructing endoluminal neoplasm).
- Atelectatic lung is hyperenhancing on contrast-enhanced CT, whereas tumor is typically hypoenhancing.

Combined Right Middle and Lower Atelectasis

- The right heart border and right hemidiaphragm are obscured (Fig. 18.5).
- Vertically oriented major fissure intersects an inferiorly displaced minor fissure.
- Right hilum is depressed, right interlobar artery is obscured, and right upper lobe pulmonary artery and right superior pulmonary vein are laterally and inferiorly displaced.
- Trachea, heart, and mediastinum shift to the right.

CT

- Allows direct visualization of atelectasis with displaced fissures as well as etiology of atelectasis such as aspiration, foreign body obstruction, or obstructing endoluminal mass.
- Atelectatic lung generally hyperenhancing on contrast-enhanced CT.

Clinical Issues

Treatment of lobar atelectasis is directed at the underlying cause:

- Proximal mucus plugging is managed with suctioning and bronchoscopy.
- Suspected foreign body aspiration is managed with bronchoscopy.
- Distal mucus plugging with proximal air bronchograms may be managed with chest physiotherapy.
- Suspected obstructing tumor should undergo staging examinations (e.g., PET/CT, mediastinoscopy, and bronchoscopy) and biopsy to determine the appropriate therapy (i.e., surgery, chemotherapy, or radiation therapy).

Key Points

- The initial sign of lower lobe atelectasis is posterior displacement of the major fissure on lateral radiography.
- Initial lower lobe atelectasis has a curvilinear convex border prior to assuming a triangular configuration.
- Obscuration of the paravertebral stripe and descending thoracic aorta may be the only radiographic markers of severe LLL atelectasis.
- Partial or complete LLL atelectasis is extremely common and of little clinical significance after open-heart surgery and should not be misdiagnosed as pneumonia or aspiration.
- Pleural effusion does not obscure the interlobar pulmonary artery, and the convexity is higher laterally than medially.
- Lower lobe atelectasis is difficult to differentiate from pneumonia or aspiration on portable inpatient chest radiography. Helpful clues in diagnosing atelectasis include signs of volume loss or opacities following surgery or extubation. Helpful clues in diagnosing aspiration or pneumonia include the absence of signs of volume loss and clinical signs or symptoms suggestive of aspiration or pneumonia. Often, the portable radiograph is suboptimal, and distinction among these three entities cannot be made.
- Atelectatic lung enhances densely on contrast-enhanced CT, whereas pneumonia is usually hypoenhancing.

Suggested Reading

Molina PL, Hiken JN, Glazer HS. Imaging evaluation of obstructive atelectasis. *J Thorac Imaging.* 1996;11:176–186.

Woodring JH, Reed JC. Radiographic manifestations of lobar atelectasis. *J Thorac Imaging.* 1996;11:109–144.

CHAPTER 19

Subsegmental and Rounded Atelectasis

Christopher M. Walker

Definition

Subsegmental atelectasis is volume loss confined to a subsegment or extending across multiple pulmonary subsegments. It is commonly described as linear, plate-like, or discoid and may extend across an entire lobe.

Rounded atelectasis (syn. folded lung, atelectatic pseudotumor, shrinking pleuritis with atelectasis, and Blesovsky syndrome) is folded collapsed lung that develops adjacent to pleural thickening, fibrosis, or effusion.

Clinical Features

Subsegmental atelectasis is seen in a wide variety of pulmonary and abdominal conditions, including pulmonary embolism, pneumonia, pulmonary edema, diaphragmatic dysfunction, prolonged shallow breathing, and any condition causing chest or abdominal pain. It is often unimpressive in appearance but may be a marker of more general respiratory impairment and often indicates more widespread atelectasis than is apparent radiographically. Patients may be asymptomatic or have symptoms related to the underlying disease causing subsegmental atelectasis.

Rounded atelectasis is usually discovered incidentally on imaging studies performed for other reasons. When affected patients are symptomatic, any pain or dyspnea is generally secondary to the pleural abnormality rather than the rounded atelectasis. Most patients have a history of asbestos exposure and are older than age 50 years. Rounded atelectasis is also associated with other conditions and can coexist with pulmonary infarction, trauma, postsurgical pleural thickening, or any condition causing pleural effusion and thickening.

Anatomy and Physiology

Subsegmental atelectasis was initially thought to occur distal to mucous plugging or small thrombosed pulmonary arteries. It is now known that subsegmental atelectasis represents flattened alveoli in the subpleural lung that develop in association with underlying pleural clefts, pleural invaginations, or accessory fissures. Collateral air drift within and between pulmonary segments allows some alveoli to remain open while others collapse. The affected lung preferentially folds in along these clefts or invaginations during periods of hypoventilation. Surfactant deficiency secondary to recent major surgery also predisposes to the development of subsegmental atelectasis.

Rounded atelectasis represents a focal round subpleural "mass" of collapsed lung adjacent to underlying pleural thickening. Similar to subsegmental atelectasis, it may develop around pleural invaginations or clefts caused by local inflammation and fibrosis. The pathogenesis of rounded atelectasis is unknown. One hypothesis suggests that pleural effusion causes atelectasis and in-folding and apposition of visceral pleura with fibrinous adhesions. Following resolution of the effusion, there is re-expansion of surrounding lung while the adherent lung remains atelectatic as a subpleural mass.

How to Approach the Image

Subsegmental atelectasis is commonly found in inpatient populations and may manifest as pulmonary opacities that may mimic early consolidation. Rounded atelectasis should be considered when a subpleural rounded opacity is detected on radiography or CT, most commonly along the posterior aspect of either lower lobe. Look for signs of volume loss and significant contact with an adjacent pleural abnormality (e.g., pleural thickening or effusion). Next, examine the periphery of the lesion for bronchovascular structures that extend from the mass and converge to the hilum. Finally, look for associated abnormalities that are more commonly present with tumor and are not seen with rounded atelectasis, including rib erosion, lymphadenopathy, or chest wall invasion.

What Not to Miss

Peripheral lung cancer may mimic rounded atelectasis. It is important to look for all imaging features of rounded atelectasis before making the diagnosis. If all criteria are not met, the diagnosis should be questioned and lung cancer should be excluded with CT/PET or biopsy. If the diagnosis is certain, close clinical and imaging follow-up is usually sufficient to avert the possibility of mistaking a lung cancer for rounded atelectasis.

Differential Diagnosis for Subsegmental Atelectasis

- Linear or fibrotic scar: Seen in lung involved by pneumonia or injury and, unlike subsegmental atelectasis, does not change over serial examinations.
- Accessory fissure: Usually pencil thin and corresponds to the location of normal accessory fissures (e.g., azygos, inferior accessory, and left minor). There is an avascular zone surrounding it on CT.
- Fluid tracking within a fissure: Follows direction of known fissure, usually has a biconvex shape, and may be associated with ipsilateral pleural effusion.
- Interlobular septal thickening or septal lines: Represents thickening of the interlobular septa that surround the secondary pulmonary lobule and is seen as short, thin horizontal lines that are best appreciated near the lung bases. It may be associated with other findings of pulmonary edema (e.g., cardiomegaly and pleural effusions) or lymphangitic carcinomatosis (e.g., mass or lymph node enlargement). Septal lines are shorter and thinner than linear opacities of subsegmental atelectasis.

Differential Diagnosis for Rounded Atelectasis

- Tumor: Lung cancer and metastatic disease can closely mimic rounded atelectasis. Generally, there is no comet tail sign, and they are usually FDG avid on PET. Percutaneous or excisional biopsy may be necessary in equivocal cases.
- Pulmonary infarction: Patients are usually acutely symptomatic and have pulmonary emboli in the arteries supplying the lung abnormality. The portion of lung that is infarcted has little or no enhancement, unlike rounded atelectasis, which enhances briskly.
- Pneumonia: There are symptoms or signs of infection. There is no comet tail sign.

Imaging Findings

Subsegmental Atelectasis

Radiography

- Horizontally or obliquely oriented linear or band-like opacity (Fig. 19.1).
- Preferentially affects the lower lobes.
- Width ranges from a few millimeters to 1 cm.
- Length can extend 1–10 cm across multiple pulmonary segments or the entire lobe.
- Commonly occurs with low lung volumes.

CT

- Horizontal or obliquely oriented linear or band-like opacity (Fig. 19.2).
- Often better appreciated on multiplanar reformatted images (e.g., coronal or sagittal reconstructions).

Rounded Atelectasis

Chest radiography is inconclusive in establishing the imaging diagnosis of rounded atelectasis, typically showing

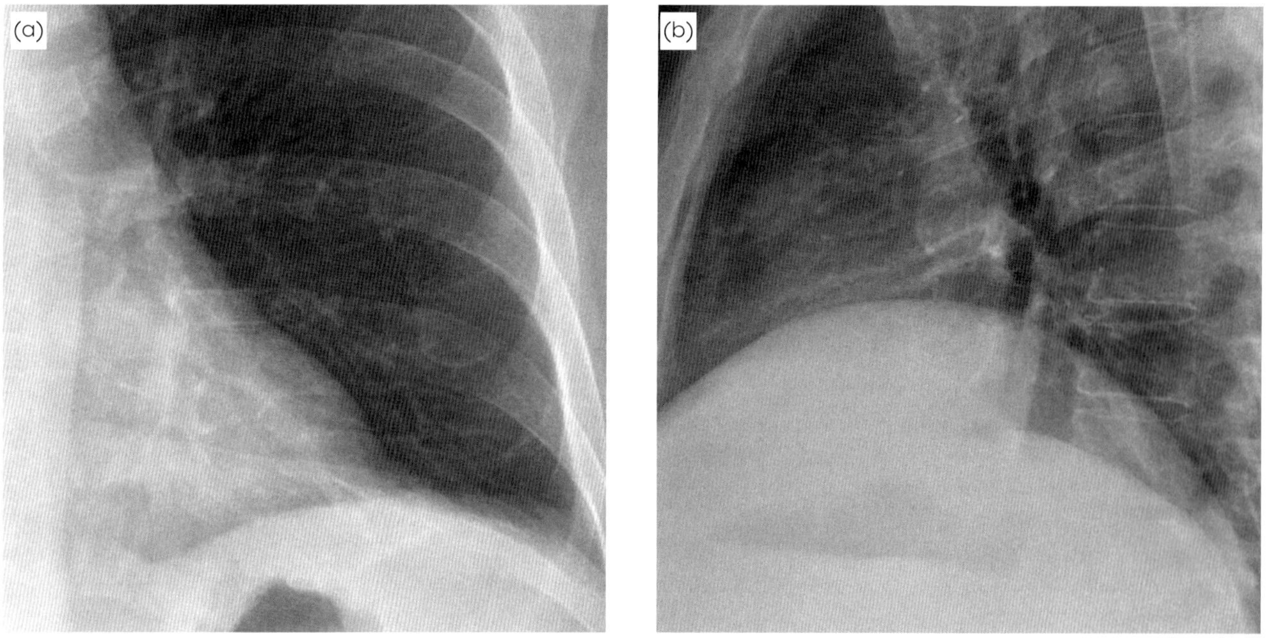

Figure 19.1. Subsegmental atelectasis. (a) Coned-down PA chest radiograph shows crowded and overlapping horizontal linear bands of subsegmental atelectasis at the left lung base. (b) Lateral chest radiograph shows band-like atelectasis in the middle lobe adjacent to an elevated right hemidiaphragm.

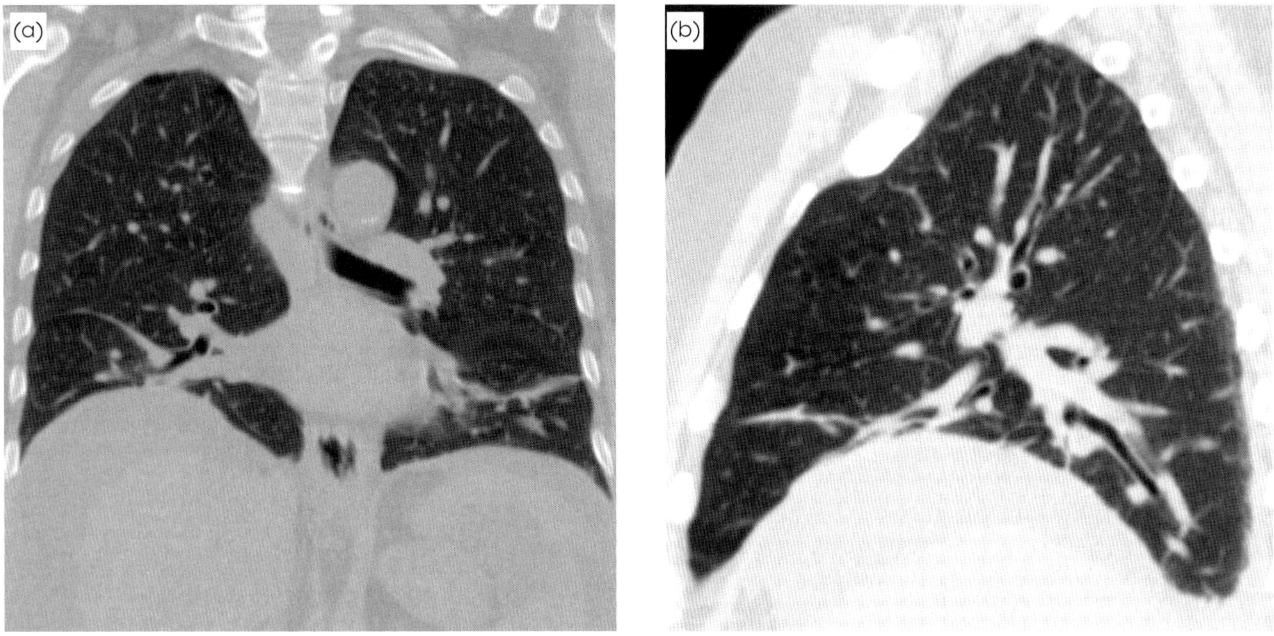

Figure 19.2. Subsegmental atelectasis. (a) Coronal unenhanced chest CT shows low lung volumes and bibasilar linear and band-like areas of subsegmental atelectasis. (b) Sagittal unenhanced chest CT of the same patient shows middle lobe horizontal band-like subsegmental atelectasis and right lower lobe vertical linear subsegmental atelectasis near the posterior costophrenic sulcus.

a rounded subpleural mass that resembles a neoplasm. There are four required CT imaging findings to confidently diagnose rounded atelectasis. If those criteria are met, CT follow-up should be sufficient. Comparison with previous CT studies may establish the chronicity of findings. The four CT features are as follows:

- Subpleural mass manifesting as a peripheral round or elliptical opacity (Fig. 19.3, top).
- The mass should be based along abnormal pleura (i.e., pleural thickening or effusion) (Fig. 19.3, top).
- Demonstration of the "comet tail sign" formed by bronchovascular structures that first diverge from the edges of the mass and then converge toward the adjacent hilum (Fig. 19.3, bottom).
- Signs of volume loss in the involved lobe, with the adjacent interlobar fissure displaced toward the opacity (Fig. 19.3, bottom).

Additional imaging features may or may not be present:

- Usually occurs in the peripheral lower lobes (Figs. 19.3 and 19.5).
- May enhance intensely following contrast administration.
- May grow, shrink, disappear, or be stable on sequential imaging studies.
- May be bilateral/multifocal (Fig. 19.5).
- The opacity often forms acute angles with the adjacent pleura, likely a manifestation of its pulmonary location.
- Most, but not all, cases are metabolically inactive on FDG-PET (i.e., uptake less than or equal to mediastinal blood pool; Fig 19.4).

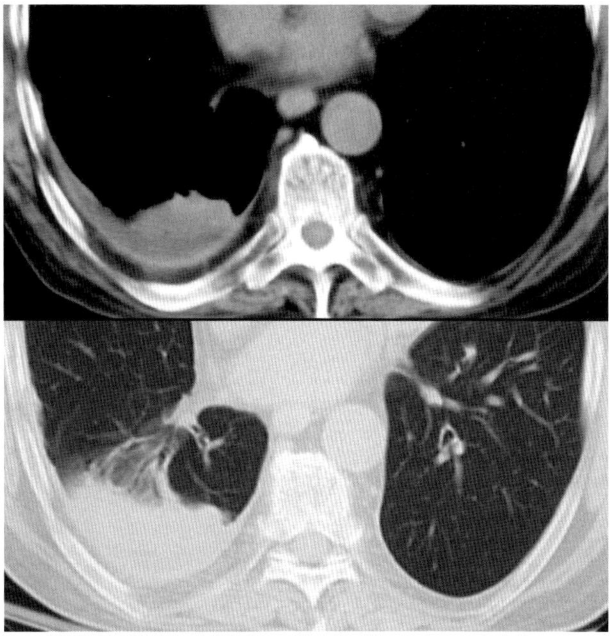

Figure 19.3. Rounded atelectasis. Composite image with axial unenhanced chest CT in soft tissue (top) and lung (bottom) window shows the four imaging features of rounded atelectasis: a subpleural mass, based along pleural thickening and/or effusion, with loss of volume in the affected lobe and a comet tail sign of bronchovascular structures converging to the hilum.

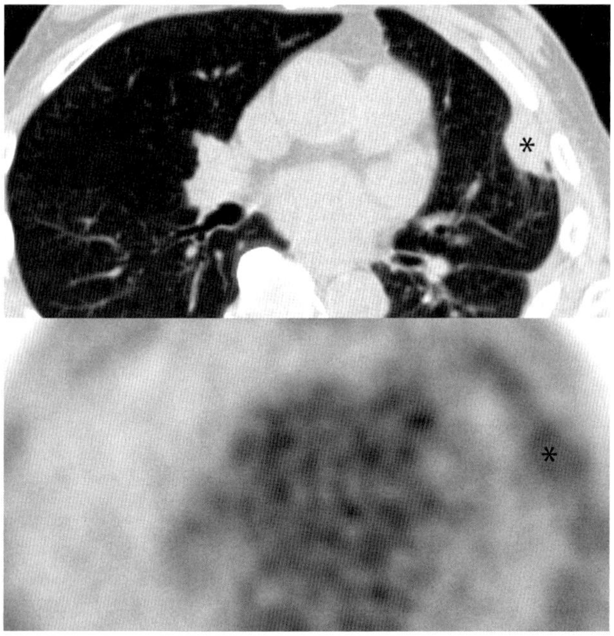

Figure 19.4. Rounded atelectasis. Composite image with unenhanced chest CT (top) and FDG-PET (bottom) shows a lingular subpleural mass (asterisks) that demonstrates low-level FDG uptake on PET imaging. Most cases of rounded atelectasis are metabolically inactive on FDG-PET imaging.

- Atypical rounded atelectasis can occasionally occur with pleural fibrosis and may exhibit unusual features, including an irregular shape, little or no pleural contact, anterior location, or no comet tail sign.

Clinical Issues

Treatment of subsegmental atelectasis is directed at its underlying cause.

Generally, no treatment is necessary for rounded atelectasis, and affected patients are followed with serial imaging to document stability. FDG-PET, needle biopsy, or excision may be performed in equivocal or atypical cases to confirm the diagnosis and exclude lung cancer.

Key Points

- Subsegmental atelectasis is a marker of more widespread ventilatory dysfunction and is seen in a variety of chest and abdominal conditions.
- Subsegmental atelectasis likely occurs adjacent to pleural clefts or invaginations that cause the overlying lung parenchyma to fold and collapse. The pathogenesis is unknown, but it is likely related to pleural effusion, adherence, and thickening.
- The four CT features required to confirm an imaging diagnosis of rounded atelectasis are (1) a subpleural mass, (2) based along pleural thickening and/or effusion, (3) a comet tail of bronchovascular structures converging toward the hilum, and (4) loss of volume in the affected lobe.
- If all features of rounded atelectasis are present, CT follow-up is usually sufficient and could be performed at 3, 6, and 12 months and 2 years.
- Comparison with prior studies may establish the chronicity of findings and obviate further evaluation.
- If some features of rounded atelectasis are absent, consider PET/CT or biopsy to confirm the diagnosis.

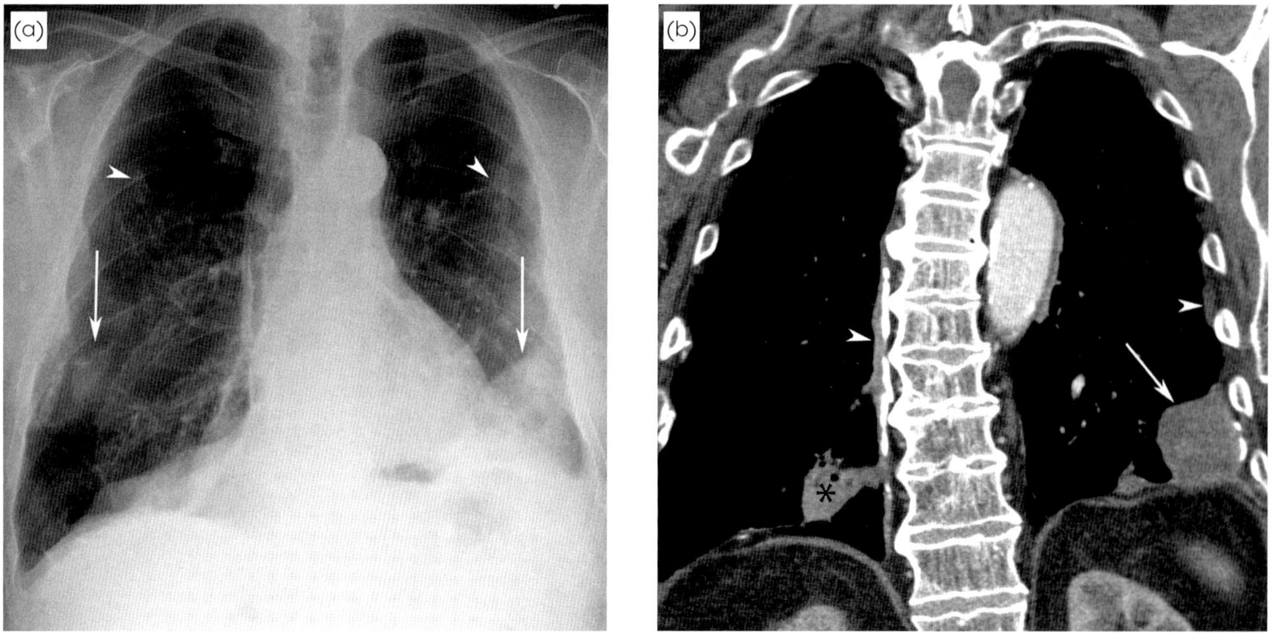

Figure 19.5. Bilateral rounded atelectasis. (a) PA chest radiograph shows bilateral indistinct rounded opacities in both lower lobes (arrows) and also calcified pleural plaques (arrowheads) indicating prior asbestos exposure. (b) Coronal contrast-enhanced chest CT shows the left rounded opacity (arrow) has significant contact with the pleura and a calcified pleural plaque. The right rounded opacity (asterisk) abuts mediastinal pleural thickening and calcification, with additional calcified and noncalcified bilateral pleural plaques (arrowheads).

Suggested Reading

Batra P, Brown K, Hayashi K, Mori M. Rounded atelectasis. *J Thorac Imaging*. 1996;11:187–197.

Gurney JW. Atypical manifestations of pulmonary atelectasis. *J Thorac Imaging*. 1996;11:165–175.

McAdams HP, Erasmus JJ, Patz EF, Goodman PC, Coleman RE. Evaluation of patients with round atelectasis using 2-[18F]-fluoro-2-deoxy-D-glucose PET. *J Comput Assist Tomogr*. 1998;22:601–604.

Woodring JH, Reed JC. Types and mechanisms of pulmonary atelectasis. *J Thorac Imaging*. 1996;11:92–108.

Section V

Emergency Radiology

CHAPTER 20

Introduction to Emergency Chest Radiology

Sanjeev Bhalla

Introduction

Perhaps the most often used imaging study in the emergency department (ED) is the chest radiograph. It is quick and fairly easy to perform. Each year, chest pain and upper respiratory infection symptoms remain among the top presenting complaints to the ED. Factor in the relatively low cost of radiography and the ease of performing a portable examination, and one can hardly be surprised at the ubiquitous nature of the chest radiograph in the ED setting.

Emergency Conditions

Emergency cardiothoracic conditions encompass a great variety of entities with variable clinical presentations. In the setting of trauma, one must look for vascular injury (most notably aortic injury), pulmonary contusion or laceration, hemothorax, pneumothorax, diaphragmatic injury, and, of course, fractures. Rarely, tracheobronchial or esophageal injuries may also be seen. In the absence of trauma, cardiovascular conditions must be considered in patients presenting with chest pain and dyspnea. Acute aortic conditions, such as aortic dissection, intramural hematoma and penetrating atherosclerotic ulcer, or pulmonary embolism, must be expeditiously excluded in patients presenting to the ED with severe chest pain in the absence of antecedent trauma. Rarely, pulmonary hypertension with its associated progressive dyspnea will result in affected patients presenting to the ED. Another frequent explanation for emergency chest radiography centers on the diagnosis and exclusion of acute airspace disease. This may take the form of pneumonia, pulmonary edema, or hemorrhage (as in the setting of vasculitis). These entities are discussed in other sections. However, an important patient group included in this section is patients with sickle cell disease. These patients often present to the ED and may be affected by a variety of conditions that may produce their symptoms.

Approach to the Emergency Chest Radiograph

The most important first step is to understand the clinical context of the ED imaging. One must know whether the patient being imaged has sustained a traumatic insult (Fig. 20.1). Understanding the type of trauma is also important. Generally, trauma can be classified as blunt trauma, such as occurs with falls and motor vehicle collisions, and penetrating trauma from knives and guns, for example. The former group may sustain injury anywhere in the chest, whereas the latter sustains injuries along the trajectory of the weapon.

A second key step in the interpretation of the emergency chest radiograph is comparison to any prior study (Fig. 20.2). A widened mediastinum takes on great importance when it is new and may be unimportant when it is unchanged from an old study. Airspace disease generates different differential diagnoses when acute (pulmonary edema, pneumonia,

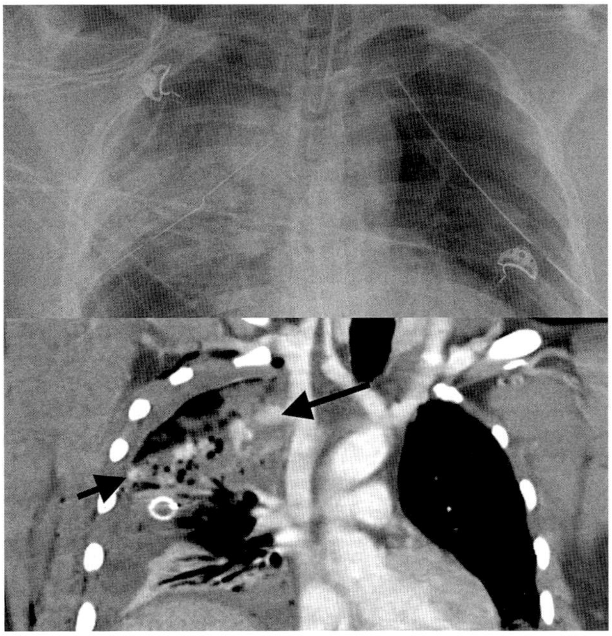

Figure 20.1. Pulmonary laceration. Composite image with portable chest radiograph (top) and coronal contrast-enhanced chest CT (bottom) of a 38-year-old man with gunshot to the right chest shows right upper lobe consolidation secondary to pulmonary contusion and laceration. Chest CT shows the projectile tract (black arrows) and contrast extravasation from the penetrating ballistic injury.

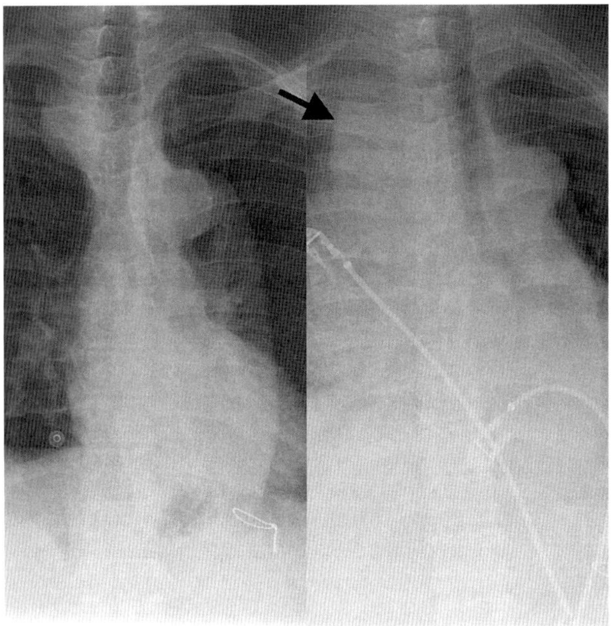

Figure 20.2. Ruptured innominate artery aneurysm. Composite images with comparison posteroanterior (PA) chest radiograph (left) and anteroposterior (AP) chest radiograph (right) of a 66-year-old man with acute chest pain show marked thickening of the right paratracheal stripe (arrow) compared to 1 month prior consistent with an acute vascular event, confirmed on chest CT (not shown).

vasculitis, or infarct) compared to chronic (neoplasm, inflammatory conditions, or structural disease).

A third useful step is to perform a dedicated survey for abnormal lucency (gas) (Fig. 20.3). Although this step forms part of all chest radiographic analyses, it is particularly helpful in the ED. One should begin by analyzing the normal gas-filled structures—the trachea, stomach, and colon—for contour and location. Once these are accounted for, the radiologist should make a conscious effort to exclude pneumothorax, pneumomediastinum, and pneumoperitoneum. Identification of these abnormalities will provide clues to possible serious underlying conditions. Rarely, pneumopericardium or pneumoretroperitoneum may be discovered.

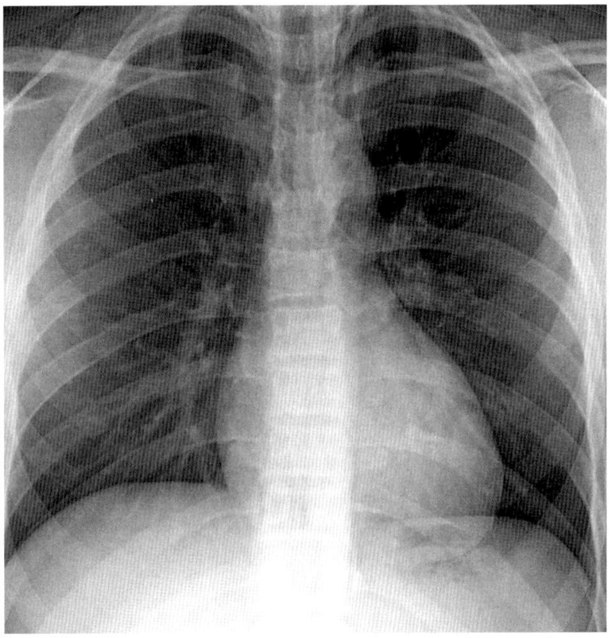

Figure 20.3. Pneumomediastinum. AP chest radiograph of an 18-year-old man with chest pain shows abnormal streaky lucencies in the mediastinum and supraclavicular regions from spontaneous pneumomediastinum secondary to multiple bouts of coughing.

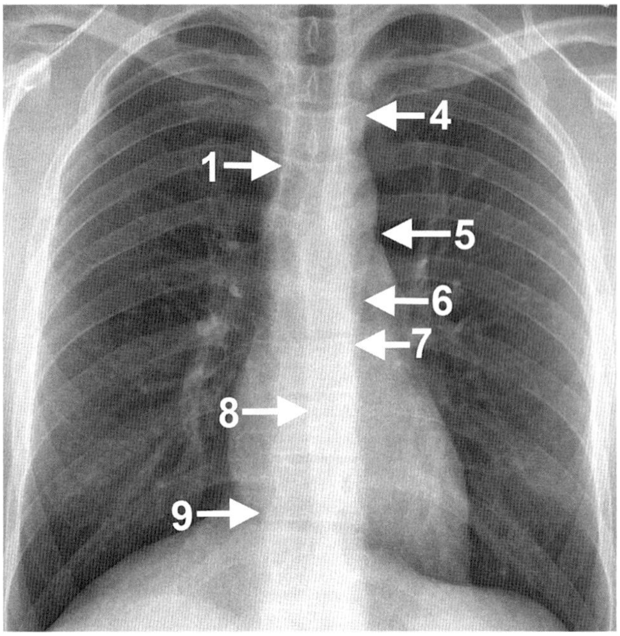

Figure 20.4. Normal mediastinal lines, stripes, and interfaces. (1) Right paratracheal stripe that should be 2 or 3 mm thick; (2) the anterior junction line (not shown), which is usually seen in patients with obstructive lung disease; (3) the posterior junction line (not shown); (4) the subclavian artery reflection, which should become more lucent cranially; (5) the aortopulmonary window, which should be concave; (6) the descending aorta or left para-aortic interface; (7) the left paravertebral stripe; (8) the azygoesophageal recess; and (9) the right paravertebral stripe.

A fourth important step is a careful analysis of nine lines, stripes, and interfaces on frontal radiography (Fig. 20.4). Although this analysis should be performed in all patients, it is very useful in the ED. These include the right paratracheal stripe (2–4 mm thick), the left subclavian artery interface (which should become more lucent as it extends cranially), and both junction lines (anterior and posterior). The fifth is the aortopulmonary window, which should be concave to the lung. Six through nine from left to right include the descending aorta, left paravertebral stripe, the azygoesophageal recess, and the right paravaretebral stripe. These nine lines, stripes, and interfaces are not seen in all patients, but consistent search for them will frequently allow for detection of abnormalities that may easily go undiscovered.

Differential Diagnosis Considerations

The high frequency of normal emergency chest radiographs and the potential great significance of the relatively

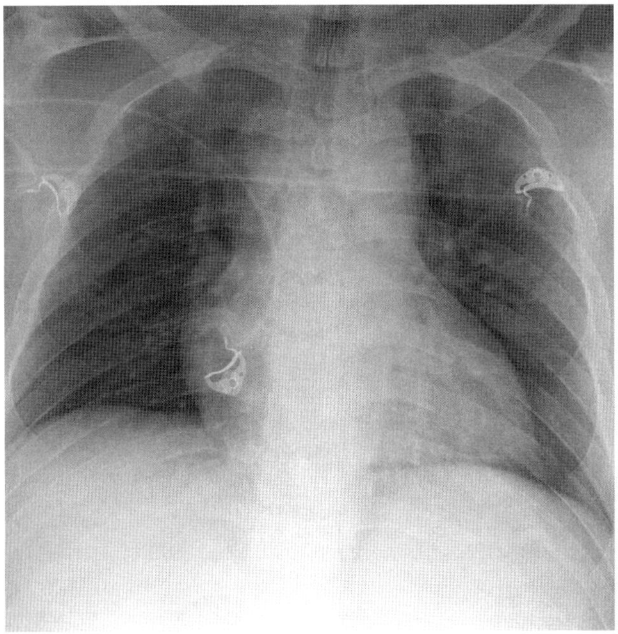

Figure 20.5. Acute traumatic aortic injury. AP portable chest radiograph of a 22-year-old man with a history of blunt chest trauma shows widening of the right paratracheal stripe, increased density of the left subclavian artery interface (apical cap), and downward displacement of the left mainstem bronchus, consistent with traumatic aortic injury confirmed on CT and at surgery.

infrequent abnormal radiograph present a challenge to the radiologist. In fact, virtually all categories of disease may produce an acute exacerbation that results in chest pain or dyspnea or a combination of the two.

Cross-sectional imaging of the thorax is often performed as a second step. However, in this era of cost and radiation awareness, these studies should be performed only when symptoms are out of proportion to the radiographic findings or when a radiographic abnormality cannot be explained. A methodical approach to chest radiographic analysis allows selection of patients in whom further imaging is both appropriate and helpful (Fig. 20.5).

Suggested Reading

Giron J, Fajadet P, Sans N, et al. Diagnostic approach to mediastinal masses. *Eur J Radiol.* 1998 Mar;27(1):21–42.

Lomoschitz FM, Eisenhuber E, Linnau KF, et al. Imaging of chest trauma: Radiological patterns of injury and diagnostic algorithms. *Eur J Radiol.* 2003 Oct;48(1):61–67.

CHAPTER 21

Thoracic Vascular Injury

Constantine Raptis

Definition

Both blunt and penetrating trauma can result in thoracic vascular injury. Injured arteries and veins may produce a hematoma from extravasated blood. Vascular injury can take place in the mediastinum, with injury to the aorta or great vessels. Injured intercostal vessels may produce a hemothorax. Chest radiographic findings, although not specific, may suggest mediastinal hematoma or hemothorax, which in turn prompt further imaging with CT for assessment of significant vascular injury.

Clinical Features

Patients with blunt or penetrating chest trauma may have a variety of presentations ranging from shock to minor or no discomfort. In fact, patients with minimal or no discomfort may have significant vascular injuries. Consideration of the mechanism of injury and interpretation of the initial chest radiograph are pivotal in determining the need for further imaging with CT. The latter should be performed when there are clinical or imaging findings of thoracic vascular injury.

Anatomy and Physiology

The normal mediastinum contains the heart, vessels, esophagus, airway, thymus, small lymph nodes, and fat. Mediastinal hematoma often results from thoracic vascular injury and replaces normal mediastinal fat. Penetrating injuries may result in direct vascular laceration, but blast forces may also produce vascular damage. In blunt trauma, several mechanisms may occur, including rapid deceleration, shearing forces, hydrostatic forces, and osseous pinch. Sternal and rib trauma may result in mediastinal and intercostal vessel injury. Vascular injury is highly variable, ranging from small intimal defects to full transections. Aortic injury can occur anywhere along the vessel course, but the most common location documented on imaging is the proximal descending thoracic aorta.

How to Approach the Image

Supine chest radiography is usually the initial study obtained in trauma cases in order to identify life-threatening conditions requiring immediate intervention, such as a tension pneumothorax or hemothorax. Careful radiographic assessment of the mediastinum (and its lines, stripes, and interfaces) and aortic contour is required to exclude underlying hematoma. Unfortunately, radiographic signs of vascular injury are neither sensitive nor specific. In fact, affected patients may have a near normal chest radiograph. Conversely, up to 40% of trauma patients with a wide mediastinum on initial supine portable anteroposterior chest radiograph have a normal mediastinum on subsequent upright posteroanterior (PA) chest radiographs. Therefore, any suspicious findings require further evaluation with either repeat PA chest radiography or CT. The decision to pursue a CT ultimately rests on the mechanism of injury and the clinical presentation.

Chest CT must be performed with contrast, and thin-section images must be evaluated. The first step in CT evaluation of the traumatized patient is determining the presence or absence of mediastinal hematoma, which manifests with high-attenuation material replacing the normal mediastinal fat. If a mediastinal hematoma is present, it is then necessary to determine whether or not it is due to an arterial injury. Mediastinal hematoma related to great vessel injury is usually in contact with the injured vessel. The injured vessel often, but not always, exhibits a contour deformity or intimal flap as direct evidence of injury. Contrast extravasation outside an injured vessel must be identified. In many cases, multiplanar reformatted images are particularly helpful.

What Not to Miss

Although the findings of blunt vascular injury are well described here, one must be very careful with regard to penetrating trauma. With bullets and knives, the trajectory must be followed because a vessel in the tract will likely be injured. At times, the injured vessel will look deceptively normal.

Differential Diagnosis

Technical Issues

- Pulsation artifact can result in a linear defect simulating an intimal flap.
- Not associated with hemorrhage.
- Should project into adjacent mediastinal fat.
- Streak artifact may arise from dense vascular contrast in the superior vena cava or from osseous structures.

Mediastinal Hematoma Unrelated to Major Vascular Injury

- May result from sternal or spine injuries, usually confined to anterior mediastinum or paravertebral region and not in contact with major vessels.
- Hematoma does not abut a major artery or vein.

Thymus

- Remnant thymus often present in anterior mediastinum of younger patients.
- Should exhibit interdigitating fat, often indistinct.

Anatomic Variants

- Aortic spindle: Mild fusiform aortic dilatation distal to ligamentum arteriosum but should appear smooth and in characteristic location on multiplanar reformats.
- Ductus diverticulum: Convex bulge along the undersurface of the aorta at the level of the isthmus with smooth, uninterrupted margins and no intimal flap.
- Branch vessel origins: Smooth conical margins of varying size, may simulate a pseudoaneurysm; small vessel identified extending from their apex.

Imaging Findings

Acute Traumatic Aortic Injury

Chest Radiography

- Wide mediastinum: >8 cm transverse or 25% of the thoracic width (Fig. 21.1)
- Obliteration of the aortopulmonary window
- Indistinct aortic arch or descending thoracic aorta
- Rightward deviation of the trachea or nasogastric tube
- Inferior displacement of the left mainstem bronchus
- Increased density of the left subclavian artery interface (apical cap)

CT

- Mediastinal hematoma that abuts the aorta
- Periaortic stranding
- Aortic contour deformity or discontinuity
- Aortic pseudoaneurysm
- Contrast extravasation (to mediastinum or pleural space)
- Aortic intimal or intimomedial flap
- Aortic caliber change
- Aortic luminal thrombus

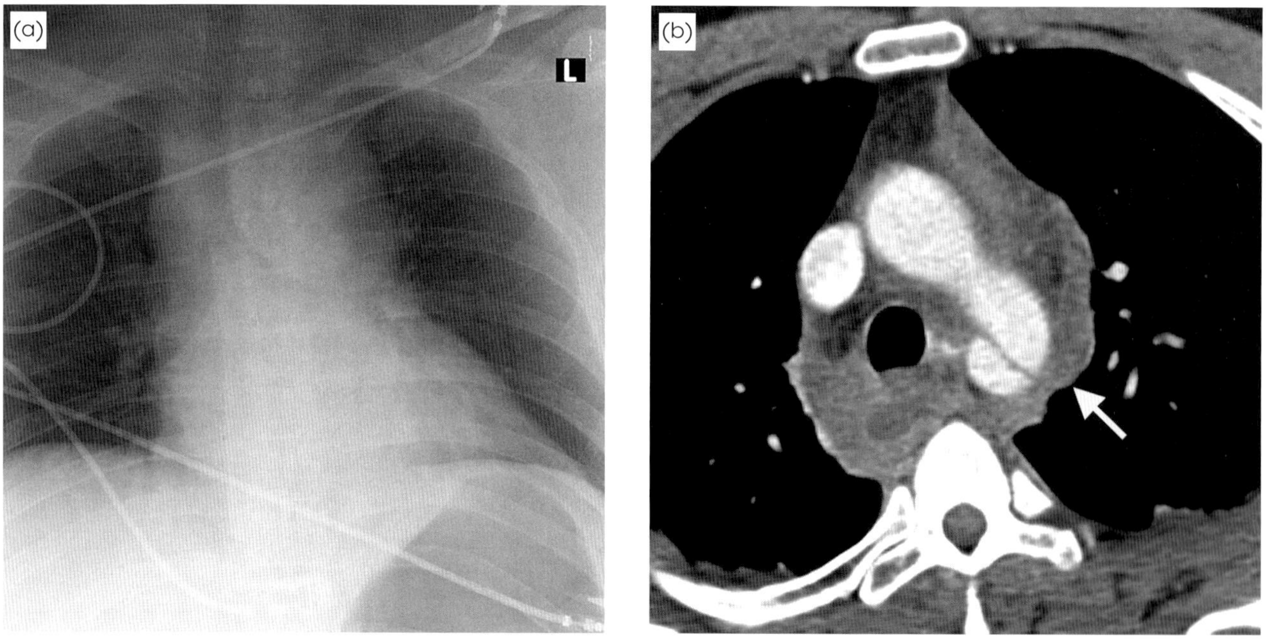

Figure 21.1. Acute traumatic aortic injury. (a) Portable chest radiograph of a 29-year-old man involved in a motor vehicle collision shows mediastinal widening, inferior displacement of the left mainstem bronchus, rightward tracheal deviation, and loss of the aortopulmonary window, concerning for mediastinal hematoma and traumatic aortic injury. (b) Contrast-enhanced chest CT shows mediastinal hematoma (arrow) abutting the proximal descending aorta, which exhibits flap indicative of aortic transection. A descending aorta pseudoaneurysm on angiography was treated with stenting.

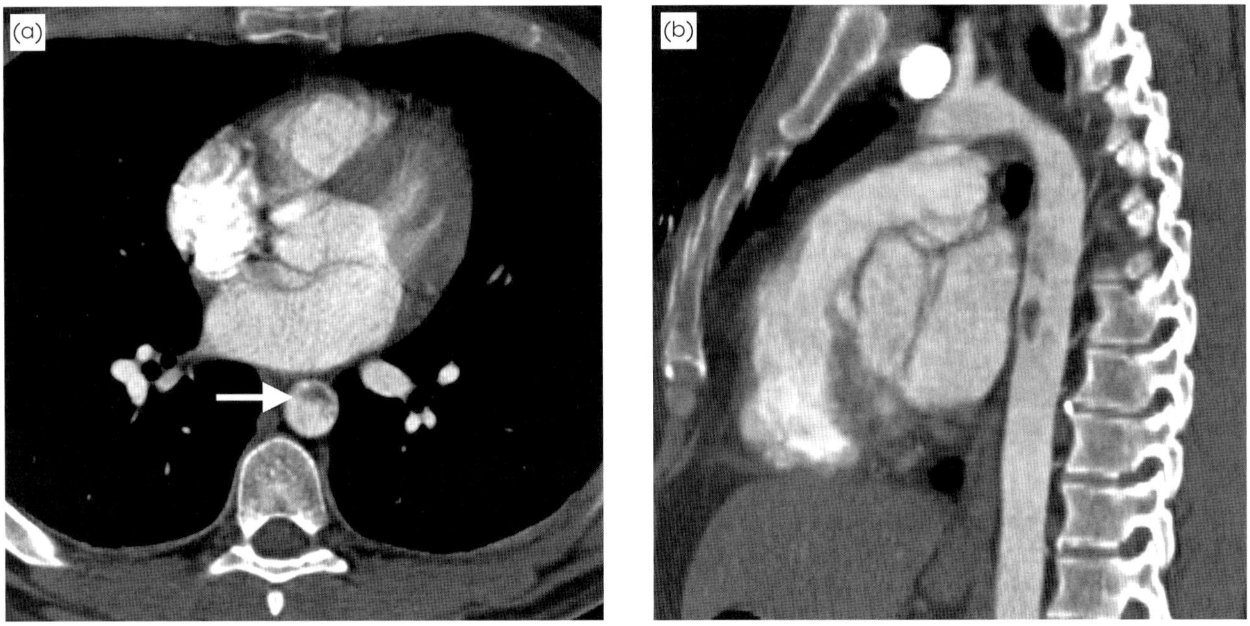

Figure 21.2. Minimal aortic injury. (a) Contrast-enhanced chest CT of a 34-year-old man after a motor vehicle collision shows a low attenuation filling defect (arrow) in the descending aorta without periaortic hematoma or aortic contour deformity. (b) Sagittal contrast-enhanced chest CT confirms the low attenuation filling defect within a normal-caliber aorta. The patient was managed conservatively, and the findings resolved on subsequent CT.

Minimal Aortic Injury

- Definition: Intimal tear <1 cm with no or minimal periaortic hemorrhage
- Not detectable on radiography
- Very short short-segment intimalirregularity or small luminal thrombus on CT with paucity of periaortic hemorrhage or stranding (Fig. 21.2)

Great Vessel Injury

Radiography

- Mediastinal hematoma located superiorly in the mediastinum
- Right paratracheal or tracheal displacement to the left, should raise suspicion for brachiocephalic artery injury (Fig. 21.3)

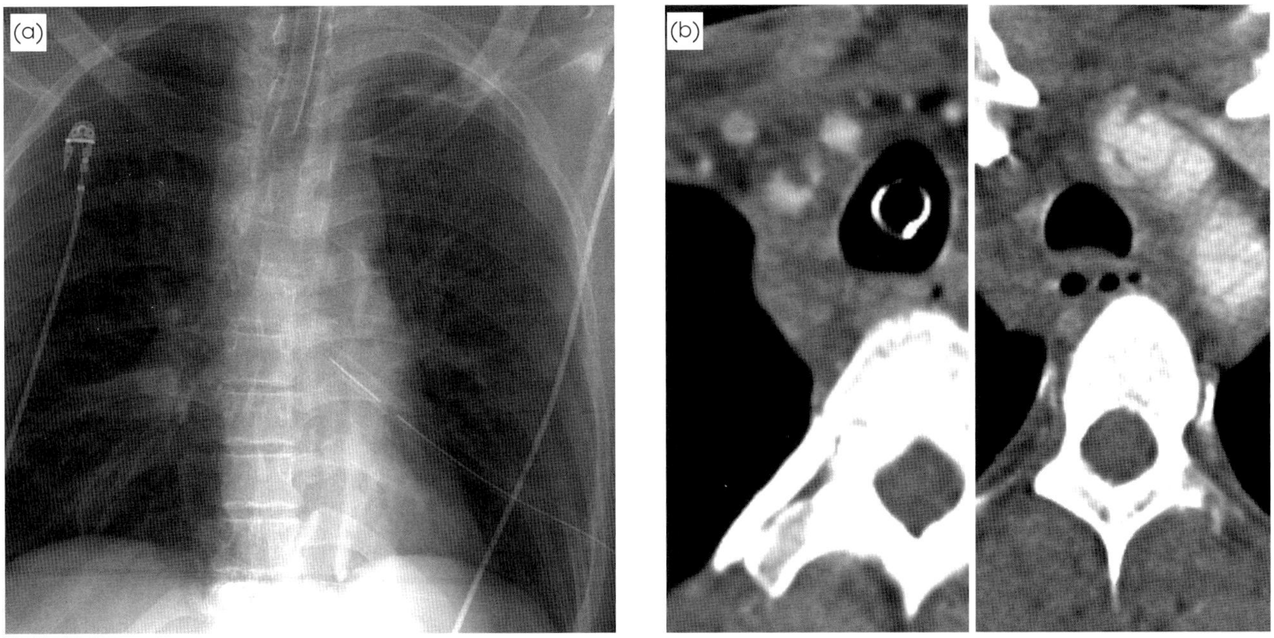

Figure 21.3. Brachiocephalic artery and subclavian injury. (a) Portable chest radiograph of a 34-year-old man after a motor vehicle collision shows superior right paratracheal widening suggesting mediastinal hematoma due to innominate artery or great vessel injury. (b) Composite axial contrast-enhanced chest CT shows right paratracheal hematoma, an eccentric thrombus in the right subclavian artery, and direct signs of brachiocephalic artery injury.

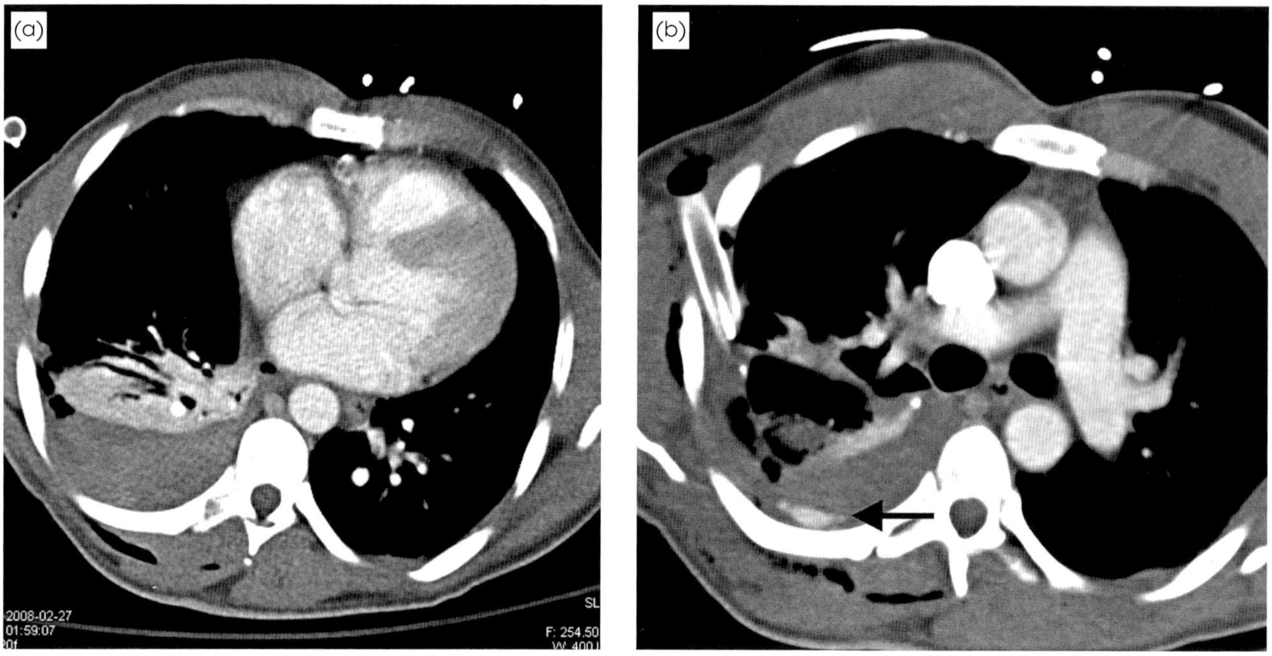

Figure 21.4. Intercostal artery injury. (a) Axial contrast-enhanced chest CT of a 37-year-old man who was stabbed in the back shows high-attenuation pleural fluid consistent with hemothorax. (b) Axial contrast-enhanced chest CT shows active contrast extravasation (arrow) manifesting as arterial contrast attenuation material posteriorly within the hemothorax, consistent with intercostal vessel injury.

CT

- Mediastinal hematoma that abuts injured vessel
- Direct signs of vascular injury
- Abnormalities may occur near margins of scan coverage

Venous Injury

- Perivascular hematoma abutting injured vessel
- Stranding adjacent to injured vessel in less severe venous injuries
- Direct signs: Luminal thrombosis, wall discontinuity, vessel caliber change, contrast extravasation

Intercostal and Internal Mammary Artery Injury

- Intercostal and internal mammary injuries account for 12% of thoracotomies after stab wounds (Fig. 21.4).
- Rapidly enlarging pleural effusion on radiography.

CT

- Hemothorax (pleural fluid with 35–70 HU or hematocrit level)
- Sentinel clot (higher density hematoma near the origin of bleeding)
- Active extravasation from injured artery manifesting with high-density material in the hematoma with attenuation equal to that of aorta and other opacified arteries

Clinical Issues

- Aortic and great vessel injuries are rare but can be lethal if missed.
- A substantial number of mediastinal hematomas detected in trauma are due to small venous injuries and osseous injuries.
- When in doubt about CT findings, consider a repeat with high pitch or electrocardiographic gating. Multiplanar images are key in the diagnosis of vascular injuries.

Key Points

- A chest radiographic mediastinal contour abnormality in the setting of trauma requires further evaluation with contrast-enhanced chest CT, but these findings have low sensitivity and specificity for thoracic vascular injuries.
- On CT, most thoracic vascular injuries are associated with hematoma or stranding that abuts the injured vessel.
- A careful interrogation of the vessels abutting a mediastinal hematoma is required to identify direct signs of vascular injury, including intimal flaps, contour deformities, pseudoaneurysms, thrombus, and active contrast extravasation.
- The radiologist must not rely only on axial images because some suspected minimal aortic injuries may

be found to exhibit greater aortic disruption when viewed in additional planes.

- Postprocessing including multiplanar reformatted images, maximum intensity projections, and volumetric reconstructions may be helpful for depicting and assessing vascular injuries.
- Minimal aortic injury must be described accurately because these lesions can often be managed conservatively.
- A thorough description of the injury on imaging may help direct the type of repair required, with particular attention to whether there is active bleeding. The caliber of the aorta above and below the injury, the proximity of the nearest branch vessels, and whether thrombus is present within the aorta are particularly helpful information if endovascular repair is pursued.
- Identifying a potential bleeding site can be helpful in directing a potential embolization.

Suggested Reading

Holly BP, Steenburg SD. Multidetector CT of blunt traumatic venous injuries in the chest, abdomen, and pelvis. *RadioGraphics*. 2011;31:1415–1424.

Mirvis SE, Shanmuganathan K. Diagnosis of blunt traumatic aortic injury 2007: Still a nemesis. *Eur J Radiol*. 2007;64(1):27–40.

Steenburg SD, Ravenel JG, Ikonomidis JS, et al. Acute traumatic aortic injury: Imaging evaluation and management. *Radiology*. 2008;248(3):248–262.

CHAPTER 22

Chest Trauma: Nonvascular Injuries

Constantine Raptis

Definition

Traumatic thoracic injuries are third in frequency after head and extremity injuries. Although the greatest source of mortality in thoracic trauma is vascular injury, nonvascular injuries are much more common and can produce substantial morbidity and mortality. All thoracic structures may be involved, resulting in a wide range of imaging abnormalities.

Pulmonary contusion results from a combination of edema and hemorrhage due to disruption of the alveolar capillary membrane and typically occurs immediately and at impact sites, although contre coup injuries may also develop. A pulmonary laceration represents lung parenchymal disruption due to a tear that forms as lung tissue pulls away because of elastic recoil. It may occur in blunt or penetrating trauma.

Clinical Features

Patients with blunt or penetrating chest trauma present with a wide range of clinical manifestations depending on the severity and location of the injury. Chest pain and dyspnea are common but nonspecific complaints. It is always helpful to review the mechanism of injury and whether injury resulted from blunt or penetrating trauma. In addition, specific sites of pain and the location of any open thoracic or abdominal wound should also be noted because such information may guide the radiologist in the search for abnormalities.

Anatomy and Physiology

In blunt trauma, the mechanism of injury and sites of maximum impact can have an important effect on what structures are most likely to be injured. Likewise, in penetrating trauma, the location of exit and entry sites, as well as wound trajectories, dictate which structures are at greatest risk.

How to Approach the Image

The chest radiograph is often the first imaging study obtained in patients with thoracic trauma and requires an expeditious interpretation. Chest radiography is principally used to exclude life-threatening abnormalities, including tension pneumothorax and large hemothorax. It also serves to verify the position of medical support devices. Findings such as airspace opacities and mediastinal widening should be reported and may indicate further evaluation with chest CT. Chest radiographs may greatly underestimate injuries, and all suspicious findings require thorough clinical and/or additional imaging investigation. When patients are able to speak, the verbalization of pain despite a normal radiograph should also prompt consideration of a chest CT. Due to its wide availability and rapid acquisition time, CT is the best imaging modality available to evaluate the full spectrum of thoracic injuries.

What Not to Miss

Because any thoracic structure may be injured, it is imperative to follow an organized and efficient search pattern. This includes a careful investigation of the mediastinum, aorta, great vessels, heart, airway, lung, diaphragm, bones, and soft tissues. In patients with penetrating trauma, outlining the wound tract is also essential because structures injured along the tract may only show subtle signs of injury or even appear normal. Patients with substantial thoracic trauma often have injuries in multiple locations, and failure to perform a detailed search may result in overlooking injuries. In the setting of trauma, a detailed analysis of the subcutaneous fat can also be helpful in preventing overlooking subtle injuries. Fat stranding is indicative of a bruise and allows a second chance for a detailed analysis of underlying structures.

Differential Diagnosis

Pulmonary Injuries

- Aspiration (Figure 22.1): Tree-in-bud poorly defined centrilobular opacities in dependent portions of the lungs, distinguished from contusion/laceration based on distribution, appearance, and lack of gas
- Atelectasis: Distinguished from contusion/laceration based on denser and homogenous appearance, greater enhancement, and findings of volume loss

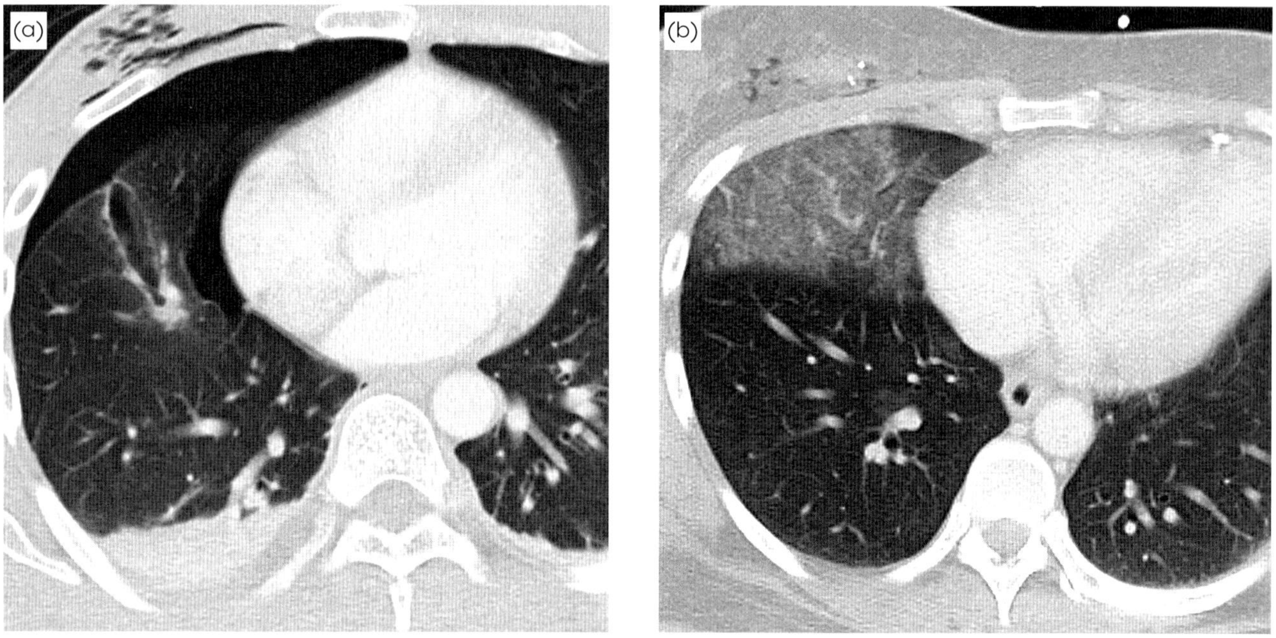

Figure 22.1. Pulmonary laceration and contusion. (a) Axial contrast-enhanced CT of a 40-year-old man stabbed in the right chest shows a middle lobe pulmonary laceration manifesting with a linear gas-filled defect in the right middle lobe. (b) Axial contrast-enhanced chest CT of a 39-year-old woman who was shot in the right breast with a bullet tract that did not penetrate the pleura shows middle lobe ground-glass opacities consistent with contusion related to blast injury.

- Pulmonary edema: Variable imaging appearance, presence of septal line thickening or underlying potential cause (volume overload, neurologic) can help to make the diagnosis
- Fat embolism syndrome: Affects patients with long bone fractures who develop mental status changes typically 24–48 hours after injury, results from local edema and pneumonitis secondary to embolized particles—CT findings of ground-glass and/or centrilobular ill-defined nodular opacities with possible septal line thickening (no zonal predilection)

Pneumomediastinum

- Usually spontaneous from a Macklin effect
- Esophageal injuries
- Tracheobronchial injuries

Imaging Findings

Pulmonary Injuries

Pulmonary Contusion

- Non-segmental focal or multifocal airspace opacities (ground glass or consolidation) (Fig. 22.2)
- May demonstrate subpleural sparing
- Air bronchograms typically (but not always) absent
- More common at lung bases
- May be occult on initial chest radiographs and become apparent during next 6 hours
- CT superior at detecting contusions

Pulmonary Laceration

- Ovoid space within injured lung that can contain blood and/or gas
- May be initially obscured by surrounding contusion
- Heals slowly over months
- Many clear but may result in persistent pulmonary opacity or lung cyst

Airway Injuries

- Rare, usually occur within 2.5 cm of carina; right bronchial injuries more common than left (Fig. 22.3).
- Chest radiograph may show pneumomediastinum, pneumothorax, subcutaneous gas.
- *Fallen lung sign*: Complete or near complete bronchial transection, results in lung falling away from hilum.
- Thin-section CT is useful for detecting airway wall defect (optimally visualized on lung window).

Pleural Injuries

- Pneumothorax: Gas collection in the pleural space
  - Upright chest radiography: White pleural line with lucent gas peripheral to it
  - Supine chest radiography: May visualize pleural line; pleural gas may collect anteriorly or inferiorly, displacing diaphragm and resulting in the *deep sulcus sign*
  - May be occult on radiograph but not on CT
  - Assessment of tension physiology: Contralateral mediastinal shift, depression or inversion of the ipsilateral hemidiaphragm, cardiac compression
- Hemothorax: Blood in the pleural space

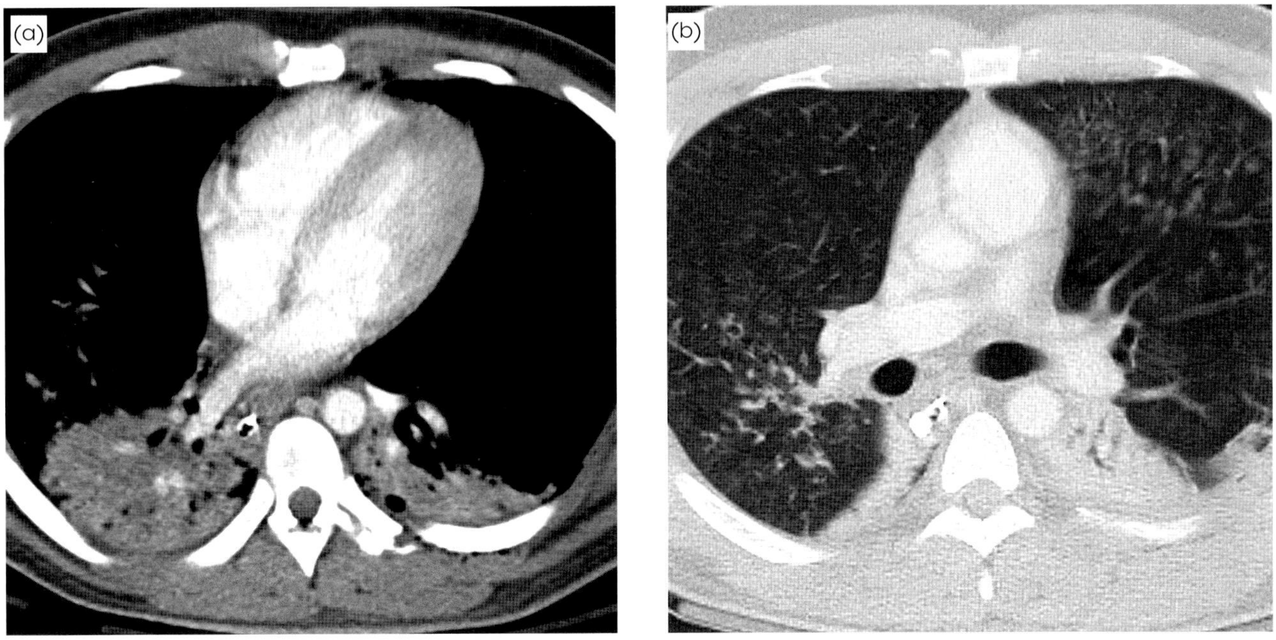

Figure 22.2. Aspiration. (a) Axial contrast-enhanced CT of a patient involved in a motor vehicle collision demonstrates weakly enhancing bilateral lower lobe consolidations, suggestive of aspiration pneumonitis. (b) Axial contrast-enhanced CT (lung window) of the same patient shows ground-glass and tree-in-bud nodules predominantly in the left upper lobe and also in the right lower lobe, consistent with aspiration.

- Pleural fluid collections on radiographs in the setting of trauma should be assumed to be hemothorax.
- Often associated with other injuries, including fractures, pneumothorax, and diaphragmatic trauma
- Increasing pleural effusion on serial radiographs should raise suspicion of active bleeding.
- CT: Increased attenuation of pleural fluid (35–70 HU) and hematocrit level

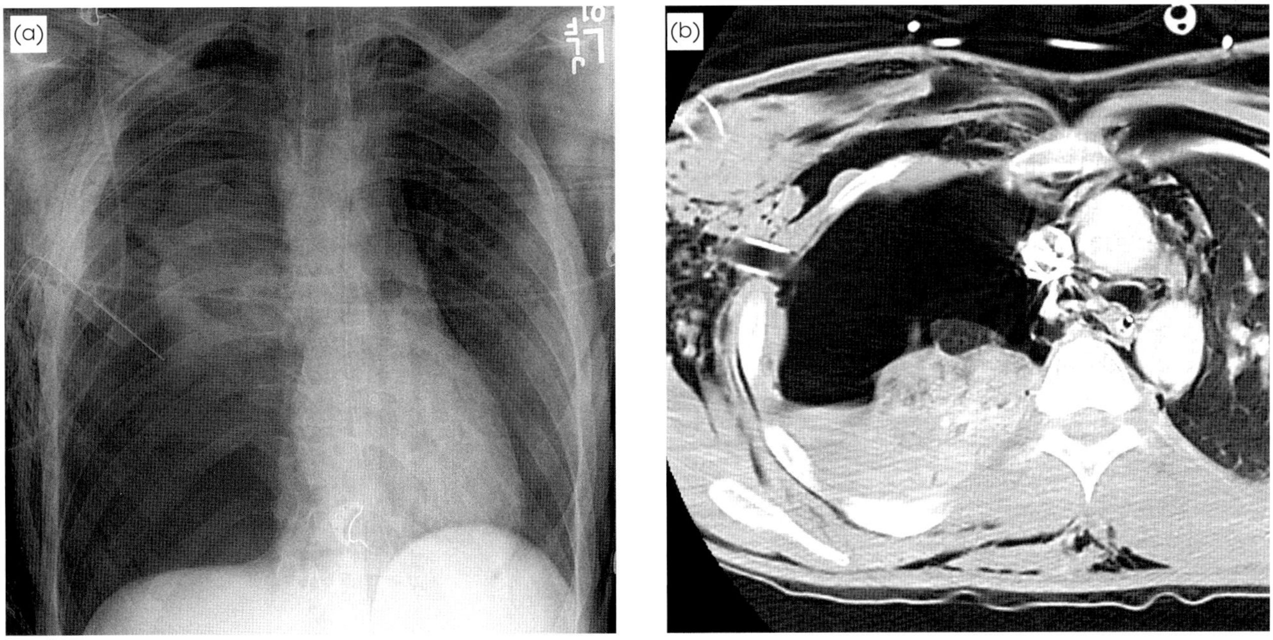

Figure 22.3. Bronchial injury. (a) Anteroposterior supine chest radiograph of a patient involved in a motorcycle collision shows a large right tension pneumothorax, a pneumomediastinum, right lung collapse, and a right chest tube. The persistent right pneumothorax despite chest tube drainage should suggest an airway injury. (b) Axial contrast-enhanced CT of the same patient shows abrupt cutoff of the right mainstem bronchus, a large right pneumothorax, and the collapsed right lung falling away posteriorly from the hilum—the "fallen lung" sign.

- CT evaluation for possible bleeding source from intercostal or internal mammary artery
- Rapidly enlarging hemothorax can cause tension.

Pneumomediastinum

- Sources include lung, tracheobronchial tree, esophagus, head/neck, and abdomen/retroperitoneum, but most are spontaneous.
- Chest radiography
  - Lucencies, most often vertically oriented, projecting over mediastinum
  - Gas outlining the pulmonary trunk on frontal view
  - *Continuous diaphragm sign*: Gas between pericardium and diaphragm allowing for interface visualization
  - *V sign of Naclerio*: Gas in the left medial lower mediastinal region, classically associated with esophageal rupture
  - *Continuous left hemidiaphragm sign*: Visualization of the left hemidiaphragm to the anterior chest wall on the lateral view
  - *Double bronchial wall sign*: Gas outlining the tracheal or bronchial wall such that both sides can be seen
- Gas outlining the heart or pericardial space may represent pneumopericardium, which can cause tamponade.

Esophageal Injuries

- May be associated with pneumomediastinum (often localized around the injury) or mediastinitis (stranding, fluid adjacent to esophagus) on CT
- Water-soluble contrast swallow can help to confirm defect
- In blunt trauma, more common in the upper esophagus where the esophagus goes from freely mobile (neck) to fixed (thorax)

Cardiac Injuries

- Hemopericardium is an indirect sign of trauma to heart but is not specific.
- Rarely, contrast extravasation can be identified.
- In penetrating trauma, a trajectory that includes the heart usually requires exploration.

Diaphragm Injuries

- Left-sided injuries more common than right (Fig. 22.4)
- Chest radiography: Abdominal viscera above expected location of diaphragm, elevated hemidiaphragm, or nasogastric tube terminating above diaphragm
- CT signs of blunt diaphragm injury: *Fallen organ sign* (abdominal organs touching posterior body wall), diaphragmatic discontinuity, *collar sign* (waist-like constriction of herniated organs)
- Increased suspicion with injuries detected on both sides of diaphragm
- In penetrating injury, wound trajectory is key because actual defect may be difficult to visualize.
- Multiplanar reconstructions are key in the evaluation of diaphragmatic injuries on CT.

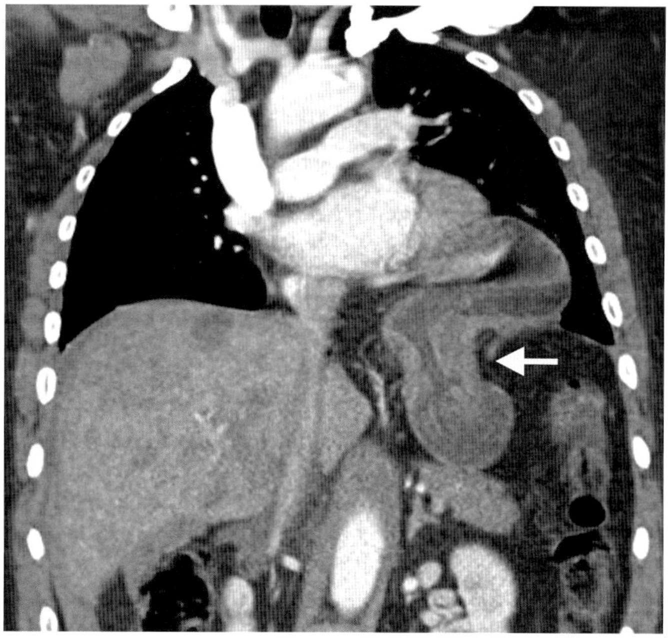

Figure 22.4. Diaphragm injury. Coronal contrast-enhanced CT of a patient involved in a high-speed motor vehicle collision demonstrates intrathoracic extension of abdominal fat and stomach and a large left hemidiaphragm defect, consistent with blunt diaphragmatic injury. The arrow marks the edge of the ruptured diaphragm. Coronal reconstructions can be very helpful in assessment of the integrity of the diaphragm in the setting of trauma.

Chest Wall Injuries

- Lung herniation (Fig. 22.5)
  - Pleural covered portion of lung extends through chest wall defect.
  - CT visualization of lung extending outside its expected contour, often at sites of rib fractures.
- Rib fractures
  - Injuries to ribs 1–3 require extreme force and can be associated with vascular and brachial plexus injuries.
  - Lower rib injuries are associated with liver and spleen injuries.
  - May be detected on radiography, but CT is superior for determination of exact number and location of rib fractures.
  - Flail chest can occur when there are two or more fractures in three or more contiguous ribs; clinical correlation of paradoxical motion with breathing is required to make diagnosis.
- Scapular fractures
  - Require large force and almost always associated with other injuries, including pneumothorax and hemothorax.
  - Can be difficult to detect on chest radiographs.
  - Dedicated inspection on CT is important because it is easy to overlook scapular fractures.
- Clavicle injuries
  - Clavicle fractures are often readily detectable on chest radiographs, but sternoclavicular dislocation can be more difficult to identify.

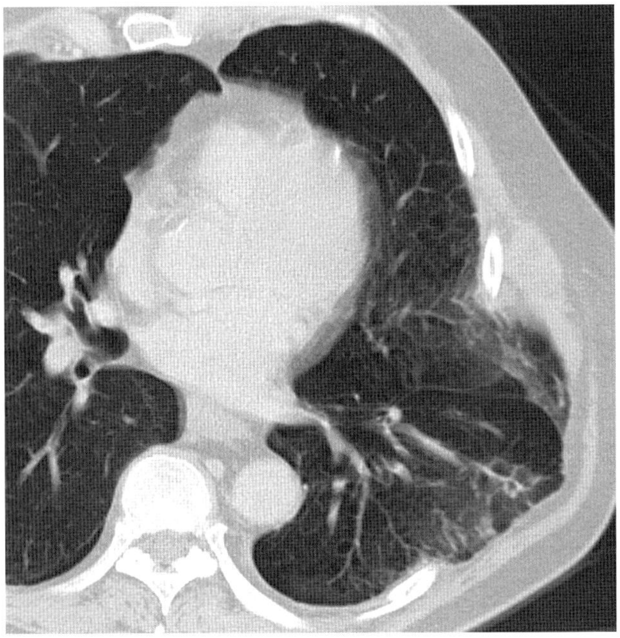

Figure 22.5. Lung herniation. Unenhanced CT of a patient status post a fall demonstrates extension of the lung outside the expected contour of the thorax in a patient with multiple rib fractures, consistent with lung herniation.

  - Most fractures demonstrate upward displacement of distal fragment.
  - Sternoclavicular dislocations may be suspected clinically and are best characterized by CT (Fig. 22.6).
  - Posterior sternoclavicular dislocations place blood vessels, trachea, and esophagus at risk—contrast is needed to fully characterize the extent of injuries.
- Sternal fractures
  - Can occur in any trauma with blunt force to chest—does not need to be high energy.
  - Often very difficult to detect on axial CT images: Sagittal reconstructions of the sternum are essential.
  - May be cause and explanation for an anterior mediastinal hematoma.
- Chest wall hematoma
  - Abnormal soft tissue in subcutaneous tissues or chest wall muscles, may exhibit intermediate to high attenuation on CT and/or hematocrit levels
  - CT assessment for active arterial extravasation that can result in rapidly enlarging hematoma and may require embolization
  - Extrapleural hematomas often associated with rib fracture and manifest as convex chest wall mass on radiography or CT

Clinical Issues

- Contusions should begin to clear 24–48 hours after injury and clear in 3–10 days: Abnormalities that develop after 24 hours or do not clear should raise suspicion for other processes.
- Rarely, lacerations require resection due to recurrent infections.
- Persistent pneumothorax after chest tube placement should suggest airway injury.
- Even when a pneumothorax is small, chest tube placement may be used due to the potential for a rapid increase in size in the setting of mechanical ventilation.
- In blunt trauma, subcutaneous gas on imaging should raise concern for pneumothorax, especially with no open wounds.
- A large hemothorax or rapid rate of drainage after thoracostomy tube drainage may prompt surgical intervention.
- Most cases of pneumomediastinum in trauma are from a Macklin effect, in which alveolar rupture results in gas tracking to the mediastinum.
- Blunt cardiac injury is usually suspected based on electrocardiogram and elevated cardiac enzymes. Patients may present with decreased function and/or pulmonary edema.
- Esophageal injuries are rare but are more common in penetrating trauma than in blunt trauma.
- Rib fractures are a common source of chest pain after trauma and should prompt assessment for pneumothorax or hemothorax.

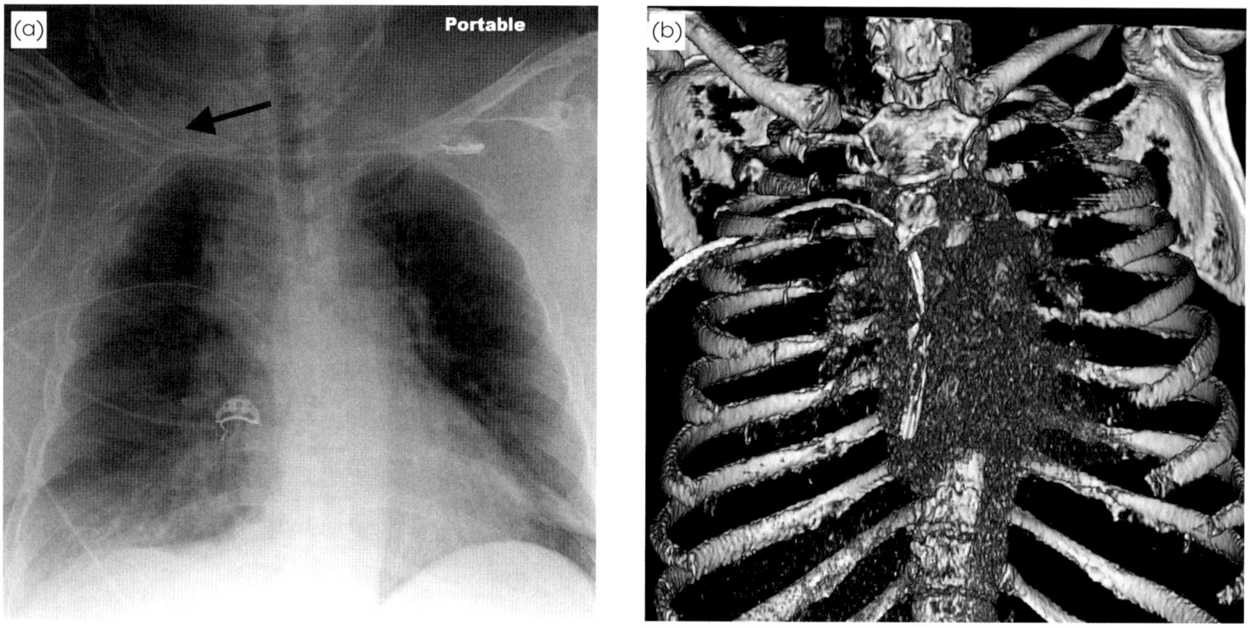

Figure 22.6. Sternoclavicular dislocation. (a) Portable chest radiograph of a patient involved in a motor vehicle collision shows asymmetric lateral and superior positioning of the right clavicular head (arrow), suspicious for sternoclavicular dislocation. Associated right paratracheal widening was worrisome for hematoma related to the injury. (b) Volume-rendered CT of the same patient confirms the superior and lateral dislocation of the right clavicular head. Some thoracic skeletal injuries may be difficult to recognize clinically, and careful imaging evaluation is required for diagnosis.

Key Points

- Chest radiographs are often the first imaging study performed and are useful in evaluating for immediately life-threatening abnormalities.
- CT is the imaging study of choice for comprehensive assessment of thoracic injuries.
- A systematic search pattern is important in trauma cases because multiple injuries often coexist in the same patient, some of which may be subtle or overlooked.
- Imaging findings of pulmonary contusion should be present in the first 24 hours after injury and should clear over 3–10 days: If this time course does not occur, suspect an additional superimposed process.
- Pneumothorax and hemothorax should be evaluated for tension physiology.
- Pneumomediastinum can be due to airway or esophageal injury, but it is more commonly due to the Macklin effect.
- Cardiac injuries are rare, but hemopericardium or a wound tract that involves the heart should raise suspicion.
- Multiplanar reconstructions are essential in the interpretation of CT examinations in trauma because they can show the diaphragm, wound trajectories, and bony injuries to advantage.
- Bony chest wall injuries can be associated with organ and vascular injuries due to proximity to adjacent structures.

Suggested Reading

Constantino M, Gosselin MV, Primack SL. The ABC's of thoracic trauma imaging. *Semin Roentgenol.* 2006;41(3):209–225.

Kaewlai R, Avery LL, Asrani AV, Novelline RA. Multidetector CT of blunt thoracic trauma. *RadioGraphics.* 2008;28: 1555–1570.

Sangster GP, Gonzalez-Beicos A, Carbo AI, et al. Blunt traumatic injuries of the lung parenchyma, pleura, thoracic wall, and intrathoracic airways: Multidetector computer tomography imaging findings. *Emerg Radiol.* 2007;14:297–310.

CHAPTER 23

Nontraumatic Thoracic Aorta

Constantine Raptis

Definition

The term acute aortic syndrome (AAS) was developed to describe nontraumatic aortic causes of chest pain. Aortic dissection (AD), intramural hematoma (IMH), and penetrating atherosclerotic ulcer (PAU) affect the aortic media and comprise the acute aortic syndromes. Although not typically included in the acute aortic syndromes, thoracic aortic aneurysms are important conditions that may manifest acutely due to rupture, instability, or infection. Additional nontraumatic diseases of the aorta, including aortic thrombus, aortic fistula, and vasculitis, are also discussed because they can be discovered on aortic imaging studies in patients with chest pain.

AD is caused by an intimal defect that allows luminal blood to access the aortic media. Blood then propagates proximally and distally, creating a false lumen that is separated from the true lumen by an intimomedial flap. In an IMH, blood (believed to be from rupture of the vast vasorum) is primarily located within the media. Connection with the lumen is usually absent (unlike with AD). In a PAU, an atherosclerotic plaque weakens the intima so that an ulcer penetrates through the intima into the media.

Clinical Features

Patients with AAS typically report sudden onset of chest or back pain in the setting of hypertension. The chest pain is often described as "tearing" and may radiate to the jaw, back, or abdomen. Chest pain, although common in patients with acute aortic pathology, is not always present, may not be severe, and may not be constant. Focal neurologic signs may occur when perfusion to the brain is compromised. There may be decreased blood pressure or pulselessness if upper extremity perfusion is compromised. If a dissection involves the aortic root, acute aortic insufficiency can occur, and it may manifest with a diastolic murmur at the cardiac apex.

Conditions associated with cystic medial necrosis (Marfan syndrome and bicuspid aortopathy) weaken the media and increase risk for AD.

Anatomy and Physiology

The thoracic aorta extends from the aortic valve to the diaphragmatic hiatus. The aortic root is composed of the sinuses of Valsalva and the aortic valve. The sinotubular junction is a waist-like narrowing that separates the aortic root from the tubular ascending aorta. Whereas the majority of the thoracic aorta is extrapericardial, the first 2 or 3 cm is intrapericardial. The descending aorta begins just distal to the takeoff of the left subclavian artery.

The intima, media, and adventitia are the three layers of the aortic wall. The inner two-thirds of the media is composed of muscular fibers oriented perpendicular to the muscular fibers in the outer third. As a result, a natural cleavage plane can develop if blood gains access to this space from an intimal breach.

How to Approach the Image

The first imaging study obtained in patients with suspected aortic pathology is the chest radiograph, which is useful for excluding other causes of chest pain, including pneumothorax and rib fractures. A change in the mediastinal contour from a prior chest radiograph should suggest acute aortic pathology (Fig. 23.1). Although mediastinal widening, displacement of aortic calcium from the aortic periphery, and effacement of mediastinal lines, stripes, and interfaces can be seen, the chest radiograph is often normal and the abnormalities can be subtle.

CT is the imaging study of choice for evaluating suspected AAS. CT protocols typically begin with a noncontrast acquisition that serves to evaluate the aortic wall for high-attenuation blood that can be seen in IMH or unstable aneurysms. Narrow windows (e.g., liver windows (width, 250 HU; center, 30 HU)) optimally display high-attenuation blood products. The noncontrast examination can also be used to identify calcium and surgical material.

The first step in evaluating the contrast-enhanced CT is selecting windows that optimize evaluation of intraluminal pathology. Setting windows for best visualization of the aortic valve is a good starting point. One should look carefully for evidence of an intimomedial flap or mural thickening. The normal fat adjacent to the aorta should be examined for stranding. Multiplanar reconstructions are essential and can display aortic pathology to advantage. To ensure consistency between readers, modalities, and studies of the same modality, all aortic measurements should be obtained in planes orthogonal to its long axis.

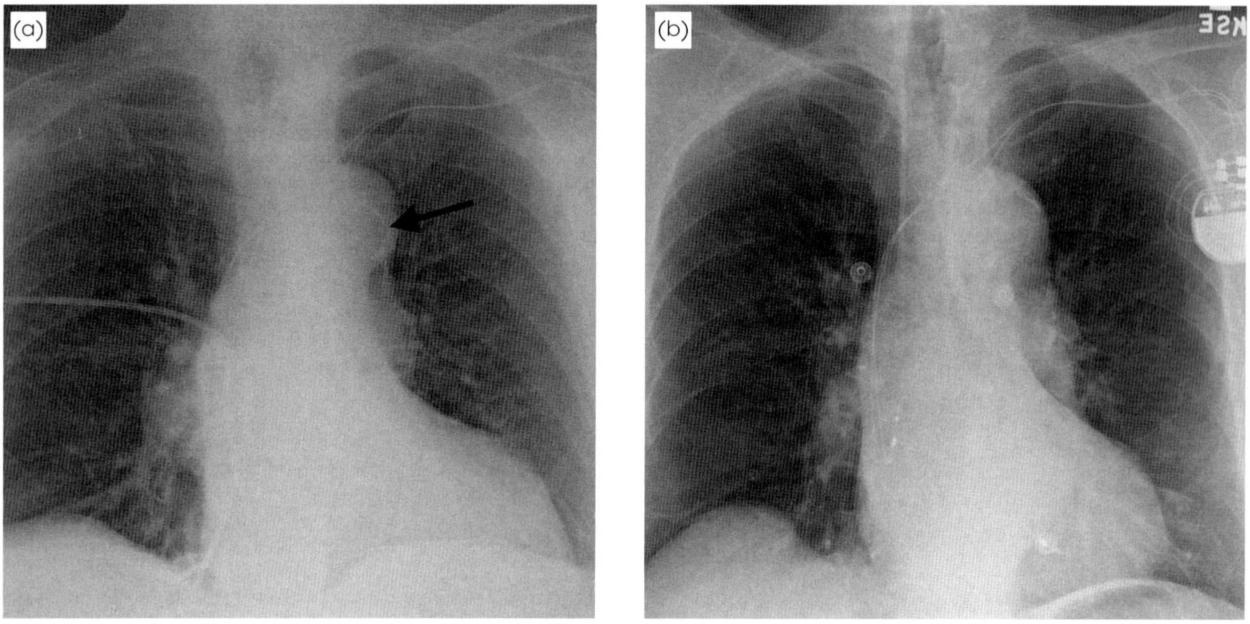

Figure 23.1. Aortic dissection. (a) Anteroposterior (AP) chest radiograph of a 78-year-old man with chest pain shows medial displacement of atherosclerotic calcification at the aortic arch (arrow) suspicious for aortic dissection (confirmed on subsequent chest CT). (b) Posteroanterior chest radiograph of the same patient obtained 1 year earlier shows peripherally located intimal atherosclerotic calcification.

MRI can be used to evaluate stable patients with suspected AAS. From a diagnostic standpoint, CT, MRI, and transesophageal echocardiography are equivalent. Drawbacks to using MRI in the setting of AAS include longer scan times, difficulty accessing an MRI from the emergency department, they are smaller than the others, and the need for screening for pacemakers and other MR-incompatible devices. MRI should be considered in patients with an iodinated contrast allergy, poor intravenous access, and borderline renal function because acute aortic syndromes can be evaluated without contrast.

Double inversion recovery (IR) black blood (BB) images can be used to interrogate the aortic wall, which should be imperceptible. Any smooth mural thickening should be suspicious for blood products. Balanced stead-state free precession (bSSFP) sequences obtained both as stack and CINE sequences are useful in evaluating the aortic wall as well as the lumen for intimomedial flaps. Noncontrast T1-weighted sequences can be used to look for blood products in the mediastinum. Although not required to diagnose the causes of AAS, contrast-enhanced MRA sequences can be used to shorten the overall exam time and better characterize abnormalities.

What Not to Miss

When AAS is encountered on imaging, one must be careful not to miss the findings that would make the lesion a surgical lesion. These mostly include any signs of rupture or instability or involvement of the ascending aorta. To minimize overlooking the former, careful analysis for mediastinal stranding should be performed. Comparison with any prior studies for change is also an important finding. Close comparison between the noncontrast and post-contrast images can be helpful to evaluate ascending aortic involvement in an IMH.

Imaging Findings

Aortic Dissection

Imaging Findings

- Visualization of intimal flap separating true and false lumens on contrast-enhanced CT
- Signs of rupture: Wall contour irregularity, mediastinal hematoma, hemothorax, or contrast extravasation
- Most patients with acute aortic syndrome have sympathetic left pleural effusion.
- Look for the intimomedial flap and any holes in the flap (fenestrations).

Classification

- Stanford type A: Ascending ± descending aortic involvement
- Stanford type B: Descending aortic involvement only
- Some dissections extend only into the distal arch and are often described as “type B with arch extension.”

Complications

- Dissection extension into pericardial sac can result in hemopericardium (high-attenuation fluid) and tamponade (Fig. 23.2).

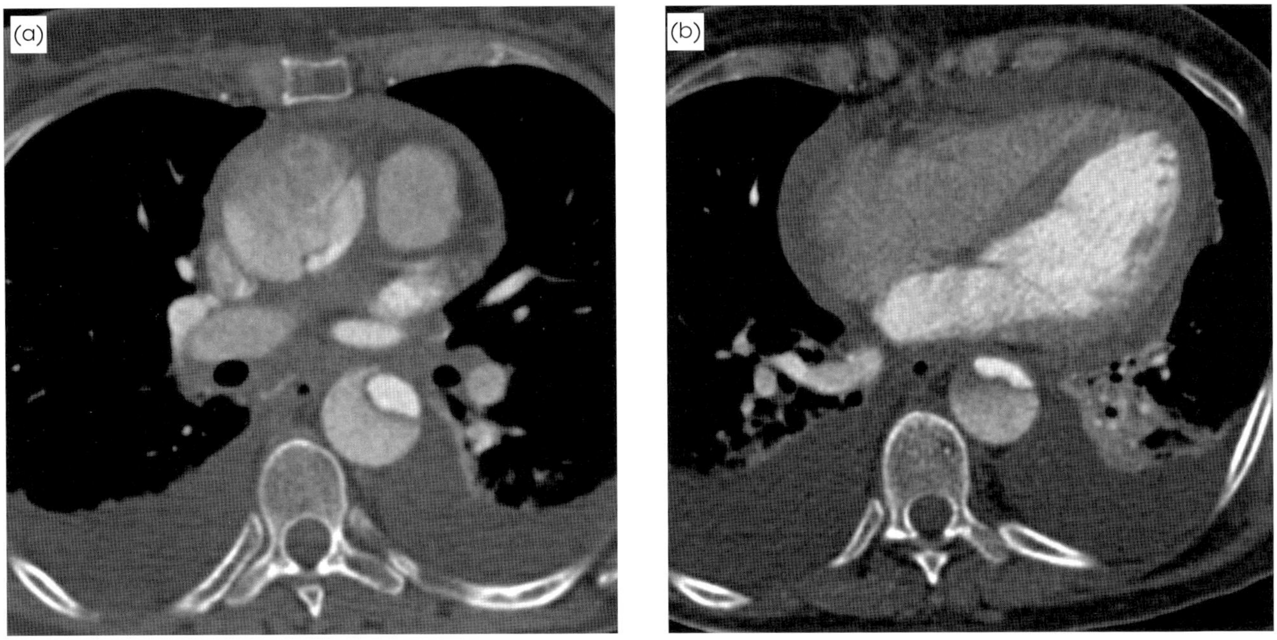

Figure 23.2. Aortic dissection with cardiac tamponade. (a) Axial contrast-enhanced CT of a 54-year-old man with chest pain shows a Stanford type A aortic dissection with medial displacement of the intimal flap by the large false lumen. (b) Axial contrast-enhanced chest CT of the same patient shows high-attenuation pericardial fluid consistent with hemopericardium. Note indentation of the anterior right ventricular wall consistent with tamponade physiology.

- Signs of ischemia in organs and bowel may be present.
  - Dynamic ischemia: Flap covers ostium of branch artery.
  - Static ischemia: Flap extends into ostium of branch artery.

Intramural Hematoma

Imaging Findings

- High-attenuation aortic wall thickening on noncontrast CT (Fig. 23.3)
- On MR, crescentic thickening of aortic wall with variable signal intensity depending on age; best sequences to evaluate for IMH on MR are double IR BB and bSSFP
- Typically does not enhance (no intimal defect)
- Contrast blush within the IMH
  - If on luminal side, may be due to an ulcer
  - If on wall side, likely due to retrograde branch artery flow (e.g., intercostal)
- Size of aorta important (>5 cm is negative prognostic indicator)

Classification

- Use of Stanford classification for categorization

Complications

- Include rupture and progression to AD but most resolve

Penetrating Atherosclerotic Ulcer

Imaging Findings

- Contrast extension into aortic wall with either eccentric outpouching or local caliber increase (Fig. 23.4)
- Distinction between ulcerating plaque and PAU: Ulcerating plaque not associated with contrast outpouching or localized lumenal expansion
- Chronic PAU common, and determination of acuity based on whether patient is symptomatic

Classification

- No classification system, but the report should include the location of the PAU and the size of the defect.

Complications

- Concomitant IMH is a negative prognostic indicator that the PAU may be unstable and rupture.
- Periaortic tissue stranding or hematoma or contrast extravasation indicate rupture.

Thoracic Aortic Aneurysm

Imaging Findings

- Thoracic aortic aneurysm is defined as enlargement of the aorta (>4 cm) or failure of aortic tapering.
- All size measurements need to be obtained orthogonal to the long axis of the aorta—requires the use of multiplanar reformatted images.
- Comparison with prior exams is helpful; interval increase in size is concerning (>0.5–1 cm during 1 year often an indication for repair).

Classification

- The relationship of the aneurysm to branch vessels should be described because this can affect the type of repair used.
- Assessment of shape is important.

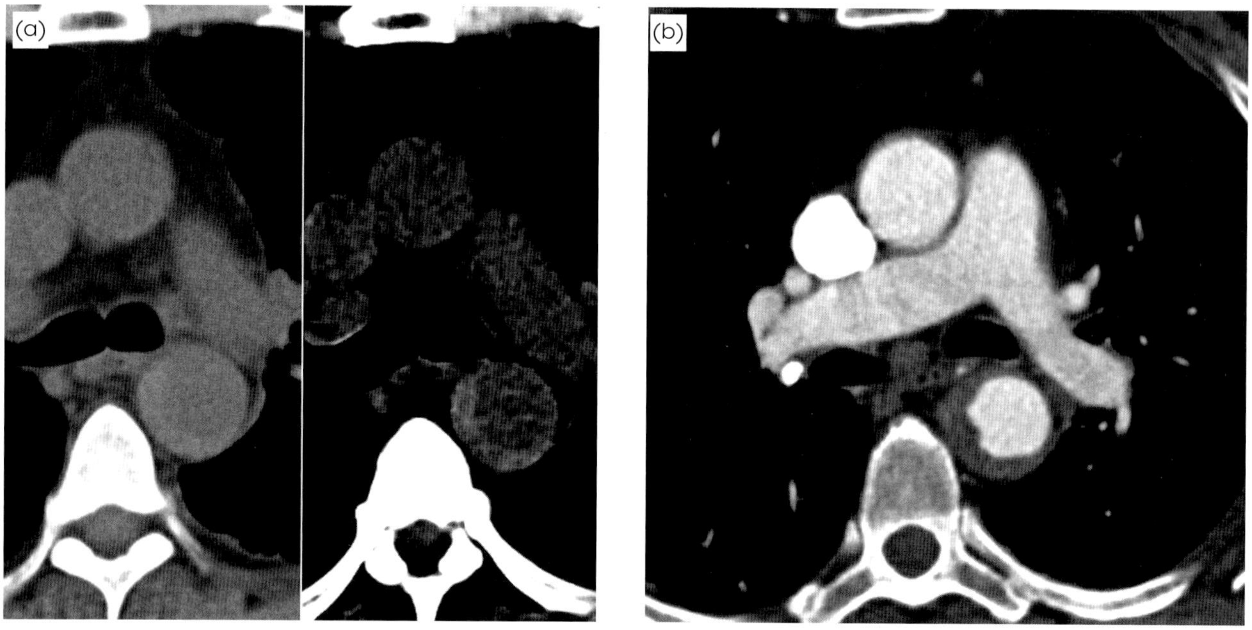

Figure 23.3. Intramural hematoma. (a) Composite image with unenhanced chest CT of 67-year-old man with chest pain and leg weakness shows crescenteric high attenuation involving the posteromedial wall of the descending aorta (left), concerning for intramural hematoma. The high attenuation is easier to see on a narrower window (right). (b) Contrast-enhanced chest CT of the same patient shows aortic wall thickening that could be mistaken for plaque because it is difficult to appreciate the mural increased attenuation.

- Fusiform aneurysms (cylindrical enlargement) are more likely due to atherosclerosis or cystic medial necrosis.
- Saccular aneurysms (or focal outpouchings) are often pseudoaneurysms due to infection, trauma, or a postoperative complication.

Complications

- The major risk is rupture. The signs of instability include high attenuation within the wall, tangential calcium, irregular shape, periaortic stranding, hemothorax, and contrast extravasation.

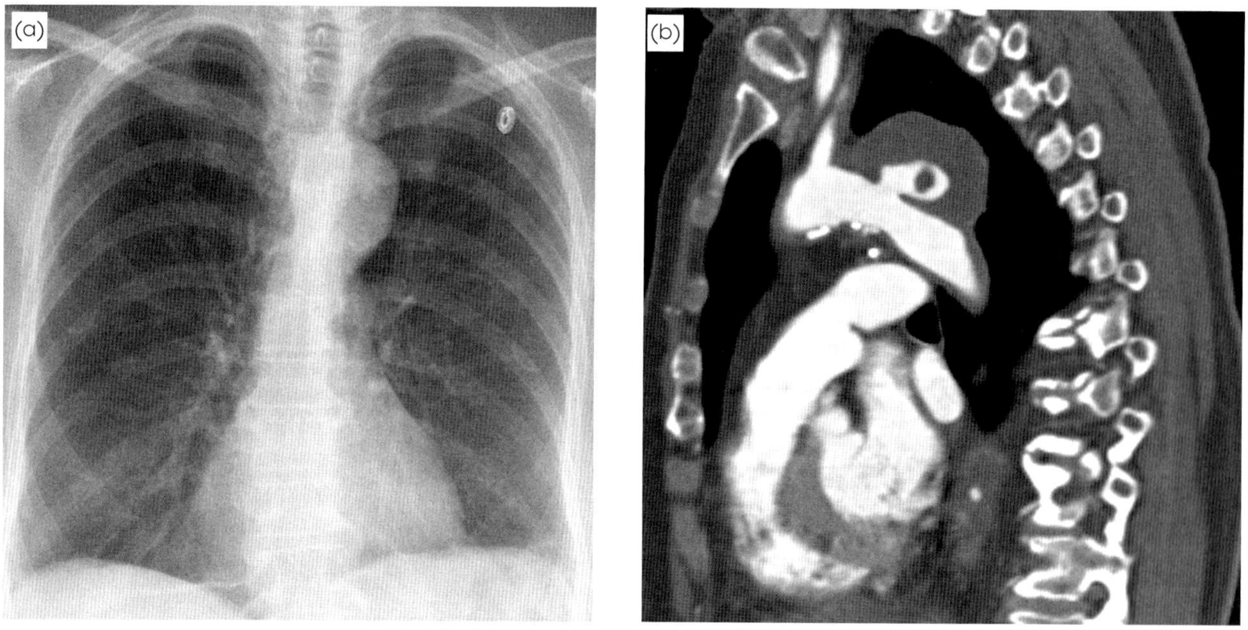

Figure 23.4. Penetrating atherosclerotic ulcer. (a) AP chest radiograph of a 75-year-old woman with chest pain shows aortic arch enlargement, new from prior studies (not shown). (b) Sagittal contrast-enhanced chest CT of the same patient shows focal contrast extension outside the aortic lumen with surrounding thrombus and local expansion of the aorta consistent with penetrating atherosclerotic ulcer. The patient was treated with endovascular stenting.

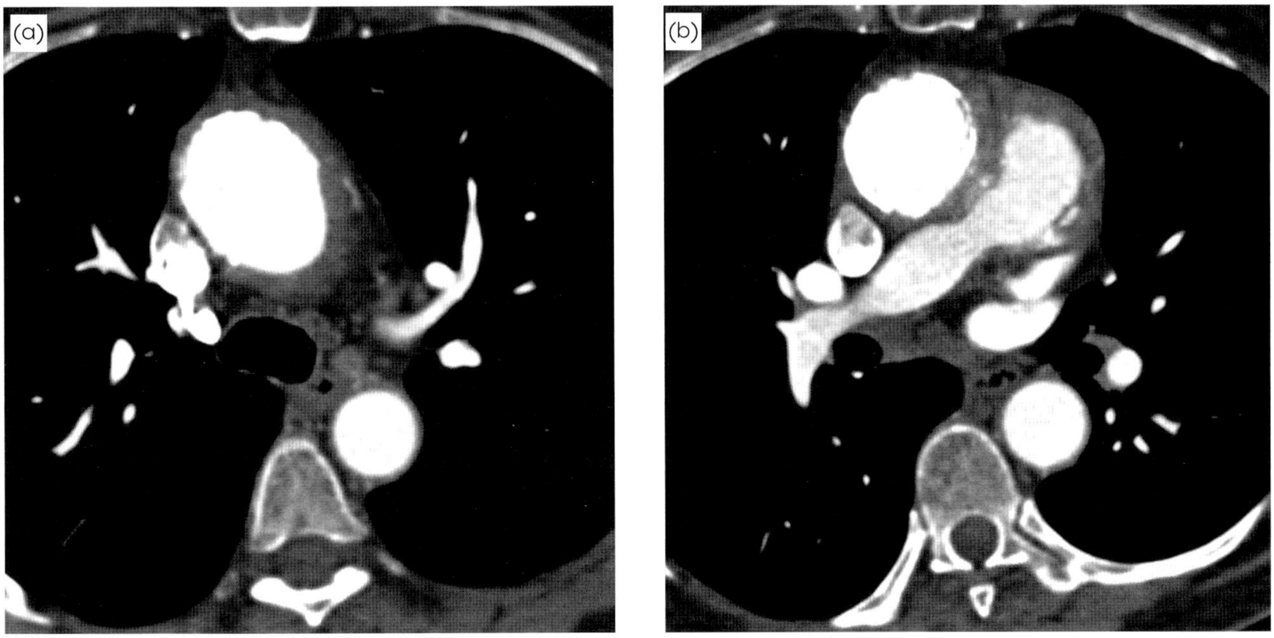

Figure 23.5. Takayasu arteritis. (a, b) Contrast-enhanced chest CT of a 65-year-old woman with chest pain shows mural thickening of the ascending aorta (a) and the pulmonary trunk (b). Note focal narrowing of the proximal right pulmonary artery. Although aortic mural thickening may suggest intramural hematoma, the pulmonary artery involvement is consistent with Takayasu arteritis.

Aortic Fistula

- Fistula can be defined as a connection between the aorta and another vessel or hollow viscus (bowel or airway).
- Findings are often very subtle on imaging or exam may be normal—clinical history of bleeding is important.
- Suspect when aorta touches another structure, particularly if there is a contour abnormality.
- Gas in the aortic lumen indicates communication with gastrointestinal tract or airway.
- Inflammation with stranding and phlegmon may occur at site of the aortic fistula.
- Contrast extravasation rarely seen because bleeding is typically intermittent.

Aortic thrombus

- Filling defect within the aortic lumen that may arise at a site of intimal irregularity (usually near the ductus).
- Evaluate for embolic phenomena in distal organs.

Vasculitis

- Typical finding is circumferential wall thickening of the aorta and branch vessels (Fig. 23.5).
- Paraaortic lymphadenopathy is more typical of vasculitis than IMH.
- Pulmonary artery involvement occurs in 50% of patients and should strongly suggest vasculitis.
- May have associated stenosis and dilatation in aorta and branch vessels.
- MRI can be used to evaluate for contrast enhancement of the wall—a sign of ongoing inflammation.

Clinical Issues

- Acute aortic syndromes present with chest pain radiating toward the back and include dissection, IMH, and PAU.
- When dissection and IMH involve the ascending aorta, they may become surgical lesions because of high risk of acute aortic valve regurgitation and myocardial infarction.
- Percutaneous treatments may be needed for end-organ ischemia from a dissection. These include fenestration for dynamic ischemia and stenting for static ischemia.
- Saccular aneurysms tend to be more unstable than fusiform aneurysms.
- Aortic fistulae are often challenging on imaging and tend to require endoscopy or bronchoscopy to confirm their presence.

Key Points

- The acute aortic syndrome includes aortic dissection, intramural hematoma, and penetrating atherosclerotic ulcer.
- Interpretation of imaging exams in patients with acute aortic syndrome requires assessment of the location and extent of pathology in addition to any signs of impending or active rupture.

- Assessment of thoracic aortic aneurysms requires measuring the aorta in planes orthogonal to its long axis.
- Other uncommon diagnoses, including aortic fistula, aortic thrombus, and vasculitis, can be encountered on exams evaluating for acute aortic syndrome.

Suggested Reading

Bhalla S, West CO. CT of nontraumatic thoracic aortic emergencies. *Semin Ultrasound CT MR*. 2005;26(5):281–304.

Litmanovich D, Bankier AA, Cantin L, et al. CT and MRI in diseases of the aorta. *AJR Am J Roentgenol*. 2009;193:928–940.

Yoo SM, Lee HY, White CS. MDCT evaluation of acute aortic syndrome. *Radiol Clin North Am*. 2010;48:67–83.

CHAPTER 24

Pulmonary Embolic Disease

Constantine Raptis

Definition

Pulmonary emboli (PE) occur when material from a distant site travels to the lungs and becomes lodged in the pulmonary arteries. The most common source arises in peripheral veins from an antecedent condition (long periods of immobility, hypercoagulability, etc.). Chronic PE represents cytokine-mediated scarring that may occur even after just one episode of acute PE. Septic emboli result from an infected source, usually thrombophlebitis or infected valve or device. This scarring increases pulmonary vascular resistance and results in pulmonary hypertension. Other material can also travel to the lungs, including fat emboli post-trauma; amniotic fluid post-delivery; tumor; gas, and iatrogenic or foreign material.

Clinical Features

Clinical diagnosis of acute PE from thromboembolic disease is difficult because patients with PE can present with a wide range of nonspecific symptoms (most commonly chest pain and dyspnea) or may be asymptomatic. Symptoms tend to overlap other life-threatening diseases, including myocardial infarction, pneumonia, and acute aortic syndrome. Consequently, clinicians often have a low threshold for using imaging to make this diagnosis. Clinical likelihood scores (e.g., Wells criteria) are often used to help stratify patients before imaging, but these have been modestly successful.

Anatomy and Physiology

The pulmonary arteries serve as the conduit of blood from the right ventricle to the lungs and are the main path of oxygenation of the circulatory system. The pulmonary trunk originates from the right ventricular outflow tract at the pulmonic valve and bifurcates into a right pulmonary artery that travels slightly posterior and inferior to the right mainstem bronchus and a left pulmonary artery that travels over the left mainstem bronchus. The pulmonary arteries divide into lobar, segmental, and subsegmental arteries, ultimately reaching a microscopic capillary level. The lungs function as a "filter" that prevents emboli from gaining access to the left heart and systemic circulation.

PE can lodge anywhere in the pulmonary arterial tree depending on the size of the embolus. Distal emboli likely produce chest pain by inciting an inflammatory response adjacent to the parietal pleura. Gas exchange distal to emboli may be abnormal due to alveolar dead space in combination with surfactant dysfunction, resulting atelectasis, and functional intrapulmonary shunting. The distal lung can hemorrhage, and in approximately 10% of patients an infarct will occur (Fig. 24.1). Larger central emboli can be devastating, impeding right ventricular outflow and resulting in acute right heart dysfunction (Fig. 24.2). Hypotension may ensue due to decreased left ventricular preload. Vasoconstriction due to hypoxia, obstruction, and inflammatory mediators may further complicate the situation. Ultimately, pulmonary pressures can exceed the compensatory abilities of the right heart, and right heart failure may occur.

How to Approach the Image

The evaluation of most patients with suspected PE should begin with a chest radiograph. Although there are radiographic signs suggestive of PE, they are not sensitive and are typically subtle. The main purpose of the chest radiograph is to exclude another explanation for the patient's symptoms (e.g., pneumothorax) that may require immediate attention. The chest radiograph can also provide valuable information that may help in choosing between the next two most commonly used imaging modalities for diagnosing PE—CT and ventilation–perfusion (V/Q) scanning.

CT is the imaging modality most commonly used to evaluate for PE. It is widely available, fast, and has excellent diagnostic performance for identifying PE to the level of the subsegmental arteries. CT can often identify alternative explanations for the patient's symptoms. PE protocol CT is performed with the intravenous contrast bolus timed to the pulmonary arteries.

What Not to Miss

Evaluation of the pulmonary arterial tree must be performed with an appropriate window setting, usually one that allows visualization of the pulmonic valve. Each arterial branch must be evaluated. A careful evaluation of the pulmonary arteries also prevents misdiagnosing a low-attenuation flow artifact in a pulmonary vein as a PE. The

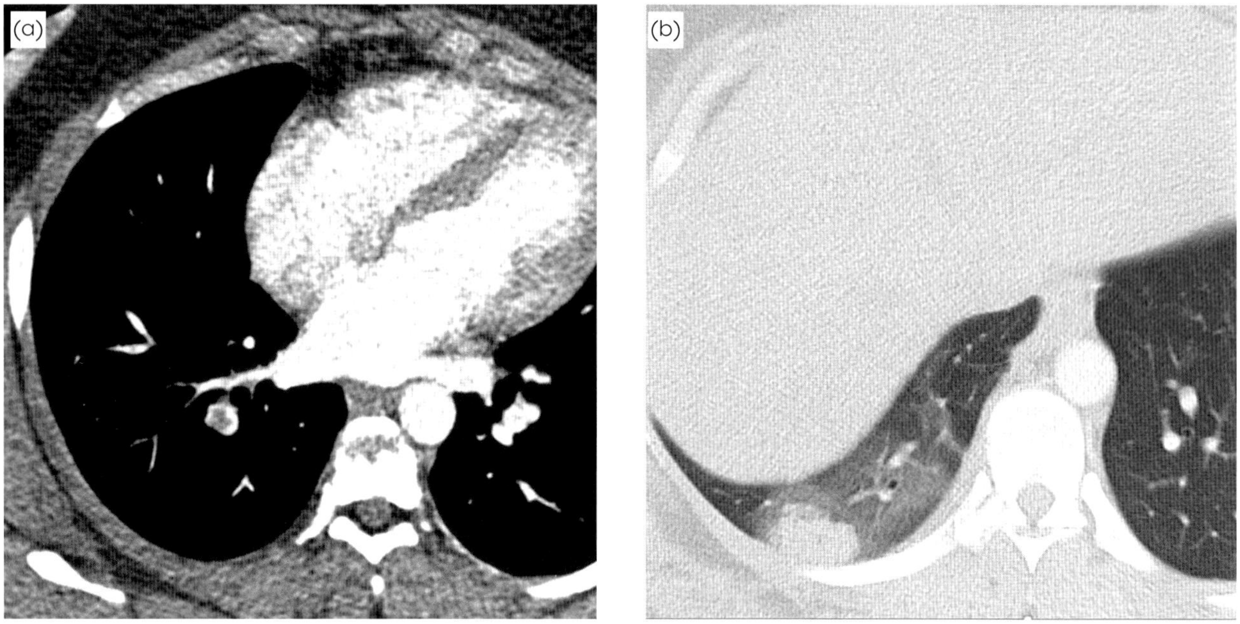

Figure 24.1. Pulmonary embolism and infarct. (a) Axial contrast-enhanced CT demonstrates a filling defect in the right lower lobe arterial tree. (b) Axial contrast-enhanced CT (lung window) of the same patient shows a nodular consolidation with surrounding ground-glass opacity in the right lower lobe consistent with an infarct.

heart should be evaluated with special attention to signs of right heart strain in patients with PE. The lungs are then examined for pulmonary infarcts. Assessment of the lungs in patients without PE may provide an alternative explanation for the patient's symptoms (Fig. 24.3). Septic emboli will usually present with no discernible intraluminal filling defects within the pulmonary arteries. The diagnosis (as in this case) will rest on the parenchymal findings on the lung windows. Septic emboli are a good reminder that not all embolic disease can be seen as filling defects in the pulmonary arteries.

The examination should conclude by completing the standard search pattern including an assessment of the aorta, airways, mediastinum, upper abdomen, and bones.

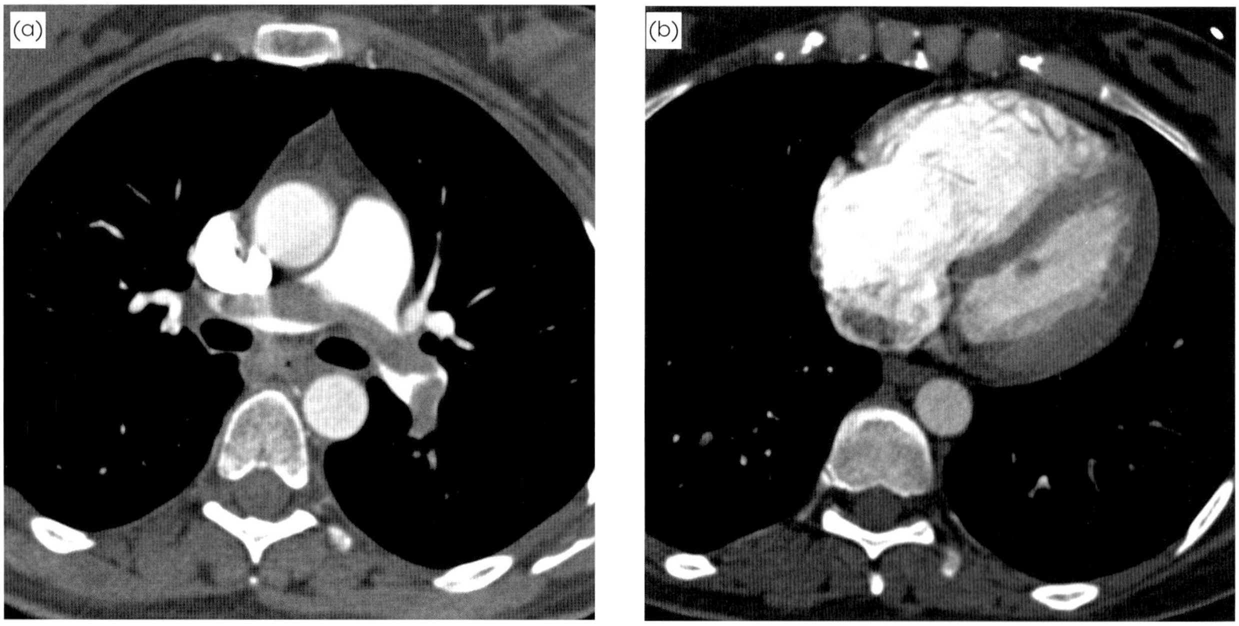

Figure 24.2. Pulmonary embolism with right heart strain. (a) Axial contrast-enhanced CT of a 33-year-old woman with chest pain shows central pulmonary emboli with saddle distribution. (b) Contrast-enhanced CT of the same patient shows enlargement of the right ventricle and straightening of the interventricular septum, concerning for right heart strain, later confirmed with echocardiography. This finding may prompt admission to an intensive care unit.

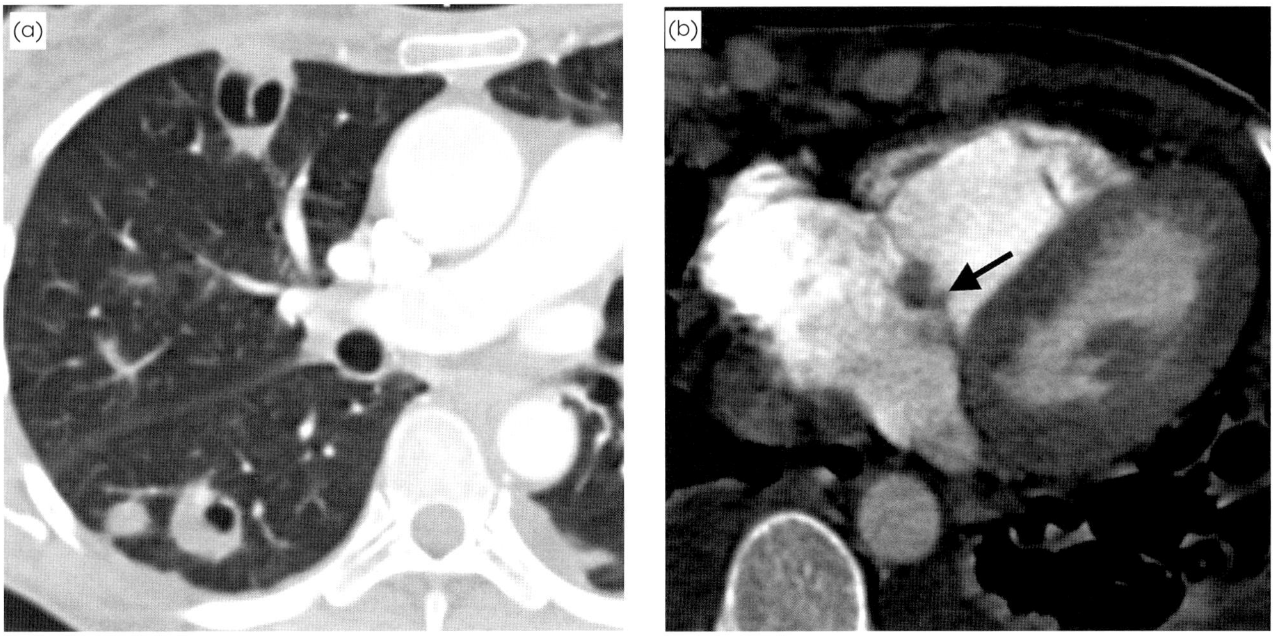

Figure 24.3. Septic emboli. (a) Axial contrast-enhanced CT of a septic patient with a history of intravenous drug use demonstrates multifocal peripheral cavitary nodules consistent with septic emboli. (b) Contrast-enhanced CT of the same patient shows low-attenuating thickening (arrow) of the tricuspid valve concerning for vegetations, which were confirmed on echocardiography.

Differential Diagnosis

- Respiratory motion: Breathing motion can produce volume averaging between the pulmonary arterial tree and the adjacent lung, simulating a filling defect; it is important to review the lung windows for areas of respiratory motion.
- Flow artifacts: Flow artifacts can simulate filling defects, particularly in the lower lobes; they typically exhibit ill-defined margins and are not as hypoattenuating as pulmonary emboli. It may be helpful to better characterize the margins of a flow artifact on coronal reconstructions.
- Streak artifact: Beam hardening streak artifact from dense contrast in the superior vena cava may simulate a filling defect but can be identified due to its non-anatomic nature.
- Transient interruption of the contrast bolus (Fig. 24.4): In some patients (usually younger, well-hydrated patients), during a deep inspiration, unopacified blood from the inferior vena cava is pushed into the right heart and pulmonary arterial tree, displacing the opacified blood from the superior vena cava. This artifact can be readily identified when there is dense contrast in the superior vena cava and aorta but decreased opacification of the right heart and pulmonary arterial tree. This artifact can be mitigated by repeating the exam and instructing the patient to suspend respiration rather than taking a deep breath in.
- Mucous-filled bronchus: Mucous-filled bronchi can appear as tubular low-attenuating structures that may resemble pulmonary emboli; these can be distinguished by their bronchial location on lung windows.
- Adjacent lymph nodes or masses: Adjacent lymph nodes or masses can lead to artifactual filling defects, particularly when there is motion leading to volume averaging. It is important to recognize that these artifactual filling defects will be eccentric and not central. Coronal reconstructions can be helpful in identifying a lymph node simulating a pulmonary embolus.
- Bronchial inflow artifact: Inflow from bronchial arteries can produce ill-defined areas of low attenuation within the pulmonary arterial tree; this can be recognized due to their ill-defined appearance.
- Malignant emboli: In cases in which there is a question of whether thrombus is bland or malignant, MRI is an excellent problem-solving tool given its superior contrast resolution and ability to do multiphase imaging with subtraction.
- Pulmonary venous flow: Flow artifacts in a pulmonary vein will occasionally stand out and have the potential to be confused for PE. The key is to recognize that the tubular structure is not an artery. The lung windows can be helpful because a pulmonary artery almost always has an accompanying bronchus.

Imaging Findings

Pulmonary Thromboembolic Disease

- Central or occlusive filling defect within pulmonary artery (vessel "cut off").

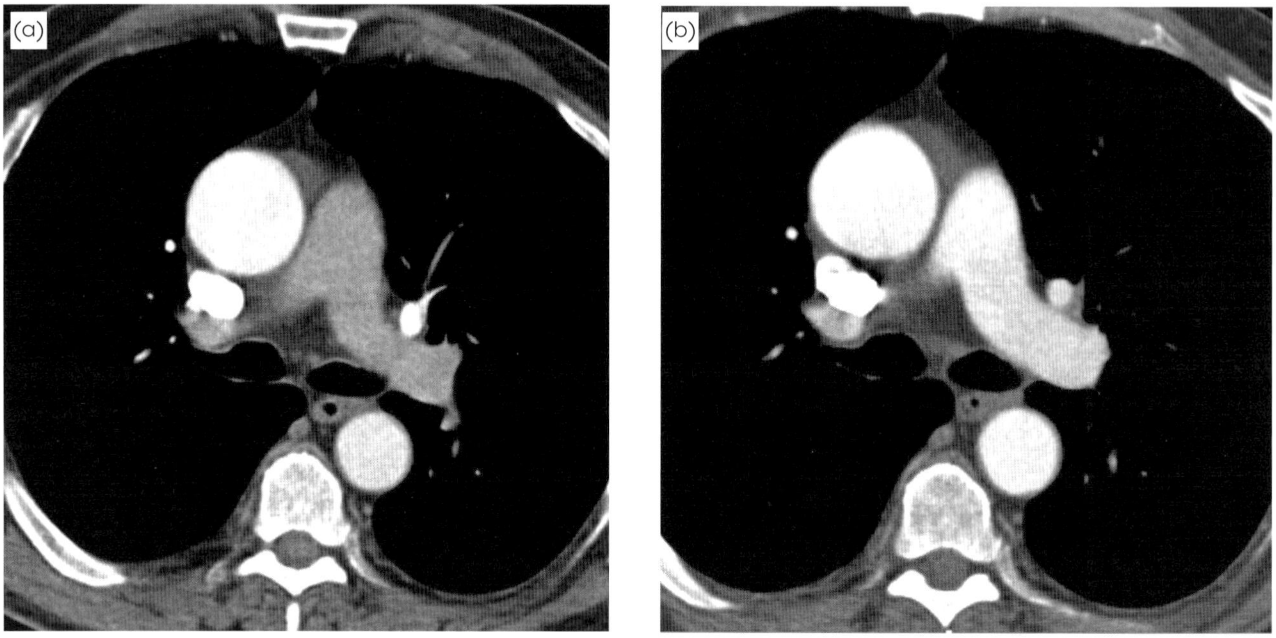

Figure 24.4. Pitfalls in pulmonary emboli imaging. (a) Contrast-enhanced PE protocol CT timed using bolus tracking software shows low attenuation in the pulmonary arteries with good opacification of the superior vena cava and aorta consistent with transient interruption of the contrast column. (b) Repeat contrast-enhanced PE protocol CT performed in exhalation shows improved enhancement of the central pulmonary arteries.

- Contrast around the embolus produces "rim" or "tram-track" sign.
- Acute PE often expand the vessel.
- It should be seen on three contiguous axial slices; if not, it is likely artifactual secondary to flow.
- Pulmonary infarcts: Peripheral nonenhancing consolidations (may rarely cavitate with time and mimic pneumonia).
- May be associated with pulmonary hemorrhage, focal oligemia, atelectasis, and small effusions.
- May cause right heart strain characterized by right heart enlargement, leftward bowing of the interventricular septum, and reflux of contrast into the inferior vena cava and/or coronary sinus; suspicion of right heart strain needs to be reported because it can be a harbinger of impending circulatory collapse.

Chronic Thromboembolic Disease

- Eccentric filling defects, beading of the pulmonary arteries, thread-like arteries, vascular webs, and vascular cutoffs
- Associated imaging findings: Central pulmonary artery enlargement, right heart hypertrophy, mosaic attenuation without air trapping (small vessel disease), and enlarged bronchial arteries

Septic Emboli

- Embolic burden is low, and septic emboli are very rarely seen within the pulmonary arterial tree.
- Most common imaging finding is peripheral cavitary opacities.
- Peripheral opacities may exhibit surrounding ground-glass opacity, producing a "dirty infarct" appearance.

Fat and Amniotic Fluid Emboli

- As with septic emboli, the embolized material is almost never seen within the arterial tree.
- Most common findings are ground-glass opacities associated with terminal arterioles ("vascular tree-in-bud") in conjunction with more confluent ground-glass and consolidation elsewhere.

Tumor Emboli

- Enhancing filling defects within the pulmonary arterial tree are indicative of macroscopic tumor emboli.
- Microscopic tumor emboli are typically not seen as filling defects in the arterial tree but, rather, as beading of the distal arterioles (often easier to detect on lung windows) producing a vascular tree-in-bud appearance. One clue will be the presence of right heart enlargement from the increased vascular resistance.
- Microscopic tumor emboli may be associated with findings of lymphangitic carcinomatosis as well as lymphadenopathy and pleural effusions.

Iatrogenic Emboli

- Embolized liquid and semisolid medications, including methlymethacrylate, manifest with dense filling defect in the pulmonary arterial tree and can be associated with an infarct (uncommon).

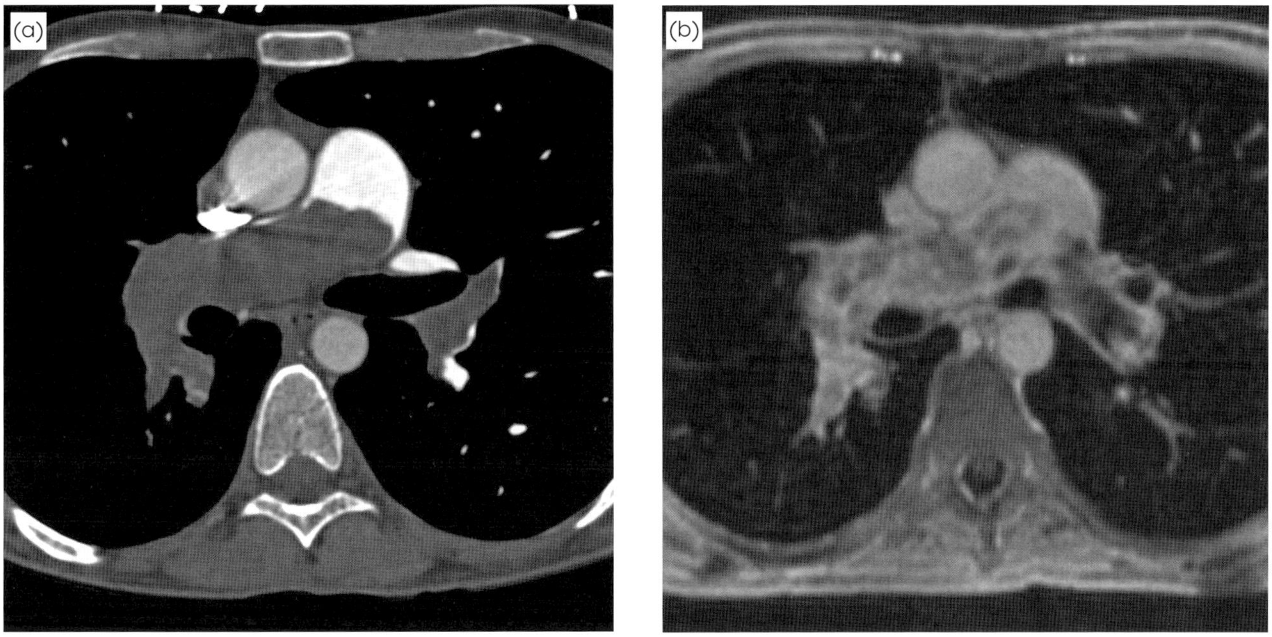

Figure 24.5. Pulmonary artery sarcoma. (a) Contrast-enhanced CT shows extensive expansile filling defects throughout the central pulmonary arterial tree. The filling defects are of higher attenuation than expected from bland emboli. There was no right heart strain or cardiac enlargement (not shown). (b) Contrast-enhanced T1-weighted MRI of the same patient shows extensive enhancement of the pulmonary artery filling defects consistent with tumor.

- Catheters may be seen within the arterial tree and are better seen when a bone window is used.

Foreign Material

- Mercury manifests on CT as very dense filling defects with a propensity for the distal arterioles.
- Talc emboli lodge in distal arterioles, resulting in visualization of the distal arterioles in a centrilobular pattern. They can be associated with increased pulmonary vascular resistance and right heart enlargement.

Primary Pulmonary Artery Angiosarcoma

- Can result in extensive filling defects (Fig. 24.5).
- Enhancement allows differentiation from bland emboli (can use MRI to confirm enhancement or increased uptake on FDG-PET if CT equivocal).
- Despite extensive filling defects, may not result in right heart strain or many symptoms clinically.
- Often associated with superimposed bland thrombus.

Clinical Issues

In some patients, CT may not be the best imaging choice. Patients with tenuous renal function or iodinated contrast allergies have relative contraindications to a PE protocol CT. A PE protocol CT carries a substantial radiation dose, and it may not be the best option in younger patients, particularly women in whom limiting radiation dose to breast tissue is desirable. In these patient groups, V/Q scans can be performed to evaluate for PE. Although V/Q scans have a high negative predictive value when read as "normal," a high number of studies are graded as "low" or "intermediate" probability for PE. To limit the number of "low" and "intermediate" probability studies that will require further workup, V/Q scans are typically reserved for patients with normal chest radiographs. To adequately triage patients, the radiologist must become familiar with the type of CT scanners available and techniques for dose reduction. These principles should be weighed against the limitations on performing V/Q scans at the time of request.

Key Points

- CT is the preferred modality for evaluating for PE.
- The most important step in evaluating for pulmonary emboli on CT is carefully tracing the course of the pulmonary arterial tree and accounting for all vessels.
- Acute PE typically manifest as central filling defects or vessels with abrupt cutoffs.
- PE may produce right heart strain, which should be reported promptly because it can portend circulatory collapse.
- Certain emboli may manifest with findings best seen on lung windows (tumor emboli, septic emboli, talc emboli, and fat and amniotic emboli). Examination of the heart for increased right heart size or vegetations may expose the vascular nature of the parenchymal abnormalities.
- Macroscopic tumor emboli may mimic PE. PET or MR may be useful in confirming.
- CT has many potential artifacts that require a high level of awareness to prevent misdiagnosis.

Suggested Reading

Kuriakose J, Patel S. Acute pulmonary embolism. *Radiol Clin North Am.* 2010;48:31–50.

Luetz PG, White CS. Acute pulmonary embolism: Imaging in the emergency department. *Radiol Clin North Am.* 2006;44:259–271.

Wittram C, Maher MM, Yoo AJ, et al. CT angiography of pulmonary embolism: Diagnostic criteria and causes of misdiagnosis. *RadioGraphics.* 2004;24:1219–1238.

Pulmonary Complications of Sickle Cell Anemia

Constantine Raptis

Definition

"Sickle cell disease" describes the spectrum of pathology in patients with abnormal hemoglobin characterized by least one HbS chain and one other abnormal hemoglobin chain. Patients who are homozygous HbSS have "sickle cell anemia," the most common and severe form of the disease, whereas others may have less severe variants, including HbSC and HbS-thal. Patients with sickle cell anemia have abnormally shaped red blood cells due to the presence of the HbS chain, which becomes insoluble, forms aggregates, and polymerizes when it is deoxygenated. In addition to increased hemolysis resulting in anemia, the abnormal red blood cells also have impaired transit through the microvasculature and increased affinity for the vascular wall. These latter set the stage for vaso-occlusive disease throughout the body. The main focus of this chapter is the acute pulmonary complications of sickle cell anemia.

Clinical Features

The hemolytic anemia and vaso-occlusive mechanisms of sickle cell anemia may produce a wide variety of clinical presentations. The most common acute manifestations are vaso-occlusive pain crises and acute chest syndrome. Vaso-occlusive pain crises result from the entrapment of abnormal red blood cells in the microcirculation. A cycle of ischemia and reperfusion drives cellular injury, infarction, and inflammation producing severe pain episodes, most commonly in the long bones, although any organ can be affected.

"Acute chest syndrome" is an acute pulmonary illness in patients with sickle cell anemia who present with a new consolidation in the setting of fever, chest pain, and respiratory symptoms (tachypnea, wheezing, and cough). It is not a disease with a distinct cause but, rather, a clinical entity that may result from several mechanisms. The most common cause is infection by a community-acquired pathogen. Patients with sickle cell disease have altered immune function (including an impaired complement system, functional asplenia, and increased susceptibility to inflammatory triggers) that allows pathogens that might cause only a mild upper respiratory infection in normal individuals to produce an excessive inflammatory response and more severe clinical symptoms.

Fat emboli are another important cause of the acute chest syndrome and are related to vaso-occlusive skeletal events that result in bone marrow infarction, edema, and necrosis. As a result, bone marrow contents, including fat, cells, and bony spicules, are released into the circulation and may embolize to the lungs, resulting in acute pulmonary hypertension, lung inflammation, and hypoxemia. Thus, acute chest syndrome is often preceded by episodes of bone pain. Bronchoscopy may reveal lipid-laden macrophages in affected patients.

A third important mechanism for acute chest syndrome is pulmonary infarction due to vaso-occlusion or in situ thrombosis. Vascular occlusion may be important in all cases of acute chest syndrome given associated regional hypoxia that causes vasoconstriction and increased sickling of red blood cells. Acute chest syndrome is the second most common reason for hospitalization and the most common cause of death in sickle cell anemia.

With increasing age, systemic and pulmonary hypertension may develop. Chronic organ complications include pulmonary fibrosis, renal failure, stroke, splenic infarction, and avascular necrosis of bone. The phenotypes exhibited by patients with sickle cell anemia demonstrate varying penetrance of potential complications.

How to Approach the Image

With the availability of newborn screening programs for sickle cell anemia in most states, the diagnosis is usually known at presentation. However, it is important to recognize the common radiographic manifestations of sickle cell disease in cases in which the history is not known or readily available (Fig. 25.1). These features include the following:

- Dense bones
- Avascular necrosis of the humeral heads
- H-shaped vertebral bodies
- Absent splenic shadow
- Enlarged heart
- Lung parenchymal scarring or fibrosis
- Enlarged pulmonary arteries
- Extramedullary hematopoeisis
- Cholecystectomy clips

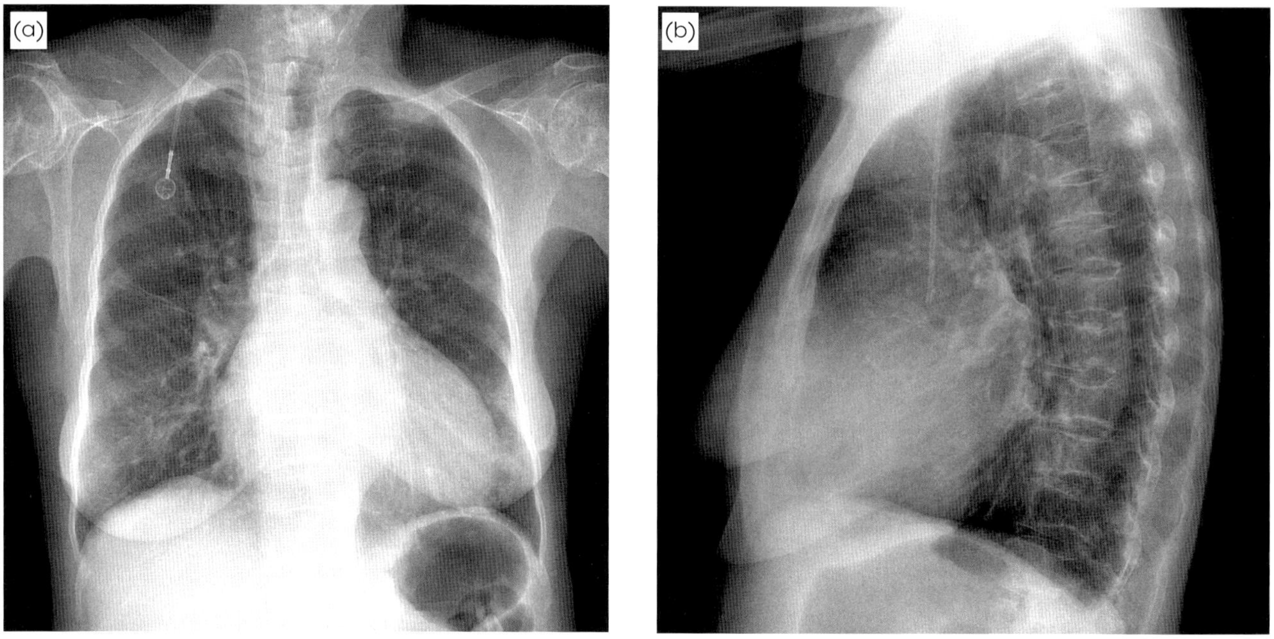

Figure 25.1. Sickle cell disease. (a) Posteroanterior chest radiograph of a patient with long-standing sickle cell disease shows cardiomegaly, enlarged pulmonary arteries, avascular necrosis of the humeral heads, and an absent splenic shadow. (b) Lateral chest radiograph of the same patient shows H-shaped vertebral bodies due to end plate osteonecrosis.

In patients with suspected acute chest syndrome, the radiologist must identify new parenchymal opacities unrelated to atelectasis that most commonly manifest as focal or multifocal airspace disease, typically involving at least an entire lung segment. Patients with sickle cell disease may present with entities that simulate acute chest syndrome, and a thorough examination of the heart, vasculature, upper abdomen, and bones is necessary in order to provide a complete interpretation.

What Not to Miss

Although a history of sickle cell may prompt consideration to one of the conditions described in this chapter, the radiologist must not forget about a simple community-acquired pneumonia because these patients are more prone to pneumonia, especially from encapsulated bacteria. Because of repeated transfusions, there is an increased risk of iron deposition in the heart, resulting in impaired cardiac function and pulmonary edema. Sickle cell disease also increases the risk of pulmonary hypertension. The latter two conditions may explain dyspnea and should not be overlooked.

Imaging Findings

Acute Chest Syndrome

- Single or multifocal airspace opacities/consolidation (typically involving at least one lung segment) (Fig. 25.2).
- Airspace opacities typically do not enhance or weakly enhance.
- Opacities may be peripheral and may cavitate, particularly when due to fat emboli.
- Lower and middle lobe involvement is more common than upper lobe involvement.
- Pleural effusions are frequently present.
- Up to 60% of patients may not have an initial imaging abnormality but may develop one later.
- Patients with repeated episodes of acute chest syndrome may develop chronic findings, including pulmonary fibrosis (septal line thickening, bronchiectasis, and architectural distortion) and pleural scarring (Fig. 25.3).

Differential Diagnosis

Rib Infarction

- Focal pain from rib infarction may simulate acute chest syndrome and may be accompanied by respiratory symptoms related to splinting and hypoventilation, resulting in atelectasis.
- Radiographic and CT findings of bone infarcts lag far behind the acute phase, and skeletal abnormalities are usually not visible in the acute setting.
- Skeletal scintigraphy may demonstrate focally increased peripheral uptake in the acute phase (typically becomes a decreased uptake cold spot after the acute phase) and may mimic osteomyelitis.
- MRI in the acute setting may show focally increased T2 marrow signal; chronic infarcts usually show signal consistent with marrow centrally with a surrounding rim of decreased T1 and T2 signal (peripheral rim may enhance).

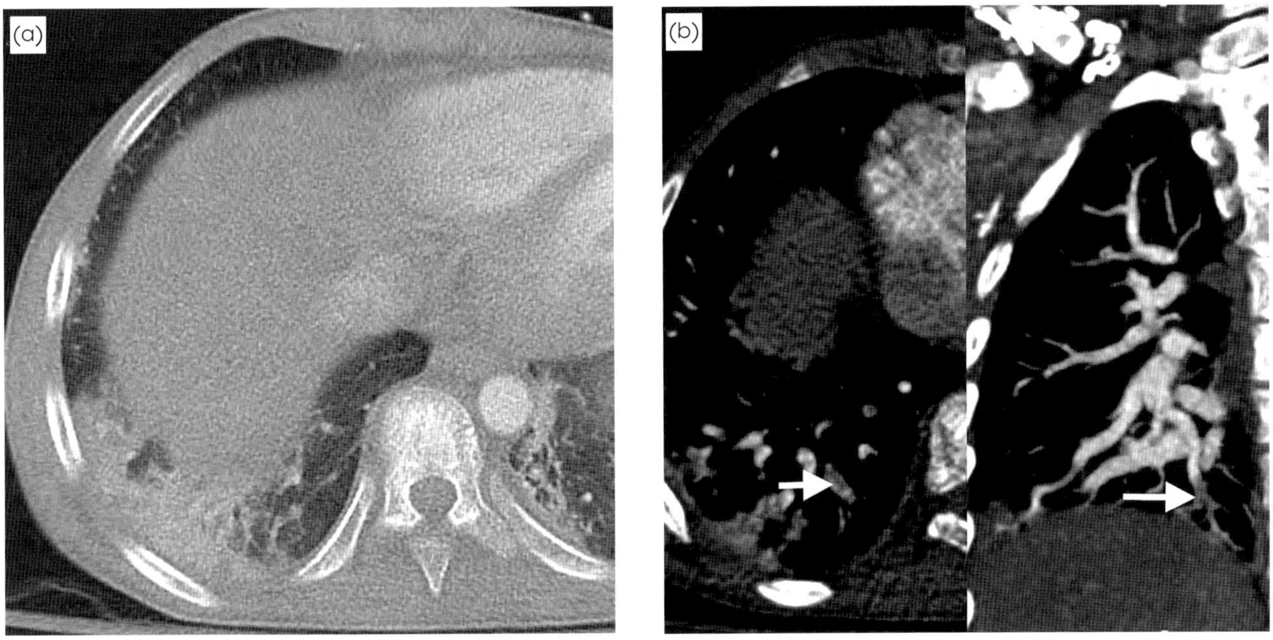

Figure 25.2. Acute chest syndrome with in situ thrombosis. (a) Contrast-enhanced chest CT of a 15-year-old patient with sickle cell disease with chest pain, fever, and dyspnea shows a peripheral right lower lobe consolidation. (b) Composite image with axial (left) and coronal maximum intensity projection (right) shows a filling defect in a right lower lobe subsegmental pulmonary artery (arrows). The pulmonary consolidation was consistent with acute chest syndrome, whereas the filling defect was thought to represent local in situ thrombosis given its distal solitary nature and a negative lower extremity Doppler ultrasound.

Cardiac and Vascular Causes

- Myocardial infarction, aortic dissection, and pulmonary thromboembolic disease may also be the cause of chest pain. The imaging features of these entities are discussed elsewhere.
- Patients with sickle cell disease may also present with pulmonary hypertension as an etiology of chest pain. The imaging features are similar to those of idiopathic pulmonary arterial hypertension described elsewhere.

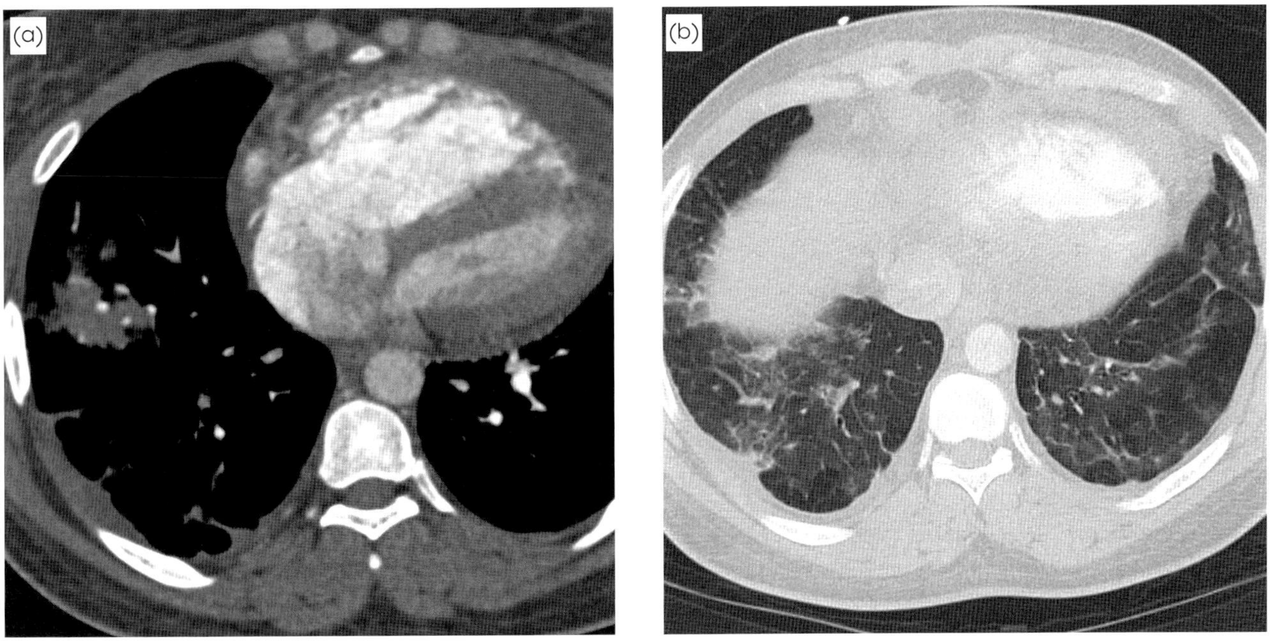

Figure 25.3. Acute chest syndrome with chronic fibrotic changes. (a) Axial contrast-enhanced CT of a patient with sickle cell anemia presenting with signs and symptoms of acute chest syndrome shows one of several nonenhancing consolidations in the right middle lobe. (b) Axial contrast-enhanced chest CT of the same patient shows basilar mosaic attenuation, architectural distortion, and interlobular septal thickening due to chronic fibrosis from repeated pulmonary insults.

Subdiaphragmatic Causes

Symptoms of subdiaphragmatic entities may mimic acute chest syndrome:

- Splenic infarction is typically asymptomatic in patients with sickle cell anemia (HbSS) and occurs progressively at a young age, producing a small, shrunken, often calcified spleen (Fig. 25.4). Massive splenic infarction with acute pain may occur in sickle disease with HbSC variant and in patients with sickle cell trait (homozygous for HbS with a normal Hb). The massively infarcted spleen is typically enlarged and may exhibit diffuse or focal nonenhancement. Infarcted spleens may rupture and/or become infected.
- Splenic sequestration syndrome is characterized by rapid pooling of blood in the spleen and results in rapidly dropping intravascular volume and hematocrit. It is almost always seen in children younger than age 8 years but has also been described in adults. The spleen is larger in size than expected (bearing in mind that most sickle patients have a very small or absent spleen). Ultrasound may show multiple hypoechoic areas in the periphery of the enlarged spleen that exhibit low attenuation on CT.
- Hepatitis may result from repeated transfusions and is common in patients with sickle cell anemia.
- Cholecystitis: Pigmented stones and sludge are common in sickle cell anemia, and many affected patients undergo cholecystectomy.

Clinical Issues

- Acute chest syndrome is more common in children with sickle cell anemia, but affected adults have a higher mortality rate.
- Adults more often present with acute chest syndrome after a pain crisis, whereas children more often present with fever and signs of infection.
- A high steady-state hemoglobin level is a risk factor for acute chest syndrome, but in acute episodes the hemoglobin may drop with an increase in markers of hemolysis.
- Treatment for acute chest syndrome involves a combination of antibiotics and supportive care including oxygen therapy, transfusion, bronchodilators, and corticosteroids. Treatment may require a high level of care with an intensive care unit stay because mechanical ventilation may be necessary.
- A substantial number of patients with sickle cell anemia develop pulmonary hypertension (up to 20% of adults with sickle cell anemia have borderline or mild pulmonary hypertension, and 10% have moderate to severe pulmonary hypertension). Although it is typically believed that the development of pulmonary hypertension is related to repeated bouts of acute chest syndrome, several studies have shown no association between the development of pulmonary hypertension and acute chest syndrome rates. The etiology of pulmonary hypertension in these patients is likely multifactorial and has been correlated with the severity of hemolytic anemia.

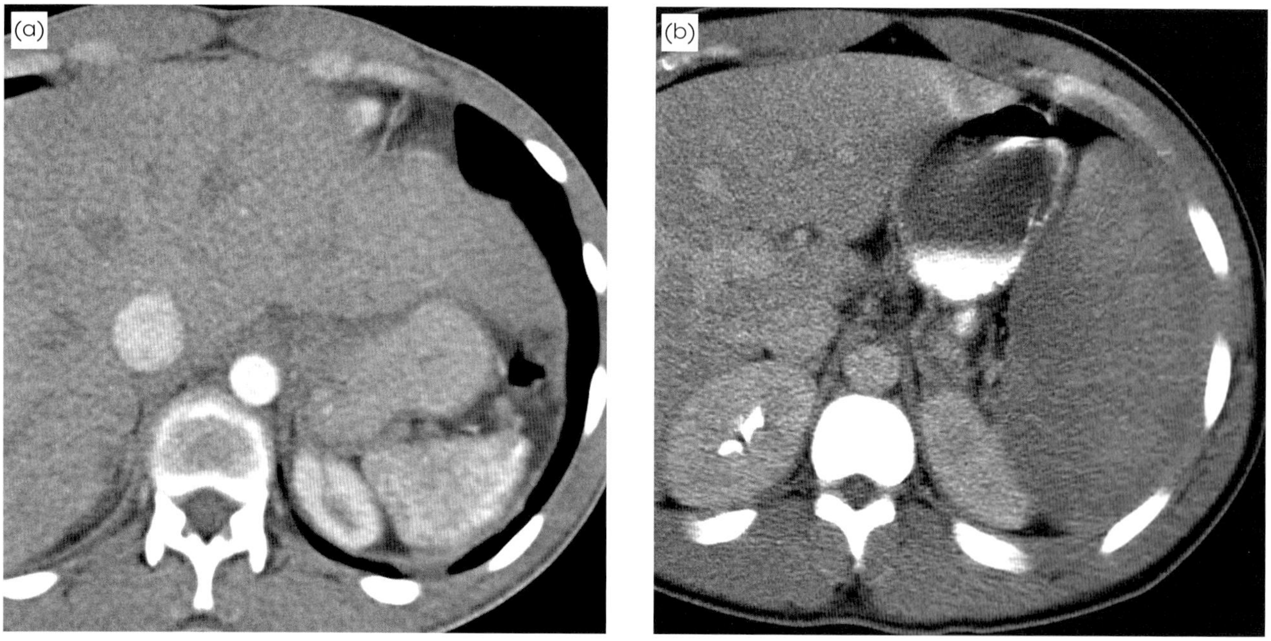

Figure 25.4. The spleen in sickle cell disease. (a) Axial contrast-enhanced CT of a patient with sickle cell anemia shows a small calcified spleen in the left upper quadrant of the abdomen due to autoinfarction. (b) Axial contrast-enhanced CT of a different patient with sickle cell anemia with acute left upper quadrant pain shows an enlarged hypoenhancing spleen consistent with acute infarction.

Key Points

- Acute chest syndrome must be considered in patients with sickle cell anemia presenting with chest pain and fever because it carries an increased mortality.
- The etiology of acute chest syndrome is multifactorial and involves a combination of infection, fat emboli, and vaso-occlusive disease.
- The key imaging feature of acute chest syndrome is focal or multifocal lung consolidation.
- Rib infarction and subdiaphragmatic pathologies may mimic acute chest syndrome.

Suggested Reading

Gladwin MT, Vichinsky E. Pulmonary complications of sickle cell disease. *N Engl J Med.* 2008;359(21):2254–2265.

Lonergan GJ, Cline DB, Abbondanzo SL. From the archives of the AFIP: Sickle cell anemia. *RadioGraphics.* 2001;21:917–994.

Siddiqui AK, Ahmed S. Pulmonary manifestations of sickle cell disease. *Postgrad Med J.* 2003;79:384–390.

CHAPTER 26

Pulmonary Hypertension

Constantine Raptis

Definition

Pulmonary hypertension (PH) is defined as elevation of pulmonary arterial pressure to greater than 25 mm Hg. Causes of PH are often divided into precapillary (pulmonary capillary wedge pressure <15 mm Hg) or post-capillary (pulmonary capillary wedge pressure >15 mm Hg). Another classification scheme, devised by the World Health Organization (WHO) and last revised in 2013 at Nice France (Nice classification), groups conditions based on shared pathophysiology and treatment. It contains five categories: class 1 pulmonary arterial hypertension (PAH) and its subtypes, class 2 PH due to left heart disease, class 3 PH due to chronic hypoxia, class 4 PH due to chronic thromboembolic disease, and class 5 PH from miscellaneous causes. The evaluation of affected patients involves a combination of imaging studies to help properly categorize the PH, giving the radiologist an important management role.

Clinical Features

Patients with PH typically present with dyspnea that is worse with exertion. Additional symptoms suggestive of an inability to increase cardiac output during activity include fatigue and syncope. If untreated, the symptoms typically worsen in a nonlinear pattern until there is dyspnea at rest. A high index of clinical suspicion can lead to early intervention. Left untreated, the mean life expectancy of patients with PH is less than 3 years.

Anatomy and Physiology

The right ventricle normally pumps against the pulmonary vascular bed, a low-pressure and low-resistance system. In patients with PH, resistance is increased. To compensate, the right ventricle dilates and hypertrophies. The normal crescentic right ventricular shape remodels to become more spherical. As dilatation worsens, tricuspid valve regurgitation may ensue. Over time, cardiac output worsens, resulting in right heart failure. The ability of the right heart to compensate for increased pulmonary pressures is the main determinant of patient symptoms and outcome.

How to Approach the Image

The purpose of imaging patients with suspected PH is twofold:(1) to evaluate for signs supporting the diagnosis of PH and (2) to look for findings that may reveal the underlying cause. The initial evaluation often begins with a chest radiograph. Radiographic signs of pulmonary hypertension include central pulmonary artery enlargement, right interlobar artery enlargement (>15 mm on a posteroanterior (PA) radiograph), vascular pruning, right heart enlargement, and oligemia (Fig. 26.1). Chest radiographs should also be assessed for potential underlying causes of PH, including emphysema, pulmonary fibrosis, and signs of left heart disease (including left heart enlargement and pulmonary edema). Rarely, severe deformities of the thoracic skeleton may be associated with PH. Many patients with suspected or confirmed PH will also undergo chest CT. CT evaluation centers on looking for evidence of PH in addition to possible underlying causes. CT findings of PH include enlargement of the pulmonary trunk (>2.9 cm from the pulmonary valve or larger than the ascending aorta), enlargement of the segmental arteries (>1.25 times the size of their accompanying bronchus), and findings of increased right heart pressure (enlarged and/or hypertrophied right ventricle (free wall >4–6 mm), bowing or straightening of the interventricular septum toward the left, and reflux of contrast into the inferior vena cava). Findings of vascular enlargement are less sensitive for detecting pulmonary hypertension in patients with interstitial lung disease. Parenchymal mosaicism and ground-glass nodules representing cholesterol granulomas are less specific findings. After evaluating for signs of PH, the typical chest CT search pattern should be employed, with emphasis on pulmonary parenchymal, cardiac, and vascular causes of pulmonary hypertension. The specific findings associated with these entities are discussed in the following sections.

What Not to Miss

A pulmonary artery that is enlarged is not diagnostic for PH. One must look to confirm that the right ventricle is enlarged and hypertrophied. If only the pulmonary artery is enlarged, then one must look for a left-to-right shunt that can increase the size of the pulmonary artery from

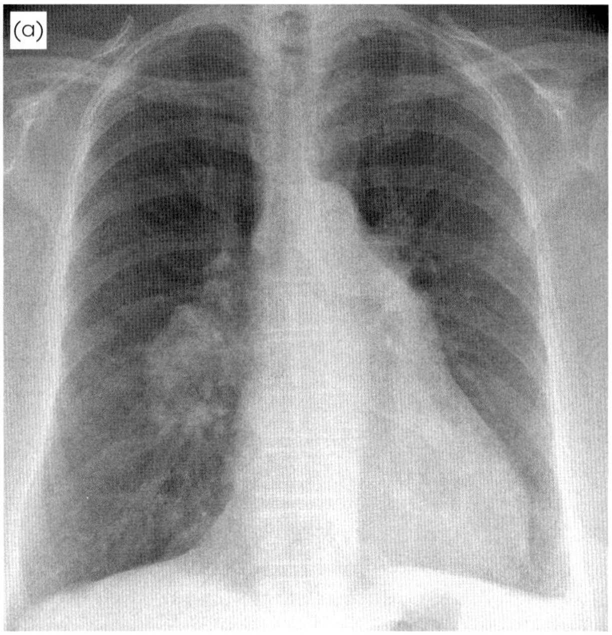

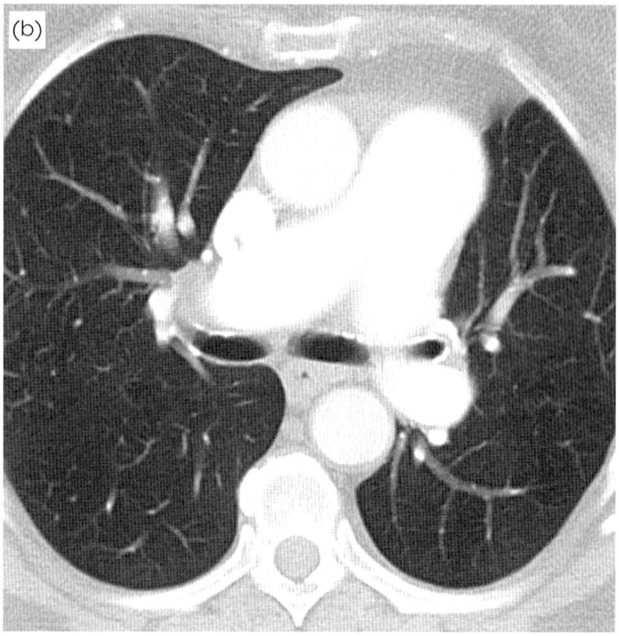

Figure 26.1. Idiopathic pulmonary arterial hypertension. (a) PA chest radiograph of a 38-year-old woman with chronic dyspnea shows cardiomegaly and enlarged pulmonary trunk and central pulmonary arteries, consistent with pulmonary hypertension. (b) Contrast-enhanced CT of the same patient confirms pulmonary trunk enlargement. Because this patient did not have any other explanation for her PH, she was diagnosed with idiopathic pulmonary hypertension (WHO category 1).

increased flow. Fibrosis may also result in enlargement of the pulmonary artery from a traction-related phenomenon. Finally, acute emboli may result in an enlarged pulmonary artery. One must confirm that no acute pulmonary emboli are present.

Differential Diagnosis

Category 1 Pulmonary Arterial Hypertension: Conditions in Which the Pathology Resides in the Pulmonary Arteries

- Includes idiopathic pulmonary arterial hypertension, heritable PH, drug- and toxin-induced PH, connective tissue diseases associated with PAH, PAH associated with HIV, PAH associated with portal hypertension, and PAH associated with congenital heart disease (Fig. 26.2), Long-standing shunts (atrial septal defect, ventricular septal defect, patent ductus arteriosus) can result in PH as can schistosomiasis

Category 1′ PH Associated with Venous Disease

- Separated from the remainder of category 1 to underscore that patients with these diseases may develop life-threatening pulmonary edema if treated with vasodilators. This category includes pulmonary veno-occlusive disease (Fig. 26.3) and pulmonary capillary hemangiomatosis.

Category 1″: Persistent PH of the Newborn

Category 2: PH Due to Left Heart Disease

- Includes causes of left heart disease, including systolic disease, diastolic disease, valvular disease, congenital left heart inflow and outflow disease, and congenital cardiomyopathies.

Category 3: PH Due to Hypoxia and Parenchymal Lung Diseases

- Caused by hypoxic vasoconstriction.
- Includes chronic obstructive pulmonary disease, interstitial lung disease (Fig. 26.4), sleep-disordered breathing, alveolar hypoventilation disorders, chronic high-altitude exposure, thoracic deformities, diseases with mixed restrictive/obstructive pattern, and developmental lung diseases.

Category 4: Chronic Thromboembolic PH

- Important cause of PH due to systemic inflammatory response to pulmonary emboli resulting in a vasculopathy of the pulmonary arterial tree.

Category 5: PH Due to Multifactorial Mechanisms

- Includes a variety of hematologic, systemic, metabolic, and other disorders that can cause PH, including lung cancer, sarcoidosis, and fibrosing mediastinitis. Also includes hemolytic anemia.

Imaging Findings

CT and/or MRI findings of some of the most important causes of PH are presented next.

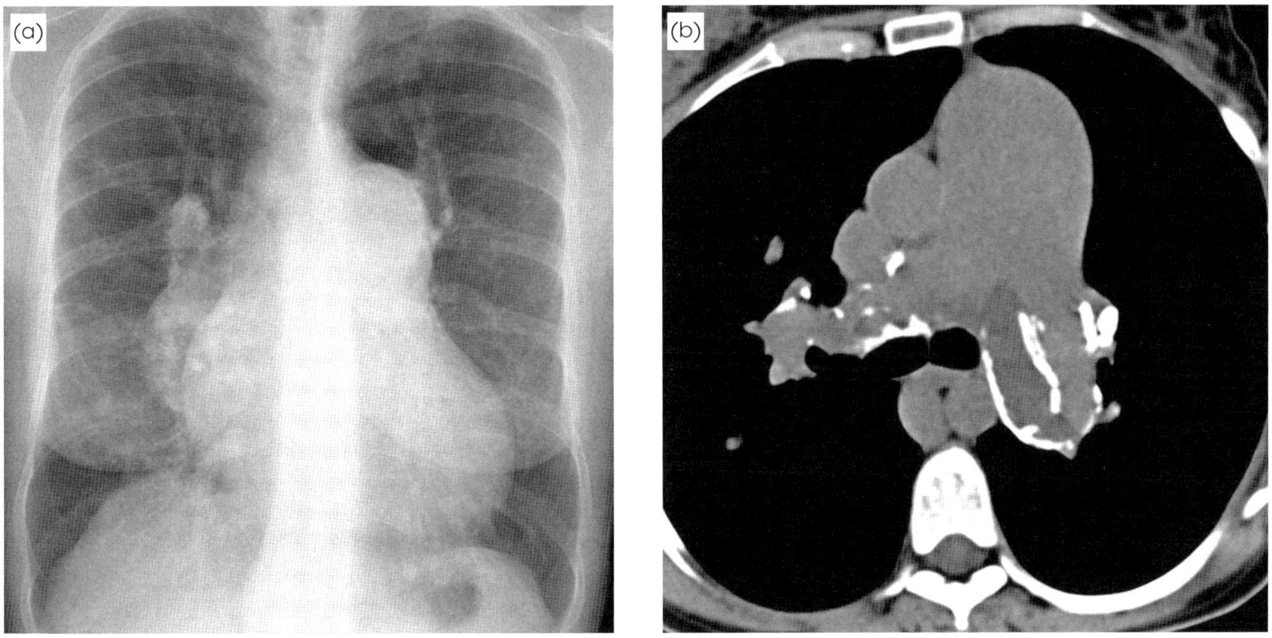

Figure 26.2. Pulmonary hypertension due to atrial septal defect. (a) PA chest radiograph of a 45-year-old woman with atrial septal defect, long-standing dyspnea, and pulmonary hypertension shows massive enlargement of the pulmonary trunk and central pulmonary arteries and mural calcification of the pulmonary arteries. (b) Unenhanced CT of the same patient shows mural calcifications and in situ thrombosis in the pulmonary arteries. This patient's PH was due to a long-standing atrial septal defect (WHO category 1).

Idiopathic Pulmonary Arterial Hypertension (Category 1)

- Central pulmonary vasculature enlargement, peripheral pruning, and right heart enlargement. Parenchymal opacities are uncommon in the untreated patient.
- In severe cases, calcification and in situ thrombi may develop along the walls of the central pulmonary arteries.
- Mosaic attenuation is usually absent in the untreated patient.

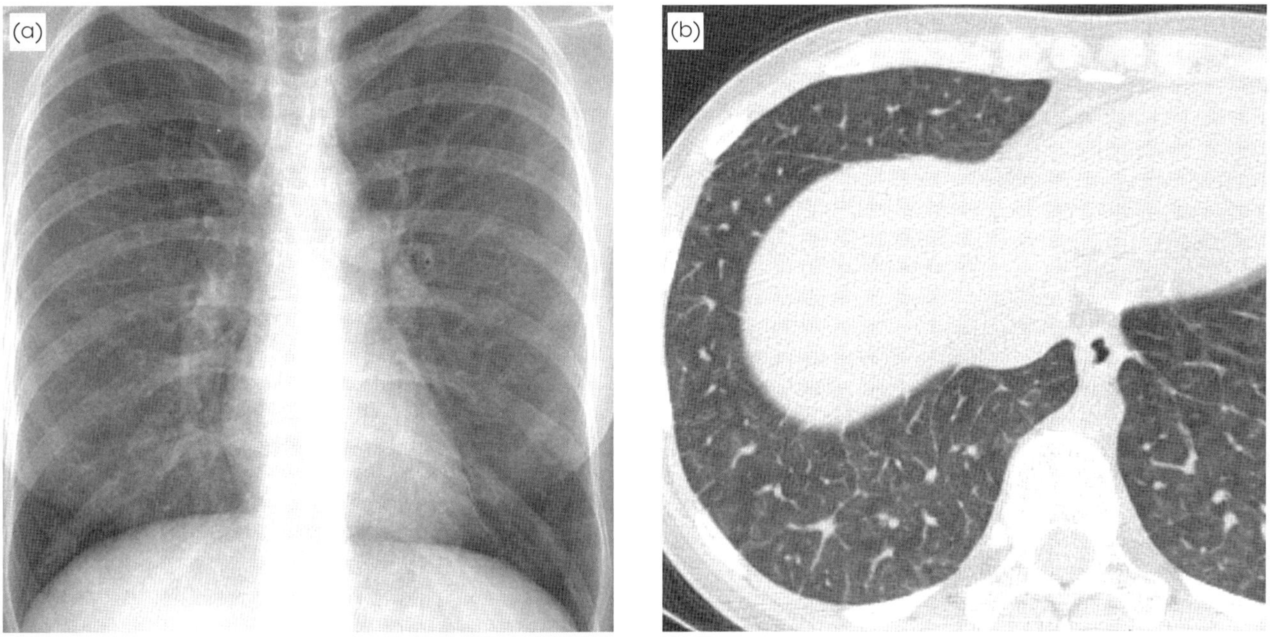

Figure 26.3. Pulmonary veno-occlusive disease. (a) PA chest radiograph of a 16-year-old woman with chronic dyspnea and mild pulmonary hypertension shows subtle bilateral lower interstitial and airspace opacities. (b) Unenhanced chest CT of the same patient shows extensive centrilobular ground-glass nodules and interlobular septal thickening. In the setting of normal left heart function, the findings suggest pulmonary veno-occlusive disease confirmed at lung biopsy (WHO category 1′).

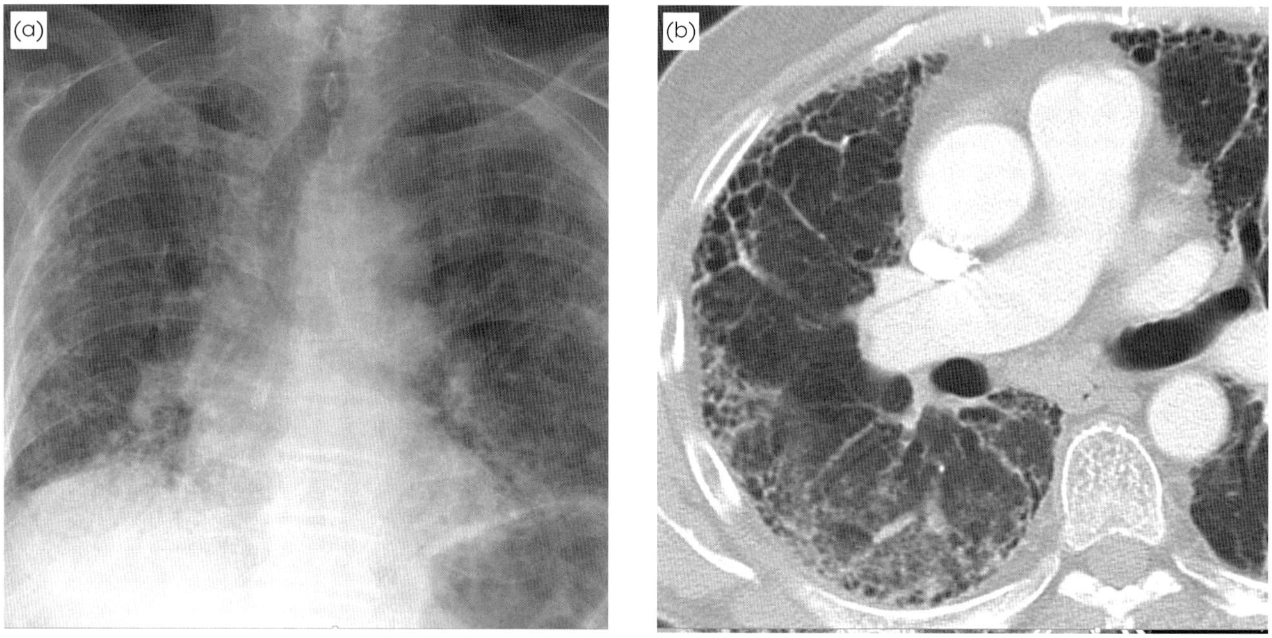

Figure 26.4. Pulmonary hypertension due to chronic lung disease. (a) Anteroposterior chest radiograph of a patient with dyspnea and pulmonary hypertension demonstrates small lung volumes and coarse interstitial opacities consistent with pulmonary fibrosis. (b) Contrast-enhanced CT of the same patient shows peripheral honeycombing consistent with usual interstitial pneumonia. This patient has WHO category 3 pulmonary hypertension due to chronic lung disease.

Congenital Heart Disease (Category 1)

- Pulmonary arterial calcification indicates prolonged exposure to high pulmonary pressures and is usually from an underlying shunt lesion.
- Atrial septal defects: Ostium primum (distal septum/endocardial cushion), ostium secundum (mid septum), sinus venosus (proximal/superior septum and associated with right upper lobe anomalous pulmonary venous drainage).
- Ventricular septal defects can occur at several locations, most commonly perimembranous type (below the aortic valve under the septal leaflet of tricuspid valve).
- Patent ductus arteriosus: Large pulmonary artery and vascular connection between the underside of the aorta and the pulmonary artery (multiplanar reformation images can be helpful to depict this connection).
- Cardiac MRI can help detect shunts both by depicting the abnormal connection (defect and/or dephasing jet across the connection) and by determining the pulmonary-to-systemic blood flow ratio (Qp:Qs) as secondary evidence of a shunt.
- Pressures in the pulmonary arterial bed may increase to the point that left-to-right flow is reversed across the shunt (Eisenmenger syndrome), resulting in cyanosis.

Pulmonary Veno-occlusive Disease (Category 1′)

- Findings of PH associated with pulmonary edema (septal line thickening and ground-glass opacities) without evidence of left heart enlargement or dysfunction.
- May be associated with small central pulmonary veins, lymphadenopathy, and pleural effusions.

Pulmonary Capillary Hemangiomatosis (Category 1′)

- Findings of PH with normal left heart associated with diffuse centrilobular ground-glass nodules.
- Septal line thickening (nodular or smooth) may be present, but typically to a lesser extent than in veno-occlusive disease, with the predominant feature being the nodules.

Pulmonary Hypertension Due to Left Heart Disease (Category 2)

- Typical features of left heart failure, including pulmonary edema (smooth septal line thickening and ground glass) and pleural effusions.
- Left heart size and function are the distinguishing factors between left heart disease and pulmonary veno-occlusive disease.

Pulmonary Hypertension Due to Chronic Hypoxia (Category 3)

- Obstructive disease such as chronic obstructive pulmonary disease/emphysema. Typical findings of these entities will be present.
- Restrictive lung diseases including usual interstitial pneumonia and nonspecific interstitial pneumonia.
- In patients with upper lobe emphysema and lower lobe fibrosis, a more specific diagnosis of combined pulmonary fibrosis and emphysema should be suggested. This condition often manifests with PH.

- Pulmonary trunk may be enlarged in the setting of fibrosis without PH, and care should be taken not to overcall PH when pulmonary trunk enlargement is seen without right ventricle enlargement in patients with fibrosis.

Pulmonary Hypertension Due to Chronic Thromboembolic Disease (Category 4)

- Vascular findings: Signs of PH with intraluminal eccentric thrombi, vascular webs, vascular beading, and vascular cutoff (Fig. 26.5).
- Collateral flow including enlarged bronchial arteries (>1.5 mm) and, less commonly, nonbronchial collaterals including inferior phrenic, intercostal, and internal mammary arteries.
- Pulmonary findings: Mosaic attenuation with features of small vessel disease (no air trapping on expiratory images) often in a segmental or subsegmental distribution is a key feature. Occasionally, peripheral ground-glass opacities or consolidations, bronchiectasis, and areas of architectural distortion may also be seen.
- PH in association with mosaicism in a small vessel pattern without vascular findings should raise the possibility of chronic thromboembolic pulmonary hypertension because the vascular findings are not always present.

Pulmonary Hypertension Due to Fibrosing Mediastinitis (Category 5)

- Fibrosing mediastinitis on CT characterized by calcified mediastinal lymph nodes/masses, vascular cutoffs (usually affecting pulmonary veins before arteries), beading or narrowing of the pulmonary vascular tree, bronchial distortion or cutoffs, and parenchymal mosaicism typically without air trapping (small vessel pattern).
- Usually bilateral, but when unilateral, it is often right-sided.
- May be difficult to distinguish from a neoplastic process, particularly when calcification is absent or minor.

Clinical Issues

- In follow-up, MRI can be used to assess changes in the right ventricle, including function, end systolic volume, end diastolic volume, and mass.
- MRI can assess pulmonary blood flow and velocities using phase contrast imaging.
- Pulmonary circulation time can also be examined using time-resolved MRI.

These values can be used to monitor changes in patients with PH; MRI is typically superior to echocardiography and unlike, CT, does not use radiation

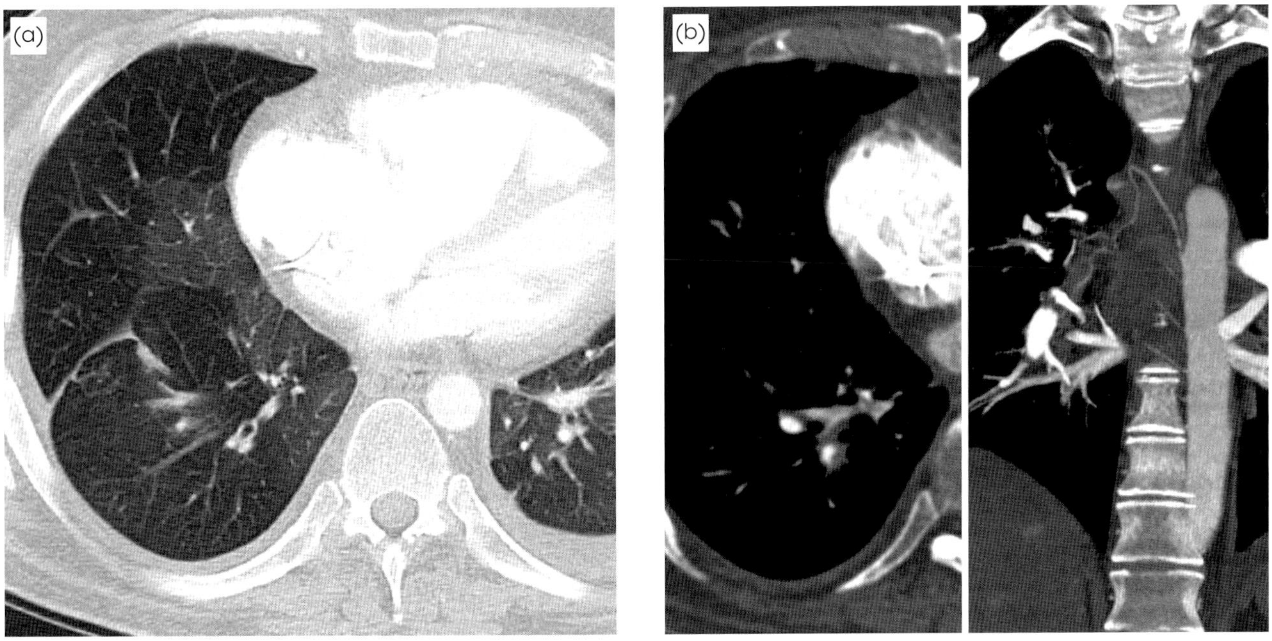

Figure 26.5. Chronic thromboembolic disease. (a) Contrast-enhanced CT shows extensive mosaic attenuation. (b) Composite image with axial (left) and coronal maximum intensity projection (right) contrast-enhanced CT shows eccentric filling defects in right lower lobe pulmonary artery and enlarged bronchial arteries. The findings together with CT signs of pulmonary hypertension confirmed PH due to chronic thromboembolic disease (WHO category 4).

Key Points

- PH is defined as a pulmonary capillary wedge pressure greater than 25 mm Hg.
- The causes of PH are classified according to the Nice classification, which groups causes of PH based on shared pathophysiology and treatments.
- Imaging plays an important role in the workup in the initial evaluation and management of patients with PH.
- In the initial workup of patients with PH, the goal of imaging is to determine if there are findings of PH and to look for clues to the underlying cause.
- Although radiography and CT are often used in the initial workup of patients with PH, MRI also has a role in the initial workup (particularly for shunts and congenital heart disease).
- MRI can be useful in the follow-up of patients with PH because it can evaluate for changes in the right ventricle.

Suggested Reading

Barbosa EJM, Gupta NK, Torigian DA, Gefter WB. Current role of imaging in the diagnosis and management of pulmonary hypertension. *AJR Am J Roentgenol.* 2012;198:1320–1331.

Grosse C, Grosse A. CT findings in diseases associated with pulmonary hypertension: A current review. *RadioGraphics.* 2010;30:1753–1777.

Lopez-Costa I, Bhalla S, Raptis C. Magnetic resonance imaging for pulmonary hypertension: Methods, applications, and outcomes. *Top Magn Reson Imaging.* 2014;23(1):43–50.

Pena E, Dennie C, Veinot J, Muniz SH. Pulmonary hypertension: How the radiologist can help. *RadioGraphics.* 2012; 32:9–32.

Section VI

Pleural Disease

CHAPTER 27

Introduction to Pleural Disease

Christopher M. Walker

Introduction

The imaging features of pleural disease include visualization of a thin visceral pleural line in patients with pneumothorax, pleural effusion that may be free or loculated, pleural thickening with or without intrinsic calcifications, and pleural nodules and/or masses that may be focal or circumferential in their growth pattern (Figs. 27.1–27.3).

The pleural space represents a potential space formed by the apposition of the visceral and parietal pleural surfaces. The pleural space surrounds the lungs from the apices to the caudal extent of the costophrenic sulci and extends into the fissures.

A small amount of fluid is normally present in the pleural space but is not detectable on imaging studies. The two apposing layers of normal visceral pleura form the interlobar fissures and manifest as a thin line on chest radiography and CT. The normal fissure may manifest as a band or as an area of the lung devoid of vascular structures on axial CT imaging. Normal visceral and parietal pleura surfaces are invisible on chest radiography but may manifest as a thin line on CT along the lung periphery, particularly in the intercostal regions.

Diseases of the Pleural Space

The imaging differential diagnosis of pleural abnormalities may be narrowed by recognizing the imaging findings discussed here.

Pneumothorax (Fig. 27.1) represents an abnormal collection of air in the pleural space. It is divided clinically into three types: primary spontaneous, secondary spontaneous, and traumatic. Primary spontaneous pneumothorax occurs in individuals without underlying lung disease; is most often seen in tall, young male smokers; and is usually secondary to rupture of a small apical bleb or bulla. Secondary spontaneous pneumothorax occurs in patients with underlying lung disease (e.g., emphysema, pneumocystis pneumonia, lymphangioleiomyomatosis, Langerhans cell histiocytosis, and cystic fibrosis). Traumatic pneumothorax occurs in patients with blunt or penetrating trauma or may follow medical procedures such as central line placement, percutaneous needle biopsy, or barotrauma. Every pneumothorax must be carefully assessed for the presence of mediastinal or diaphragmatic displacement (i.e., tension) because these findings may indicate the risk of impending cardiopulmonary arrest.

Pleural effusion is an abnormal collection of fluid in the pleural space that manifests with imaging features that vary with the size of the collection. The most common radiographic manifestation is blunting of a costophrenic sulcus in an upright patient or a veil-like opacity within the involved hemithorax in a supine patient. Less commonly, pleural fluid may accumulate in a subpulmonic location and mimic elevation of the ipsilateral hemidiaphragm. Lateral decubitus radiography may detect as little as 5 cc of pleural fluid, whereas frontal radiography detects only collections of 200 cc of fluid or more. Clinically, pleural effusions are categorized as transudative or exudative based on Light's criteria. Transudative pleural effusions have low protein and lactate dehydrogenase (LDH) content and occur in patients

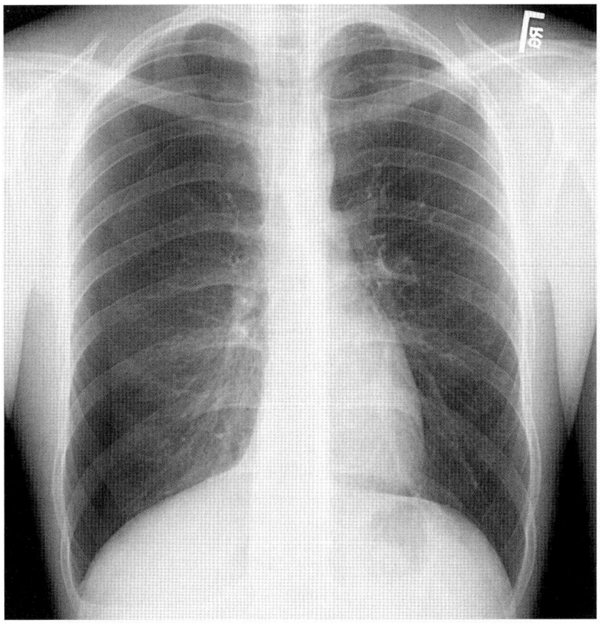

Figure 27.1. Spontaneous tension pneumothorax. Posteroanterior (PA) chest radiograph of an otherwise healthy 22-year-old man demonstrates a right pneumothorax. The visceral pleura of the right lung manifests as a thin pleural line. The bronchovascular structures in the right lung are crowded, and there is mild shift of the trachea and other mediastinal structures to the left in this hypotensive patient with tension pneumothorax.

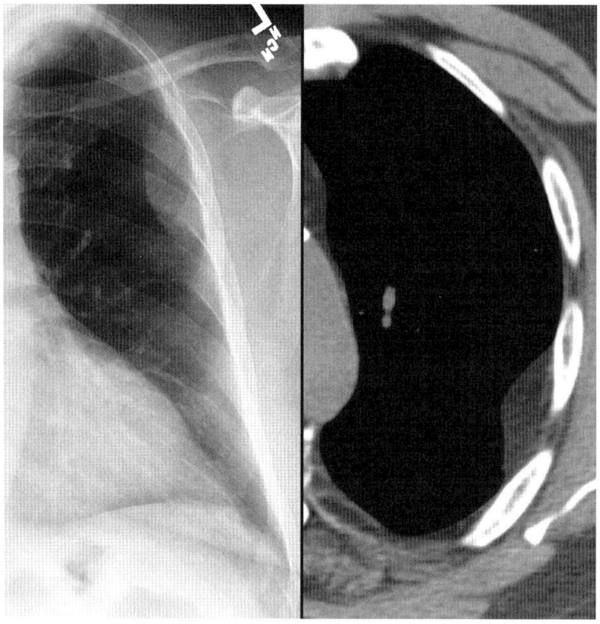

Figure 27.2. Features of pleural lesions. Composite image with PA chest radiograph and axial unenhanced chest CT shows a pleural metastasis (left) and a chest wall lipoma (right). The metastasis is lenticular in shape, forms obtuse angles with the adjacent pleura, and exhibits the incomplete border sign. The chest wall lipoma exhibits fat attenuation and forms obtuse angles with the adjacent pleura.

with heart failure, renal failure, and cirrhosis. Exudative pleural effusions have high protein and LDH content and are seen with inflammatory disorders such as pneumonia, malignancy, and collagen vascular disease. Pleural effusion with high attenuation on CT should suggest hemothorax, which is typically related to trauma but may be associated with acute aortic syndrome or an underlying coagulopathy.

Pleural mass, nodule, or *thickening* may indicate metastatic disease, most often from breast or lung cancer. Four CT features of pleural thickening are suggestive of malignant pleural thickening, whether detected in isolation or in combination:

1. Pleural thickening greater than 1 cm in thickness
2. Pleural nodules or masses
3. Circumferential pleural involvement
4. Involvement of mediastinal pleura

Mesothelioma is the most common primary malignant pleural neoplasm and is indistinguishable from pleural metastases based on imaging features alone. Although strongly associated with asbestos exposure, only 20% of patients with mesothelioma exhibit pleural plaques as a marker of prior exposure. Benign pleural thickening (fibrothorax) is usually secondary to an inflammatory process that causes focal or diffuse thickening and fusion of the visceral and parietal pleural surfaces. It is typically unilateral, may blunt the costophrenic sulcus, and may extend across multiple ribs and intercostal spaces. When the inciting inflammation is severe, pleural thickening may extend over the entire costal and diaphragmatic pleural surfaces to encase the lung and cause restrictive lung physiology. Fibrothorax spares the mediastinal pleura in 88% of cases, but it may be involved by some infectious etiologies (e.g., tuberculosis).

Diffuse pleural thickening with calcification most commonly follows tuberculous empyema or hemothorax. Talc

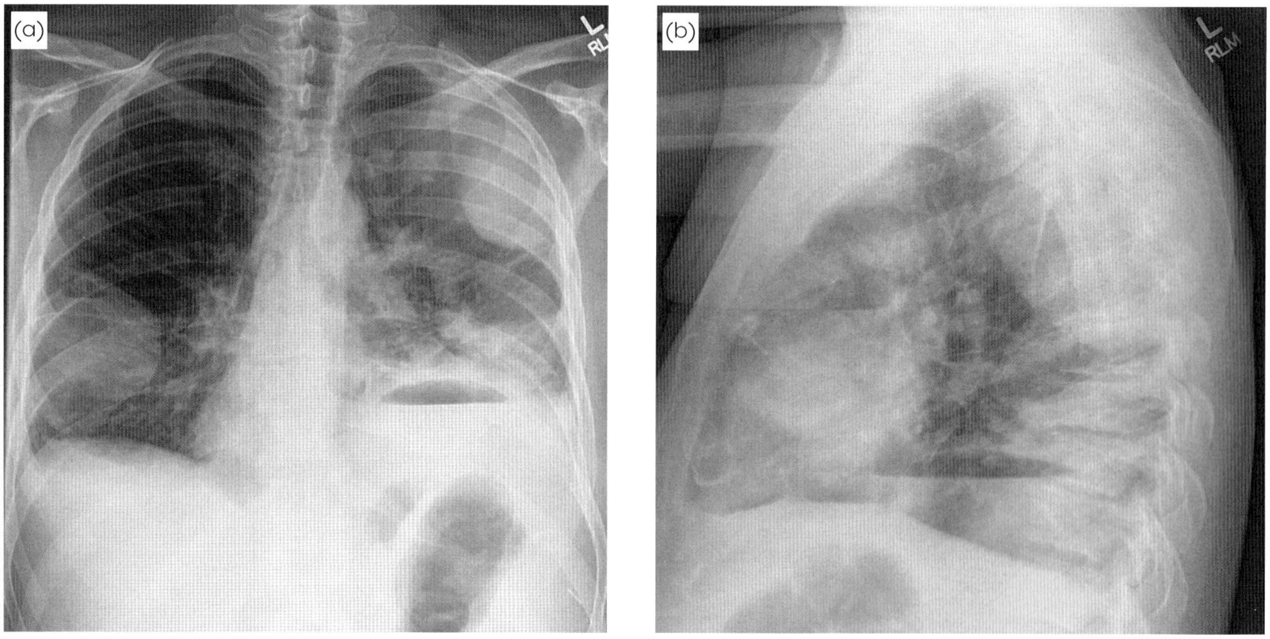

Figure 27.3. Multifocal empyema (*Staphylococcus aureus*). (a, b) AP and lateral chest radiographs show bilateral rounded and lenticular pleural fluid collections. Two fluid collections show an air–fluid level and a disparity of their length when compared on the two orthogonal views, consistent with pleural rather than a parenchymal process.

is a chemical irritant used to treat refractory pleural effusion and pneumothorax by pleurodesis, and it manifests as high-density material in the pleura mimicking pleural calcification. Malignant neoplasms such as mesothelioma or metastasis may uncommonly exhibit calcification when there is osteocartilagenous differentiation (rare) or when tumor engulfs preexisting calcified pleural plaques.

Approach to Pleural Abnormalities

An important first step in chest radiographic analysis is determining whether an abnormality is pulmonary or extrapulmonary in location. Several radiographic and CT features suggest a pleural or chest wall origin of a mass or fluid collection:

1. Pleural (and chest wall) abnormalities may manifest with incomplete borders on orthogonal radiographs when part of the lesion border has no tangential relationship to the x-ray beam (Fig. 27.2).
2. Pleural lesions often exhibit obtuse angles or smooth tapering margins with the adjacent chest wall or mediastinum (Fig. 27.2). However, large pleural masses often form acute angles with the adjacent pleural and chest wall.
3. Pleural lesions are always adjacent to a pleural surface (costal, mediastinal, diaphragmatic, or fissural).
4. Pleural lesions tend to displace rather than engulf adjacent pulmonary structures on cross-sectional imaging.
5. Air within a loculated pleural collection indicates the presence of empyema with bronchopleural fistula in the absence of prior intervention. Air–fluid level length in a lenticular-shaped empyema with bronchopleural fistula is typically unequal on PA and lateral radiographs (Fig. 27.3), in contrast to the equal length exhibited in a spherical cavitary lung abscess.

Suggested Reading

Kuhlman JE, Singha NK. Complex disease of the pleural space: Radiographic and CT evaluation. *RadioGraphics.* 1997 Jan–Feb 1997;17(1):63–79.

Walker CM, Takasugi JE, Chung JH, et al. Tumorlike conditions of the pleura. *RadioGraphics.* 2012 Jul–Aug 2012;32(4):971–985.

CHAPTER 28

Pneumothorax

Christopher M. Walker

Definition

Pneumothorax is an abnormal collection of air within the pleural space. It is divided clinically into three types: primary spontaneous, secondary spontaneous, and traumatic:

- *Primary spontaneous pneumothorax* occurs in the absence of visible lung pathology and is frequently secondary to rupture of a small apical bleb or bulla. It is most often seen in tall, young male smokers (Fig. 28.1).
- *Secondary spontaneous pneumothorax* occurs in patients with preexisting lung pathology.
- *Traumatic pneumothorax* occurs in penetrating or blunt chest trauma or may be iatrogenic caused by positive pressure ventilation or following medical procedures such as central line placement or biopsy.

Clinical Features

Dyspnea and chest pain, frequently exacerbated by deep inspiration, are the most common presenting symptoms in patients with pneumothorax. However, affected patients may be asymptomatic if the pneumothorax is small or if there are distracting conditions such as a skeletal fracture. Physical examination is often normal but may reveal hypoxia, decreased breath sounds, and hyperresonance to chest percussion on the side of the pneumothorax.

Pneumothorax is divided clinically into three types.

Primary Spontaneous Pneumothorax

- Usually caused by rupture of an apical bleb or bulla.
- Ipsilateral recurrence is common, occurring in approximately 50% of patients.
- Contralateral recurrence occurs in 15% of patients.

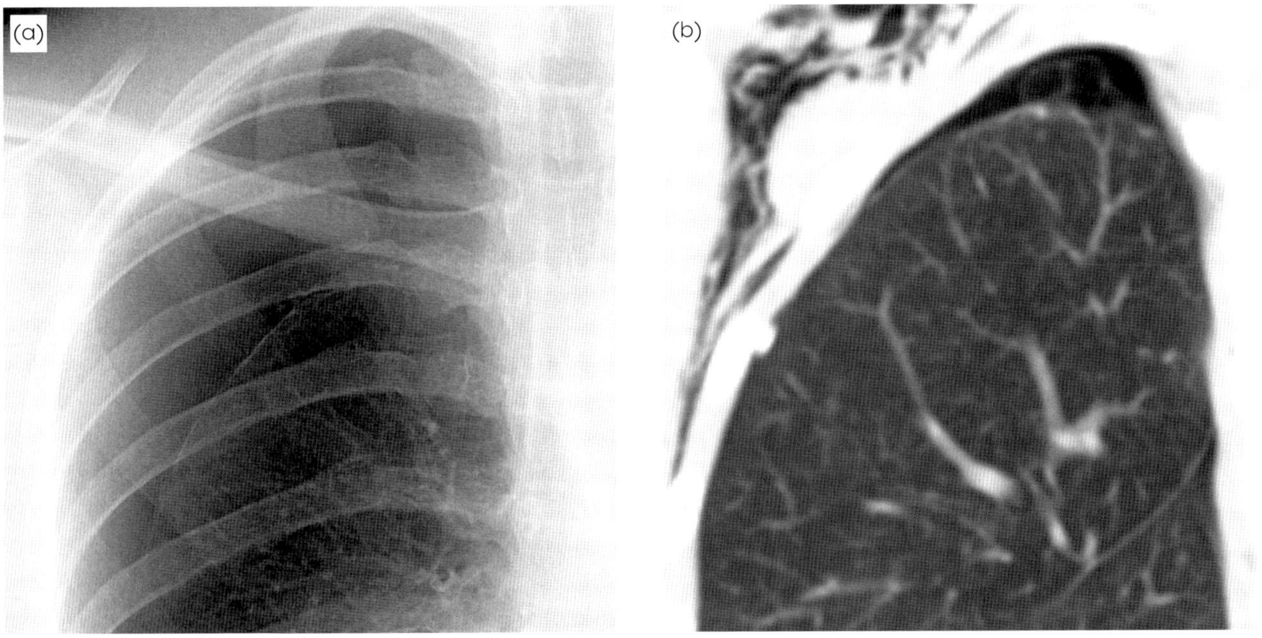

Figure 28.1. Spontaneous pneumothorax in a 22-year-old athlete. (a) Coned-down posteroanterior (PA) chest radiograph shows a right apical pneumothorax manifesting as a thin white pleural line representing the visceral pleura of the atelectatic right upper lobe and peripheral lucency in the apicolateral right hemithorax. (b) Coronal chest CT of the same patient shows a right chest tube in place laterally and apical blebs or bullae projecting from the visceral pleural surface. The small right apical pneumothorax outlines the outer walls of the apical blebs.

- CT is usually obtained after recurrent pneumothorax to look for an underlying cause (e.g., apical bleb or bulla) prior to operative intervention.

Secondary Spontaneous Pneumothorax

- Airway disorder: Asthma, cystic fibrosis, emphysema
- Infection: *Pneumocystis jiroveci, Staphylococcus aureus*
- Malignancy: Cystic metastasis, osteosarcoma metastasis
- Cystic lung disease: Langerhans cell histiocytosis, lymphangioleiomyomatosis
- Interstitial lung disease: Usual interstitial pneumonia, lymphocytic interstitial pneumonia
- Catamenial pneumothorax: Recurrent pneumothorax caused by thoracic endometriosis. It almost always affects the right pleural space, and patients present with pneumothorax and symptoms within 48 hours of the menstrual cycle. Rarely, CT may show small nodules along the diaphragm or other pleural surfaces in the right lower hemithorax that represent endometriosis deposits.

Traumatic Pneumothorax

- Seen in 15–40% of patients following blunt trauma
- 10–50% missed at initial chest radiography due to basal or subpulmonic location
- Usually caused by rib fracture or alveolar rupture

Anatomy and Physiology

Intrapleural air moves to the least dependent portion of the pleural space, which varies depending on the patient position at the time of imaging. In upright patients, pneumothorax generally collects over the lung apices. In semierect or supine patients, air first collects in the inferior and anterior pleural space (e.g., anteromedial and subpulmonic pleural spaces) and may be difficult to visualize on portable radiography.

Tension pneumothorax is a special situation in which intrapleural pressure is equal to or exceeds atmospheric pressure, potentially leading to impaired venous return to the heart and eventually to cardiopulmonary arrest. It is a clinical diagnosis and is most commonly seen in traumatic pneumothorax or in pneumothorax occurring in ventilated patients. Although certain radiologic signs have been associated with tension, it is important to remember that many patients with pneumothorax lack these findings. Conversely, patients with these findings may not exhibit tension physiology.

How to Approach the Image

It is important to search every radiograph using magnification with panning because the imaging findings of pneumothorax may be subtle. After detection, measurement of the interpleural distance (visceral to parietal) is useful for documentation of size and for determining whether there are any signs that suggest tension. The radiologist must look for clues to explain the cause of the pneumothorax (i.e., rib fracture and underlying lung disease). Following diagnosis of pneumothorax, the finding should be communicated to the referring clinician, and the communication should be documented in the radiology report.

What Not to Miss

Subpulmonic or basal pneumothorax is frequently overlooked in intubated patients or in patients with traumatic injuries. Unfortunately, these patients are at the greatest risk for developing tension physiology. Traumatic pneumothorax is often seen in conjunction with other injuries, including rib and sternal fractures, pulmonary laceration and contusion, aortic transection, and solid organ injury (especially liver, spleen, and kidneys).

Differential Diagnosis

Skin Fold

- Curvilinear opaque edge that often crosses the chest wall (pneumothorax typically manifests as a thin pleural line) (Figs. 28.2 and 28.3).
- Lung markings are visible distal to opaque edge.
- If indeterminate, obtain repeat radiography; skin folds frequently change shape or position or resolve.

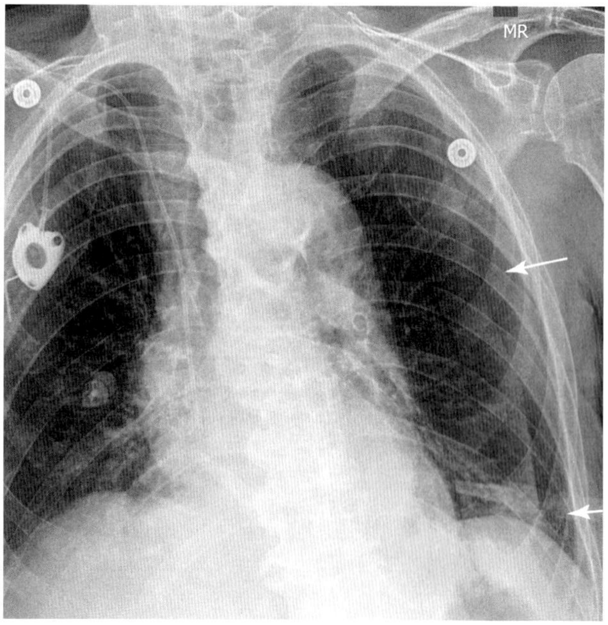

Figure 28.2. Skin fold. AP chest radiograph shows a broad opaque edge along the lateral aspect of the left with an adjacent radiolucent band formed by a skin fold with vascular structures visible peripheral to the opaque edge.

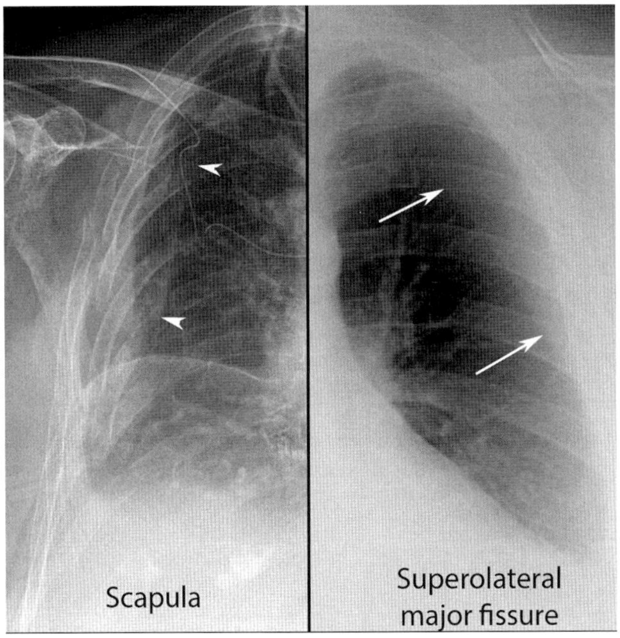

Figure 28.3. Pneumothorax mimics. Composite image with AP chest radiographs shows a scapular edge (arrowheads) (left) and a curvilinear opacity (arrows) caused by extrapleural fat extending into the major fissure (right).

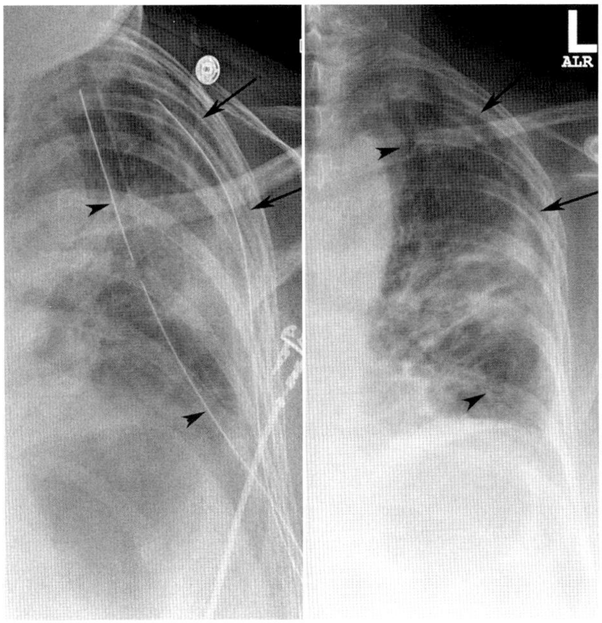

Figure 28.4. Chest tube tracks. Composite image with AP radiographs obtained before and after chest tube removal shows two lucent chest tube tracks (right; arrowheads and arrows) at the location of the recently removed chest tubes (left; arrowheads and arrows). Chest tube tracks represent loculated pneumothorax or hydropneumothorax and should be differentiated from a free pneumothorax.

Chest Tube Track

- Immediately following removal, air or fluid may remain in the track created by the chest tube (technically this represents a loculated pneumothorax or hydropneumothorax of no clinical significance) (Fig. 28.4).
- Chest tube tracks do not require further monitoring.
- Chest tube tracks are more common in patients with chest tubes in place for longer than 3 days and typically resolve within days.
- Comparison with previous radiographs that document chest tube position allows correct identification of chest tube tracks.

Bullae

- Bullae are rounded intrapulmonary air collections, whereas a pneumothorax typically has a crescentic shape.
- May require CT for definitive diagnosis.

Superolateral Major Fissure

- Extrapleural fat may be drawn into the outer aspect of a major fissure, causing a curvilinear edge or opacity on chest radiography.
- Edge merges with chest wall inferiorly.
- Vascular markings are seen distal to edge.

Pneumomediastinum

- Medial pneumothorax may simulate pneumo mediastinum.
- On CT, pneumomediastinum may dissect outward and simulate an anterior pneumothorax.

Imaging Findings

Pneumothorax in Upright Patient

- Apicolateral thin pleural line is characteristic; may manifest as an edge when adjacent to dense lung consolidation (Fig. 28.1a).
- No lung markings distal to pleural line/edge.
- Pneumothorax typically appears larger on expiratory chest radiography.
- CT and lateral decubitus radiography (normal side down) are the most sensitive examinations.
- Pneumothorax is best identified on CT using lung windows manifesting as air interposed between the visceral and parietal pleura.

Pneumothorax in Supine Patient

- Increased basal lucency.
- Sharp delineation of ipsilateral hemidiaphragm or mediastinal structures (e.g., heart border, pericardial fat pad or tag, and inferior vena cava).
- Air lucency may extend inferiorly, deep within ipsilateral costophrenic sulcus (deep sulcus sign) (Figs. 28.5 and 28.6).
- Double diaphragm sign may occur (air within the pleural space outlines the anterior costophrenic

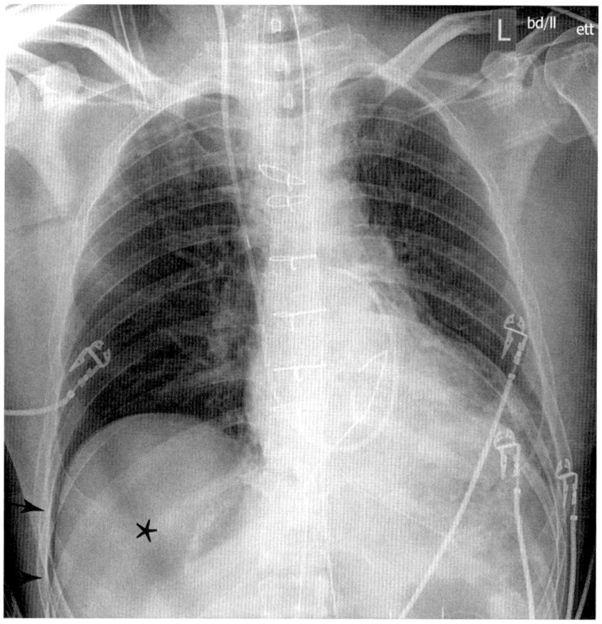

Figure 28.5. Deep sulcus sign. Anteroposterior (AP) supine chest radiograph shows a right basal pneumothorax manifesting as abnormal basal hyperlucency extending inferolaterally into the lateral costophrenic sulcus (deep sulcus sign). A faint visceral pleural line is visible along the lateral chest wall.

sulcus, allowing visualization of the diaphragmatic dome and anterior costophrenic sulcus).
- Ultrasound is increasingly utilized to detect pneumothorax at the bedside in European countries.

Tension Pneumothorax

- Tension pneumothorax is a clinical diagnosis and may show some, all, or none of the following findings:
  - Ipsilateral hemidiaphragm depression or inversion
  - Contralateral mediastinal shift
  - Ipsilateral rib interspace widening
  - Complete lung collapse

Pneumothorax Ex Vacuo

- Most frequently seen with right upper lobe atelectasis but can accompany any sudden lobar collapse (Fig. 28.1).
- Caused by a drop in intrapleural pressure adjacent to a collapsed lobe, which causes air to enter the pleural space from adjacent tissue and blood.
- Pneumothorax ex vacuo resolves with treatment of the lobar collapse and does not require chest tube drainage.
- Trapped lung is similar to pneumothorax ex vacuo and occurs in patients with visceral pleural thickening secondary to chronic pleural effusion. After drainage of the effusion, the lower lobe fails to re-expand, resulting in a basal pneumothorax.

Clinical Issues

- The decision to treat pneumothorax is generally based on patient symptoms and hemodynamic status.

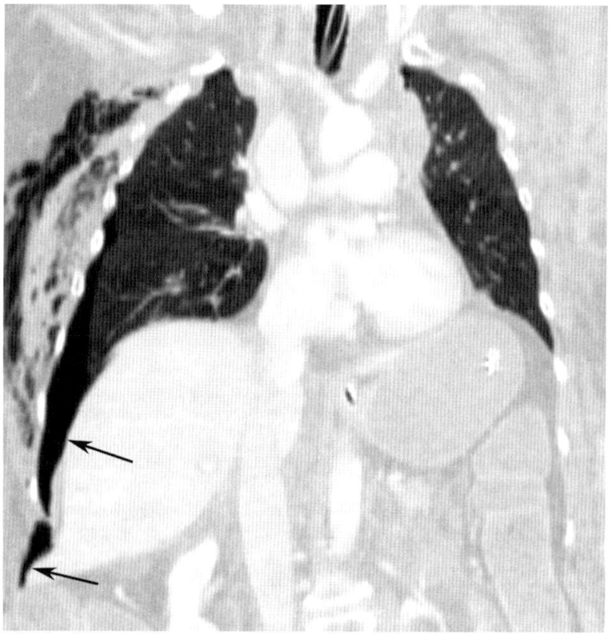

Figure 28.6. Deep sulcus sign. Coronal chest CT shows a pneumothorax extending inferiorly into the right lateral costophrenic sulcus, demonstrating the basis of the radiographic deep sulcus sign (arrow) of pneumothorax in a supine patient. The anteromedial pleural space is the least-dependent portion of the pleural space in a supine patient.

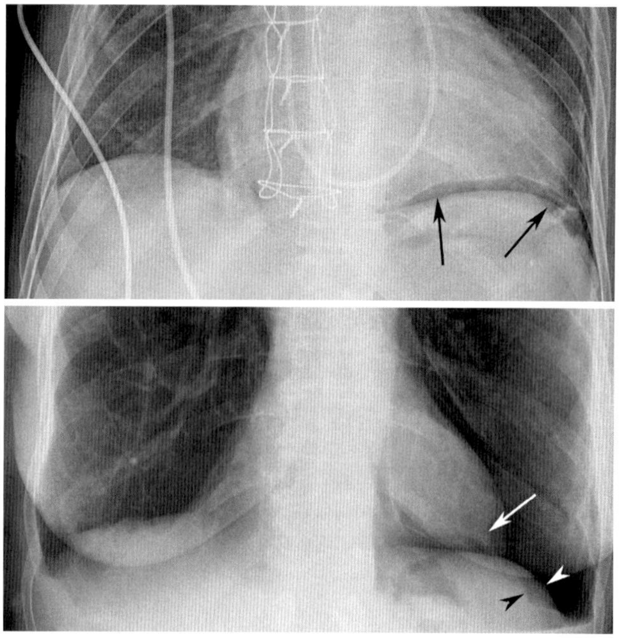

Figure 28.7. Signs of basal pneumothorax. Composite image with PA chest radiographs from two different patients shows left basilar hyperlucency (top; black arrows), mediastinal tag or prominent fat pad (bottom; white arrow), and a double diaphragm sign (bottom; arrowheads).

- A small pneumothorax is often observed and treated with supplemental oxygen, which increases the rate of resorption of air from the pleural space.
- In the setting of trauma or endobronchial intubation, pneumothorax is often treated with chest tube drainage to prevent tension pneumothorax.
- Patients with recurrent pneumothorax may require talc pleurodesis or bullectomy.
- Patients should avoid air travel for at least 6 weeks following resolution of a pneumothorax and should never engage in scuba diving.
- Small changes in pneumothorax size should be interpreted with caution because size may vary up to 1 cm or more based solely on the level of inspiration or on patient rotation.
- Pneumothorax ex vacuo is rare, caused by a sudden drop in intrapleural pressure that may accompany lobar collapse (Fig. 28.1).
- Treatment of pneumothorax ex vacuo is aimed at the lobar collapse; this type of pneumothorax does not require chest tube drainage.

Key Points

- Basal pneumothorax is common in intubated patients and in those who have sustained chest trauma.
- Signs of basal pneumothorax (Fig. 28.7) include increased basal hyperlucency, a sharp outline of the hemidiaphragm and/or mediastinal structures, and the deep sulcus sign (Fig. 28.5).
- Tension pneumothorax is a clinical diagnosis, but suggestive radiographic signs include hemidiaphragm inversion, contralateral mediastinal shift, and rib interspace widening.

Suggested Reading

Fisher JK. Skin fold versus pneumothorax. *AJR Am J Roentgenol.* Apr 1978;130(4):791–792.

Kaewlai R, Avery LL, Asrani AV, Novelline RA. Multidetector CT of blunt thoracic trauma. *RadioGraphics.* Oct 2008; 28(6):1555–1570.

Panicek DM, Randall PA, Witanowski LS, Raasch BN, Heitzman ER. Chest tube tracks. *RadioGraphics.* Mar 1987;7(2):321–342.

Ziter FM, Westcott JL. Supine subpulmonary pneumothorax. *AJR Am J Roentgenol.* Oct 1981;137(4):699–701.

CHAPTER 29

Pleural Effusion

Christopher M. Walker

Definition

Pleural effusion is an abnormal collection of fluid in the pleural space caused by a variety of conditions, including pleural and pulmonary disorders, organ dysfunction, systemic disease, and drug exposure. Pleural effusions are classified clinically as transudative or exudative based on pleural fluid analysis using Light's criteria. Less common causes of pleural effusion include hemothorax, chylothorax, and accidental infusion of parenteral fluid or contrast material (infusothorax).

Clinical Features

Patients with pleural effusion may be asymptomatic or may present with dyspnea, chest pain, cough, or fever. Symptoms may relate to the size of the pleural fluid collection. Symptoms related to the underlying medical condition causing the pleural effusion are often present.

Anatomy and Physiology

Pleural fluid is normally formed in the parietal pleura and reabsorbed by lymphatics in the inferior and medial parietal pleura. Pleural effusion occurs when there is increased fluid production and/or reduced fluid resorption. This may be due to an imbalance between capillary hydrostatic or osmotic pressures, an increase in capillary permeability, or lymphatic obstruction.

Free pleural fluid collects in the most dependent part of the pleural space due to gravity. Lateral decubitus radiography is the most sensitive radiographic examination for detecting small quantities of pleural fluid and may demonstrate effusions as small as 5 ml. The lateral chest radiograph is the next most sensitive examination and can detect effusions of 50 ml or more. The frontal chest radiograph detects a minimum of 200 ml of fluid, and effusions of 500 ml or more may obscure the ipsilateral hemidiaphragm.

A large pleural effusion may cause flattening or even inversion of the adjacent hemidiaphragm, more commonly on the left than on the right—where the liver provides resistance to diaphragmatic inversion. This may be appreciated on radiography by inspecting the liver shadow or by identifying inferior displacement of the gastric bubble. In this setting, the radiographic appearance of a pleural effusion may not change significantly following a large-volume thoracentesis.

How to Approach the Image

The earliest manifestation of pleural effusion on chest radiography is a meniscus sign on the lateral and frontal chest radiographs. Subpulmonic pleural effusion may be present when there is lateral displacement of the apex of the ipsilateral hemidiaphragm. A lateral decubitus chest radiograph, with the affected side down, is the most sensitive radiographic examination for detecting small quantities of pleural fluid.

A large unilateral pleural effusion should suggest malignancy. Contrast-enhanced CT is helpful in diagnosing an exudative effusion and in distinguishing benign from malignant pleural thickening. Ultrasound may be used at the bedside and has been found to be more sensitive than CT in detecting pleural septations and loculations.

What Not to Miss

Pleural effusion is caused by a variety of disorders. It is important to search for associated findings that may provide clues to the underlying cause of the pleural effusion. These include pulmonary embolism, consolidation from pneumonia, lymphadenopathy from lymphoma or malignancy, and pleural nodules or masses from pleural metastasis or mesothelioma.

Differential Diagnosis

Transudative Pleural Effusion

- Low serum protein and lactate dehydrogenase (LDH) content.
- Most commonly occurs in patients with heart failure, cirrhosis, and renal failure.
- Less common causes include pericardial disease, hypoalbuminemia, and pregnancy.

Exudative Pleural Effusion

- High serum protein and LDH content ("inflammatory fluid").

- Most commonly associated with pneumonia (parapneumonic effusion), empyema, malignancy, and pulmonary embolism.
- Less common causes include collagen vascular disease (e.g., lupus and rheumatoid arthritis), asbestos-related pleural effusion, radiation therapy, and endometriosis.

Hemothorax

- Pleural fluid with a hematocrit greater than 50% of blood hematocrit (Fig. 29.1).
- High-attenuation fluid representing acute blood (35–70 HU).
- Usually a result of trauma (penetrating, blunt, or iatrogenic).
- Nontraumatic causes include aortic dissection, ruptured aortic aneurysm, coagulopathy, and thoracic endometriosis.

Chylothorax

- Most commonly occurs from iatrogenic injury to the thoracic duct during thoracic surgery (esophageal > lung) or in patients with malignancy (lymphoma, metastatic cancer, or mediastinal mass). Other causes include blunt or penetrating trauma, mediastinal fibrosis, lymphangioleiomyomatosis, and congenital pulmonary lymphangiectasia.
- Fluid contains a high level of protein and fatty acid.
- Imaging features similar to those of pleural effusion from any cause (cannot reliably distinguish chylous effusion from other pleural effusion based on CT HU).
- Due to its anatomic course, injury to the lower thoracic duct results in a right chylothorax, whereas injury to the upper thoracic duct results in left chylothorax.

Imaging Findings

Findings Favoring an Exudative Effusion

- Parietal pleural thickening and enhancement is typically seen with exudative effusions (sensitivity of 60%).
- Pleural septations indicate an exudative effusion and are better appreciated with ultrasound and MRI than with CT. Septations may be indirectly inferred when multiple locules of air or multiple air–fluid levels are detected within a pleural fluid collection.
- Pleural fluid loculation usually indicates an exudative effusion.
- CT attenuation levels (HU) are not helpful in distinguishing exudative from transudative pleural effusions.

Pleural Effusion in an Upright Patient

- "Meniscus configuration" with concave, upward sloping contour across the costophrenic sulcus on frontal and lateral chest radiographs (Figs. 29.2 and 29.3).

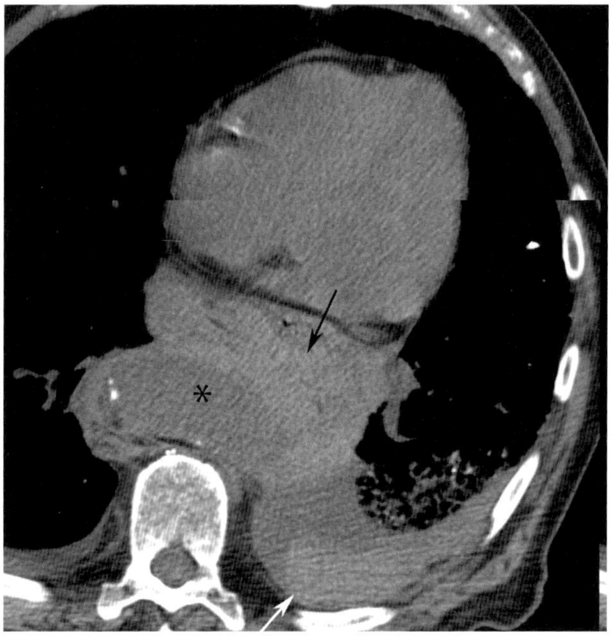

Figure 29.1. Hemothorax and mediastinal hemorrhage. Unenhanced chest CT shows a left pleural fluid collection that exhibits increased attenuation (white arrow) indicating hemothorax. High-attenuation mediastinal hemorrhage (black arrow) is secondary to a ruptured thoracic aortic aneurysm (asterisk).

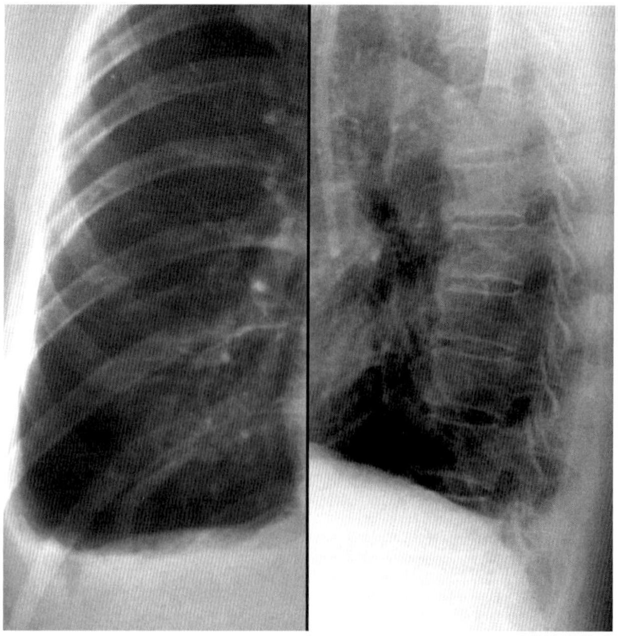

Figure 29.2. Bilateral small pleural effusions (upright patient). Composite image with posteroanterior (PA) (left) and lateral (right) chest radiographs shows a meniscus of pleural fluid in the costophrenic sulcus. Free pleural fluid typically manifests with a meniscus configuration in upright chest radiography.

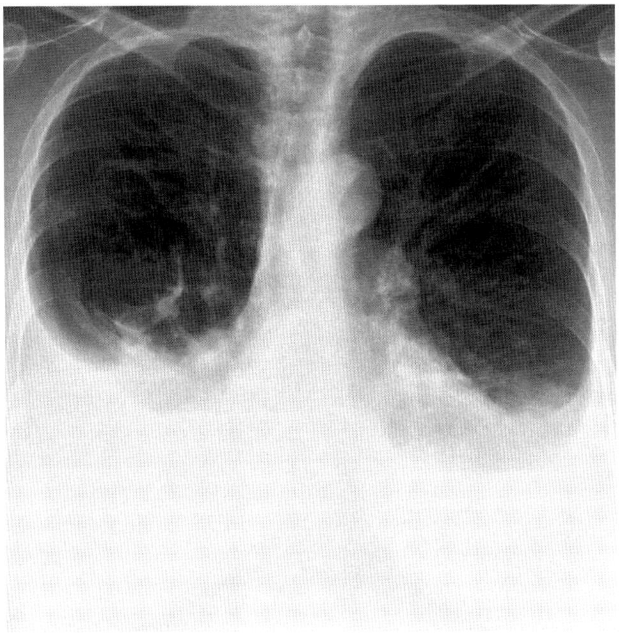

Figure 29.3. Bilateral moderate pleural effusions (upright patient). PA chest radiograph shows bilateral dense opacities with hazy upper borders and meniscus configuration that obscures both hemidiaphragms, the heart borders, and the costophrenic sulci. The effusions cause relaxation (compressive) atelectasis of both lung bases.

- Loculated pleural effusion manifests with more defined convex borders, sometimes within the hazy opacity of surrounding free pleural fluid (Fig. 29.4).

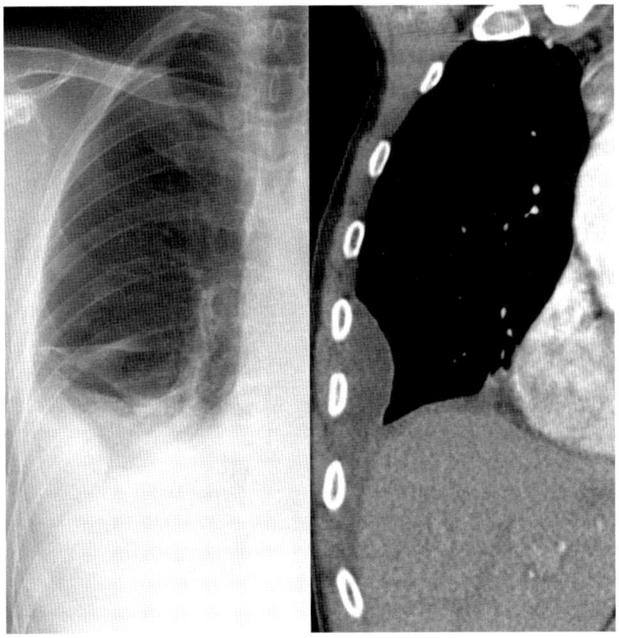

Figure 29.4. Loculated pleural effusion. Composite image with PA chest radiography (left) and coronal chest CT (right) shows the more defined convex border of a loculated pleural effusion within the hazy opacity of an adjacent free right basilar pleural effusion. CT shows the characteristic lenticular shape of loculated pleural fluid, with inferior extension of fluid deep in the lateral costophrenic sulcus.

Pleural Effusion in a Supine Patient

- Homogeneous increased opacity (veil-like) over affected hemithorax with normal visibility of bronchovascular structures through the opacity.
- Apical pleural "cap" (the apical pleural space is the most dependent portion of the pleural space in a supine patient).
- Elevation or loss of contour of ipsilateral hemidia phragm.
- Blunt lateral costophrenic sulcus.
- Decreased visibility of lower lobe vasculature through ipsilateral hemidiaphragm.
- Thick minor fissure.
- Supine chest radiography may miss approximately 35% of all pleural effusions; when a pleural effusion is detected, its size is often underestimated.

Subpulmonic Pleural Effusion

- Lateral displacement of the apex of the hemidiaphragm (i.e., the diaphragm is in its normal position but appears elevated by overlying subpulmonic pleural fluid) (Fig. 29.5).
- Pulmonary vessels are not visible through the pseudodiaphragmatic contour.
- Left-sided subpulmonic effusions may manifest as increased distance between the gastric air bubble and the pseudodiaphragmatic contour (more readily detected when comparison films are available).
- Pseudodiaphragmatic contour has a flattened contour posteriorly on the lateral radiograph and then slants

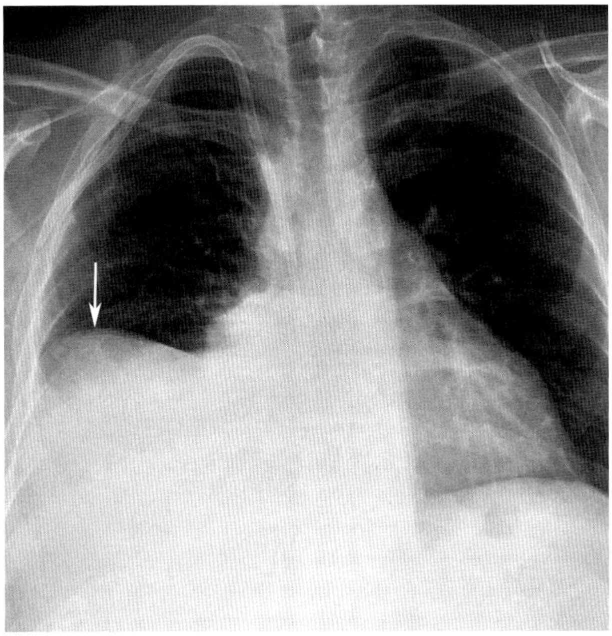

Figure 29.5. Subpulmonic pleural effusion. AP chest radiograph shows apparent elevation of the right hemidiaphragm (pseudodiaphragm formed by caudal lung resting on the pleural fluid collection) with lateral displacement of the apex of the pseudohemidiaphragm (arrow).

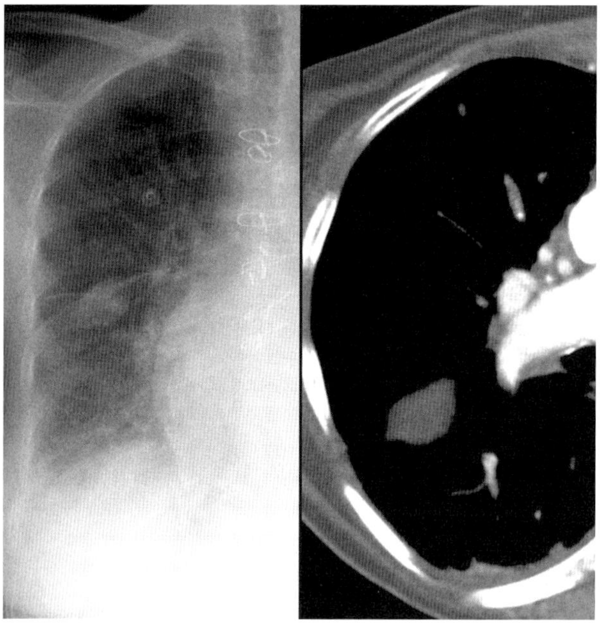

Figure 29.6. Pseudotumor (supine patient). Composite image with anteroposterior (AP) supine chest radiograph (left) and contrast-enhanced chest CT (right) shows a well-defined lenticular opacity within the right major fissure on radiography that correlates with a lenticular fluid attenuation collection on CT. The free pleural effusion manifests as a faint veil-like opacity in the right hemithorax with normal visibility of overlying bronchovascular structures.

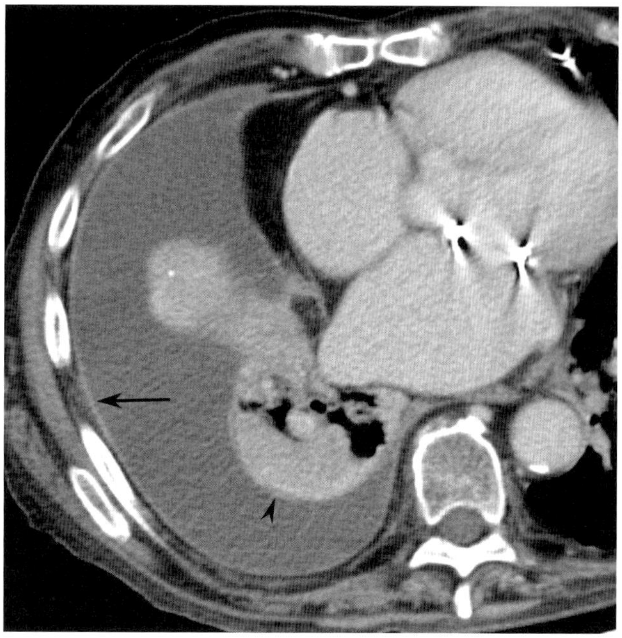

Figure 29.7. Exudative effusion. Axial contrast-enhanced CT shows abnormal parietal (arrow) and visceral (arrowhead) pleura thickening and enhancement in a patient with a malignant pleural effusion. Thickening and enhancement of the parietal pleura indicates the presence of an exudative effusion and must be correlated with clinical findings to establish an accurate diagnosis.

abruptly downward at its interface with the major fissure, with fluid often extending into the major fissure.

Loculated Pleural Effusion

- Lenticular or elliptical fluid collection; often in a nondependent location; may exhibit septations (Figs. 29.4 and 29.6).
- Fluid accumulated in an interlobar fissure may or may not be loculated.
- Fluid trapped within the fissure may mimic a lung neoplasm (pseudotumor).
- Pleural pseudotumor does not necessarily indicate a loculated pleural effusion because fluid may be pulled into a nondependent location within the fissure caused by the elastic recoil of lung toward the hilum.

Unilateral Large Pleural Effusion

- Homogeneous opacification of a hemithorax with contralateral mediastinal shift and inferior displacement of ipsilateral hemidiaphragm.
- Differential diagnosis of a large unilateral pleural effusion includes malignant pleural effusion, empyema, hemothorax, and chylothorax (Fig. 29.7).

Clinical Issues

- Treatment of pleural effusion is usually directed at the underlying cause. In patients with heart failure, diuretic therapy and salt restriction are generally sufficient.

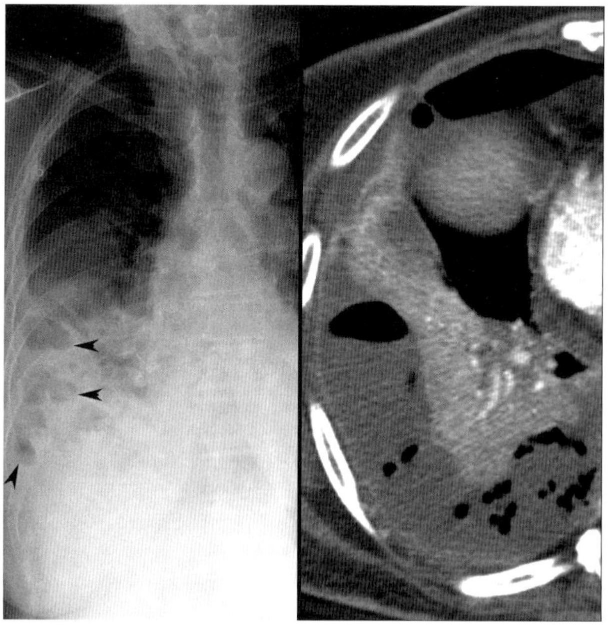

Figure 29.8. Empyema with bronchopleural fistula. Composite image with PA chest radiograph (left) and contrast-enhanced chest CT (right) shows opacification over the mid and lower right hemithorax with multiple air–fluid levels (arrowheads). CT shows parietal pleural thickening and enhancement and a loculated pleural effusion with multiple air collections from bronchopleural fistula. The air collections are separated by septations not directly visualized on CT.

- Ultrasound is increasingly used to guide therapeutic and diagnostic thoracentesis, lowering the risk of complications such as pneumothorax and organ injury.
- Occasionally, large pleural effusions and those occurring after surgery may require chest tube drainage.
- Recurrent pleural effusions may require chemical pleurodesis or insertion of a long-term indwelling pleural catheter.

Key Points

- Parietal pleural thickening and enhancement almost always indicates the presence of an exudative pleural effusion.
- Heart failure most commonly causes bilateral or right-sided pleural effusions. A unilateral left-sided pleural effusion should suggest an alternate diagnosis.
- The differential diagnosis of a large, unilateral pleural effusion includes malignant pleural effusion, empyema, hemothorax, and chylothorax.
- Air in a pleural fluid collection suggests the presence of a bronchopleural fistula, unless a recent thoracentesis has been attempted or performed (Fig. 29.8).
- Ultrasound is more sensitive than CT in detecting loculations and septations in a pleural fluid collection.

Suggested Reading

Aquino SL, Webb WR, Gushiken BJ. Pleural exudates and transudates: Diagnosis with contrast-enhanced CT. *Radiology*. Sep 1994;192(3):803–808.

Blackmore CC, Black WC, Dallas RV, Crow HC. Pleural fluid volume estimation: A chest radiograph prediction rule. *Acad Radiol*. Feb 1996;3(2):103–109.

Federle MP, Mark AS, Guillaumin ES. CT of subpulmonic pleural effusions and atelectasis: Criteria for differentiation from subphrenic fluid. *AJR Am J Roentgenol*. Apr 1986;146(4):685–689.

Halvorsen RA, Fedyshin PJ, Korobkin M, Foster WL, Thompson WM. Ascites or pleural effusion? CT differentiation: Four useful criteria. *RadioGraphics*. Jan 1986;6(1):135–149.

Maskell NA, Butland RJ; Pleural Diseases Group, British Thoracic Society. BTS guidelines for the investigation of a unilateral pleural effusion in adults. *Thorax*. May 2003;58(Suppl 2):ii8–ii17.

Raasch BN, Carsky EW, Lane EJ, O'Callaghan JP, Heitzman ER. Pleural effusion: Explanation of some typical appearances. *AJR Am J Roentgenol*. Nov 1982;139(5):899–904.

Stark DD, Federle MP, Goodman PC, Podrasky AE, Webb WR. Differentiating lung abscess and empyema: Radiography and computed tomography. *AJR Am J Roentgenol*. Jul 1983;141(1):163–167.

CHAPTER 30

Empyema

Christopher M. Walker

Definition

Empyema (syn. pyothorax) represents the accumulation of pus or an abscess in the pleural space. The evolution of empyema occurs in three stages (exudative, fibropurulent, and organizing) that form a continuous spectrum.

Clinical Features

Most patients with empyema have symptoms referable to pneumonia (cough, fever, chest pain, and shortness of breath). Occasionally, empyema is unassociated with pneumonia and occurs in patients with traumatic injuries.

Patients with chronic empyema—often caused by anaerobic infection—may have no pulmonary symptoms but may instead present with anemia and weight loss.

Anatomy and Physiology

Pneumonia may irritate the visceral pleura, causing increased capillary permeability and an exudative pleural effusion. Pleural fluid in the first (exudative) stage of empyema (i.e., simple parapneumonic effusion) is generally free flowing, culture-negative, and has normal pH and glucose levels. If the patient does not seek treatment or receives inadequate therapy, the pleural effusion may progress to the fibropurulent stage, in which pleural fluid is typically thicker, culture-positive, has low pH and glucose levels, and becomes progressively more difficult to treat due to increasing loculation (Figs. 30.1 and 30.2). If inadequately treated, empyema may progress to the organizing stage in which fibroblasts enter the collection from the visceral and parietal pleura to deposit collagen and produce a thick pleural rind that may encase the lung and prevent normal lung expansion (Figs. 30.3 and 30.4).

How to Approach the Image

Associated pleural effusion should always be excluded in patients with radiographic evidence of pneumonia. Lateral decubitus radiography may be useful for identifying

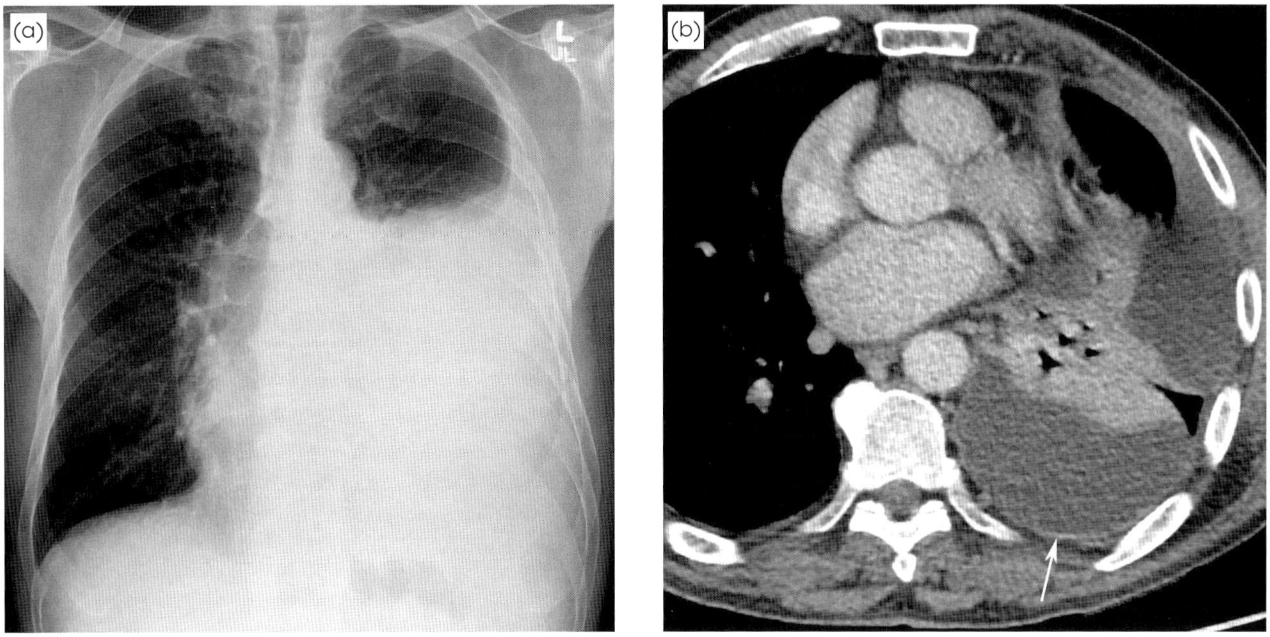

Figure 30.1. Empyema (tuberculosis). (a) PA chest radiograph shows a large left pleural effusion with mass effect on the heart and mediastinum. (b) Contrast-enhanced chest CT of the same patient shows a multiloculated left pleural effusion with parietal pleural thickening (arrow) indicating the effusion is exudative. There is no split pleura sign, a finding absent in approximately half of all empyemas.

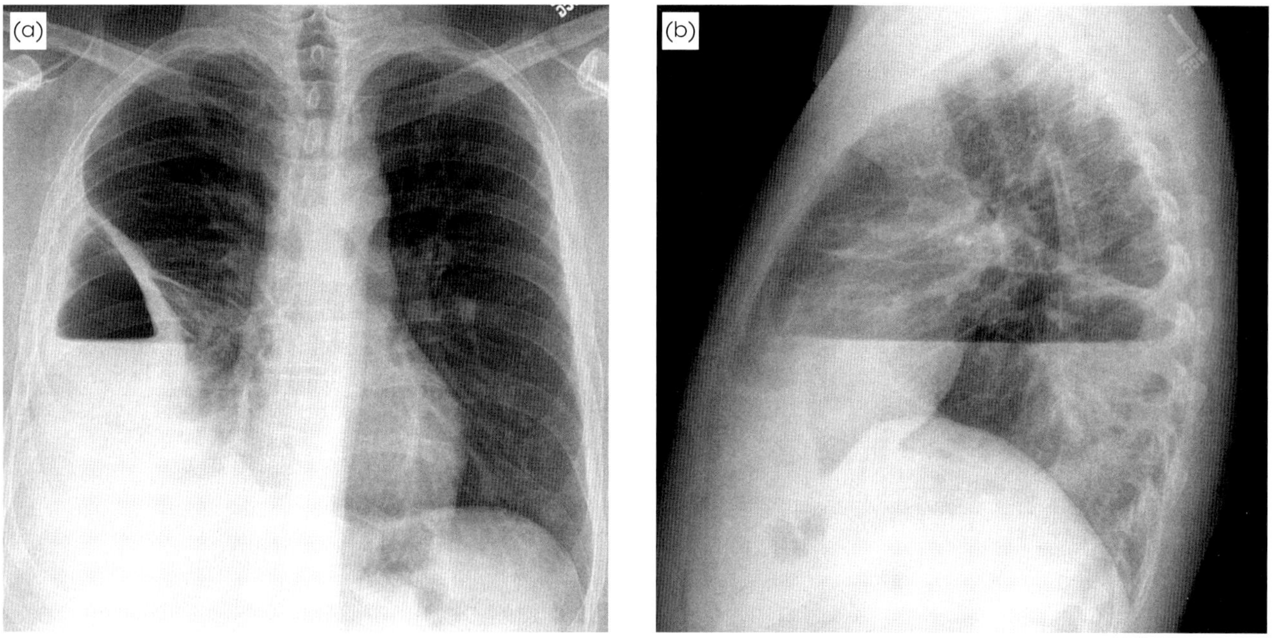

Figure 30.2. Empyema with bronchopleural fistula. (a) PA chest radiograph shows a large loculated right pleural effusion that contains an air–fluid level and compresses the adjacent lung. (b) Lateral chest radiograph of the same patient shows marked disparity between the air–fluid level lengths shown on the lateral radiograph compared to the PA, a finding consistent with empyema rather than lung abscess.

free-flowing pleural fluid and offering clinicians the option of performing thoracentesis. A pleural effusion must be greater than 1 cm in thickness on lateral decubitus radiography before thoracentesis will be attempted by most clinicians.

Pleural effusions should be evaluated for loculations or septations because this may change the method used for pleural fluid drainage. Ultrasound and CT are useful modalities to guide therapeutic and diagnostic thoracentesis.

What Not to Miss

Consider CT and/or ultrasound to evaluate patients with suboptimal response to chest tube drainage of pleural effusions. Both modalities can identify malpositioned chest tubes or undrained fluid collections that may explain a patient's persistent fever or leukocytosis.

Differential Diagnosis

Pneumonia with Parapneumonic Effusion (Exudative Stage)

- 20–40% of hospitalized patients with pneumonia have a parapneumonic pleural effusion.
- Parapneumonic pleural effusions are associated with a higher mortality rate.

Empyema (Fibropurulent Stage)

- Infected pleural fluid collections are usually seen in association with pneumonia.
- Such pleural effusions may progress from the fibropurulent to the organizing stage (i.e., thick pleural rind) within days to weeks.

Exudative Effusion Without Infection

- Exudative effusion from any cause may exhibit the "split pleura sign" or parietal pleural thickening and enhancement on CT. The split pleura sign is not diagnostic of empyema but, rather, indicates an effusion is exudative.
- Other imaging findings may suggest an alternate diagnosis (e.g., lung mass in lung cancer, bilateral pulmonary nodules in metastatic disease, or pericardial thickening/enhancement in Dressler syndrome).

Peripheral Lung Abscess

- Must be distinguished from empyema because lung abscess is generally treated with antibiotics, not by drainage.
- Imaging features that favor lung abscess include (1) spherical shape, (2) ill-defined borders, (3) thick irregular or ill-defined wall, and (4) engulfment of pulmonary vessels and bronchi (Fig. 30.3b).
- Air–fluid level length in a spherical cavitary lung abscess is typically equal on posteroanterior (PA) and lateral radiographs, in contrast to a characteristic disparity in length on orthogonal radiography in patients with empyema and bronchopleural fistula.

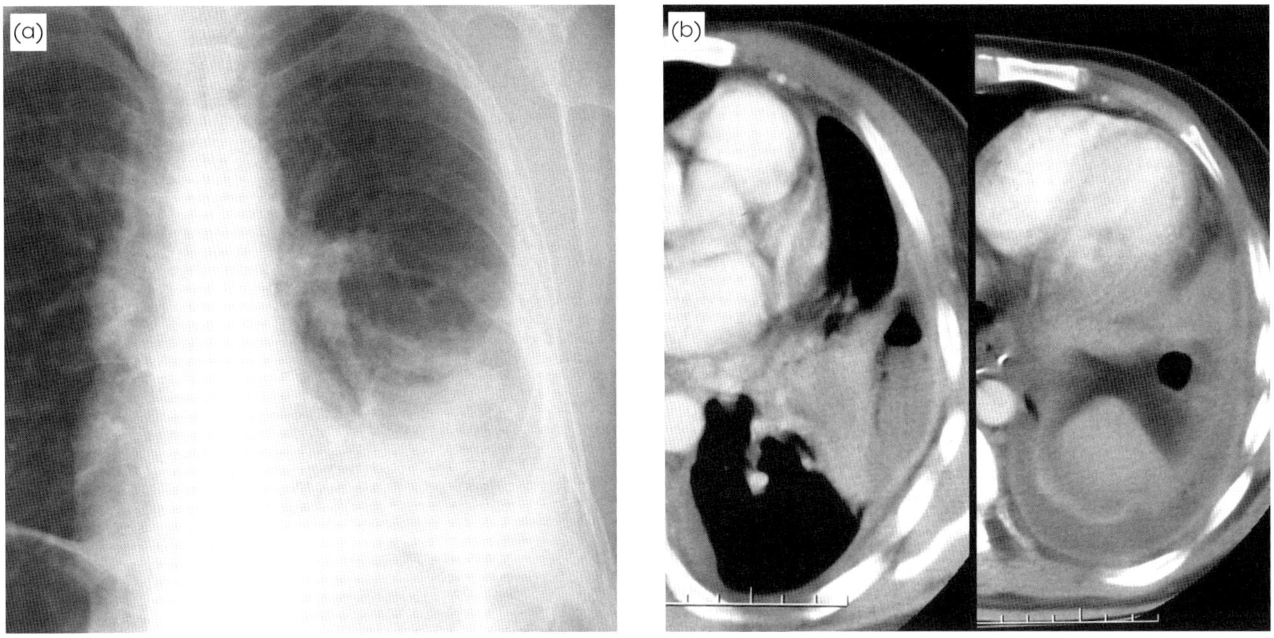

Figure 30.3. Empyema with bronchopleural fistula. (a) Coned-down PA chest radiograph shows a left pleural effusion with a subtle air–fluid level along its upper aspect suggestive of empyema and bronchopleural fistula. (b) Composite image of the same patient with contrast-enhanced chest CT shows thickening and enhancement of costal (left) and visceral (right) pleura separated or "split" by a loculated lenticular empyema (split pleura sign). Subtle low attenuation in the atelectatic left lower lobe (left) represented a lung abscess. Air within the loculated pleural fluid is due to bronchopleural fistula. The split pleura sign is suggestive—but not diagnostic of—an empyema.

Imaging Findings

Simple Parapneumonic Effusion

- Small to moderate-sized dependent pleural effusion without loculation
- Meniscus-shaped on radiography and crescent-shaped on CT
- May manifest on CT as thickening and enhancement of visceral and parietal pleura

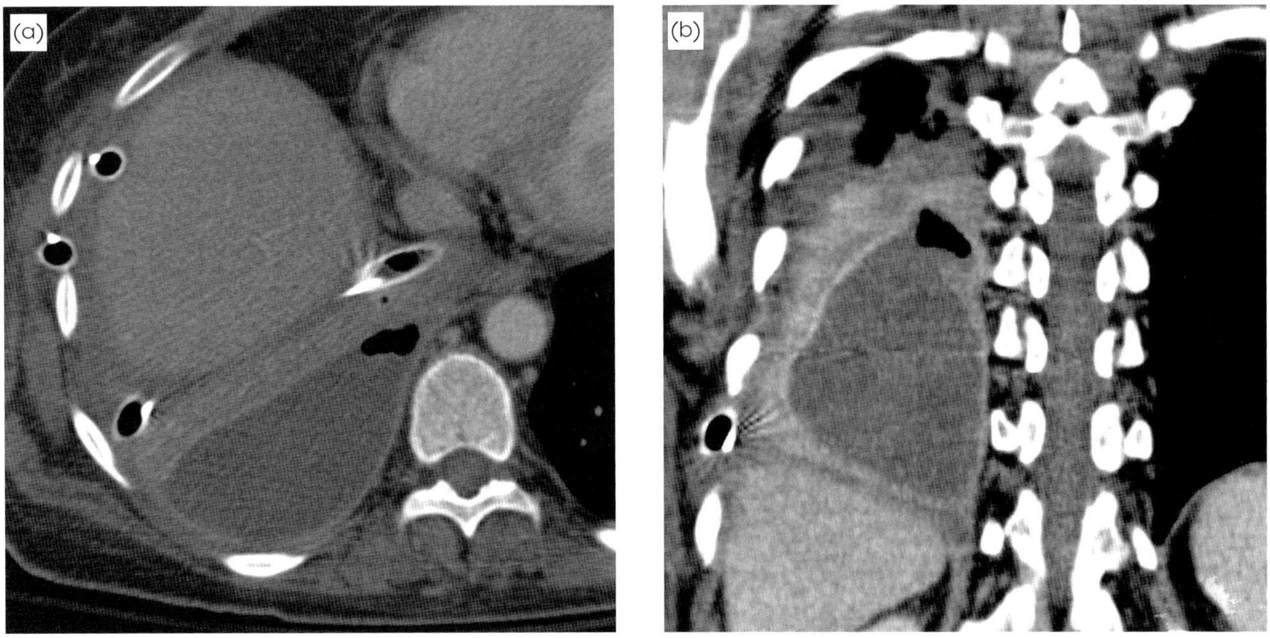

Figure 30.4. Empyema, split pleura sign. (a) Contrast-enhanced chest CT shows a right pleural effusion surrounded by thickened and enhancing visceral and parietal pleura. A right chest tube introduced air into the pleural fluid collection. (b) Coronal contrast-enhanced chest CT of the same patient shows thick, enhancing visceral and parietal pleura surrounding the pleural fluid collection, the split pleura sign—a CT imaging finding that is suggestive of empyema.

Empyema

- Loculated small to large pleural effusion
- May or may not be associated with pneumonia
- Most manifest with smooth pleural thickening and pleural enhancement surrounding loculated pleural fluid; displacement and compression of adjacent lung (Figs. 30.3 and 30.4)
- 50% exhibit split pleura sign (i.e., parietal and visceral pleural thickening and enhancement surrounding a pleural fluid collection) (Figs. 30.3 and 30.4)
- Pleural septations not typically seen on CT but may be inferred when multiple locules of air or multiple air–fluid levels are present within the pleural space
- Thickening and increased attenuation of adjacent extrapleural fat on CT

Complications of Empyema

- *Bronchopleural fistula* should be suspected when locules of air or air–fluid levels occur within a pleural effusion (in the absence of recent pleural intervention). The underlying fistulous communication with lung or bronchus is not usually seen on CT. Gas-forming organisms could theoretically produce air within the pleural space, but that phenomenon is exceedingly rare.
- *Empyema necessitatis or necessitans* represents chest wall involvement by empyema and most commonly occurs in those caused by tuberculosis. (A useful mnemonic for recalling infections that may cross fascial planes is BATMAN: *b*lastomycosis, *a*ctinomycosis, *Mycobacterium tuberculosis*, *m*ucormycosis, *a*spergillosis, and *n*ocardiosis.)
- *"Trapped" lung* is characterized by the inability of lung to expand when encased by a restricting fibrous rind of thickened visceral pleura. It most commonly occurs in the setting of an inadequately treated empyema.
- *Malignant transformation* is a rare complication of chronic empyema that may occur with long-standing inflammation (>5 years). Associated malignancies include lymphoma, squamous cell carcinoma, mesothelioma, and sarcoma. Malignant transformation is most commonly associated with chronic tuberculous empyema and should be considered in the differential diagnosis when imaging shows a new soft tissue mass or chest wall extension associated with an empyema.

Clinical Issues

- Pneumonia with complicated parapneumonic effusion or empyema generally requires percutaneous or open pleural drainage in addition to systemic antibiotics.
- Simple parapneumonic effusion is treated conservatively with antibiotics directed toward treating underlying pneumonia.
- Symptomatic organized empyema and trapped lung are usually treated with surgical decortication that involves stripping the fibrous pleural peel from the surface of the lung.
- Distinguishing empyema from lung abscess is important because their treatments are different. Empyema is treated with percutaneous chest tube drainage, whereas lung abscess is treated with antibiotics alone.

Key Points

- The lateral decubitus radiograph is helpful for identifying a free pleural effusion.
- The "split pleura sign" is specific for an exudative effusion and may indicate the presence of an empyema in the correct clinical setting.
- Consider bronchopleural fistula when locules of air or air–fluid levels are seen within an empyema in the absence of prior intervention.
- Imaging features favoring empyema include an elliptical shape, smooth borders, discrepant air–fluid level length on orthogonal chest radiographs, displacement of bronchovascular structures, and the split pleura sign
- Imaging features favoring abscess include a spherical shape, thick and irregular wall, similar air–fluid level length on orthogonal chest radiographs, and engulfment of underlying bronchovascular structures.
- Organized empyema with trapped lung is not effectively treated with tube drainage and usually requires decortication.

Suggested Reading

Kuhlman JE, Singha NK. Complex disease of the pleural space: Radiographic and CT evaluation. *RadioGraphics*. 1997 Jan–Feb 1997;17(1):63–79.

Light RW. Parapneumonic effusions and empyema. *Proc Am Thorac Soc*. 2006;3(1):75–80.

Minami M, Kawauchi N, Yoshikawa K, et al. Malignancy associated with chronic empyema: Radiologic assessment. *Radiology*. Feb 1991;178(2):417–423.

Stark DD, Federle MP, Goodman PC, Podrasky AE, Webb WR. Differentiating lung abscess and empyema: Radiography and computed tomography. *AJR Am J Roentgenol*. Jul 1983;141(1):163–167.

Waite RJ, Carbonneau RJ, Balikian JP, Umali CB, Pezzella AT, Nash G. Parietal pleural changes in empyema: Appearances at CT. *Radiology*. Apr 1990;175(1):145–150.

CHAPTER 31

Pleural Thickening and Calcification

Christopher M. Walker

Definition

The normal pleura is only a few cell layers thick and is barely visible on standard imaging. Pleural thickening may be visible on chest radiography and readily visualized on cross-sectional imaging. Malignant pleural thickening should be distinguished from benign causes of pleural thickening. This chapter focuses on benign causes of pleural thickening and calcification. Malignant pleural thickening is discussed elsewhere.

Clinical Features

Patients with conditions that manifest with benign focal pleural thickening or multifocal nodularity are often asymptomatic. Patients with diffuse pleural thickening may present with dyspnea, cough, and restrictive lung physiology on pulmonary function testing.

Anatomy and Physiology

Several normal anatomic structures may be mistaken for pleural thickening on cross-sectional imaging. The transversus thoracis muscle is almost always seen beneath the anterior second through sixth ribs and costochondral junctions, where it attaches to the sternum. The subcostalis muscle is located at the same levels but is seen beneath the posterior ribs. Unlike pleural thickening or pleural plaque, these muscles are bilaterally symmetric, of uniform thickness, and only a few millimeters thick. Intercostal veins travel adjacent to the vertebral bodies and may be confidently identified when they opacify with contrast or are seen to drain into the azygos or hemiazygos veins.

How to Approach the Image

Pleural thickening should be characterized as focal or diffuse. Benign pleural thickening must be differentiated from malignant pleural thickening. Benign diffuse pleural thickening most commonly follows either empyema (Fig. 31.1) or hemothorax. Several imaging findings associated with pleural thickening suggest benignity, including adjacent healed rib fractures (Fig. 31.2) and pleural calcification. Pleural plaques commonly produce multifocal discontinuous pleural thickening and almost always indicate a history of occupational asbestos exposure (Figs. 31.3–31.5).

What Not to Miss

- Malignant pleural thickening should not be mistaken for a benign condition.
- Pleural thickening should be assessed for the four CT features of malignant pleural thickening.
- If a specific diagnosis cannot be made, short-interval follow-up imaging should be performed or the finding should be assessed with FDG-PET imaging or needle biopsy.

Differential Diagnosis

Extrapleural Fat

- Common finding along lateral chest wall (Fig. 31.6)
- Usually bilateral and symmetric
- Distinguished from pleural thickening by its smooth, wavy borders; its sparing of the costophrenic angle pleura; and the absence of adjacent lung scarring or atelectasis

Pleural Plaque

- Most common manifestation of asbestos exposure (Figs. 31.3–31.5)
- Occur 15–20 years following first exposure
- Asbestos fibers reach the parietal pleural from the lung and incite an inflammatory reaction causing hyaline pleural fibrosis
- Affected patients are asymptomatic, and there is no risk of malignant degeneration.

Diffuse Pleural Thickening

- Usually follows or is associated with hemothorax, empyema, connective tissue diseases, and asbestos exposure (Fig. 31.2)
- Caused by an inflammatory pleuritis that fuses the visceral and parietal pleura
- Affected patients may have restrictive lung physiology.

Pleural Mouse

- Synonyms: fibrin body, fibrin ball, thoracolith, and pleural stone
- Exudative pleural effusion or resolving hemothorax may leave behind a fibrin clot within the pleural space that resembles a solitary nodule.

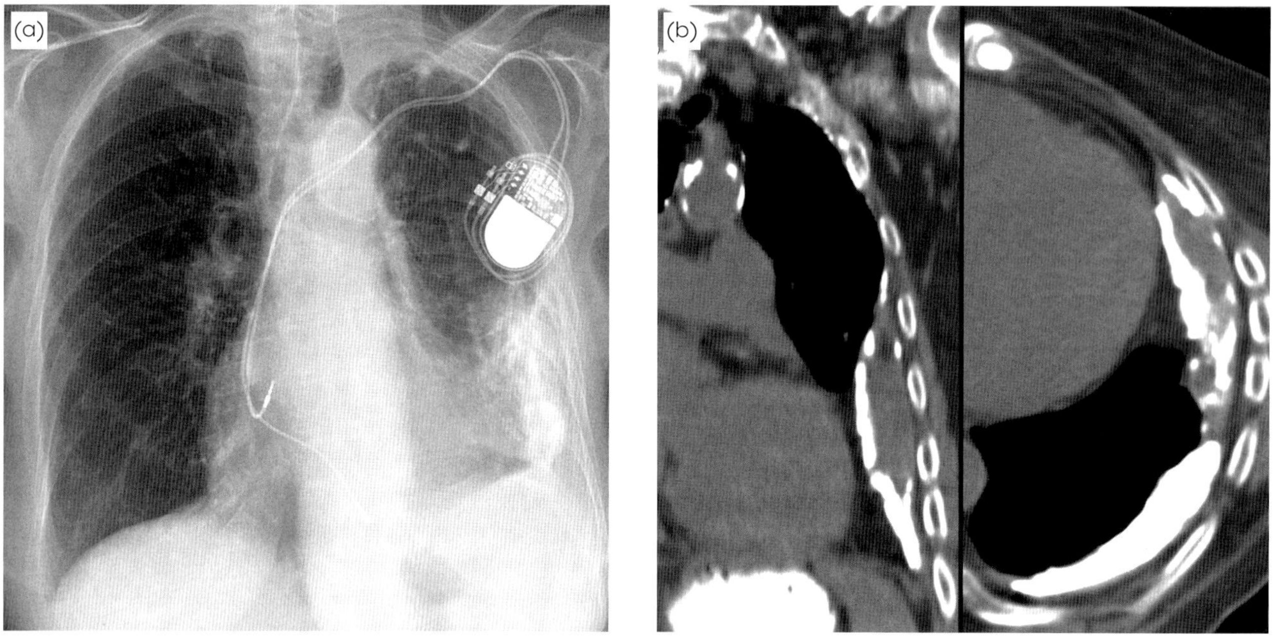

Figure 31.1 Fibrothorax (healed empyema). (a) Posteroanterior (PA) chest radiograph shows thickening and calcification of the left mid to lower pleura with associated left basilar volume loss. (b) Composite image with unenhanced coronal (left) and axial (right) chest CT shows extensive pleural thickening with calcification resulting from a healed empyema. The coronal image demonstrates the lenticular shape characteristic of pleural masses (e.g., loculated effusion, healed empyema, and pleural mass). The underlying lung parenchyma was displaced (not shown) by the healed, calcified empyema, a characteristic CT feature of pleural masses of any nature.

- The clot may calcify and is often mobile within the pleural space.
- May resolve, remain stable, or enlarge over time
- May be solitary or multiple

Thoracic Splenosis

- Autotransplantation of splenic tissue into the pleural space following traumatic injury (penetrating > blunt)
- Splenic tissue gains access through a diaphragmatic tear or congenital defect.

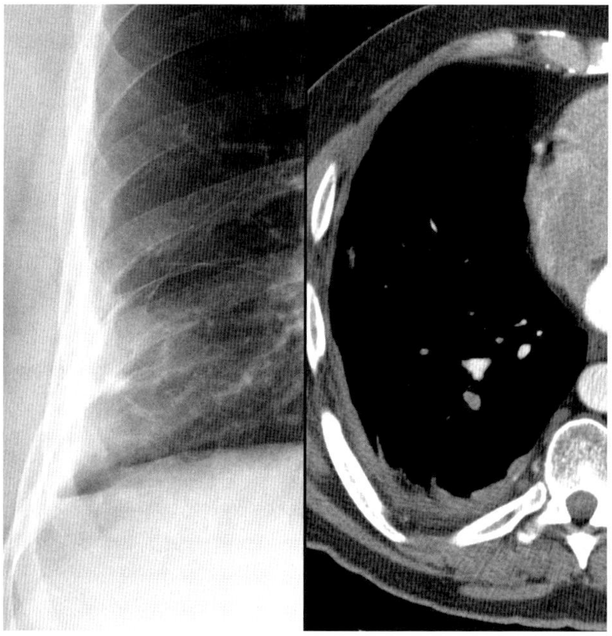

Figure 31.2 Pleural thickening, post-traumatic. Composite image with PA chest radiograph (left) and contrast-enhanced axial chest CT (right) shows a continuous band of pleural thickening extending along the lateral, posterior, and medial aspects of the right lower hemithorax adjacent to a healed rib fracture related to remote trauma. Post-traumatic pleural thickening may result from blunt or penetrating thoracic trauma or iatrogenic causes (e.g., thoracotomy).

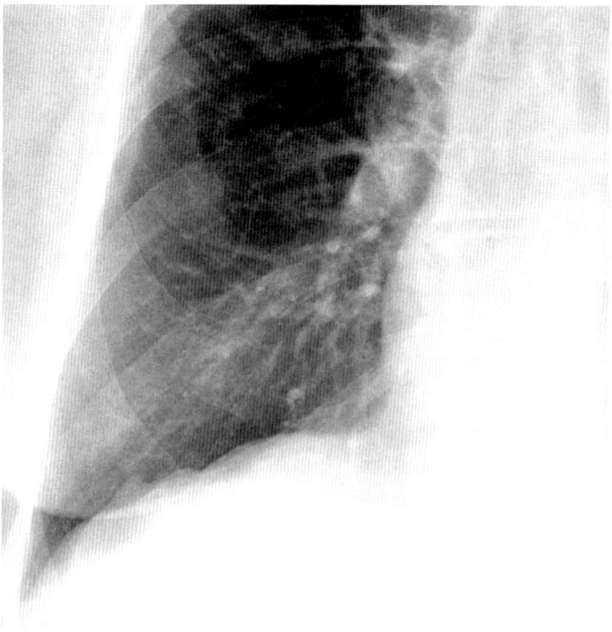

Figure 31.3 Pleural plaques, noncalcified. Coned-down PA chest radiograph shows indistinct nodular opacities that exhibit the incomplete border sign and represent noncalcified pleural plaques in a characteristic distribution along rib margins. Pleural plaques occur most commonly in asbestos-exposed individuals 15–20 years after exposure.

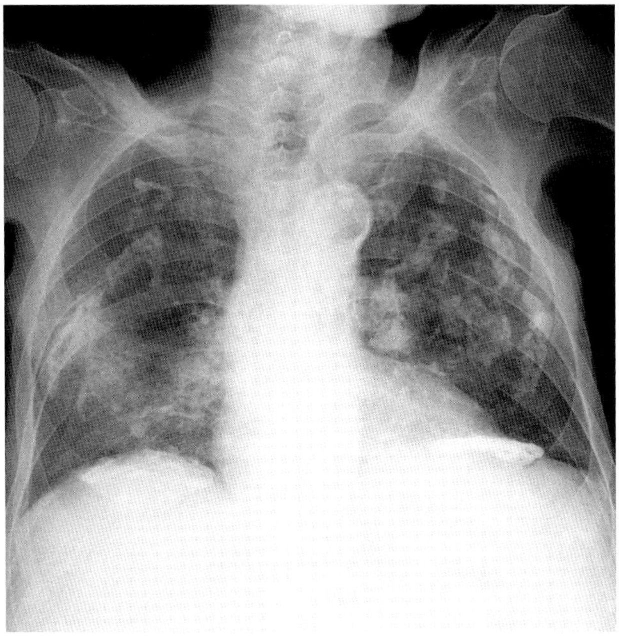

Figure 31.4 Pleural plaques, calcified. PA chest radiograph shows extensive multifocal calcified pleural plaques in a characteristic distribution along the costal and diaphragmatic pleural surfaces, obscuring most of the underlying lung parenchyma. The patient had an occupational history of asbestos exposure.

- Affected patients are generally asymptomatic but may rarely present with hemoptysis.

Extrapleural Hematoma

- Most common in elderly men following blunt or iatrogenic trauma

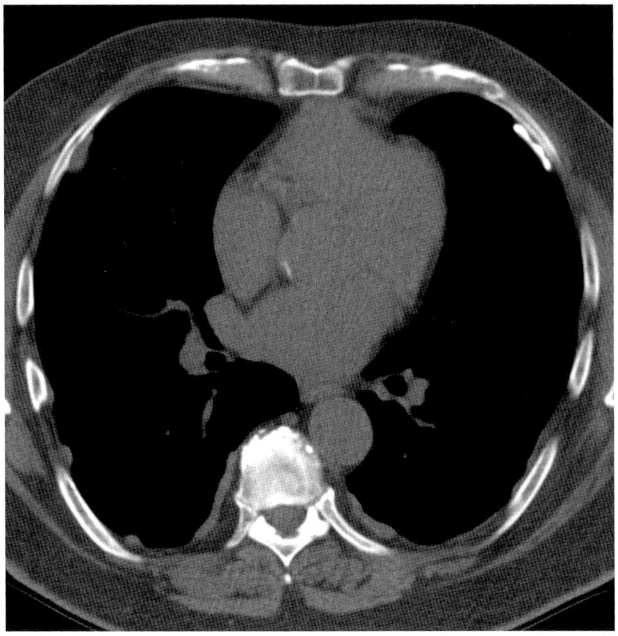

Figure 31.5 Pleural plaques (CT). Unenhanced chest CT shows calcified and noncalcified pleural plaques, manifesting as discontinuous pleural thickening and nodularity, some of which exhibit an elongated morphology along the inner rib surfaces. The patient had a documented occupational history of asbestos exposure.

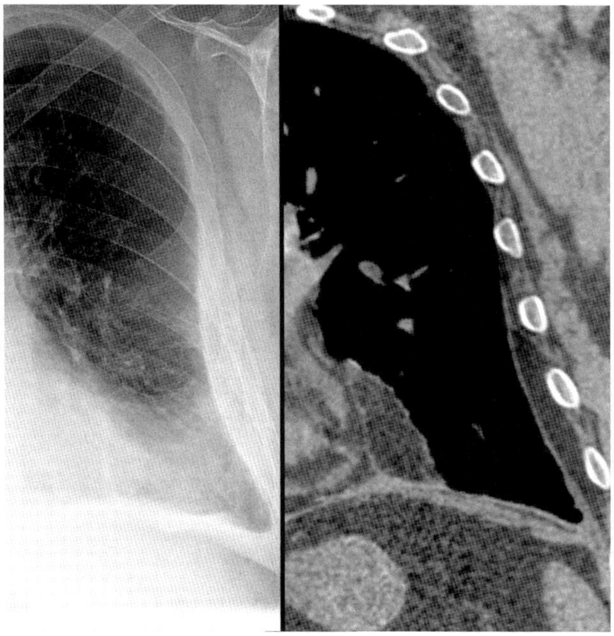

Figure 31.6 Extrapleural fat mimics pleural thickening. Composite image with PA radiograph (left) and coronal unenhanced chest CT (right) shows smooth extrapleural fat deposition along the lateral chest wall that is distinguished from pleural thickening by its symmetric appearance compared to the opposite hemithorax (not shown), sparing of the costophrenic sulci, and the absence of adjacent parenchymal scarring or atelectasis.

- Vascular disruption with an intact parietal pleura allows blood to remain in the extrapleural space rather than causing hemothorax.
- High-density fluid collection inwardly displaces the extrapleural fat (extrapleural fat sign).
- Often associated with rib fracture(s)
- Biconvex hematoma is suggestive of arterial bleeding and may require surgery or percutaneous embolization.
- Nonconvex hematoma is suggestive of venous bleeding and may be treated conservatively.

Talc Pleurodesis

- Talc may be instilled into the pleural space to treat recurrent pleural effusion or pneumothorax (Fig. 31.7).
- Talc is a chemical irritant that causes pleural inflammation and fibrosis.
- Mimics pleural calcification given its high density
- Often clumps posteriorly in the dependent pleural space and may be transported to mediastinal lymph nodes causing high attenuation
- Causes intense FDG uptake in the pleura that may persist for more than a decade following the procedure

Erdheim–Chester Disease

- Rare non-Langerhans cell histiocytosis
- Majority of patients have osseous manifestations consisting of symmetric long bone sclerosis most commonly in the distal femoral metadiaphyses

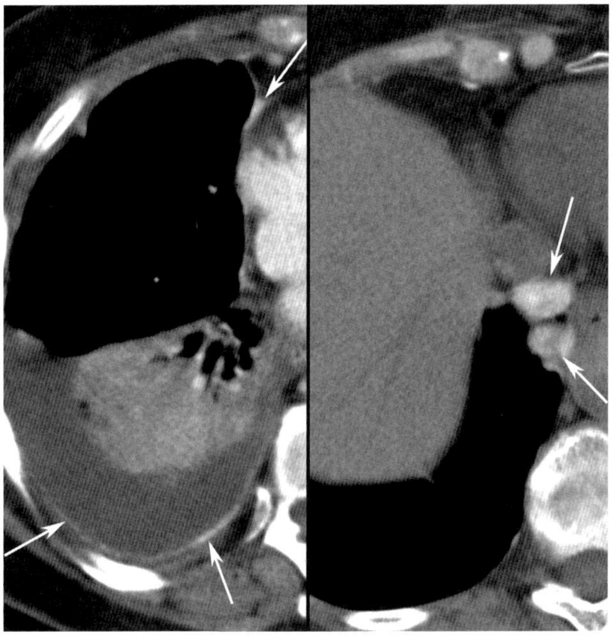

Figure 31.7 Talc pleurodesis. Composite image with contrast-enhanced chest CT of a patient 1 year status post talc pleurodesis shows linear high attenuation along the right posteroinferior parietal pleural surface (left; arrows) adjacent to a chronic right malignant pleural effusion. Talc may be transported to regional lymph nodes that may become hyperdense (right; arrows).

- Extraosseous disease manifests in approximately half of affected patients and may affect nearly any organ (pulmonary involvement in 14–23%).

Imaging Findings

Pleural Plaques

- Predilection for diaphragmatic pleura, undersurface of lower posterolateral ribs at costal margin (Figs. 31.3–31.5)
- Always spare the apical and costophrenic sulci pleura; occasionally seen in the visceral pleura of the interlobar fissures.

Radiography

- Localized, sharply marginated calcified pleural thickening with geographic configuration
- Plaques may resemble a holly leaf when viewed en face.
- Approximately 15–20% of plaques calcify, with more plaques calcifying with advancing age.

CT

- Bilateral, multifocal discontinuous pleural thickening
- Mesa or rectangular shaped
- CT better demonstrates pleural plaque calcification compared to radiography.

Diffuse Pleural Thickening

- Usually unilateral, causes blunting of costophrenic angle, is ill-defined and irregular in shape, and spans across multiple ribs (Fig. 31.2)
- May calcify and may be associated with volume loss in the affected lung (so-called fibrothorax)
- Extrapleural fat hypertrophy is a common associated finding on CT.

Thoracic Splenosis

- Manifests on CT with small pleural nodules (<3 cm) typically in the left lower and posterior pleural space
- Signs of remote trauma (e.g., absent spleen or multiple splenules in left upper quadrant and healed left rib fractures)
- MRI signal intensity of nodules follows splenic tissue on all pulse sequences
- Tc-99m heat-damaged red blood cell scintigraphy is imaging study of choice for confirming thoracic splenosis; Tc-99m sulfur colloid is less specific but more widely available.

Erdheim–Chester Disease

- Thoracic involvement manifests on CT with smooth, circumferential pleural, subpleural lung, and pericardial thickening; interlobular septal thickening; peribronchovascular thickening; and centrilobular nodules.
- Perirenal and periaortic soft tissue encasement may accompany thoracic findings and is a helpful ancillary clue that may suggest the diagnosis.

Clinical Issues

- Pleural plaque, thoracic splenosis, pleural mouse, and diffuse pleural thickening generally require no clinical intervention.
- Extrapleural hematoma is usually managed conservatively unless there is rapid expansion or if the patient is hemodynamically unstable.
- Erdheim–Chester disease is treated with combination therapy (e.g., surgery, chemotherapy, radiation therapy, and corticosteroids).

Key Points

- Extrapleural fat should not be misdiagnosed as pleural thickening. It is bilateral and symmetric, spares the costophrenic angles, and is smoothly marginated.
- Fibrothorax represents diffuse pleural thickening with calcification and adjacent volume loss. It usually follows tuberculous empyema or hemothorax and may cause restrictive lung physiology.
- Thoracic splenosis should be considered when multiple left-sided pleural nodules are seen in association with signs of remote trauma such as rib fracture

or abdominal splenosis. The diagnosis may be confirmed with either Tc-99m heat-damaged red blood cell or sulfur colloid scintigraphy.

- Talc pleurodesis produces an inflammatory pleural reaction and is associated with intense linear FDG uptake that should not be mistaken for pleural metastases.
- Erdheim–Chester disease is rare but should be considered when circumferential pleural and pericardial thickening is seen in conjunction with soft tissue thickening that surrounds the aorta and kidneys.

Suggested Reading

Kuhlman JE, Singha NK. Complex disease of the pleural space: Radiographic and CT evaluation. *RadioGraphics*. 1997 Jan–Feb 1997;17(1):63–79.

Qureshi NR, Gleeson FV. Imaging of pleural disease. *Clin Chest Med*. Jun 2006;27(2):193–213.

Walker CM, Takasugi JE, Chung JH, et al. Tumorlike conditions of the pleura. *RadioGraphics*. 2012 Jul–Aug 2012;32(4): 971–985.

CHAPTER 32

Pleural Neoplasms

Christopher M. Walker

Definition

The most common pleural neoplasm is metastatic disease. Primary pleural neoplasms are rare, and they include malignant mesothelioma and localized (syn. solitary) fibrous tumor of the pleura. Pleural neoplasms manifest as pleural thickening that may be nodular or mass-like and are often accompanied by pleural effusion.

Clinical Features

Patients with a malignant pleural tumor may present with dyspnea and localized pain, but some affected patients are asymptomatic or have nonspecific symptoms, including anorexia, weight loss, and nausea. Patients with benign pleural tumors are often asymptomatic but may present with symptoms when a large tumor causes mass effect on adjacent structures. Localized fibrous tumor uncommonly presents with paraneoplastic syndromes, including hypoglycemia and hypertrophic osteoarthropathy.

Anatomy and Physiology

The normal pleura consists of two serosal membranes, the visceral and parietal pleura. The visceral pleura covers the lungs and forms the interlobar fissures, whereas the parietal pleura lines the costal, mediastinal, and diaphragmatic thoracic surfaces. Lymphatic drainage from the visceral pleura flows centrally to the hilum, whereas lymphatic drainage from the parietal pleura flows to diaphragmatic, intercostal, and internal mammary lymph nodes. The normal parietal pleura is not apparent on chest radiography or CT, whereas the normal visceral pleura is visible as the interlobar fissures, formed by two apposing layers of pleura. Benign and malignant pleural tumors usually manifest as focal or diffuse pleural thickening that may form nodules or masses (Figs. 32.1), often with associated pleural effusion (Figs. 32.2 and 32.3).

How to Approach the Image

The first step in formulating an imaging diagnosis in the thorax is determining whether a lesion is pulmonary or extrapulmonary in location. Several radiographic and CT features suggest a pleural or chest wall lesion location:

- Pleural tumors are always associated with a pleural surface (costal, mediastinal, diaphragmatic, or fissural).
- Pleural tumors often form interfaces that exhibit obtuse angles with the adjacent pleural surface.
- Pleural abnormalities may exhibit borders that exhibit the incomplete border sign on radiography.
- The lesion borders are indistinct when there is no tangential relationship to the x-ray beam (incomplete border sign; Fig. 32.1a) and sharp when the x-ray beam is tangential to the lesion border.
- Pleural tumors may displace—but will not engulf—pulmonary vessels on cross-sectional imaging.

What Not to Miss

Four CT features of pleural thickening are highly suggestive of malignant pleural disease (Figs. 32.1b and 32.4):

- Pleural thickening greater than 1 cm (specificity 94%)
- Nodular pleural thickening (specificity 94%)
- Circumferential pleural thickening (specificity nearly 100%)
- Mediastinal pleura involvement (specificity 88%)

These findings have a moderate degree of sensitivity, and their absence does not exclude malignant pleural disease.

Differential Diagnosis

Metastatic Disease

- Most common malignant pleural neoplasm
- Affected patients often present with dyspnea.
- Adenocarcinomas of lung, breast, and gastrointestinal origin are the most common tumors to metastasize to the pleura.
- Thymoma may spread to the pleura via direct extension or "drop metastases."

Mesothelioma

- Most common primary malignant pleural tumor
- Highly associated with occupational asbestos exposure (e.g., ship builders, construction, and plumbing)
- Latency period of 20–40 years after asbestos exposure
- Patients typically present with chest pain and dyspnea.

Lymphoma

- The pleura may be involved as a secondary site of systemic lymphoma and may be a site of tumor recurrence.

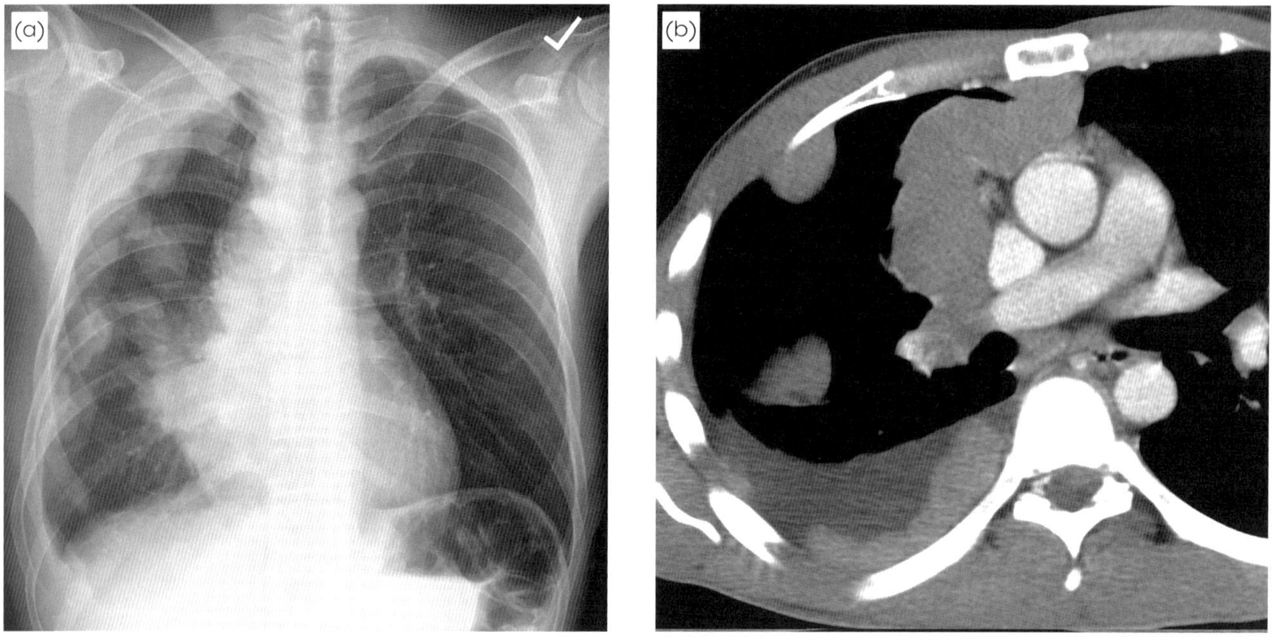

Figure 32.1 Malignant pleural thickening (invasive thymoma). (a) Posteroanterior (PA) chest radiograph shows right nodular pleural thickening with characteristic features suggestive of pleural malignancy, including pleural thickening greater than 1 cm in thickness, nodularity, a circumferential growth pattern within the involved hemithorax, and mediastinal pleural involvement. (b) Contrast-enhanced CT of the same patient shows multiple pleural masses involving the costal and mediastinal pleura that measure greater than 1 cm and exhibit nodularity.

- Rarely, lymphoma originates in the pleural space (primary pleural lymphoma).

Localized (Solitary) Fibrous Tumor of the Pleura

- Most are benign, but 15–20% may be malignant.
- Affect men and women older than age 40 years
- Affected patients may be asymptomatic (54%) or may present with chest pain, cough, or dyspnea.
- May be associated with hypertrophic osteoarthropathy (reported in 0–35% of patients) or episodic hypoglycemia (<5% of patients); also reported with mesothelioma and lung cancer
- Most arise from visceral pleural surface and may be attached by a pedicle.

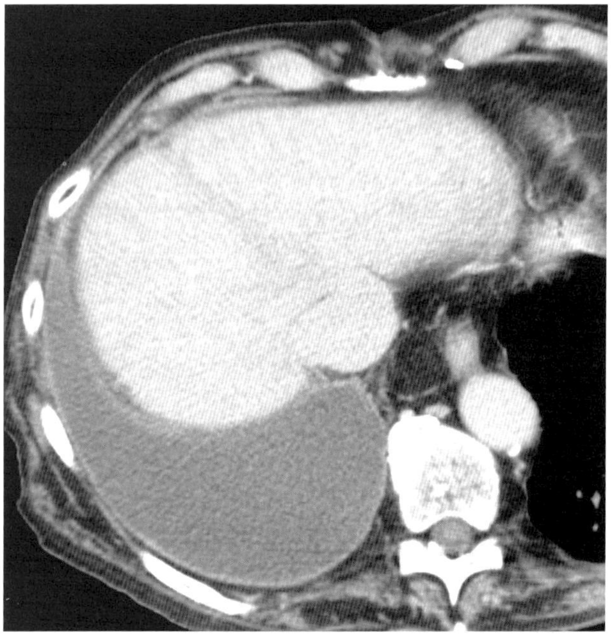

Figure 32.2 Malignant pleural effusion and pleural thickening. Contrast-enhanced chest CT shows a large right pleural effusion and smooth enhancing pleural thickening (arrows). Thoracentesis was positive for malignancy.

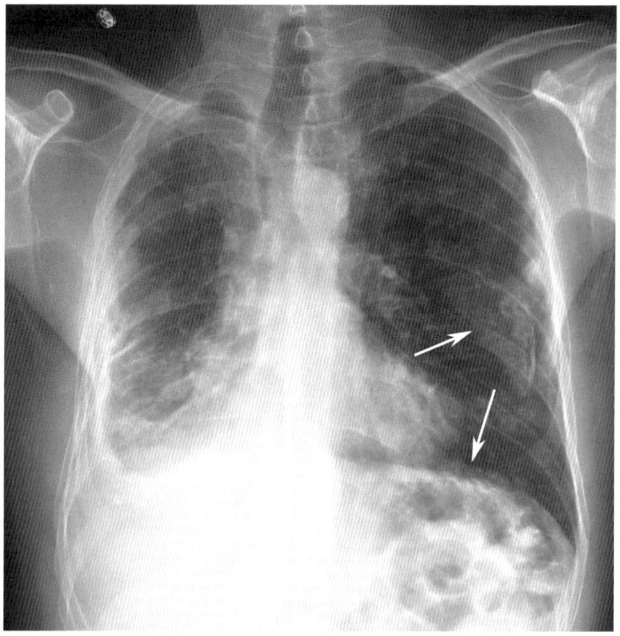

Figure 32.3 Mesothelioma and pleural plaques. PA chest radiograph shows bilateral calcified pleural plaques along the costal and left diaphragmatic pleura (arrows) and a moderate right pleural effusion that partially obscures right pleural nodules and masses. Pleural biopsy revealed mesothelioma.

Lipoma

- Benign chest wall tumor that may produce mass effect on the adjacent pleura; characteristic CT fat attenuation
- Usually discovered incidentally on imaging performed for other reasons

Pleural Plaque

- Most common manifestation of asbestos exposure
- Mesa- or rectangular-shaped, discontinuous pleural thickening that may exhibit calcification

Imaging Findings

Metastatic Disease

- Pleural effusion is the most common imaging manifestation; effusions may be large and obscure most of the involved hemithorax (Figs. 32.1 and 32.2).
- Solitary or multiple pleural nodules/masses or diffuse pleural thickening on radiography or CT.
- Thymoma is an anterior mediastinal mass that may be invasive, with a propensity for pleural spread; it may cause diffuse pleural thickening and/or multiple drop metastases better appreciated on CT.

Mesothelioma

- Multifocal and/or circumferential nodular pleural thickening and/or pleural effusion (Figs. 32.3 and 32.4)
- Involved hemithorax often has a reduced volume.
- Pleural effusion may be the only imaging finding.
- Propensity for fissural involvement better appreciated on CT
- Hilar and mediastinal lymph node metastases
- 20% of affected patients have calcified pleural plaques indicating prior asbestos exposure.
- Tumor spreads by direct extension to chest wall, diaphragm, and mediastinum.
- May contain calcification when tumor engulfs calcified pleural plaques, or rarely with osteocartilagenous differentiation.
- MRI has better capability than CT in detection of chest wall and diaphragmatic invasion.
- Signs of mediastinal, chest wall, or diaphragmatic invasion on CT or MRI include infiltration or obliteration of normal fat planes.

Lymphoma

- Manifests as a solitary pleural nodule or diffuse pleural thickening usually in association with pleural effusion (Fig. 32.5)
- Usually associated with mediastinal, axillary, or retroperitoneal lymphadenopathy on CT

Localized (Solitary) Fibrous Tumor of the Pleura

- May mimic diaphragmatic elevation or cardiomegaly on chest radiography (Figs. 32.6 and 32.7)
- Well-defined lobular mass in the mid or lower hemithorax that abuts a pleural surface or fissure
- May exhibit positional mobility within pleural space by virtue of pedicle attachment

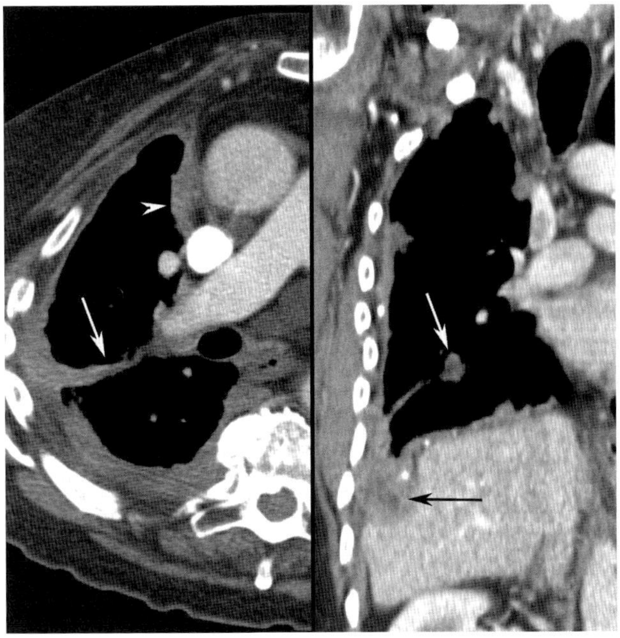

Figure 32.4 Mesothelioma. Composite image with contrast-enhanced chest CT from different patients demonstrates nodular and circumferential pleural thickening that extends along the lateral, diaphragmatic, and mediastinal pleura and into the major fissure (white arrows). Tumor engulfs calcified pleural plaques along the costal and diaphragmatic pleura (black arrow). The lesions exhibit circumferential and fissural involvement and thickening greater than 1 cm (arrowhead).

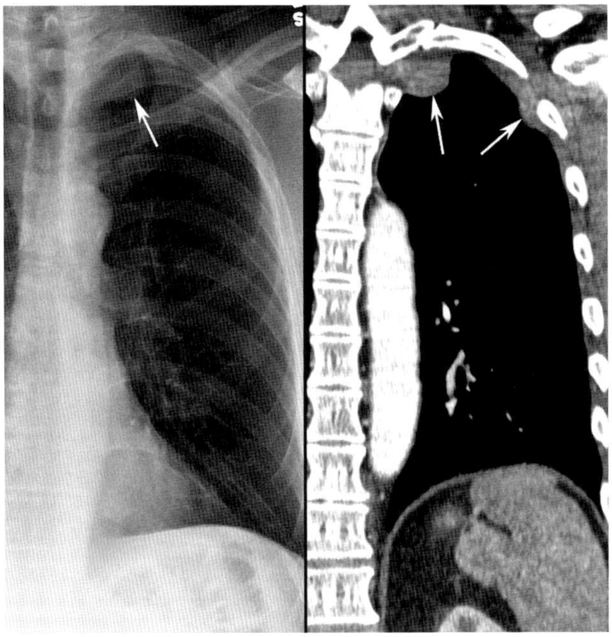

Figure 32.5 Pleural lymphoma. Composite image with PA chest radiograph (left) and coronal contrast-enhanced chest CT (right) shows two left apical pleural masses (arrows) that form obtuse angles with the adjacent pleura and represented pleural lymphoma.

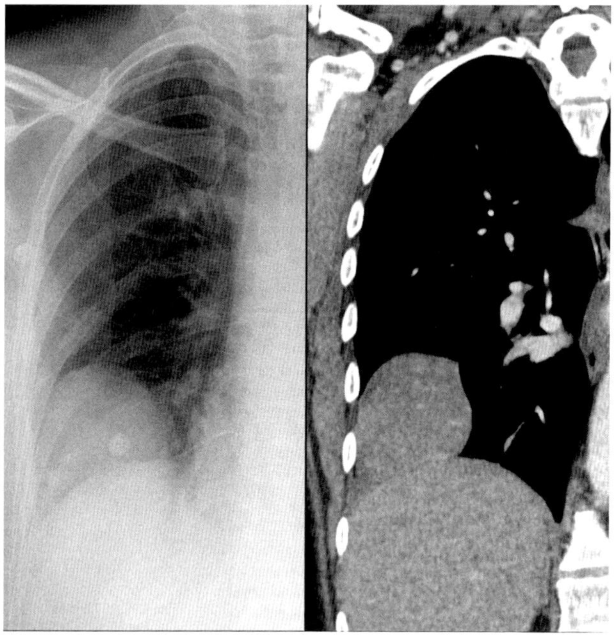

Figure 32.6 Localized fibrous tumor of the pleura. Composite image with PA chest radiograph (left) and contrast-enhanced CT (right) shows a well-defined, smooth mass in the right inferior hemithorax.

- Often large at diagnosis (>10 cm) with internal heterogeneity on CT and MRI
- 10% may recur following surgical resection.
- Lymphadenopathy, hematogenous metastases, and chest wall invasion are rare and better demonstrated on CT and MRI.
- Large lesions may form acute angles with pleura.

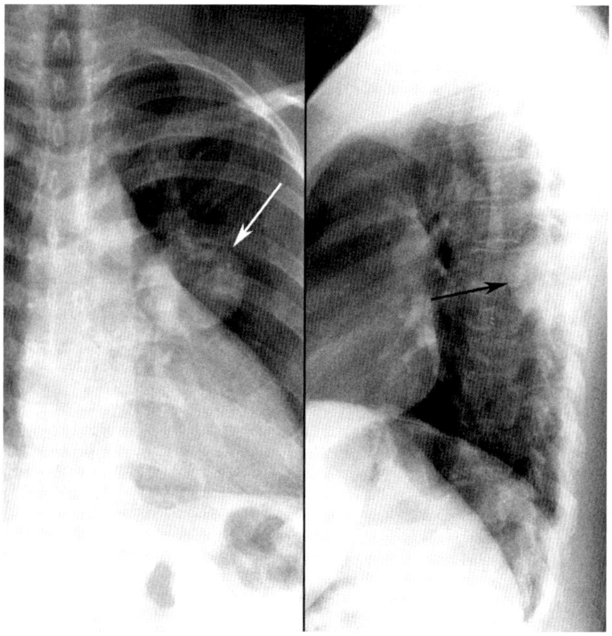

Figure 32.7 Localized fibrous tumor of the pleura. Composite image of a PA and lateral radiograph shows a round mass (arrows) abutting the posterior left pleural surface. The mass is well-defined on the PA radiograph, but only the anterior margin is visualized on the lateral radiograph.

Clinical Issues

- Metastatic pleural disease generally indicates incurable disease, and affected patients are treated with chemotherapy or palliative measures (e.g., talc pleurodesis, pleural drainage, and tumor debulking).
- Mesothelioma has a poor prognosis, with a median survival of 12 months from diagnosis. Multimodality therapy consisting of extrapleural pneumonectomy followed by adjuvant chemoradiation is the treatment of choice for patients without distant disease or extensive chest wall, mediastinal, or diaphragmatic spread. Most cases are unresectable, and treatment is supportive.
- Localized fibrous tumor of the pleura requires complete surgical excision. Long-term follow-up is performed to look for metastatic or recurrent disease that manifests as ipsilateral pleural or pulmonary nodules.

Key Points

- Imaging features suggestive of a pleural mass include obtuse interfaces with the adjacent pleura or chest wall, demonstration of the incomplete border sign, and displacement of adjacent pulmonary vessels.
- CT features of pleural thickening that are highly suggestive of pleural malignancy include thickening measuring greater than 1 cm, nodular and/or circumferential pleural thickening, and mediastinal pleural involvement.
- Lung and breast adenocarcinomas and lymphoma are the most common malignancies to metastasize to the pleura.
- Thymoma should be considered when an anterior mediastinal mass is associated with multiple pleural nodules.
- Mesothelioma is often indistinguishable from metastatic pleural disease based on imaging features alone.
- Localized fibrous tumors of the pleura may be mistaken for pulmonary or mediastinal masses because they may lack obvious signs of their pleural origin. Consider the diagnosis when a large, heterogeneous mass abuts the pleura without mediastinal lymphadenopathy, chest wall invasion, or distant metastases.

Suggested Reading

Dynes MC, White EM, Fry WA, Ghahremani GG. Imaging manifestations of pleural tumors. *RadioGraphics.* Nov 1992;12(6):1191–1201.

Leung AN, Müller NL, Miller RR. CT in differential diagnosis of diffuse pleural disease. *AJR Am J Roentgenol.* Mar 1990;154(3):487–492.

Rosado-de-Christenson ML, Abbott GF, McAdams HP, Franks TJ, Galvin JR. From the archives of the AFIP: Localized fibrous tumor of the pleura. *RadioGraphics.* 2003 May–Jun 2003;23(3):759–783.

Sharma A, Fidias P, Hayman LA, Loomis SL, Taber KH, Aquino SL. Patterns of lymphadenopathy in thoracic malignancies. *RadioGraphics.* 2004 Mar–Apr 2004;24(2):419–434.

Wang ZJ, Reddy GP, Gotway MB, et al. Malignant pleural mesothelioma: Evaluation with CT, MR imaging, and PET. *RadioGraphics.* 2004 Jan–Feb 2004;24(1):105–119.

Section VII

Pulmonary Infections

CHAPTER 33

Pulmonary Infections

Santiago Martínez-Jiménez

Introduction

Pneumonia is the leading cause of death among children worldwide. Approximately 1.1 million children younger than age 5 years die of pneumonia every year, constituting a mortality higher than that of AIDS, malaria, and tuberculosis combined. Among adults, pneumonia is one of the top 10 causes of mortality. Pneumonia can be classified as community-acquired pneumonia (CAP), hospital-acquired pneumonia (HAP), ventilator-associated pneumonia (VAP), health care-associated pneumonia (HCAP), and pneumonia in immunosuppressed patients. Although these types of pneumonia are similar pathologically, they are very different from a clinical perspective.

Definitions

CAP is defined as pulmonary infection acquired outside the hospital or extended-care facilities. HAP occurs 48 hours or more after admission to the hospital. VAP occurs 48–72 hours after endotracheal intubation. HCAP occurs in nonhospitalized patients with extensive health care contacts. Well-recognized risk factors for HAC, VAP, and HCAP include age older than70 years, chronic lung disease, decreased level of consciousness, aspiration, chest surgery, intracranial pressure monitor or nasogastric tube use, H2 blocker or antacid therapy, transport from the intensive care unit for additional procedures, previous antibiotic exposure, reintubation or prolonged intubation, hospitalization during the fall or winter, mechanical ventilation for acute respiratory distress syndrome, certain ventilator parameters, paralytic agents, and underlying illness.

Treatment

All pneumonias, regardless of severity or management on an outpatient or an inpatient basis, are treated with antibiotics. Recommendation regarding use of specific antibiotics is beyond the scope of this work. However, it is important to determine which patients with CAP require hospitalization.

Several guidelines have been developed to determine the management of patients with CAP and whether or not they require hospitalization for treatment purposes. The most accurate is the pneumonia severity index (PSI), which requires assessment of 20 variables. The CURB-65 is a more practical approach based on five parameters: confusion, urea greater than 20 md/dl, respiratory rate 30 per minute or greater, low systolic (<90 mm Hg) or diastolic (≤60 mm Hg) blood pressure, and age 65 years or older. Each parameter is assigned a value of 0 if absent or 1 when present. A total of 0 or 1 points is considered low severity, and outpatient treatment is appropriate; a total of 2 points is considered moderate severity, and hospitalization should be considered; and a total of 3–5 points is considered high severity, and hospitalization is indicated.

When considering antibiotic treatment in patients with HAC, VAP, and HCAP, it is important to recognize the higher likelihood of drug resistance (both multidrug and pan-resistance), one of the main reasons why these entities are considered different from other types of pneumonia.

Differential Diagnosis, Follow-Up, and Further Imaging

The terms consolidation and airspace disease are traditionally linked to pulmonary infection. This is probably because pneumonia is by far the most common cause of pulmonary consolidation. However, it is important to recognize that airspace consolidation may be produced by any substance filling the alveoli, such as water (e.g., pulmonary edema), blood (e.g., alveolar hemorrhage and pulmonary infarct), inflammatory cells (e.g., drug pneumonitis and granulomatosis with polyangiitis), and neoplastic cells (e.g., lung cancer with lepidic growth). For this reason, patients with suspected pneumonia should undergo radiographic follow-up 4–6 weeks after the onset of treatment to document resolution and exclude other etiologies, specifically malignancy (Fig. 33.1). Although clinical response to treatment often occurs within days after initiation of the appropriate antibiotic, radiographic resolution of infectious consolidations is slower. Thus, imaging patients before 4–6 weeks after the onset of treatment may lead to the erroneous conclusion that patients are not responding to treatment. In addition, pulmonary infections with certain microorganisms (e.g., *Legionella pneumophila, Staphylococcus pneumoniae*, and *Streptococcus pneumoniae*) are well-known to exhibit initial radiographic worsening despite appropriate

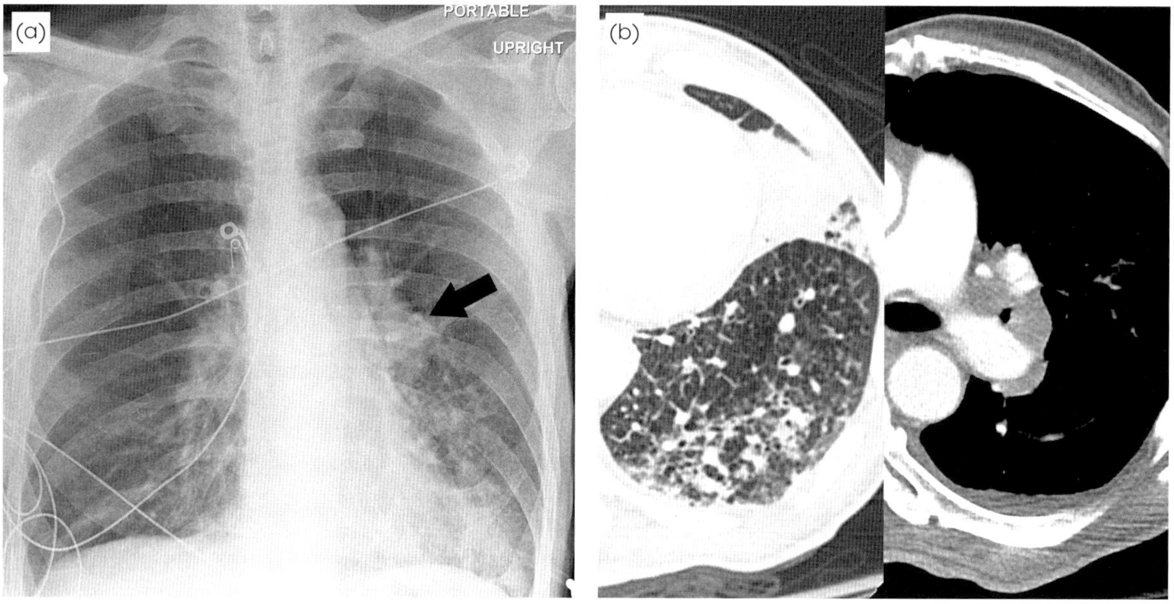

Figure 33.1 Lung cancer simulating pneumonia. (a) Posteroanterior (PA) chest radiograph of a 71-year-old man with dyspnea shows lingular and, to a lesser extent, left lower lobe airspace disease and left hilar enlargement (arrow). (b) Composite image from a contrast-enhanced chest CT shows dense lingular consolidation, left lower lobe ground-glass opacities, and ipsilateral left hilar lymphadenopathy.

clinical response (Fig. 33.2). Nevertheless, earlier follow-up chest radiography should be obtained when complications of pneumonia are suspected (e.g., pulmonary abscess, empyema, and bronchopleural fistula).

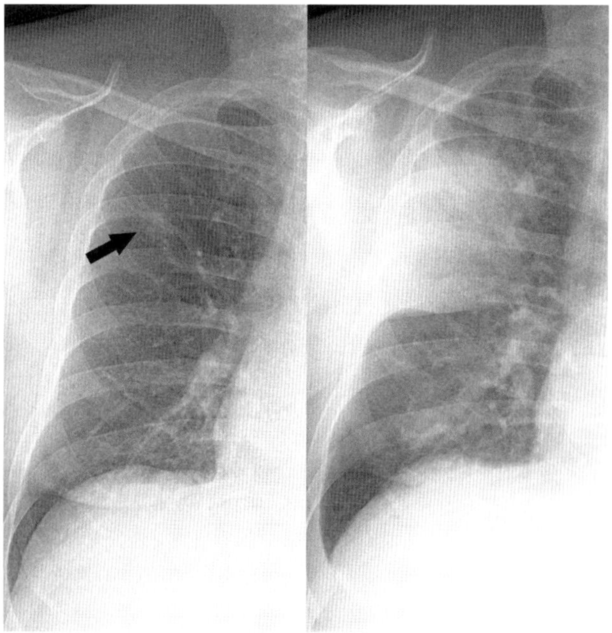

Figure 33.2 *Streptococcus pneumoniae* pneumonia. Composite image with PA chest radiographs of a 35-year-old woman with pneumonia at initial onset of symptoms (left) and after 48 hours (right) shows a small focus of airspace disease (arrow). Despite a favorable clinical response after initiation of antibiotics, the follow-up radiograph shows marked progression of the consolidation. This case highlights the importance of appropriate follow-up only after 4–6 weeks or when complications are suspected.

In theory, any patient with airspace disease that persists beyond 6 weeks must be further assessed with chest CT to exclude underlying malignancy, but several factors must be taken into consideration before making this decision. Potential causes of nonresolving consolidation may be broadly divided into infectious and noninfectious. Infectious causes include resistant, unusual (*Mycobacterium tuberculosis*, fungi, and atypical organisms such as *Nocardia* and *Actynomyces*), and nosocomial microorganisms. Severe cases of pneumonia may require more than 10 weeks for resolution. Consolidations associated with certain microorganisms may resolve slowly (e.g., *Legionella pneumophila* and *Staphylococcus aureus*). Noninfectious etiologies that may affect resolution of infectious airspace disease include chronic obstructive pulmonary disease, alcoholism, neurologic disease, heart failure, chronic kidney disease, HIV infection, and diabetes. Immunosuppression, particularly that due to chronic corticosteroid treatment, may also contribute to slow resolution of consolidation. Increasing age is also associated with slowly resolving infectious airspace disease. If none of these factors are present and the chest radiograph remains abnormal after 6 weeks, the next appropriate step is further evaluation with chest CT. Although chest CT is the first step in evaluating such patients, bronchoscopic assessment with culture and biopsy may be required. Patients with consolidation due to malignancy often exhibit bronchial obliteration, hilar/mediastinal lymphadenopathy, and/or lytic osseous lesions that help support the diagnosis. Other etiologies of nonresolving airspace disease include organizing pneumonia, chronic eosinophilic pneumonia, sarcoidosis, drug pneumonitis, and lymphoma.

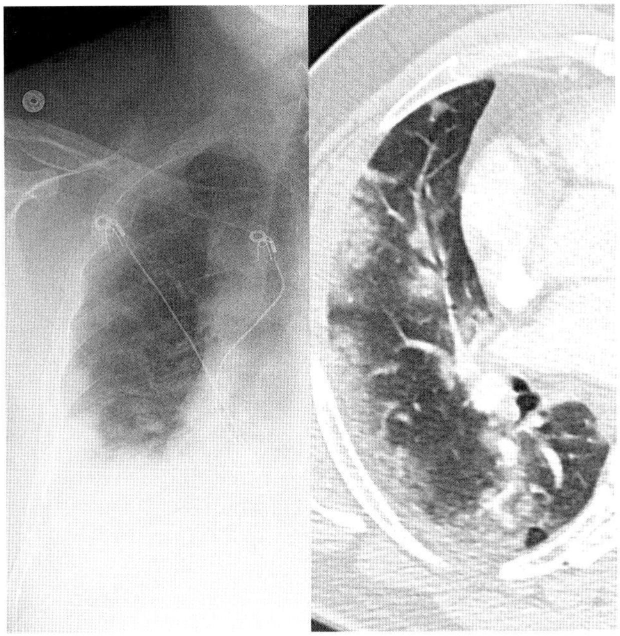

Figure 33.3 Influenza A pneumonia. Composite image of a 52-year-old man with pneumonia with PA chest radiograph (left) and CT (right) shows multifocal peripheral opacities. Serology was positive for influenza A, and PCT levels were low. PCT is frequently positive in bacterial infections and tends to be negative in viral infections. Low PCT levels in patients with pneumonia often correlate with a better prognosis.

Biomarkers

The role of biomarkers in patients with pneumonia is beyond the scope of this work. However, radiologists should be aware that this is an emerging area of study. Procalcitonin (PCT) is the most commonly used new biomarker in clinical practice. Theoretically, PCT is elevated in bacterial but not in viral infections, and it may help predict the presence of radiographic airspace disease in patients with CAP and the need for antibiotic therapy. Its use is limited because it may be elevated in patients with severe influenza, a viral infection (Fig. 33.3). When serially measured, PCT may correlate with prognosis (i.e., lower levels correlate with better prognosis) and may be helpful in assessing response to treatment and in patient management (e.g., low levels of PCT may require a lesser dose and shorter duration of antibiotics).

Summary

Pneumonia is a clinical diagnosis. Chest radiography is often performed to support the diagnosis and to determine the extent of involvement prior to the onset of therapy. Radiography should not be performed in the short term in patients who are improving clinically because it can lead to the misdiagnosis of treatment failure. Chest radiography in patients treated for pneumonia should be obtained before 4–6 weeks after the onset of therapy only if there is a failure of clinical response or if complications of pneumonia are clinically suspected. The majority of pneumonia cases will resolve after 6 weeks of appropriate antibiotic therapy.

Suggested Reading

Nair GB, Niederman MS. Community-acquired pneumonia: An unfinished battle. *Med Clin North Am.* 2011 Nov;95(6):1143–1161.

Nair GB, Niederman MS. Nosocomial pneumonia: Lessons learned. *Crit Care Clin.* 2013 Jul;29(3):521–546.

Sialer S, Liapikou A, Torres A. What is the best approach to the nonresponding patient with community-acquired pneumonia? *Infect Dis Clin North Am.* 2013;27(1):189–203.

Weyers CM, Leeper KV. Nonresolving pneumonia. *Clin Chest Med.* 2005;26(1):143–158.

CHAPTER 34

Community-Acquired Pneumonia

Sonia L. Betancourt

Definition

The term pneumonia refers to acute inflammation of the lower respiratory tract and lung parenchyma. Community-acquired pneumonia (CAP) refers to pneumonia acquired outside of hospitals or long-term care facilities in patients without known inherited or acquired immunodeficiency or active cancer or within 48 hours after hospital admission. This is in contrast to nosocomial pneumonia (hospital-acquired pneumonia) that develops more than 48 hours after hospital admission and involves a different set of microorganisms.

Clinical Features

Pneumonia remains the most common cause of death from infection in the United States. Classic clinical features of CAP include cough, fever, pleuritic pain, dyspnea, and sputum production. However, CAP can be clinically subtle in elderly individuals who may present with altered mental status or weakness. Microorganisms related to CAP include *Streptococcus pneumoniae, Haemophilus influenzae, Staphylococcus aureus, Mycoplasma pneumoniae, Chlamydia pneumoniae, Klebsiella pneumoniae*, and *Legionella pneumophila*. Gram-negative bacteria are common in elderly patients, alcoholics, and patients with chronic debilitating illnesses. Empyema and lung abscesses may complicate CAP secondary to any microorganism, but they are frequent complications in patients with aspiration pneumonia.

Anatomy and Physiology

Although CAP most commonly results from inhalation of infectious droplets, approximately 10% of cases may occur in the setting of aspiration of oropharyngeal or gastric secretions. Classically, patterns of pneumonia are classified as lobar pneumonia, bronchopneumonia (lobular pneumonia), and interstitial pneumonia. Lobar pneumonia results from spread of infection throughout the acini, the pores of Kohn, and canals of Lambert, involving partial or complete pulmonary segments or an entire lobe. The bronchopneumonia (lobular) pattern relates to infection centered on larger airways. Finally, interstitial pneumonia is characterized by an inflammatory cellular process with preferential involvement of the interlobular and peribronchovascular interstitium.

How to Approach the Image

Chest radiography remains the imaging study of choice in the evaluation of CAP. Although the diagnosis of CAP is entirely clinical, chest radiographic abnormalities help support the clinical diagnosis and may help direct treatment. Some imaging abnormalities may alter treatment (e.g., multifocal pneumonia, empyema, and bronchopleural fistula). The absence of consolidation and normal chest radiographs are not uncommon in patients with CAP.

CT is useful to identify early infection in patients with normal chest radiographs. CT also allows evaluation of associated complications (e.g., empyema) and to exclude pneumonia mimickers such as lung cancer.

What Not to Miss

Patients with CAP should always be evaluated for complications such as abscess, empyema, and bronchopleural fistula.

Differential Diagnosis

Several noninfectious processes may manifest acutely with fever and respiratory symptoms:

- Pulmonary hemorrhage is characterized by diffuse consolidation in a patient with a dropping hematocrit. Hemoptysis is common but not always present. Etiologies including granulomatosis with polyangiitis should be considered.
- Pulmonary edema is characterized by interlobular septal thickening, diffuse airspace opacities, bilateral pleural effusions, and cardiomegaly in the setting of elevated capillary wedge pressures.
- Pulmonary infarcts manifest with peripheral, lower lung zone wedge-shaped opacities (Hampton hump).
- Gastric aspiration manifests with pulmonary opacities that preferentially affect the posterior segments of the upper lobes and/or superior segments of the lower lobes. There may be predisposing conditions, such as esophageal motility disorders and altered consciousness.
- Acute eosinophilic pneumonia affects young patients with severe acute febrile illness with associated hypoxemic respiratory failure and manifests with

patchy consolidation, ground-glass opacities, and small bilateral pleural effusions. There is marked elevation of eosinophils in bronchoalveolar lavage fluid.

Imaging Findings

Several radiologic patterns of pneumonia (i.e., lobar, lobular, and interstitial) have been associated with different microorganisms. Lobar pneumonia is usually of bacterial origin and most commonly due to *S. pneumoniae* or *K. pneumoniae.* Bronchopneumonia is very common in *Staph. aureus* infection. Interstitial pneumonia may be associated with *M. pneumoniae.*

Lobar Pneumonia Pattern

- Most commonly caused by *S. pneumoniae.* Chest radiographs may show nonsegmental, homogeneous consolidations with air bronchograms that involve one or multiple lobes (Fig. 34.1).
- *Klebsiella pneumoniae* pneumonia more commonly affects patients with chronic debilitating illness or alcoholism. Chest radiographs show homogeneous nonsegmental consolidation that spreads rapidly. Bulging of fissures has been classically described. Cavitation from abscess formation may occur in 30–50% of cases.
- *Legionella pneumophila* infection may result from contaminated air-conditioning systems, cooling towers, and showerheads. Chest radiographs show airspace consolidation that may initially be peripheral and segmental and rapidly evolves to lobar consolidation.

Bronchopneumonia Pattern

- *Staphylococcus aureus* may cause CAP particularly in elderly individuals and infants, often complicating influenza. Chest radiographs show patchy segmental consolidation with volume loss, which may spread rapidly and become confluent. Intrinsic cavitation may relate to necrosis and abscess formation. Pneumatocele formation is common in children. Empyema is a frequent complication (Fig. 34.2).
- *Haemophilus influenzae* exhibits variable imaging manifestations, including a bronchopneumonia pattern with patchy, segmental, or lobar airspace disease.
- Other microorganisms include *Streptococcus pyogenes, Escherichia coli, Pseudomonas aeruginosa,* anaerobic bacteria, and viruses.

Interstitial Pattern

- *Mycoplasma pneumoniae* results in pulmonary infection with a clinical presentation that resembles a systemic viral infection. The chest radiograph shows linear opacities that may progress to unilateral or bilateral segmental consolidations (Fig. 34.3).
- *Chlamydia pneumoniae* infection often manifests with sore throat and nonproductive cough. The radiographic appearance includes reticular opacities and airspace consolidation. Airway dilation and bronchovascular thickening are frequent.

Aspiration pneumonia (Fig. 34.4) is thought to be responsible for 5–15% of cases of CAP, and it may result from neurologic abnormalities affecting deglutition or altered mental status (common in alcoholic and trauma

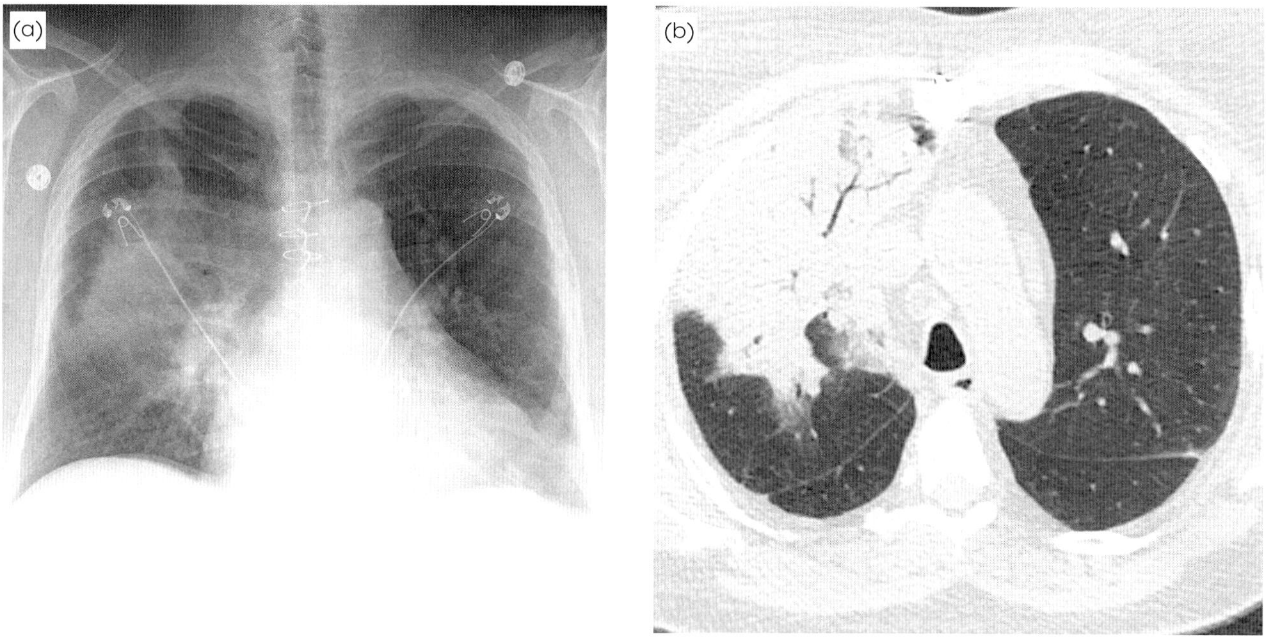

Figure 34.1 Lobar pneumonia due to *S. pneumoniae.* (a) Posteroanterior (PA) chest radiograph of a 58-year-old man with fever and dyspnea shows a right upper lobe consolidation. (b) Unenhanced chest CT of the same patient shows a dense right upper lobe consolidation with air bronchograms.

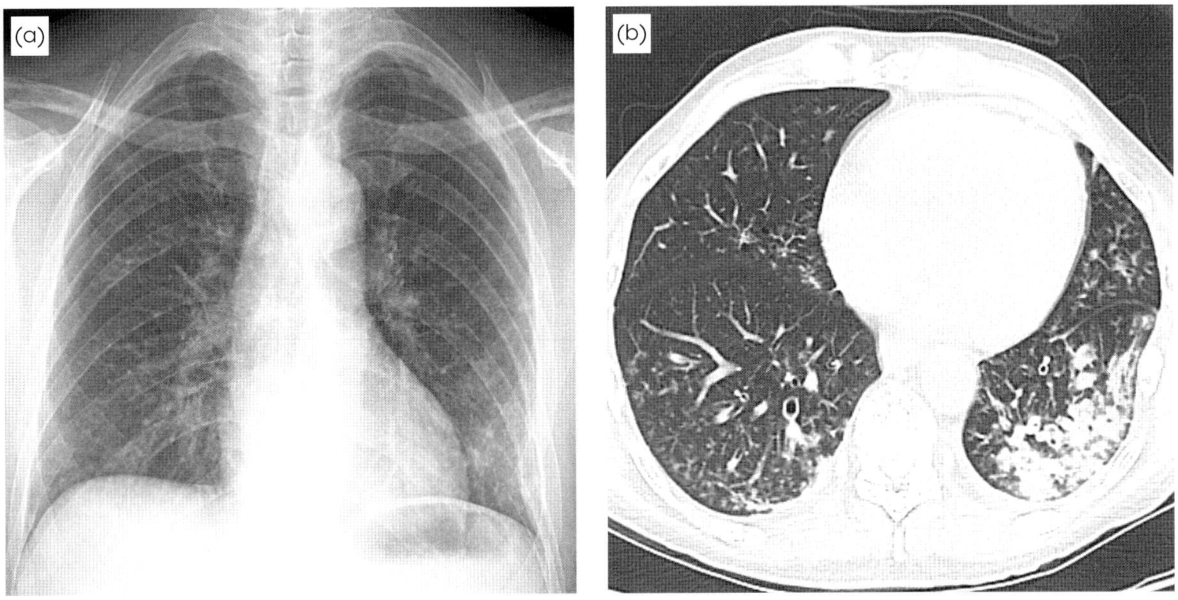

Figure 34.2 Bronchopneumonia due to *Staphylococcus aureus*. (a) PA chest radiograph of a 32-year-old man with fever, chills, cough, and dyspnea shows bilateral ill-defined pulmonary opacities, more confluent in the left lower lobe. (b) Unenhanced chest CT of the same patient shows scattered centrilobular and tree-in-bud opacities with coalescence left lower lobe consolidation.

patients). Lobar pneumonia, bronchopneumonia, lung abscess, and empyema are common. Anaerobes and gram-negative bacteria are the most common pathogens.

Round pneumonia (Fig. 34.5) occurs more frequently in children and may mimic a neoplastic nodule or mass in all age groups. The most common pathogen is *S. pneumoniae*. Chest radiographic findings vary from a small, dense nodule to a large, spherical or ovoid mass. Air bronchograms may be identified on radiographs or CT. Follow-up radiographs are helpful to verify resolution and exclude neoplastic process.

Lung abscess (Fig. 34.6) manifests with air–fluid levels in association with consolidation. Compared to empyema, which exhibits obtuse angles, a lung abscess typically forms acute angles with the adjacent chest wall. On CT, lung abscess manifests as single or multiple masses with intrinsic low attenuation (i.e., fluid and/or air) and peripheral enhancement.

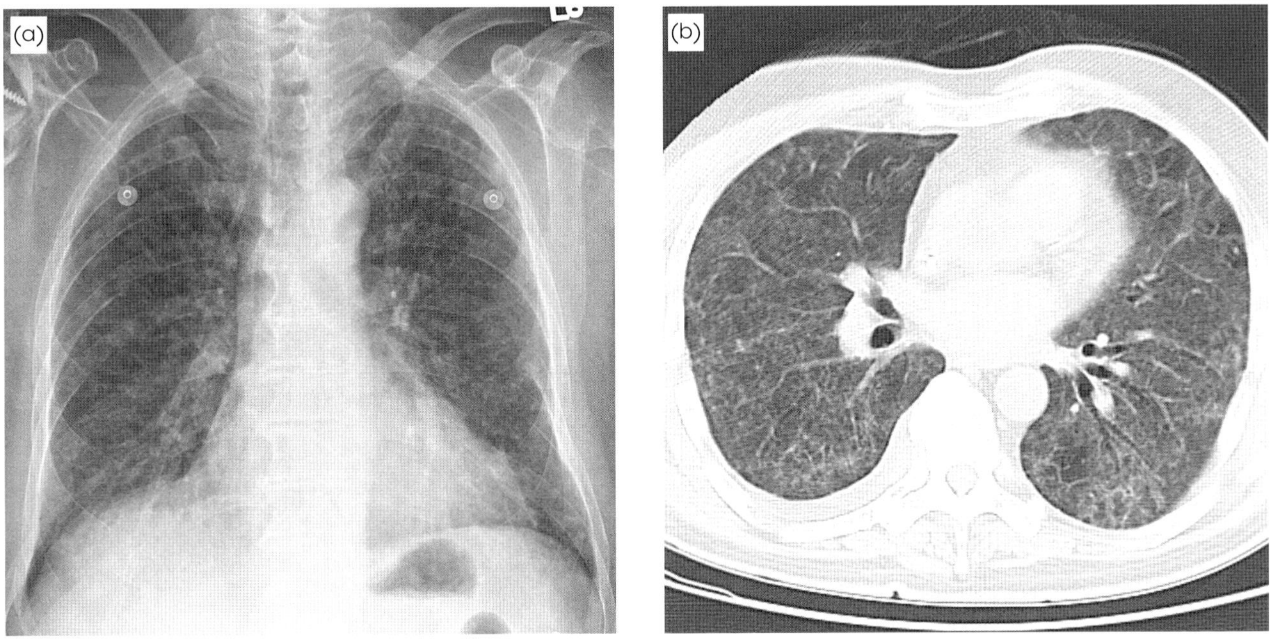

Figure 34.3 Interstitial pneumonia due to *M. pneumoniae*. (a) AP chest radiograph of a 60-year-old man with fever and cough shows diffuse bilateral ill-defined reticulonodular opacities. (b) Unenhanced chest CT of the same patient shows diffuse bilateral ground-glass and centrilobular nodular opacities and a small right pleural effusion.

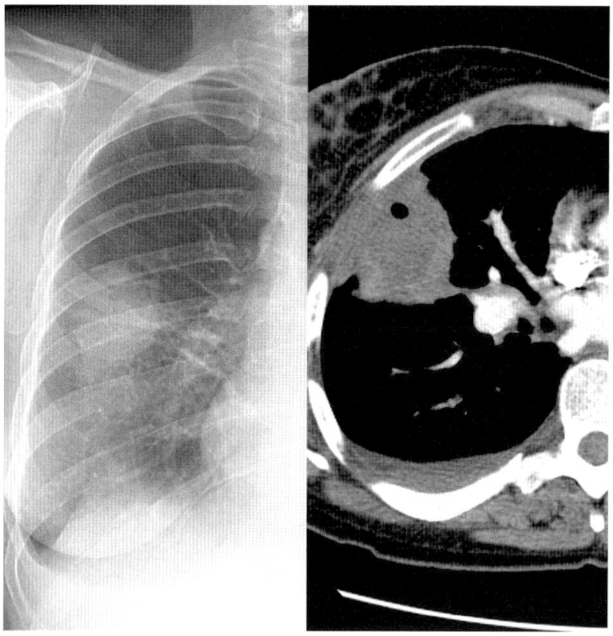

Figure 34.4 Lung abscess from aspiration pneumonia due to gram-negative organisms. Composite image with PA chest radiograph (left) and contrast-enhanced chest CT (right) of a 44-year-old woman with persistent fever shows a right mid lung zone mass that exhibits central low attenuation, intrinsic air, and surrounding consolidation consistent with lung abscess.

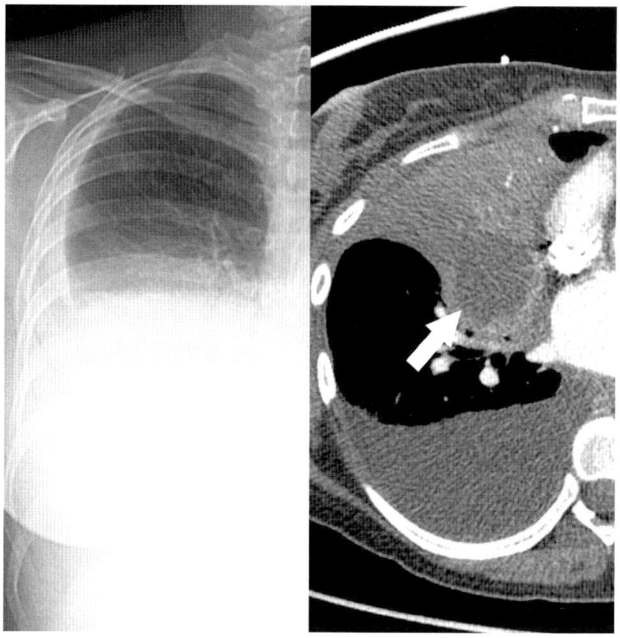

Figure 34.6 Lung abscess due to *S. pneumoniae*. Composite image with PA chest radiograph (left) and contrast-enhanced chest CT (right) of a 28-year-old woman with persistent fever despite antibiotic treatment for pneumonia shows right basilar airspace disease and a moderate right pleural effusion. CT shows middle lobe consolidation with a rounded low-attenuation area (arrow) adjacent to the hilum that represented a lung abscess and a right pleural effusion.

Necrotizing pneumonia can complicate CAP from associated vascular thrombosis. *Streptococcus pneumoniae* and *K. pneumoniae* are common etiologies in immunocompetent patients. Radiographically, pulmonary gangrene manifests with lobar consolidation that develops intrinsic cavitation on follow-up imaging.

Empyema (Fig. 34.7) occurs when parenchymal infection spreads to the pleural space and manifests with a

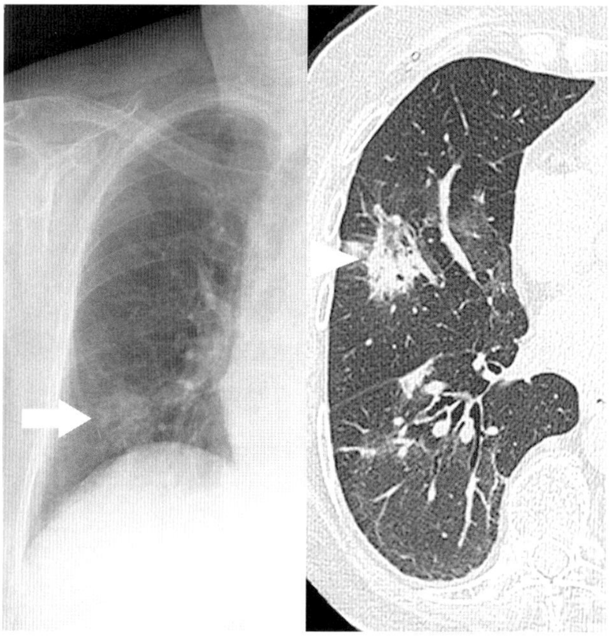

Figure 34.5 Round pneumonia due to *S. pneumoniae*. Composite image with PA chest radiograph (left) and unenhanced chest CT (right) of a 69-year-old man with dyspnea and fever shows a poorly defined right lower lung zone nodular consolidation that exhibits spiculated borders, air bronchograms, and surrounding ground-glass opacities on CT.

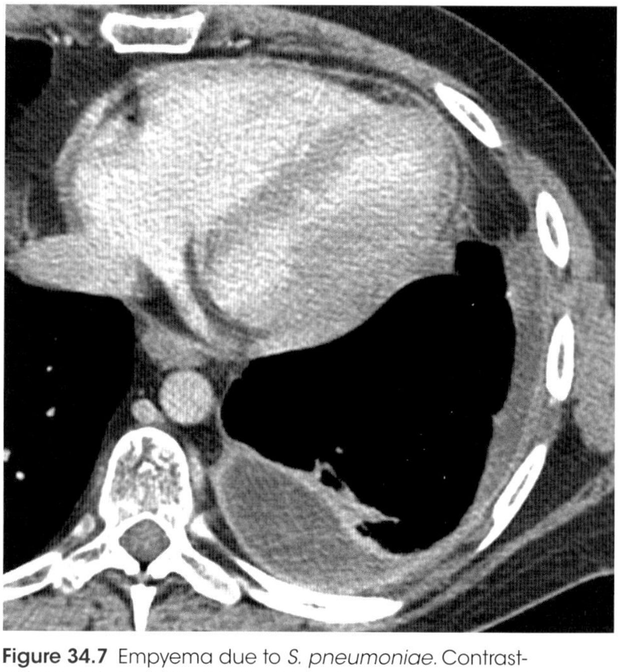

Figure 34.7 Empyema due to *S. pneumoniae*. Contrast-enhanced chest CT of a 34-year-old man with fever and chest pain shows a loculated right pleural effusion with pleural thickening and enhancement—the so-called split pleural sign.

loculated effusion on chest radiography. Development of hydropneumothorax typically signifies bronchopleural fistula. CT may show parietal and visceral pleural thickening that may enhance the so-called "split pleura sign" (Fig. 34.6) typical but not diagnostic of empyema.

Pneumatoceles can occur in association with *Staphylococcus aureus, E. coli,* and *S. pneumoniae* infections. They manifest radiographically as single or multiple thin-walled gas-filled spaces within areas of consolidation. They may increase in size over days to weeks and often resolve.

Clinical Issues

- Lung cancer, organizing pneumonia, and eosinophilic pneumonia may mimic pneumonia.
- Consolidations should be followed with chest radiography in 4–6 weeks or until complete resolution. Nonresolving consolidations require further evaluation with CT to exclude underlying malignancy.

Key Points

- The most common organisms that cause CAP are *S. pneumoniae, H. influenzae, M. pneumoniae, C. pneumoniae, K. pneumoniae*, and *L. pneumophila.*
- CAP is diagnosed based on clinical features. Chest radiographic demonstration of airspace disease helps support the diagnosis in the appropriate clinical setting.
- Patients with CAP are treated with antibiotics regardless of chest radiography findings. Further evaluation with CT, bronchoscopy, pleural fluid analysis, etc. is reserved for patients who do not respond to treatment or in whom complications are suspected.
- CT is useful in assessing complications such as empyema, bronchopleural fistula, abscess, and necrotizing pneumonia.
- Lung abscesses and empyema are frequently associated with aspiration pneumonia.

Suggested Reading

Franquet T. Imaging of pneumonia: Trends and algorithms. *Eur Respir J.* 2001;18:196–208.

Nair GB, Niederman MS. Community-acquired pneumonia: An unfinished battle. *Med Clin North Am.* 2011 Nov;95(6): 1143–1161.

Tarver RD, Teague SD, Heitkamp DE, et al. Radiology of community-acquired pneumonia. *Radiol Clin North Am.* 2005;43:497–512.

Vilar J, Domingo ML, Soto C, Cogollos J. Radiology of bacterial pneumonia. *Eur J Radiol.* 2004;51(2):102–113.

CHAPTER 35

Cavitation

Sonia L. Betancourt

Definition

Cavitation is defined by the Fleischner Society as low attenuation or lucency within a consolidation, nodule, or mass. Although infection is the most common etiology of cavitation, other entities should also be considered (e.g., vasculitides and pulmonary infarct).

Clinical Features

Cavitation is frequent in pulmonary infections. Cavitary consolidation can occur in community-acquired pneumonia (CAP) secondary to *Staphylococcus aureus, Klebsiella pneumoniae*, and *Streptococcus pneumoniae.* Presenting symptoms and signs include acute fever, cough, sputum production, pleuritic chest pain, and hemoptysis. Tuberculosis (TB) is a common cause of cavitation and may manifest with progressive fatigue, malaise, weight loss, chills, and night sweats. In patients with AIDS, TB is a common cause of pulmonary cavitation, especially if CD4 count is greater than 200 CD4 cell/mm^3. As the CD4 count decreases, cavitary infections are less common in the patient compromised immune status.

Septic embolism typically results from bacterial endocarditis, infected peripheral or central venous lines or pacemaker wires, or septic thrombophlebitis. Affected patients often present with sepsis typically from *Staphylococcus aureus* infection, although *Pseudomonas aeruginosa* infection is common in patients with burns and nonthyphoid *Salmonella* is seen in severely immunocompromised patients. Lemierre syndrome refers to septic embolism from anaerobic infection associated with suppurative jugular vein thrombosis.

Opportunistic infections frequently affect immunocompromised patients with acute or subacute symptoms who are infected with fungi such as *Aspergillus* spp. and *Pneumocystis jirovecii* or bacteria such as *Nocardia* spp. Knowledge of the patient's immune status, pathologic condition, and epidemiological factors is helpful for the formulation of a focused differential diagnosis.

Aspiration pneumonia with abscess formation is a frequent cause of cavitary opacities in hospitalized patients with altered state of consciousness. Anaerobes and enterobacteria are common etiologic agents.

Pulmonary infarcts occasionally cavitate. Cavitation may develop with time, and a diagnosis of thromboembolic disease has usually been established in the majority of cases.

Vasculitis such as granulomatosis with polyangiitis, discussed in detail elsewhere, is a common cause of cavitary nodules, masses, and consolidations.

Anatomy and Physiology

Cavitation may result from caseous necrosis (e.g., TB and fungal infection), suppurative necrosis (e.g., abscess), and ischemic necrosis (e.g., pulmonary infarction from angioinvasive infection). Pneumatocele formation (e.g., *Pneumocystis jirovecii* and *Staphylococcus aureus*) is thought to result from a combination of necrosis and a check-valve mechanism.

How to Approach the Image

Chest radiography is the imaging study of choice to evaluate pulmonary infection. Although diagnosis of CAP is clinical, chest radiography allows identification of complications such as abscess, pleural effusion, or bronchopleural fistula. Identification of associated cavitation is important, but it may be subtle and not visible on radiography. CT is superior to radiography for identification of subtle pulmonary opacities and cavitation.

Image interpretation should always include a thorough review of the medical record for assessment of clinical findings and immune status.

What Not to Miss

Cavitation is a common complication of severe infection. Multifocal and/or cavitary consolidations should suggest a life-threatening infection.

Identification of cavitation may allow diagnosis of abscess formation.

Differential Diagnosis

Pulmonary infection is a common cause of cavitation. Cavitation in the setting of pneumonia often indicates a complicated infection. Any microorganism can produce cavitation due to abscess formation. *Streptococcus pneumoniae* and *Haemophilus influenzae* are common causes of CAP.

- Infection with *K. pneumoniae* may be a hospital- or community-acquired pneumonia. Risk factors include alcoholism, corticosteroid use, and hematologic malignancy.
- *Staphylococcus aureus* may be a hospital- or community-acquired pneumonia, more commonly seen in debilitated hospitalized patients with extrapulmonary infections and intravenous drugs users.
- *Actinomyces israelii* is a normal habitant of the oral cavity that may cause pneumonia particularly in male alcoholics with poor oral hygiene.
- Infection with *P. aeruginosa* is often a hospital-acquired pneumonia and may occur in the setting of mechanical ventilation.
- Nocardiosis is an opportunistic infection caused by *Nocardia asteroides* and is more common in patients with chronic obstructive pulmonary disease, corticosteroid use, HIV/AIDS, malignancy, and transplantation.
- *Mycobacterium tuberculosis* is more prevalent in developing countries. Risk factors include diabetes mellitus, hematologic malignancy, HIV/AIDS, head and neck cancer, and immunosuppressive therapy. Atypical mycobacterial infection may manifest with upper lobe cavitary disease on imaging and mimic TB.
- *Aspergillus fumigatus* is a saprophytic fungus that may cause infection in patients with hematologic malignancy and severe neutropenia, HIV/AIDS, immunosuppressive therapy, and both hematologic and solid-organ transplanation.
- *Pneumocystis jirovecii* affects patients with HIV/AIDS, hematologic malignancy, and transplantation. It rarely causes cavitary disease.

Septic embolism and vasculitis should always be considered in the differential diagnosis of multifocal cavitary nodules, masses, and/or consolidations.

Pulmonary metastases may rarely cavitate; common examples include particularly squamous cell carcinomas and sarcomas.

Imaging Findings

There are no specific imaging features that help differentiate cavitation from infection, infarction, or vasculitis.

Cavitary consolidation is commonly due to infection. Differential considerations are based on clinical presentation, immune status, and microbiologic and serologic assessment.

The following should be considered in evaluating cavitary pulmonary infection (Figs. 35.1–35.5):

- All microorganisms can cause multifocal consolidation and/or cavitation.
- *Klebsiella pneumoniae* may exhibit bulging fissures on imaging.
- *Staphylococcus aureus* may exhibit rapid progression clinically and on imaging (i.e., within hours to a few days).
- *Mycobacterium tuberculosis* characteristically manifests with upper lobe cavitary disease. In the United States, atypical mycobacterial infection is more likely. However, always assume TB until a final microbiologic diagnosis is established.
- *Aspergillus fumigatus* produces angioinvasive fungal infection in a very specific patient population characterized by neutropenia (i.e., hematologic malignancies, transplantation, chronic corticosteroid therapy, and advanced HIV). Cavitation may manifest with the "crescent" sign during recovery. The CT halo sign (a halo of ground-glass opacity) and the reverse halo sign (ground-glass opacity surrounded by consolidation) are frequent findings at early stages of disease. Other fungal infections may exhibit similar imaging findings.
- *Pneumocystis jirovecii* pneumonia is characterized by bilateral and diffuse perihilar ground-glass opacities. Pneumatoceles and pneumothorax can occasionally occur.

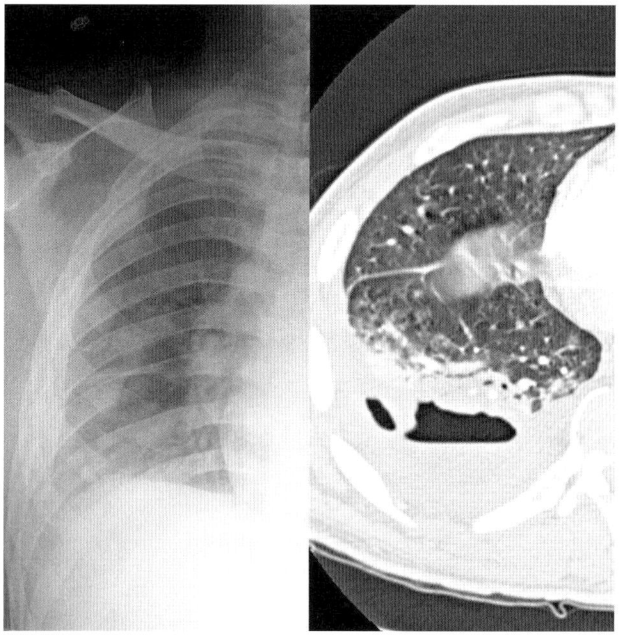

Figure 35.1 Necrotizing pneumonia due to *Staphylococcus aureus*. Composite image with anteroposterior (AP) chest radiograph (left) and contrast-enhanced chest CT (right) of a 53-year-old man with acute dyspnea, chest pain, and hemoptysis shows a small right pleural effusion and right lower lung zone lucency that corresponds to a right lower lobe abscess with extension into the right pleural space (i.e., empyema) that exhibits a small pneumothorax from a bronchopleural fistula.

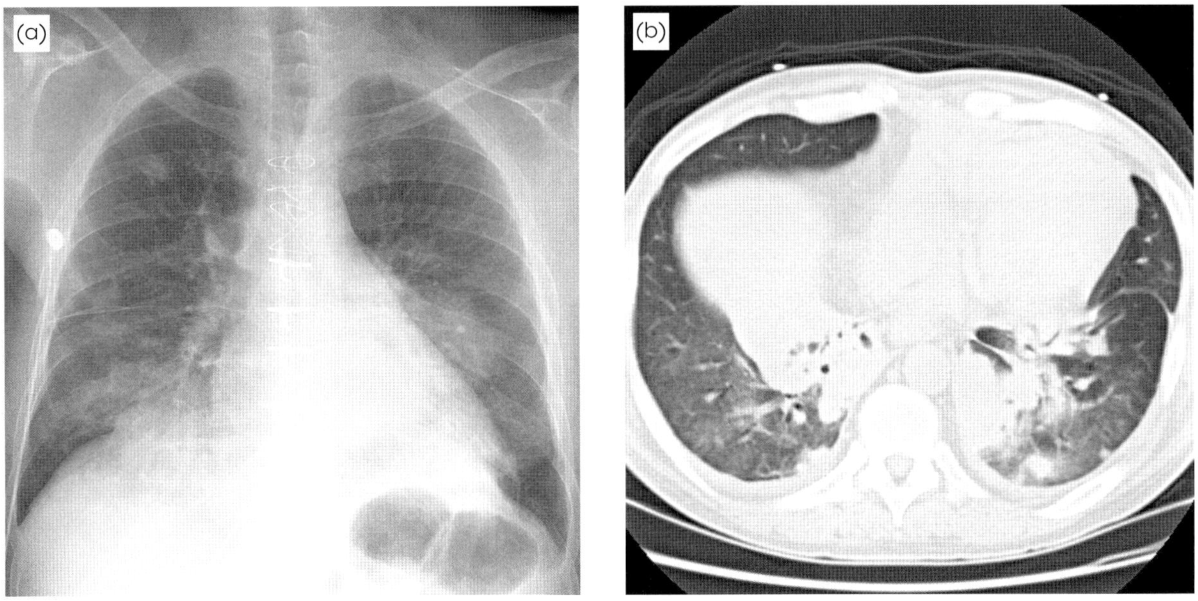

Figure 35.2 Multifocal pneumonia due to *N. asteroides*. (a) Posteroanterior (PA) chest radiograph of a 57-year-old man with HIV, malaise, fever, and dyspnea shows extensive bilateral lower lobe airspace disease. (b) Unenhanced chest shows bibasilar ground-glass opacities and consolidations with intrinsic cavitation in the right lower lobe.

- *Actinomyces israelii* may manifest with airspace disease with intrinsic low attenuation from necrosis and adjacent pleural thickening. Chest wall involvement with abscess formation and bone destruction are common.
- Mucormycosis may manifest with cavitary mass or consolidation in a diabetic patient.
- Septic embolism: Multiple 1- to 3-cm nodules that are often cavitary. CT is superior to radiography for detecting pulmonary nodules and demonstrating intrinsic cavitation and other findings, such as surrounding ground-glass (halo sign), peripheral wedge-shaped opacities (from

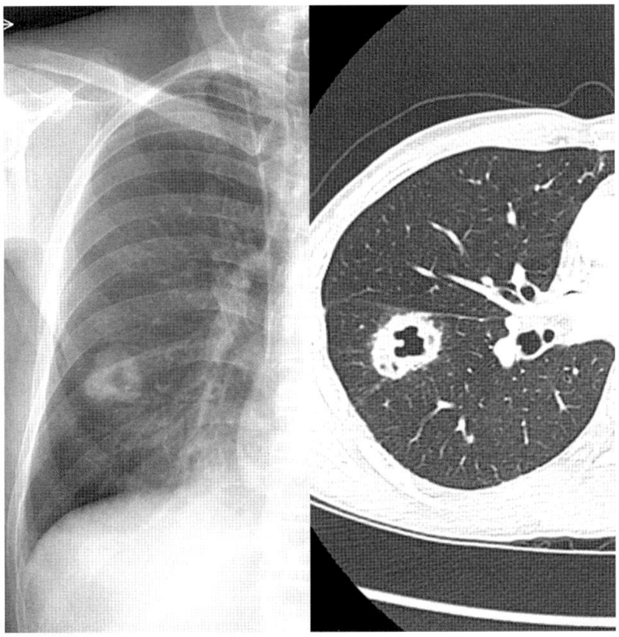

Figure 35.3 Cavitary nodule due to *N. asteroides*. Composite image with PA chest radiograph (left) and unenhanced chest CT (right) of a 43-year-old man with lymphoma shows a cavitary right lower lobe nodule with thick nodular cavity walls.

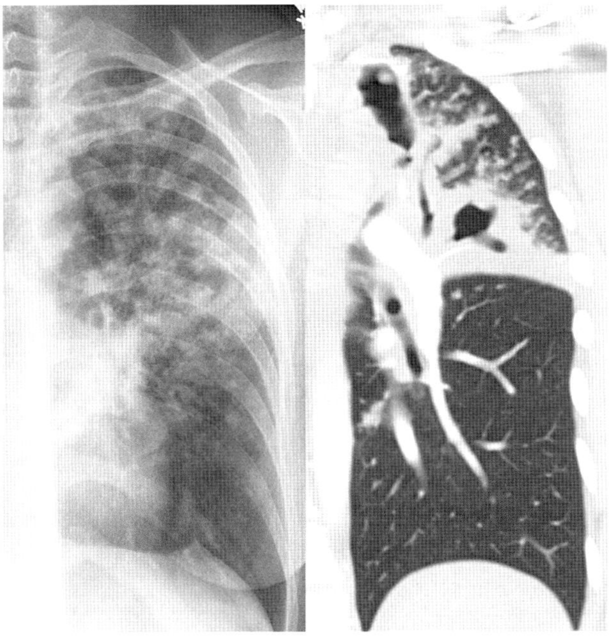

Figure 35.4 Active cavitary tuberculosis. Composite image with PA chest radiograph (left) and contrast-enhanced chest CT (right) of a 37-year-old woman with fever, chronic cough, and sputum production shows heterogeneous nodular opacities in the left mid and upper lung zones that exhibit cavitation and extensive tree-in-bud opacities on chest CT (right).

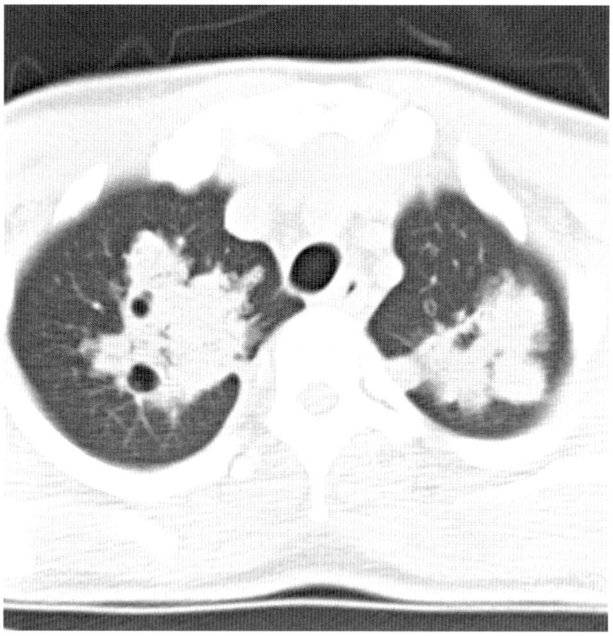

Figure 35.5 Multifocal pneumonia due to *Pneumocystis jirovecii*. Unenhanced chest CT of a 43-year-old man with HIV, dyspnea, and cough shows bilateral upper lobe consolidations with intrinsic lucencies from pneumatoceles.

infarction), and the feeding vessel sign (vessel coursing into a nodule or wedge-shaped opacity) (Fig. 35.6).

Granulomatosis with polyangiitis (i.e., Wegener granulomatosis) may exhibit nodules, masses, and consolidations that typically cavitate (Fig. 35.7).

Cavitary infarction is an unusual manifestation of thromboembolic disease and typically manifests as a peripheral wedge-shaped consolidation with intrinsic lucency (Fig. 35.8). Contrast-enhanced chest CT may show coexistent endoluminal filling defects consistent with thromboembolic disease.

Clinical Issues

- Imaging features do not allow differentiation among infectious agents.
- Some patients (e.g., patients with neutropenic fever) may be treated empirically based on history, symptoms, and laboratory and imaging findings suggestive of a particular organism.
- Fiber-optic bronchoscopy with bronchoalveolar lavage, transbronchial biopsy, and transthoracic needle aspiration may be required for definitive diagnosis but is not always possible.

Key Points

- Cavitation of nodules, masses, or consolidations is often related to infection, but it can also occur in septic embolism, vasculitides, and pulmonary infarction.
- Aspiration pneumonia may manifest with cavitation and is common in institutionalized patients with altered state of consciousness. Anaerobes and enterobacteria are common etiologic agents.
- *Mycobacterium tuberculosis* should always be considered in patients with upper lobe cavitary disease.

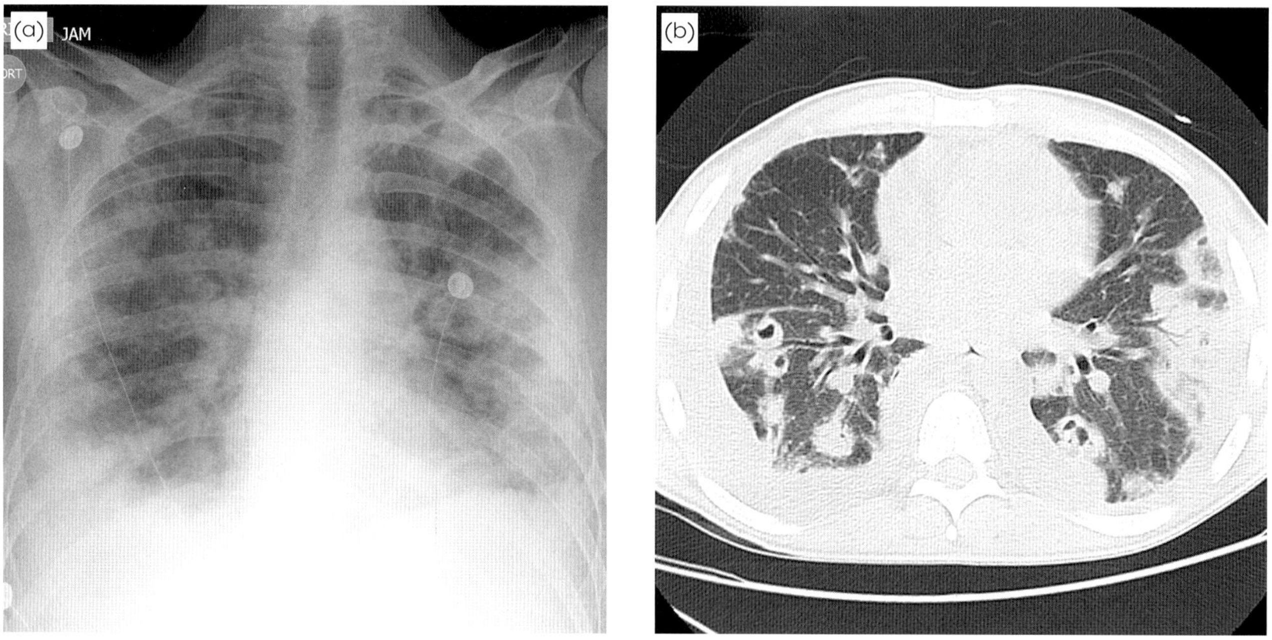

Figure 35.6 Septic embolism due to *Staphylococcus aureus*. (a) AP chest radiograph of a 27-year-old patient with a history of intravenous drug use, fever, and chills shows scattered heterogeneous opacities with apparent cavitation. (b) Unenhanced chest CT demonstrates multiple cavitary nodules and peripheral wedge-shaped consolidations and bilateral pleural effusions.

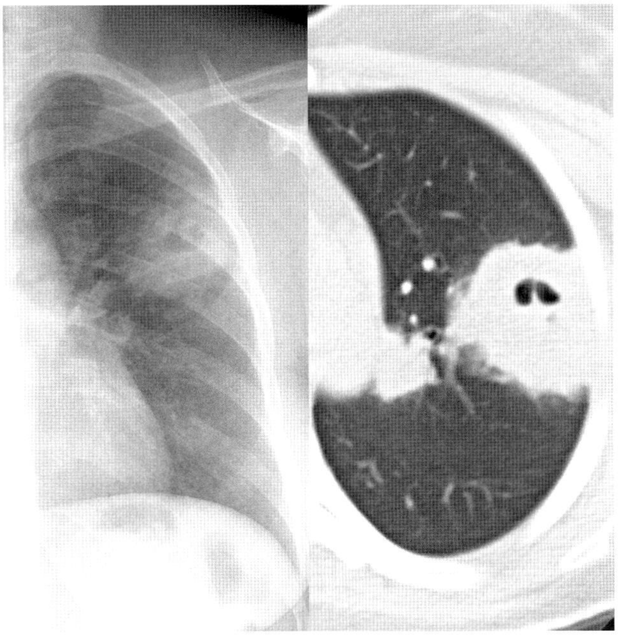

Figure 35.7 Cavitary masses in granulomatosis with polyangiitis (Wegener granulomatosis). Composite image with PA chest radiograph (left) and unenhanced chest CT (right) of a 32-year-old man with chest pain and dyspnea shows a cavitary left upper lobe mass.

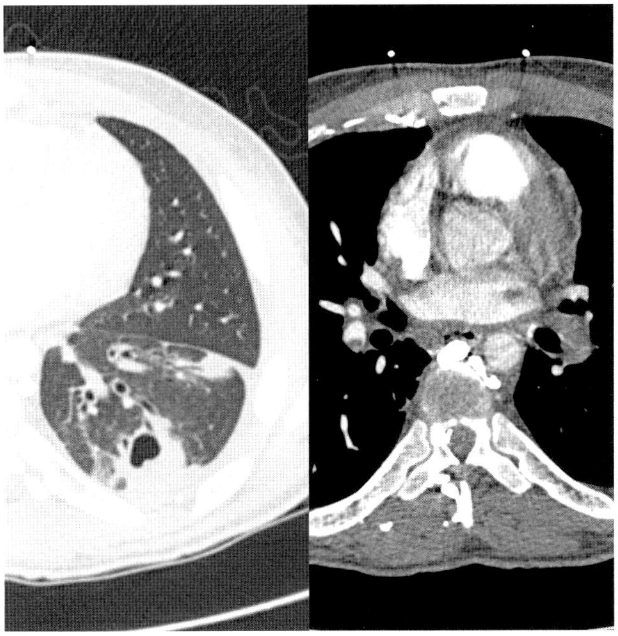

Figure 35.8 Cavitary pulmonary infarct. Composite image of a 39-year-old patient with chest pain and dyspnea shows a peripheral, left lower lobe; wedge-shaped consolidation with intrinsic cavitation (left); and bilateral pulmonary emboli (right).

These patients should be isolated until etiology is proven.

- *Aspergillus* spp., *nocardia* spp., and *Pneumocystis jiroveci* should be considered in immunocompromised patients.
- *Staphylococcus aureus* is the most common cause of septic emboli.
- In patients without clinical evidence of infection, granulomatosis with polyangiitis and metastatic disease should be considered.

Suggested Reading

Gadkowski LB, Stout JE. Cavitary pulmonary disease. *Clin Microbiol Rev*. 2008;21:305–333.

Kwon WJ, Jeong YJ, Kim KI, Lee IS, Jeon UB, Lee SH, et al. Computed tomographic features of pulmonary septic emboli: Comparison of causative microorganisms. *J Comput Assist Tomogr*. 2007;31(3):390–394.

Martinez F, Chung JH, Digumarthy SR, Kanne JP, Abbott GF, Shepard JA, et al. Common and uncommon manifestations of Wegener granulomatosis at chest CT: Radiologic–pathologic correlation. *RadioGraphics*. 2012;32(1):51–69.

Vilar J, Domingo ML, Soto C, Cogollos J. Radiology of bacterial pneumonia. *Eur J Radiol*. 2004;51:102–113.

Washington L, Palacio D. Imaging of bacterial pulmonary infection in the immunocompetent patient. *Semin Roentgenol*. 2007;42:122–145.

CHAPTER 36

Endemic Fungal Infection

Sonia L. Betancourt

Definition

The term endemic refers to a disease or condition found in a particular geographic area. Common endemic fungi, including *Histoplasma capsulatum*, *Coccidioides immitis*, and *Blastomyces dermatitidis*, are found in the soil and may produce infection in healthy individuals who live in or have visited certain areas. However, disseminated life-threatening disease may affect immunocompromised patients (e.g., AIDS patients).

Clinical Features

Most patients with endemic fungal (EF) infection are asymptomatic. Patients with acute infection may present with nonspecific self-limited symptoms and signs, including fever, headaches, chills, and cough. Immunocompromised individuals may develop fulminant acute or chronic disease with or without dissemination. Patients with coccidiodomycosis and blastomycosis may present with cutaneous lesions.

The diagnosis of EF infection requires familiarity with the epidemiology and spectrum of radiologic findings. History of travel to or residence in endemic regions should raise suspicion. Definitive diagnosis requires culture or pathologic demonstration of the microorganism. Radioimmunoassay for *H. capsulatum* polysaccharide antigen is useful in the diagnosis of disseminated histoplasmosis. Serologic tests for antibodies are widely used and useful in diagnosing *C. immitis* infection. *Blastomyces dermatitidis* antigen can be detected in serum, urine, and bronchoalveolar lavage fluid.

Histoplasmosis is endemic in the Ohio, Mississippi, and Missouri River valleys. *Histoplasma capsulatum* is found in soil contaminated with fecal material from chickens, pigeons, and bats. It frequently affects farmers, construction workers, and outdoor enthusiasts. Patients with acute pulmonary histoplasmosis may be asymptomatic or may present with nonspecific upper respiratory tract symptoms. Chronic histoplasmosis is common in middle-aged men with emphysema who often present with cough, fever, hemoptysis, dyspnea, and weight loss. Chronic mediastinal histoplasmosis (i.e., fibrosing mediastinitis) is a severe fibrous reaction due to immunologic stimulation by *H. capsulatum* antigens that may compress regional structures and result in focal occlusive vascular disease and narrowing of the airways.

Coccidioides immitis is endemic in the desertic and semidesertic southwestern United States and northern Mexico. Patients with acute coccidioidomycosis may be asymptomatic or may present with flu-like symptoms. Valley fever (named after one of the earliest descriptions in the San Joaquin Valley in California) is a manifestation of acute coccidioidomycosis characterized by pneumonitis, erythema nodosum, and arthralgias. Chronic coccidioidomycosis affects a minority of patients who are frequently asymptomatic or have mild constitutional symptoms. Disseminated coccidioidomycosis complicates less than 1% of immunocompetent patients and more frequently complicates immunocompromised patients.

Blastomyces dermatitidis is endemic in the southeastern and southwestern United States, mostly the Ohio and Mississippi River valleys and the Great Lakes area. Verrucous and ulcerative cutaneous lesions are helpful when infection is suspected. Extrathoracic dissemination affects the skin, musculoskeletal structures, and genitourinary tract. Pleuritic chest pain, chills, fever, and productive cough commonly occur in acute blastomycosis. Chronic blastomycosis may manifest with constitutional symptoms. Disseminated infection typically affects patients with chronic blastomycosis.

Anatomy and Physiology

After inhalation, spores convert into yeast forms. In healthy individuals, yeasts cause an intense inflammatory reaction leading to the development of caseous necrosis and calcification. Involvement of hilar and/or mediastinal lymph nodes follows due to invasion of pulmonary lymphatics. Systemic dissemination affects elderly patients or those with impaired T-cell immunity.

How to Approach the Image

Imaging findings of EF infection may mimic those of other infections (e.g., tuberculosis [TB]) and neoplasms (e.g., lung cancer). The initial diagnosis is generally challenging. Often, the final diagnosis emerges unsuspectedly during the workup of a pulmonary nodule or mass or in patients presumed to have cavitary TB.

What Not to Miss

EF infection should be suspected in patients from endemic areas who present with pulmonary opacities and/or cavitary disease on imaging.

EF infection should be considered in patients with pneumonia or bronchopneumonia that does not improve despite medical treatment.

Differential Diagnosis

- Nodules or masses with associated hilar and/or mediastinal lymphadenopathy: Frequent findings in acute histoplasmosis; they are also characteristic of lung cancer. Radiologic differentiation is often impossible and may require pathologic sampling and/or follow-up imaging.
- Upper lobe cavitary disease: Frequent radiologic manifestation of EF infection that should also suggest cavitary TB. In fact, cavitary disease should be presumed to be TB until proven otherwise.
- Miliary nodules: Manifestation of disseminated EF infection mimics miliary TB, miliary metastases, and sarcoidosis. EF infection may also affect the meninges, brain, skeleton, skin, spleen, and kidneys.
- Chronic mediastinal histoplasmosis (fibrosing mediastinitis) may simulate a mediastinal infiltrative process such as lymphoma or lung cancer.

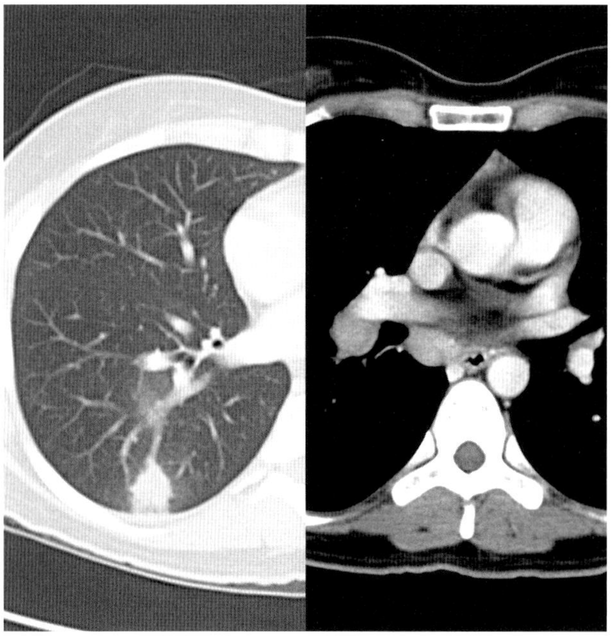

Figure 36.1 Acute histoplasmosis. Contrast-enhanced chest CT of a 28-year-old man with fever, cough, and malaise shows a spiculated right lower lobe nodule with surrounding ground-glass opacities and right hilar and subcarinal lymphadenopathy.

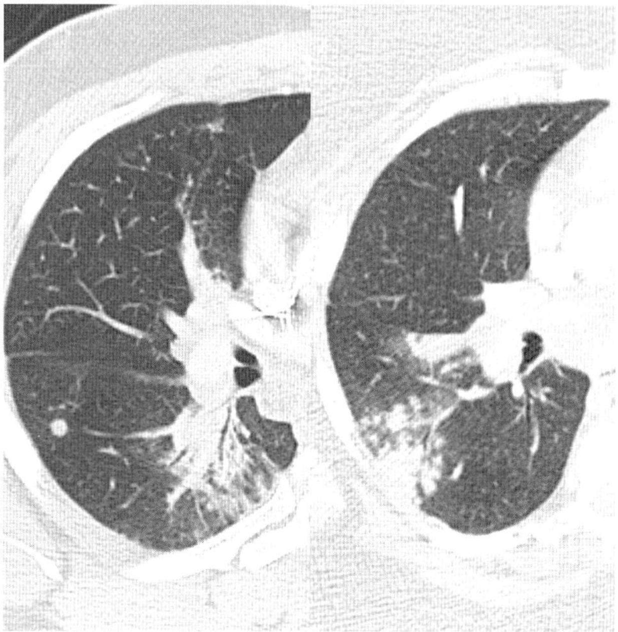

Figure 36.2 Acute histoplasmosis. Composite image with chest CT of two different patients with acute histoplasmosis shows a right lower lobe consolidation (left) and clustered centrilobular nodules associated with nodular consolidations (right).

Imaging Findings

Histoplasmosis

- Patients with acute histoplasmosis may have a normal chest radiograph.
- Typically, there are airspace opacities that can simulate community-acquired pneumonia (Fig 36.1).

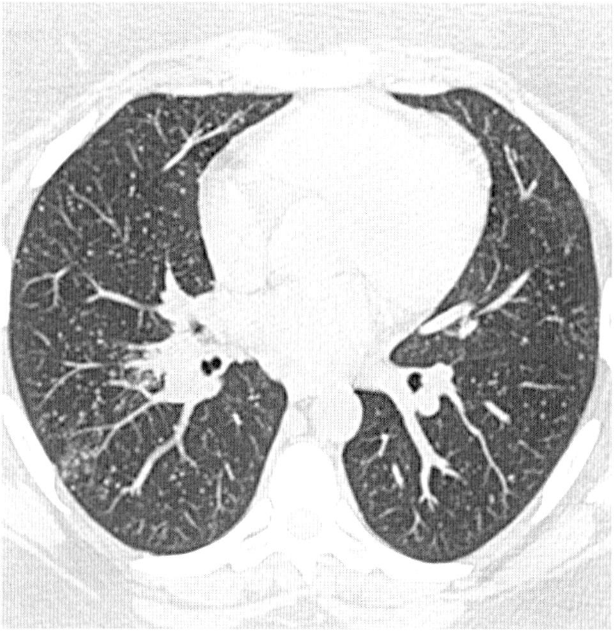

Figure 36.3 Miliary histoplasmosis. Unenhanced chest CT of a 43-year-old woman with recent diagnosis of acute histoplasmosis shows innumerable bilateral micronodules with random distribution.

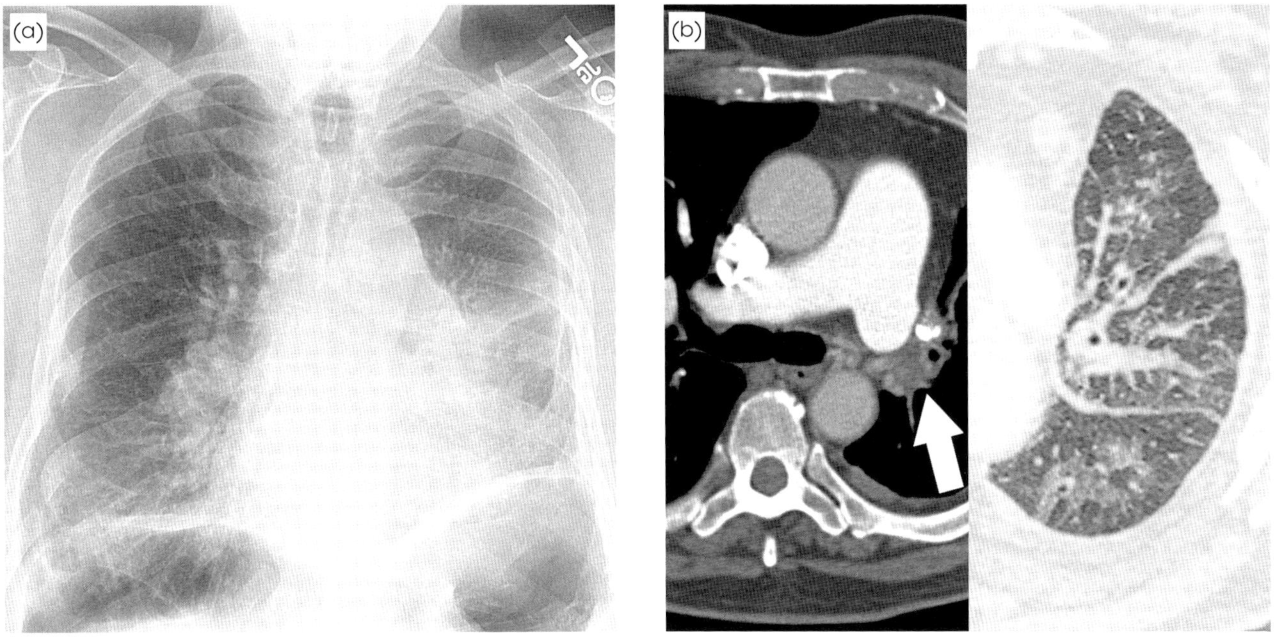

Figure 36.4 Chronic mediastinal histoplasmosis. (a) Anteroposterior (AP) chest radiograph of a 63-year-old woman with chronic obstructive pulmonary disease shows left lower lobe volume loss and an ill-defined left hilar mass that had remained stable for years. (b) Contrast-enhanced chest CT shows a left hilar mass (arrow) with intrinsic calcification that obstructs the left pulmonary artery (left) and ground-glass opacities with associated interlobular septal thickening consistent with pulmonary veno-occlusive disease (right).

- Solitary or multiple pulmonary nodules may develop with healing and may be associated with mediastinal and hilar lymphadenopathy (Fig 36.2). Intrinsic calcification of nodules and/or lymph nodes is common.
- Chronic histoplasmosis may exhibit upper lobe airspace disease with intrinsic cavitation.
- Chronic mediastinal histoplasmosis (i.e., fibrosing mediastinitis) manifests as mediastinal or hilar soft tissue masses with intrinsic high attenuation and/or calcification that may produce airway narrowing, vascular compression (pulmonary veins and arteries), and esophageal obstruction. Involvement of a pulmonary vein may result in atelectasis, ground-glass opacities, and interlobular septal thickening in the affected lung as a manifestation of focal veno-occlusive disease (Fig. 36.4).

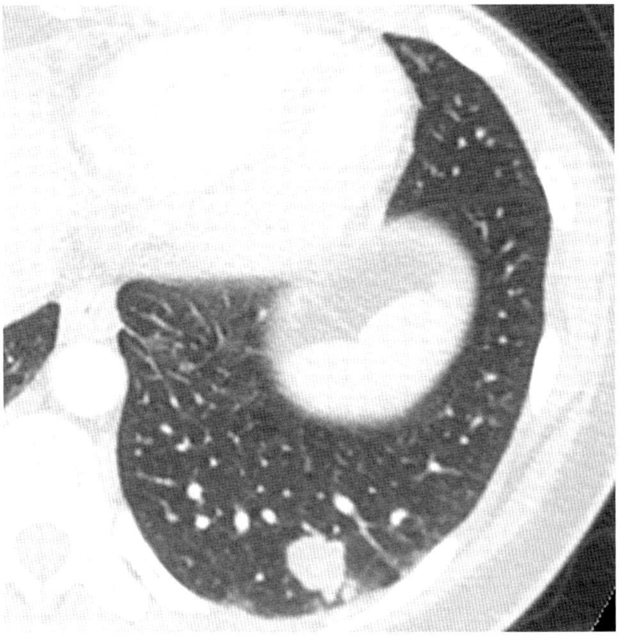

Figure 36.5 Acute coccidiodomycosis. Unenhanced chest CT of a 28-year-old man with recent respiratory symptoms shows a left lower lobe polylobular nodule.

- Disseminated histoplasmosis manifests with diffuse randomly distributed micronodules (i.e., miliary pattern) that may progress to diffuse airspace opacities (Fig 36.1).
- Histoplasmoma is a lung nodule measuring up to 3 cm that may exhibit soft tissue attenuation or intrinsic calcification with central, diffuse, or laminated ("bullseye" or "target") patterns. Satellite or clustered centrilobular micronodules are common on CT.

Coccidioidomycosis

- Acute coccidioidomycosis may exhibit focal or multifocal airspace disease or nodules/masses (Fig 36.5). Hilar and mediastinal lymphadenopathy and satellite nodules are common. With healing, nodules can become calcified (Figs. 36.5 and 36.6).
- Chronic coccidioidomycosis manifests with progressive upper lobe predominant consolidation with intrinsic cavitation that may be complicated by spontaneous pneumothorax or bronchopleural fistula.
- Disseminated coccidioidomycosis often manifests with miliary nodules that may rapidly coalesce in immunocompromised patients (Fig 36.6).

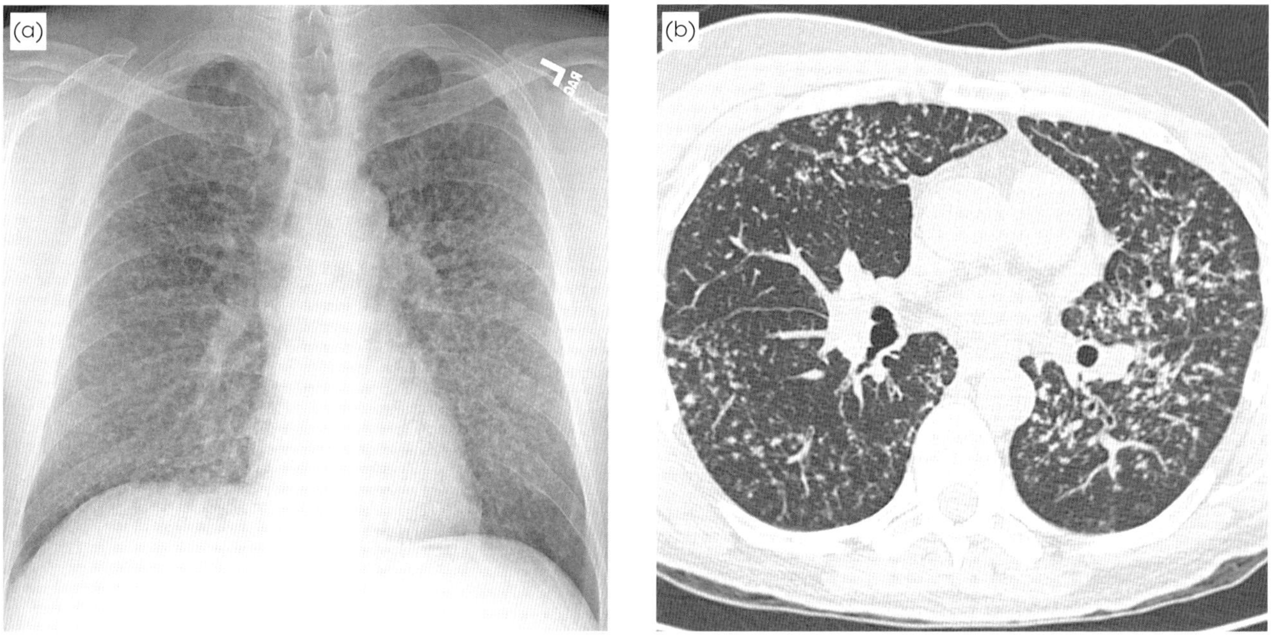

Figure 36.6 Miliary coccidiodomycosis. (a) Posteroanterior (PA) chest radiograph of a 37-year-old man with dyspnea and low-grade fever demonstrates diffuse bilateral pulmonary micronodules. (b) Unenhanced chest CT of the same patient shows diffuse randomly distributed bilateral pulmonary micronodules.

North American Blastomycosis

- Frequent imaging findings include airspace opacities, masses, and nodules that may exhibit cavitation (Figs. 36.7 and 36.8).
- Pleural thickening is more common than pleural effusion.
- Rib erosion, associated with a chest wall mass or fistulae, may complicate chronic and disseminated disease.

EF infection is a known cause of false-positive FDG-PET/CT studies and often manifests with FDG avid

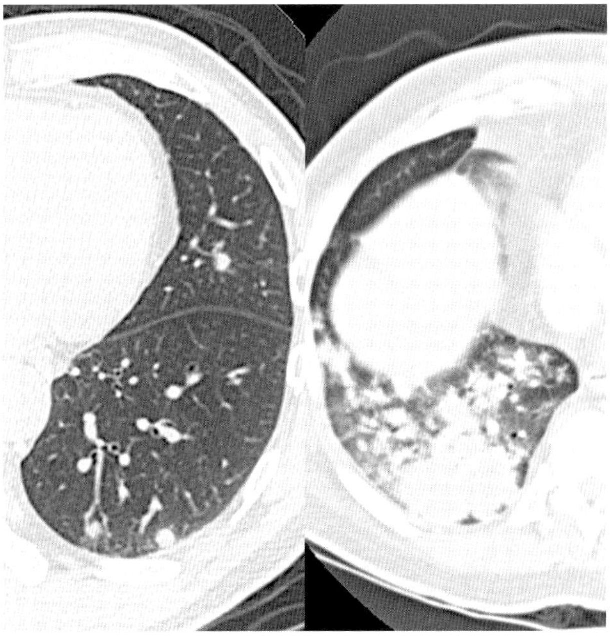

Figure 36.7 Acute blastomycosis. Composite image with unenhanced chest CT of two different patients with acute blastomycosis shows small left lower lobe pulmonary nodules (left) and right lower lobe consolidation and surrounding small nodules (right).

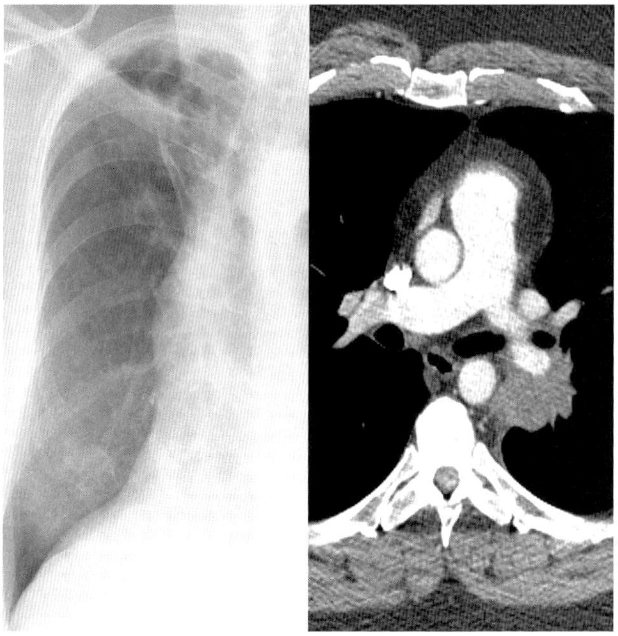

Figure 36.8 Chronic blastomycosis. Composite image with PA chest radiograph (left) and contrast-enhanced chest CT (right) of two different patients with chronic blastomycosis shows right upper lobe heterogeneous opacities and volume loss (left) and a soft tissue mass encasing the left pulmonary artery (right).

nodules/masses. In these cases, biopsy may be required for definitive diagnosis.

Clinical Issues

- The diagnosis of EF infection may be challenging. Initial diagnosis may be delayed due to low clinical suspicion because these entities are rather uncommon compared to other infections. Lung opacities that do not improve with antibiotics should raise suspicion for EF infection. Hilar and mediastinal lymphadenopathy with or without associated lung opacities or nodules in a patient from or with a history of travel to an endemic area should suggest the possibility of EF infection.
- Skin manifestations such as erythema nodosum, necrotic nodules, and ulcers associated with lung abnormalities should raise consideration of EF infection.

Key Points

- Endemic fungi live in soil as saprophytes, infect humans when their spores are inhaled, and often affect healthy individuals.
- Consider EF infection in patients with bronchopneumonia associated with lymphadenopathy that does not respond to antibiotics. Fungal infection may mimic TB, metastatic disease, and lung cancer.
- Immunosuppression is frequently associated with disseminated EF infection.
- Chronic mediastinal histoplasmosis is a common benign etiology of superior vena cava syndrome.

Suggested Reading

Fang W, Washington L, Kumar N. Imaging manifestations of blastomycosis: A pulmonary infection with potential dissemination. *RadioGraphics*. 2007;27(3):641–655.

McAdams HP, Rosado-de-Christenson M, Lesar M, et al. Thoracic mycoses from endemic fungi: Radiologic–pathologic correlation. *RadioGraphics*. 1995;15:255–270.

Panackal AA, Hajjeh RA, Cetron MS, et al. Fungal infection among returning travelers. *Clin Infect Dis*. 2002:35:1088–1095.

Tarver R, Teague SD, Heitkamp DE, et al. Radiology of community-acquired pneumonia. *Radiol Clin North Am*. 2005;43:497–512.

CHAPTER 37

Opportunistic Fungal Infection

Sonia L. Betancourt

Definition

Opportunistic fungal infections are caused by fungi that are nonpathogenic in the immunocompetent host, many of which are part of the normal upper respiratory tract flora. These organisms may cause pulmonary infection in immunocompromised hosts. Some of the most common opportunistic fungi are *Aspergillus* spp., *Pneumocystis jirovecii*, *Candida* spp., *Cryptoccoccus neoformans*, and Zygomycetes (i.e., *Mucor, Rhizopus*, and *Absidia*).

Clinical Features

Opportunistic fungi affect patients with congenital or acquired immunodeficiency (e.g., AIDS), chemotherapy-induced neutropenia, or immunosuppression after bone marrow or solid organ transplantation. Fever is a common presenting sign, but symptoms and signs may be absent.

In patients with allogenic bone marrow transplant, *Aspergillus* spp. are the most common cause of fungal pneumonia. In hematologic malignancies, *Aspergillus* spp. are the primary cause of infection, but *P. jirovecii* and *Candida* spp. are also of concern. Cryptococcosis, aspergillosis, and mucormycosis are common after renal transplantation. *Aspergillus* spp. and *Candida* spp. are common after heart transplantation. *Aspergillus* spp. and *P. jirovecii* are common after lung transplantation.

Angioinvasive and airway-invasive aspergillosis occurs in severe immunosuppression (e.g., severe neutropenia, prolonged corticosteroid therapy, graft-versus-host disease after allogeneic bone marrow transplant (BMT), and late-stage AIDS). It can also occur in the first 6 months after solid organ transplant (5% of patients). Following BMT, it usually occurs in the pre-engraftment period (i.e., 0–30 days); however, it can occur beyond 6 months in patients with impaired graft function that required high levels of immunosuppressive therapy.

Semi-invasive aspergillosis occurs in mild immunosuppression (e.g., low-dose corticosteroid therapy, diabetes mellitus, malnutrition, and lung disease such as chronic obstructive pulmonary disease (COPD) and pneumoconiosis).

Pneumocystis jirovecii pneumonia is the most common pulmonary fungal infection in patients with AIDS and CD4 counts less than 200 cell/mm^3.

After *P. jirovecii*, cryptococcosis is the second most common fungal infection in patients with AIDS. It may affect the central nervous system and is a known cause of meningitis.

Candidiasis is common in patients with hematologic malignancies and may occur as hematogenous dissemination from an extrapulmonary source or, less frequently, from oropharyngeal aspiration. Co-infection with other pathogens is common. *Candida* spp. rarely cause pneumonia in patients with AIDS in the absence of disseminated disease.

Zygomycosis is common in transplantation, hematologic malignancy, diabetes, and renal failure, and it has a propensity for invading the pulmonary arteries.

Anatomy and Physiology

Mononuclear cells are the primary defense against bacteria and fungi. Neutropenia occurs in patients with acute leukemia undergoing chemotherapy and receiving high doses of steroids. Thus, these patients are at risk for angioinvasive fungal infections, typically *Aspergillus*. AIDS patients, who have decreased T-cell immunity, are predominantly affected by intracellular pathogens, including *P. jirovecii*, *C. neoformans*, and *Histoplasma capsulatum*.

How to Approach the Image

Chest radiography and CT are important in the diagnosis of opportunistic fungal infections. Because imaging findings are nonspecific, full knowledge of the patient's disease is required. Although normal chest radiographs are frequent, common radiographic abnormalities include nodules, masses, and consolidations.

Thin-section CT may demonstrate more specific abnormalities, such as the "CT halo" sign, the "reverse halo" sign (i.e., ground-glass opacity surrounded by a crescentic or complete ring of consolidation), and cavitation. These findings should suggest opportunistic fungal infection in the appropriate clinical setting.

What Not to Miss

Immunocompromised patients and patients with febrile neutropenia with opportunistic fungal infections may have normal chest radiographs. Thus, chest CT should be performed for further evaluation. Imaging abnormalities in this patient population should raise suspicion for opportunistic infection.

Differential Diagnosis

The "CT halo" sign denotes ground-glass opacity surrounding a pulmonary nodule and is a classic finding of angioinvasive fungal infections (e.g., aspergillosis and zygomycosis). However, this sign has been described in other infections (e.g., viral pneumonia), vasculitides (e.g., granulomatosis with polyangiitis), and hemorrhagic metastases (e.g., angiosarcoma).

Lung nodules and masses in patients with COPD are frequently related to lung cancer. However, *semi-invasive aspergillosis* may mimic lung cancer clinically and on imaging, even exhibiting increased FDG uptake on PET/CT.

Ground-glass opacities is a nonspecific pattern on CT that may be present in atypical infections, alveolar hemorrhage, and pulmonary edema. *Pneumocystis jirovecii* pneumonia is a common cause of diffuse ground-glass opacities and should be suspected in patients with HIV and low CD4 counts.

Several opportunistic fungi may exhibit a miliary pattern on imaging (e.g., *P. jirovecii* pneumonia and cryptococcosis). Tuberculosis and metastatic disease should also be considered in the differential diagnosis.

Imaging Findings

Angioinvasive Aspergillosis

- Chest radiograph: Single or multiple peripheral pulmonary nodules, masses, or consolidations (Figs. 37.1a).
- Chest CT: "halo" sign and "reverse halo" sign. In the recovery phase (i.e., improved neutropenia), cavitation may produce the "air crescent" sign (i.e., a crescentic peripheral lucency within a nodule or mass) (Figs. 37.1b–37.3).

Airway Invasive Aspergillosis

- Bronchopneumonia
- Bronchial wall thickening (Fig. 37.4)

Semi-invasive Aspergillosis

- Chest radiograph: Upper lobe consolidation, nodular opacities and cavitation (mimicking tuberculosis and malignancy), and apical pleural thickening (Fig 37.5a)
- Chest CT: Multiple upper lobe pulmonary nodules, segmental or lobar consolidation, and cavitation (Fig 37.5b).

Candidiasis

- Chest radiograph: Nonsegmental, segmental, or lobar consolidation, often bilateral (Fig. 37.6)
- Chest CT: Lower lobe predominant nodules ranging from 3 to 30 mm; "halo" sign may be present; may colonize preexisting tuberculous cavities or cystic spaces (Fig 37.6)

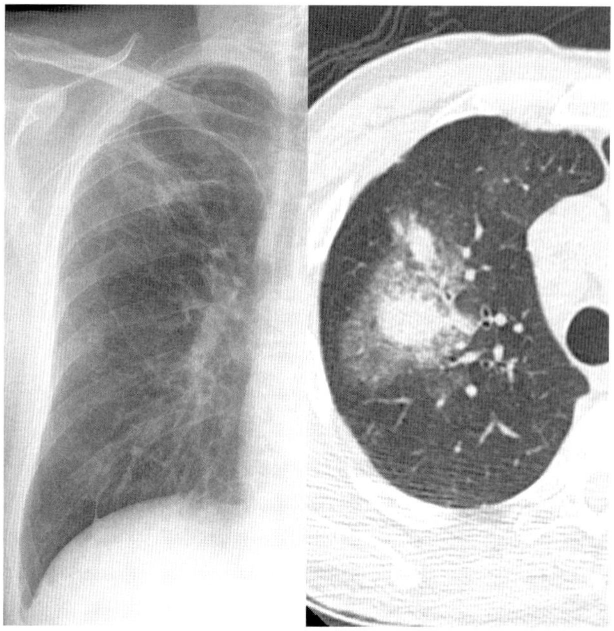

Figure 37.1 Angioinvasive aspergillosis. Composite image of a 45-year-old neutropenic man with recent history of bone marrow transplant with posteroanterior (PA) chest radiograph (left) and unenhanced chest CT (right) shows an irregular right upper lobe nodular opacity that demonstrates the "CT halo" sign manifesting as pulmonary nodules with surrounding ground-glass opacities.

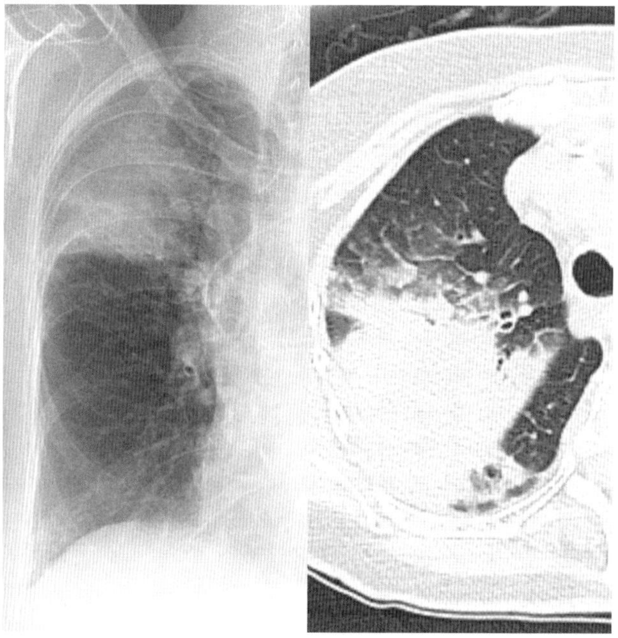

Figure 37.2 Angioinvasive aspergillosis. Composite image of a 55-year-old neutropenic woman with chronic lymphoblastic leukemia with PA chest radiograph (left) and unenhanced chest CT (right) shows a dense right upper lobe consolidation with surrounding ground-glass opacities.

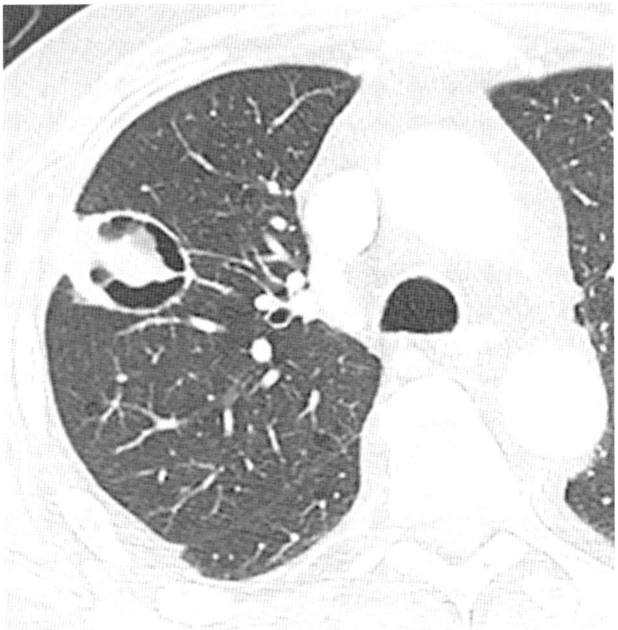

Figure 37.3 Angioinvasive aspergillosis. Chest CT of a 50-year-old man with recent bone marrow transplantation shows a right upper lobe nodule with surrounding crescentic air attenuation lucency, the so-called "air crescent" sign.

Mucormycosis

Imaging findings mimic those of invasive aspergillosis, given angioinvasive behavior (Fig. 37.7):

- Chest radiograph: Lobar consolidation; solitary or multiple nodules or masses, with or without cavitation

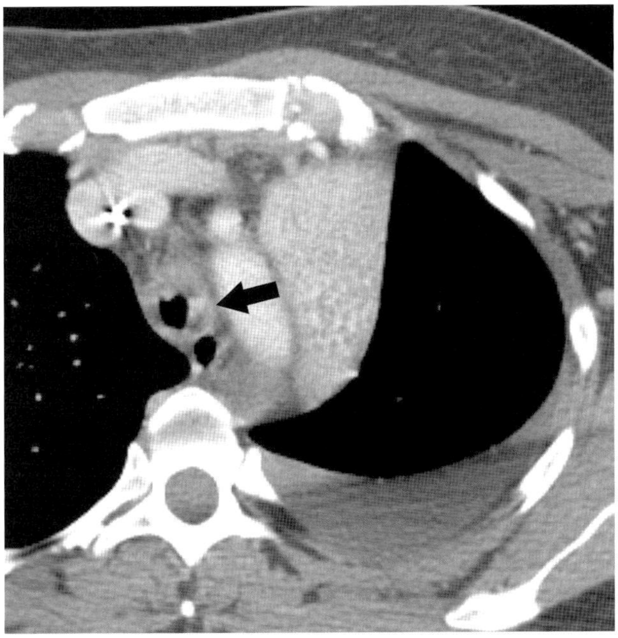

Figure 37.4 Airway-invasive aspergillosis. Contrast-enhanced chest CT of a 37-year-old woman with acute myeloid leukemia demonstrates circumferential tracheal wall thickening (arrow), left upper lobe atelectasis, and a small left pleural effusion.

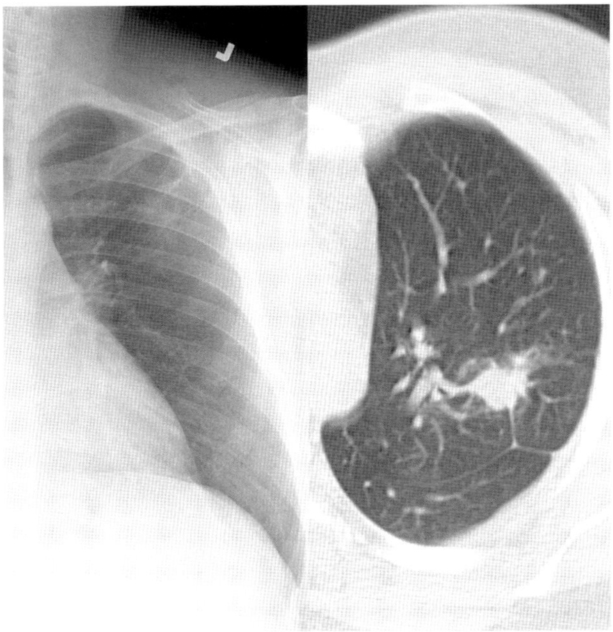

Figure 37.5 Semi-invasive aspergillosis. Composite image with PA chest radiograph (left) and unenhanced chest CT of a 59-year-old male smoker with COPD shows an irregular left upper lobe nodule that exhibits spiculated margins on CT. Surgical resection was performed given concern for lung cancer, and it showed findings of semi-invasive aspergillosis.

- Chest CT: Nodules or masses with the "halo" or "reverse halo" sign; cavitation may produce an "air crescent" sign; rarely, bronchial occlusion and pulmonary pseudoaneurysms (Fig 37.7)

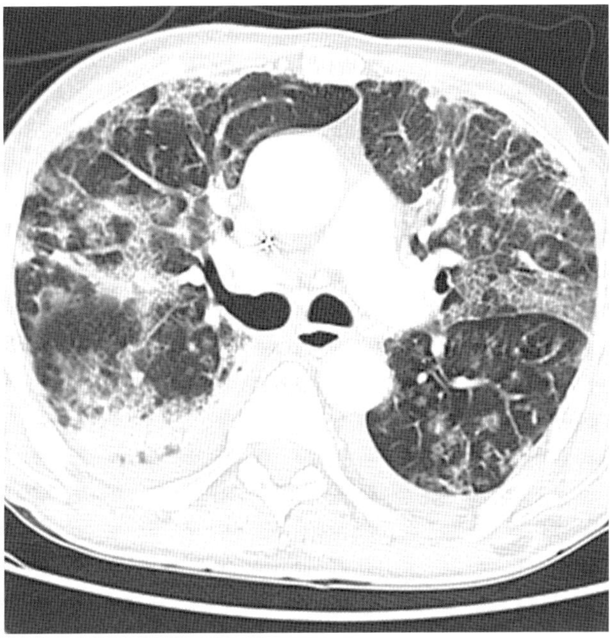

Figure 37.6 Pulmonary candidiasis. Chest CT of a 62-year-old man with chronic lymphocytic leukemia shows multifocal bilateral nodular ground-glass opacities and consolidations. Bronchoalveolar lavage showed *Candida albicans*.

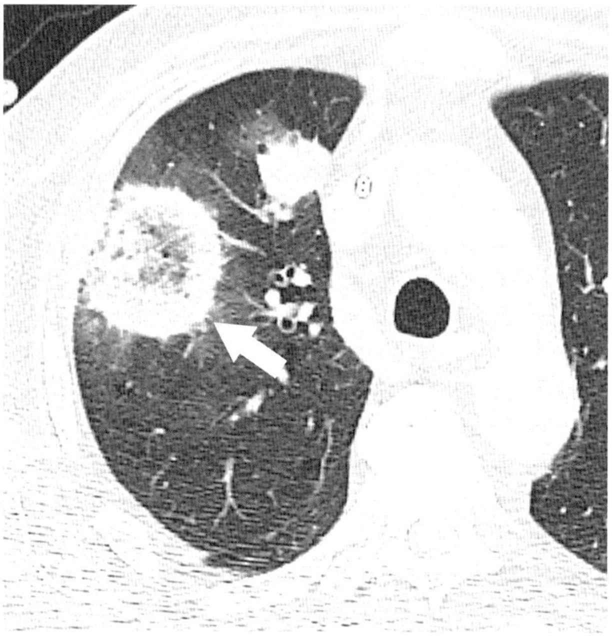

Figure 37.7 Mucormycosis. Chest CT of a 48-year-old man with acute lymphoblastic leukemia shows a right upper lobe mass (arrow) with central ground-glass attenuation surrounded by a dense ring of consolidation (i.e., "reverse halo" sign) and an adjacent solid nodule. Mucormycosis was diagnosed on percutaneous biopsy.

Cryptococcosis

Frequently coexists with other opportunistic infections (Figs. 37.8 and 37.9).

- Chest radiograph: Diffuse heterogeneous or reticulonodular opacities; solitary or multiple lung nodules or masses

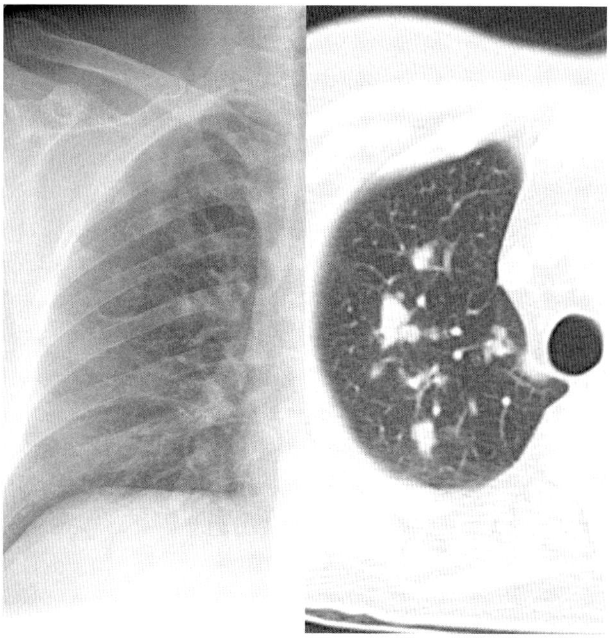

Figure 37.8 Cryptococcosis. Composite image with PA chest radiograph (left) and unenhanced chest CT of a 34-year-old healthy individual with remote history of melanoma shows multiple bilateral nodules, with several appearing spiculated on unenhanced chest CT. Sublobar resection demonstrated cryptococcosis.

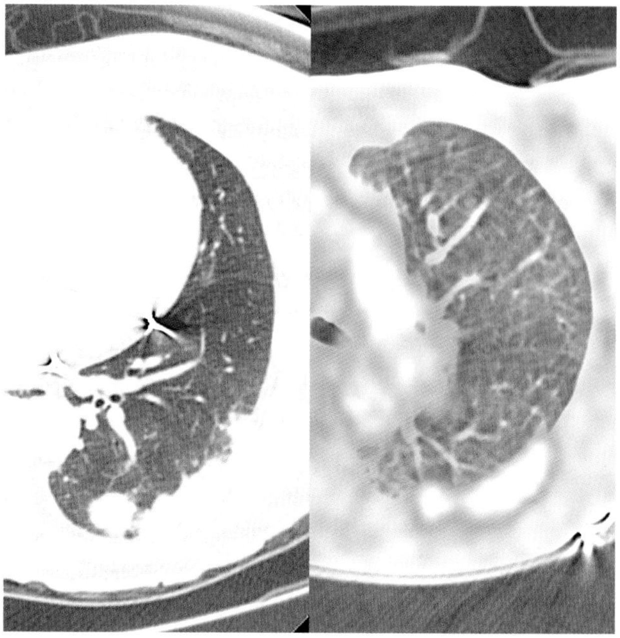

Figure 37.9 Cryptococcosis. Composite image with unenhanced chest CT (left) and PET/CT of a 45-year-old healthy individual with abnormal chest pain showing spiculated nodules with intense FDG uptake. Sublobar resection demonstrated cryptococcosis.

- Chest CT: Nodules/masses that may exhibit cavitation; miliary pattern; hilar/mediastinal lymphadenopathy and pleural effusion less common

Clinical Issues

Fungal infections in immunocompromised hosts are life-threatening because they tend to be angioinvasive and disseminated.

Although definitive diagnosis requires identification of the organism in body fluids or tissue samples, a presumptive diagnosis and management plan may be established based on imaging findings in patients with febrile neutropenia.

Immunocompromised patients with AIDS and patients undergoing intensive immunomodulation may develop pulmonary infection caused by endemic fungi such as histoplasmosis, coccidioidomycosis, and blastomycosis.

Opportunistic fungal lung infections caused by unfamiliar species have recently increased, and many are resistant to antifungal agents. These emerging opportunists include *Fusarium* spp. (Fig. 37.10), *Scedosporium* spp., *Penicillium marnaffei, Trichosporon beigelii, Blastoschizomyces capitatus*, and *Dematiaceous fungi.*

- *Fusarium* is common in hematologic malignancies and lung and hematopoietic stem cell transplantation. It is an angioinvasive fungus causing hemorrhagic tissue infarcts, disseminated disease, and fungemia. The presence of multiple skin lesions is a useful clinical clue.

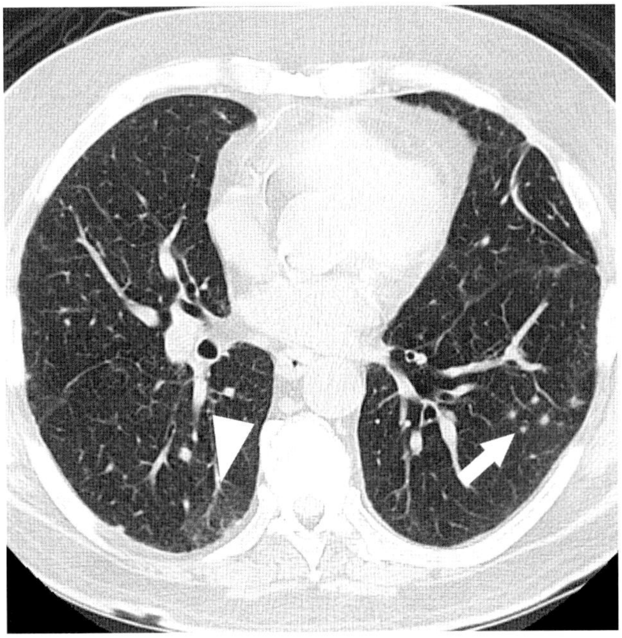

Figure 37.10 Fusariosis. Contrast-enhanced chest CT of a 69-year-old woman with acute myeloid leukemia shows multiple small bilateral pulmonary nodules (arrow) and focal right lower lobe ground-glass opacity (arrowhead). Sublobar resection demonstrated disseminated fusariosis.

- *Scedosporium* is common in hematologic malignancies and bone marrow transplantation. More than 50% of patients have disseminated disease at presentation. Immunocompetent individuals may develop *Scedosporium* pneumonia following inhalation during near drowning and may present with synchronous lung and brain abscesses.
- *Penicillium* causes cavitary consolidation and airspace and reticular opacities in patients with AIDS.
- Tissue sampling for histopathology and culture and PCR-based identification are fundamental in the diagnosis of these emerging unusual pathogens.

Key Points

- Opportunistic fungal lung infections are diagnosed with increasing frequency because of the increasing immmunocompromised population.
- Aspergillosis is the most common opportunistic infection in patients with hematologic malignancy and bone marrow transplantation.
- Neutropenia is the most important risk factor for aspergillosis.
- *Aspergillus* spp., *Candida* spp., and *Cryptococcus* spp. are the most common causes of fungal infections in patients with solid organ transplantation.
- *Pneumocystis jirovecii* is the most common cause of fungal infection in AIDS patients with CD4 counts less than 200 cells/mm^3. Cryptococcal pneumonia is also common in this population.
- There has been a recent increase in uncommon fungal pathogens causing invasive pulmonary disease.

Suggested Reading

Franquet T. Imaging of pneumonia: Trends and algorithms. *Eur Respir J*. 2001;18:196–208.

Marchiori E, Zanetti G, Hochhegger B, Irion KL, Carvalho AC, Godoy MC. Reversed halo sign on computed tomography: State-of-the-art review. *Lung*. 2012;190(4):389–394.

Tarver RD, Teague SD, Heitkamp DE, et al. Radiology of community-acquired pneumonia. *Radiol Clin North Am*. 2005;43:497–512.

Vilar J, Domingo ML, Soto C, et al. Radiology of bacterial pneumonia. *Eur J Radiol*. 2004;51:102–113.

CHAPTER 38

Tuberculosis

Sonia L. Betancourt

Definition

Tuberculosis (TB) is an airborne infection caused by *Mycobacterium tuberculosis*, an obligate aerobe, nonmotile, non-spore-forming bacillus. TB is a major cause of morbidity and mortality, especially in developing countries. In 2013, there were 8.6 million new cases of active TB and 1.3 million deaths related to the disease. TB is the second leading cause of death from infectious disease worldwide after HIV.

Clinical Features

Risk factors for developing TB include elderly and immunocompromised subjects and individuals in congregate settings. Also, in the United States, a significant proportion of affected patients are from endemic areas. Classic symptoms and signs of active pulmonary TB include cough, fever, weight loss, night sweats, hemoptysis, chest pain, and fatigue. Elderly individuals may not exhibit typical signs and symptoms because they may have impaired immune response. In such cases, a high index of suspicion is necessary for a timely diagnosis. Additional clinical manifestations of TB may relate to extrathoracic disease or the development of complications involving the lungs, airways, vessels, and/or pleura. Acute respiratory distress syndrome (ARDS) secondary to TB is seen in association with miliary or endobronchial spread of TB. Early diagnosis is essential to prevent transmission of disease and provide timely treatment.

Anatomy and Physiology

TB is transmitted from person to person via airborne bacilli containing droplets. The number and virulence of bacilli in the droplets and the duration of the exposure influence TB transmission. Common risk factors include impaired cellular immunity, including HIV; malnutrition; diabetes; age older than 65 years; chronic disease; and immunosuppressive therapy. Mycobacteria grow until development of cellular immunity limits multiplication and results in granuloma formation.

The primary site of infection is called the Ghon focus. The combination of the Ghon focus and affected lymph nodes is known as Ranke complex. In approximately 5% of infected individuals, immunity is inadequate and widespread dissemination occurs.

Increasing evidence challenges the classic concepts of primary and postprimary TB. The primary pattern of TB (consolidation and lymphadenopathy) occurs more frequently in children. The postprimary pattern of TB (i.e., upper lobe opacities and/or cavitary disease) relates to a better immune response rather than reinfection or reactivation, and it is often a manifestation of initial infection in healthy young individuals.

Activity of disease implies microbiologic confirmation and cannot be established on chest radiography. However, certain findings on CT should suggest active TB. Interferon-γ release assays (IGRAs) have been proven useful to diagnose latent TB with a specificity greater than 95%; however, IGRAs cannot differentiate between active and latent TB. Xpert MTB/RIF assay is another helpful test that simultaneously assesses for TB and rifampin resistance with high accuracy; it has been endorse by the World Health Organization since 2010.

How to Approach the Image

In patients with clinical suspicion for TB, consolidation, lymphadenopathy, upper lobe opacities, and/or cavitary disease should suggest the diagnosis. Any patient with upper lobe cavitary disease should be presumed to have active TB and placed in isolation pending final diagnosis.

What Not to Miss

- Upper lobe opacities should always be analyzed for cavitation as a hallmark of active TB.
- Miliary nodules, mediastinal/hilar lymphadenopathy, and subtle parenchymal abnormalities are features of TB commonly missed on chest radiographs.

Differential Diagnosis

- Bacterial pneumonia: Hilar or mediastinal lymphadenopathy is not a common finding.
- Lung abscess and cavitary malignancy: May mimic TB on imaging; associated tree-in-bud opacities on CT suggest TB.
- Miliary fungal infection, sarcoidosis, and metastases: May mimic miliary TB.

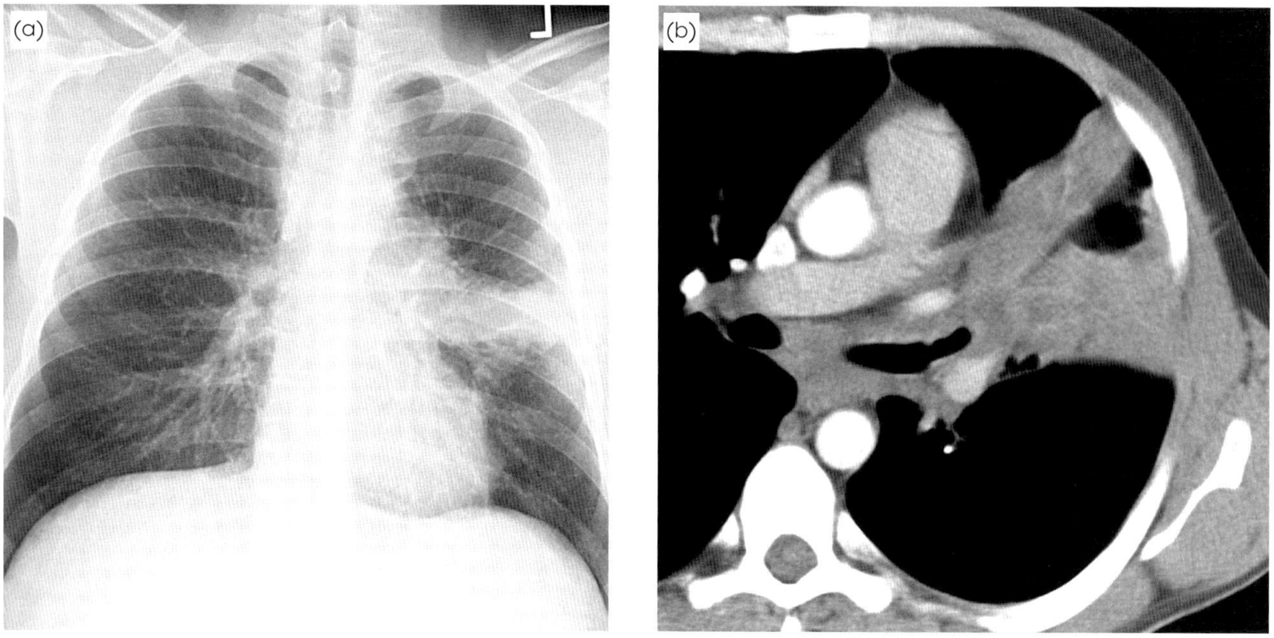

Figure 38.1 Primary pattern of TB. Posteroanterior (PA) chest radiograph (a) and contrast-enhanced chest CT (b) of a 25-year-old man with acute productive cough show left upper lobe consolidation and ipsilateral mediastinal lymphadenopathy. Chest CT confirms left upper lobe consolidation and subcarinal lymphadenopathy.

- Mediastinal/hilar lymphadenopathy with central low attenuation (necrosis) and peripheral enhancement: Characteristic of TB, but it may occur in benign conditions (e.g., Whipple and Crohn disease) and in malignancy (e.g., lymphoma and metastases).

Imaging Findings

- Primary childhood infection often manifests with consolidation and/or mediastinal/hilar lymphadenopathy (the primary pattern of TB) (Fig. 38.1). Ipsilateral hilar and paratracheal lymph nodes are commonly affected. CT may demonstrate peripheral rim enhancement and central low attenuation (Fig. 38.2). Calcification is common in chronically enlarged lymph nodes.
- Initial infection in immunocompetent subjects may be self-limited and may lead to parenchymal calcification (Ghon focus) or coexistent parenchymal and hilar calcification (Ranke complex). If immune response is not appropriate, hematogenous dissemination can occur (e.g., miliary TB).
- Initial infection in immunocompetent healthy adults may manifest with upper lobe predominant opacities and cavitary disease, also seen in reactivation or reinfection and often designated as the postprimary pattern of TB (Figs. 38.3 and 38.4). Upper lobe cavitary disease correlates with a relatively successful cellular immunity. However, individuals with cavitary disease are highly infectious and should be isolated.
- Although chest radiographic findings may suggest active TB, microbiologic confirmation is required for diagnosis. However, CT findings of discrete nodules, tree-in-bud opacities, and cavitation are signs of active TB.
- Pleural effusion is typically unilateral, occurs in 12–20% of patients, and may be the only manifestation

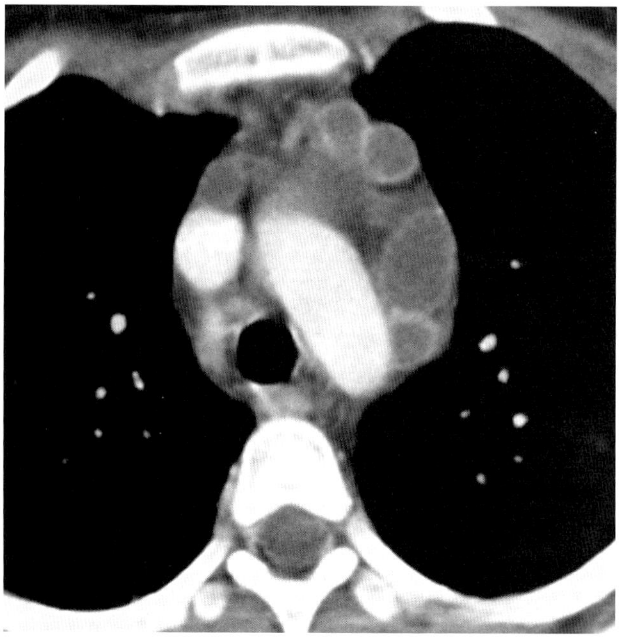

Figure 38.2 Lymphadenopathy in primary disseminated TB. Contrast-enhanced chest CT of an 11-year-old child with progressive fever, cough, and malaise shows mediastinal lymphadenopathy with intrinsic hypoattenuation and peripheral rim enhancement.

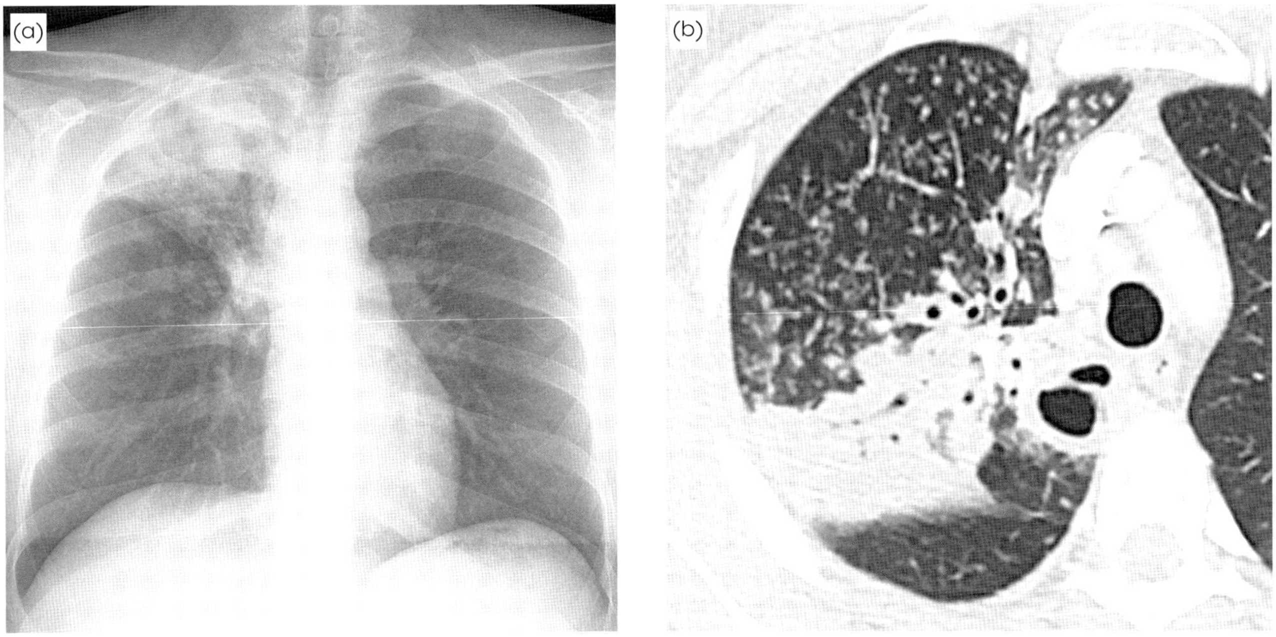

Figure 38.3 Upper lobe cavitary TB. PA chest radiograph (a) and unenhanced chest CT (b) of a 37-year-old woman with chronic cough and malaise show extensive right upper lobe airspace disease and volume loss. CT shows consolidation and cavitation with associated tree-in-bud opacities consistent with endobronchial dissemination of TB.

of TB. Known complications of pleural TB include empyema, bronchopleural fistula, chest wall invasion, and pleurocutaneous fistulae (Fig. 38.5).

- Miliary TB results from hematogenous dissemination, may be subtle on chest radiography, and manifests with diffuse micronodular opacities or randomly distributed 2- to 3-mm micronodules on CT (Figs. 38.6 and 38.7). Superimposed consolidation may indicate ARDS.
- Imaging findings in patients with AIDS relate to the level of immunosuppression. CD4 lymphocyte counts less than 200/mm^3 have a high association with mediastinal/hilar lymphadenopathy and miliary disease. Patients with CD4 lymphocyte counts greater than 200/mm^3 tend to have airspace disease (Fig. 38.8) that can be cavitary.

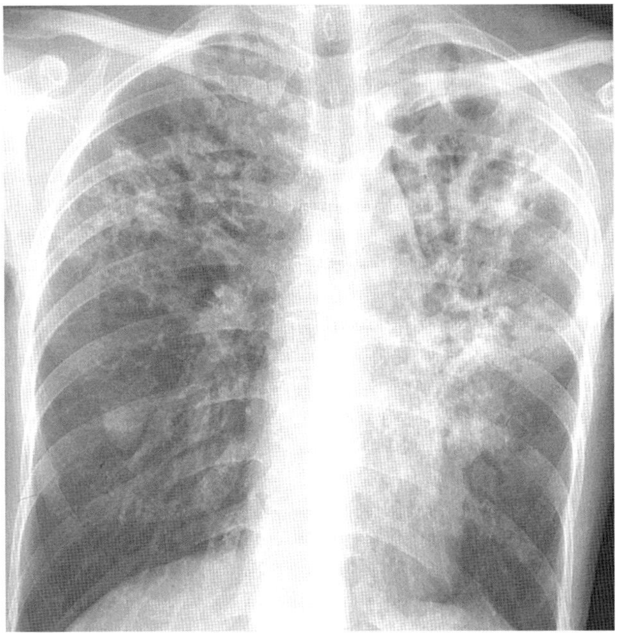

Figure 38.4 Upper lobe cavitary TB. AP chest radiograph of a 48-year-old man shows bilateral upper lobe and left lower lobe superior segment opacities with extensive multifocal cavitation.

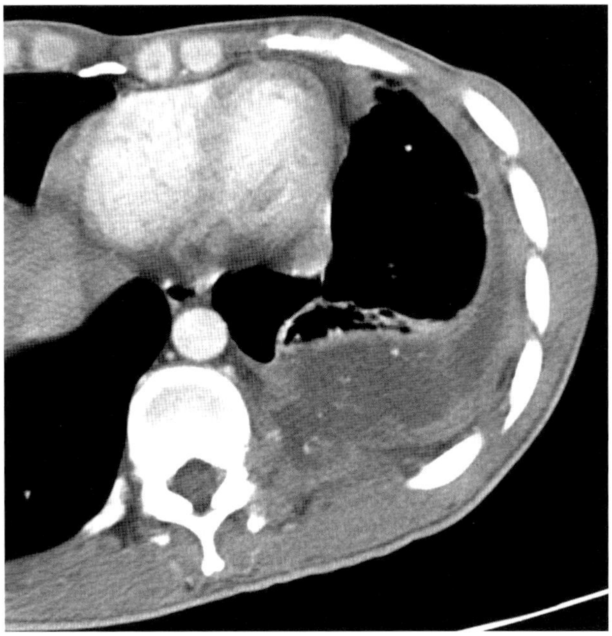

Figure 38.5 Tuberculous empyema. Contrast-enhanced chest CT of a 28-year-old man with pleuritic chest pain shows a left loculated pleural effusion enhancing pleural thickening and extension into the soft tissues of the adjacent chest wall.

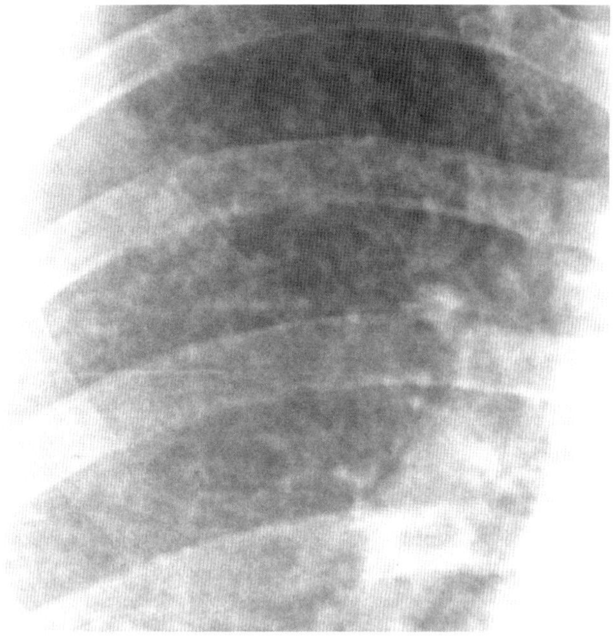

Figure 38.6 Miliary TB. Coned-down AP chest radiograph of a 34-year-old patient with chronic renal failure and fever demonstrates diffuse micronodular pulmonary opacities.

- Tracheobronchial TB manifests with irregular luminal narrowing, airway wall thickening with contrast enhancement, and peribronchial cuffing.
- Broncholithiasis is due to erosion of a bronchus by calcified peribronchial lymph nodes. It may cause cough, hemoptysis, and wheezing.
- A positive tuberculin test often prompts screening chest radiography. Any parenchymal, nodal, or pleural abnormality should be interpreted as disease of indeterminate activity and require clinical and microbiologic analysis to diagnose active disease. If there is no clinical or microbiological evidence of disease, latent TB is presumed and may be treated with isoniazid.

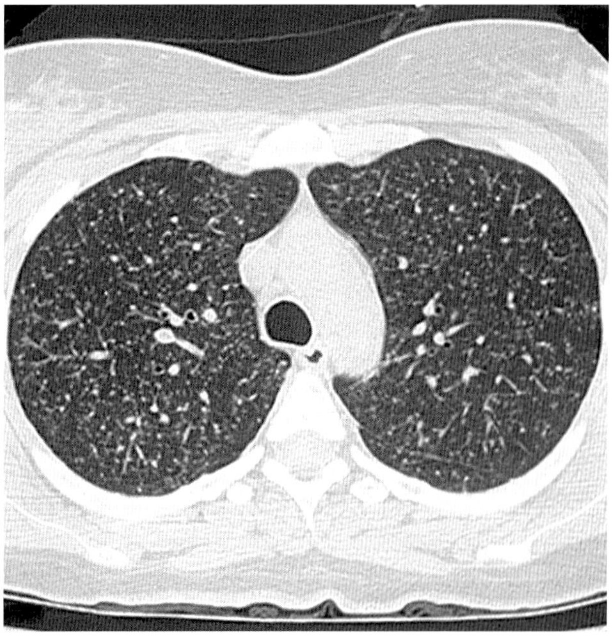

Figure 38.7 Miliary TB. Thin-section chest CT of a 28-year-old woman with a spontaneous septic abortion shows profuse bilateral randomly distributed pulmonary micronodules.

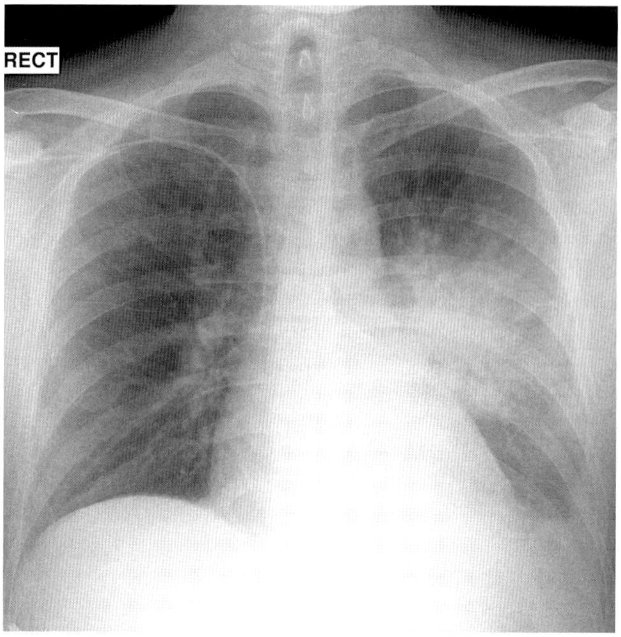

Figure 38.8 Primary pattern of TB. AP chest radiograph of a 28-year-old man with HIV infection and a CD4 count <200 cell/mm mm^3 demonstrates consolidation in the superior segment of the left lower lobe and a small left pleural effusion.

Clinical Issues

- Bronchiectatic and residual upper lobe cavities may be colonized by *Aspergillus* species, with formation of a fungus ball (or mycetoma). Such patients often have hemoptysis, which may be life-threatening.
- A Rasmussen aneurysm is a pseudoaneurysm of a pulmonary artery caused by erosion from an adjacent cavity and may result in massive life-threatening hemoptysis.
- Empyema necessitatis results in involvement of the adjacent chest wall by tuberculous empyema.
- Tuberculous pericarditis may manifest as pericardial effusion or pericardial thickening and may be complicated by constrictive pericarditis.

Key Points

- Patients with impaired cellular immunity including HIV (positive), elderly, prisoners, indigents, and homeless patients have an increased susceptibility for active TB disease.
- Primary infection usually resolves without complications in immunocompetent patients.
- The most common radiologic manifestations of primary TB in children are consolidation and lymphadenopathy.

Progressive primary TB with widespread hematogenous dissemination may rarely occur.

- Patchy or nodular opacities in the upper lobes with associated cavitation are characteristic radiologic findings of active infection. Although this pattern often correlates with relatively spared immunity, it denotes highly infectious individuals who require isolation.
- CT is very sensitive for the detection of bronchogenic spread of infection manifesting with discrete nodules, tree-in-bud opacities, and cavitation.
- Miliary TB refers to hematogenous spread of infection.

Suggested Reading

Jeong YJ, Lee KS. Pulmonary tuberculosis: Up-to date imaging and management. *AJR Am J Roentgenol.* 2008;191:834–844.

Marais BJ, Parker SK, Verver S, van Rie A, Warren RM. Primary and postprimary or reactivation tuberculosis: Time to revise confusing terminology? *AJR Am J Roentgenol.* 2009 Apr;192(4):W198; Author Reply, W199–W200.

Saurborn DP, Fishman JE, Boiselle PM. The imaging spectrum of pulmonary tuberculosis in AIDS. *J Thorac Imaging.* 2002;17:28–33.

World Health Organization. *Global Tuberculosis Report 2013.* Geneva: World Health Organization; 2013.

CHAPTER 39

Nontuberculous Mycobacterial Infection

Santiago Martínez-Jiménez

Definition

Nontuberculous mycobacteria (NTM) other than *Mycobacterium tuberculosis* (TB) may produce pulmonary infection. Some of these organisms include *Mycobacterium avium-intracellulare* (MAC), *Mycobacterium kansasii, Mycobacterium gordonae, Mycobacterium fortuitum, Mycobacterium xenopi*, and *Mycobacterium malmoense.*

Clinical Features

When approaching nontuberculous mycobacterial infection (NTMI), it is helpful to recognize that NTMI tends to present with certain clusters or specific clinical features and demographic groups. Although this approach is not perfect, especially because it is common for NTMIs to share features of several clusters, it remains helpful to understand pathophysiology and imaging manifestations. The American Thoracic Society has published diagnostic criteria for pulmonary NTMI.

Cavitary or Classic Form

Affected patients present with symptoms similar to those of active TB. White men with underlying chronic pulmonary disease (e.g., chronic obstructive pulmonary disease (COPD) and interstitial lung disease) are more frequently affected, and MAC and *M. kansasii* are the most commonly recovered organisms.

Bronchiectatic or Nonclassic Form

Affected patients are typically elderly white women presenting with chronic cough often without predisposing factors. MAC and *M. kansasii* are the most frequent causative organisms.

HIV-Infected Patients

These patients typically present with disseminated disease, particularly if the CD4 count is less than 200 cells/mm^3. Symptoms and signs are nonspecific and include fever, weight loss, abdominal pain, diarrhea, lymphadenopathy, and hepatosplenomegaly. Extensive lymphadenopathy simulating lymphoma may occur in the setting of immune reconstitution syndrome after initiation of highly active antiretroviral therapy (HAART). In these cases, MAC is the most common causative organism, but *M. xenopi* and *M. kansasii* are also implicated. NTMI may coexist with other infections (e.g., *Pneumocystis jirovecii* and *Candida* spp.) or neoplasms (e.g., Kaposi sarcoma).

Immune Compromise Other Than HIV

NTMI may affect patients on chemotherapy or chronic corticosteroid therapy, patients with solid organ transplantation, and those with leukemia and lymphoma. Symptoms are nonspecific and include fever, weight loss, and malaise. In these patients, MAC is the most common cause of NTMI; other causes are *M. gordonae, M. chelonei*, and *M. fortuitum.*

Asymptomatic Patients with Discrete Nodules and Masses

These patients may exhibit pulmonary lesions that may mimic lung cancer. MAC is the typical causative organism.

Patients with Impaired Deglutition

Patients with achalasia, hiatus hernia, stroke, and Parkinson disease may develop NTMI that is typically caused by *M. chelonei* and *M. fortuitum.* Clinical manifestations include cough, dyspnea, and constitutional symptoms.

Hypersensitivity Pneumonitis

Hypersensitivity pneumonitis may be related to NTMI or allergic reaction to these organisms and results from inhalation of MAC colonizing various water sources, including indoor hot tubs (i.e., "hot tub lung"), or fluids used in the metalworking and automotive industries. Affected patients present with dyspnea, cough, and fever.

Difficult-to-Control Asthma

NTMI is a diagnostic consideration in adult patients with difficult-to-treat asthma. These patients are typically in the sixth and seventh decades, have severe airflow obstruction, and are exposed to inhaled or systemic corticosteroid therapy. The most commonly implicated organisms are MAC, *Mycobacterium xenopi*, and *Mycobacterium abscessus*.

Anatomy and Physiology

NTM are ubiquitous organisms, and their presence in sputum does not necessarily imply disease. In bronchiectatic NTMI, the presence of predominant middle lobe and lingular involvement is postulated to result from voluntary cough suppression (i.e., Lady Windermere syndrome) and impaired mucociliary and lymphatic drainage in these areas, which may allow engraftment of NTM.

How to Approach the Image

Chest radiographs of patients with NTMI are often normal. When present, radiographic abnormalities are often subtle, consisting of bronchiectasis and small lung nodules. However, NTMI can often be suggested based on CT and high-resolution CT findings (including expiratory imaging).

What Not to Miss

- In the United States, upper lobe cavitary disease is often related to NTMI. However, patients with such findings must first be presumed to have active cavitary TB and placed in isolation until a definitive bacteriologic diagnosis is made.
- Elderly White women with right middle lobe syndrome (chronic atelectasis and/or airspace disease) very often have bronchiectatic NTMI that may be an incidental finding.

Differential Diagnosis

Imaging findings of solid pulmonary micronodules are seen in infectious bronchiolitis caused by other organisms and in aspiration bronchiolitis. Imaging findings of tree-in-bud opacities may be seen in aspiration, endobronchial spread of infection, follicular bronchiolitis, allergic bronchopulmonary aspergillosis, and diffuse panbronchiolitis.

Active Cavitary Tuberculosis

Cavitary NTMI is referred to as classic because it mimics active cavitary TB. These infections are indistinguishable from each other based on imaging.

Other Infections

Many other infections can cause cavitary disease, including nocardiosis, cryptoccocosis, and bacterial pneumonias with abscess formation. Semi-invasive aspergillosis may also manifest with upper lobe cavitary disease.

Aspiration

Aspiration may mimic NTMI in a few different settings:

- Acute aspiration of anaerobic bacteria can result in pulmonary abscess and may mimic cavitary or classic NTMI.
- Chronic aspiration bronchiolitis may mimic bronchiectatic NTMI. The presence of known esophageal dysmotility, hiatus hernia, achalasia, tight gastric ring, or other obstructive distal esophageal procedure helps suggest aspiration.

Diffuse Post-infectious Bronchiectasis

- Bronchiectasis is often the sequela of prior infection(s) and may mimic bronchiectatic NTMI.
- Patients with clinical and imaging findings of bronchiectasis may have recurrent infections with *Pseudomonas aeruginosa*, an important differential consideration for the imaging features of bronchiectatic NTMI.

Diffuse Panbronchiolitis

Severe cases of bronchiectatic NTMI may mimic diffuse panbronchiolitis. However, the latter is uncommon in the United States and typically affects the Asian population.

Imaging Findings

Cavitary or Classic Form

- Chest radiography: Upper lobe cavitary disease often associated with preexisting pulmonary disease such as COPD or interstitial lung disease. Multifocal small pulmonary nodules may also be seen (Fig. 39.1).
- Chest CT: Thin-walled upper lobe predominant pulmonary cavity(ies) with associated discrete nodules, centrilobular and tree-in-bud opacities, and bronchiectasis.

Bronchiectatic or Nonclassic Form

- Chest radiography: Scattered nodules; bronchiectasis typically in the middle lobe and lingula; persistent right middle lobe/lingular atelectasis or consolidation. Ancillary findings include pectus excavatum and scoliosis (Fig. 39.2).

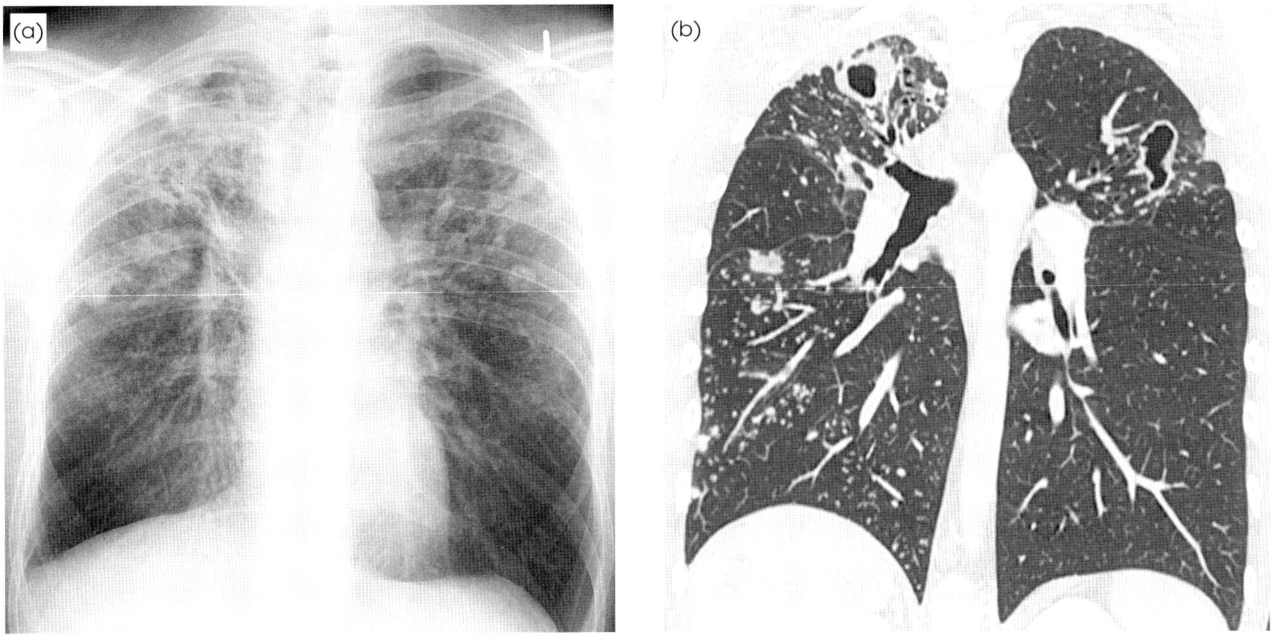

Figure 39.1 Classic NTMI. (a) Posteroanterior chest radiograph of a 62-year-old man with COPD shows heterogeneous and nodular upper lobe opacities with intrinsic cavitation indistinguishable from active cavitary TB. (b) Unenhanced coronal chest CT of the same patient shows bilateral upper lobe cavities and multifocal discrete small nodules and centrilobular micronodules.

- CT: Tree-in-bud opacities, bronchiectasis with or without mucus plugging, volume loss in the middle lobe and/or lingula, and mosaic attenuation (or frank air trapping if expiratory imaging is performed)

NTMI in Immune Compromise

- Chest radiography and CT: Consolidation, nodules, and mediastinal/hilar lymphadenopathy (Figs. 39.3 and 39.4)
- Immune reconstitution syndrome: Extensive lymphadenopathy that may exhibit hypoattenuating centers secondary to necrosis on CT

Discrete Nodules and Masses in Asymptomatic Patients

Radiologically similar to lung cancer. PET/CT may demonstrate increased FDG uptake (Fig. 39.5).

NTMI in Patients with Impaired Deglutition

Reticular or reticulonodular opacities in patients with predisposing factors or in association with esophageal dilatation, hiatus hernia, or gastric banding (Fig. 39.6).

Hypersensitivity Pneumonitis

- Chest radiography: May be normal or show diffuse hazy opacities (Fig. 39.7)
- Chest CT: Centrilobular ground-glass nodules, diffuse ground-glass opacities, and air trapping on expiratory imaging

Clinical Issues

- NTM may be difficult to culture.
- Cultures can be falsely positive in patients with preexistent lung disease and falsely negative in infected patients.

Key Points

- NTMI is typically an indolent infection except in immunocompromised and HIV-infected patients. Imaging plays a crucial role in suggesting NTMI as a possible diagnosis in this patient population.
- Always consider classic or cavitary NTMI in patients with upper lobe cavitary disease similar to active cavitary TB. However, in such cases, TB must always be excluded.
- In elderly White women, persistent right middle lobe/lingular atelectasis, bronchiectasis, or consolidation should suggest the diagnosis of bronchiectactic NTMI.
- In patients with imaging findings of subacute hypersensitivity pneumonitis, the radiologist must review the history and consult with the clinician to identify the triggering allergen, including NTM, which is associated with indoor hot tubs.

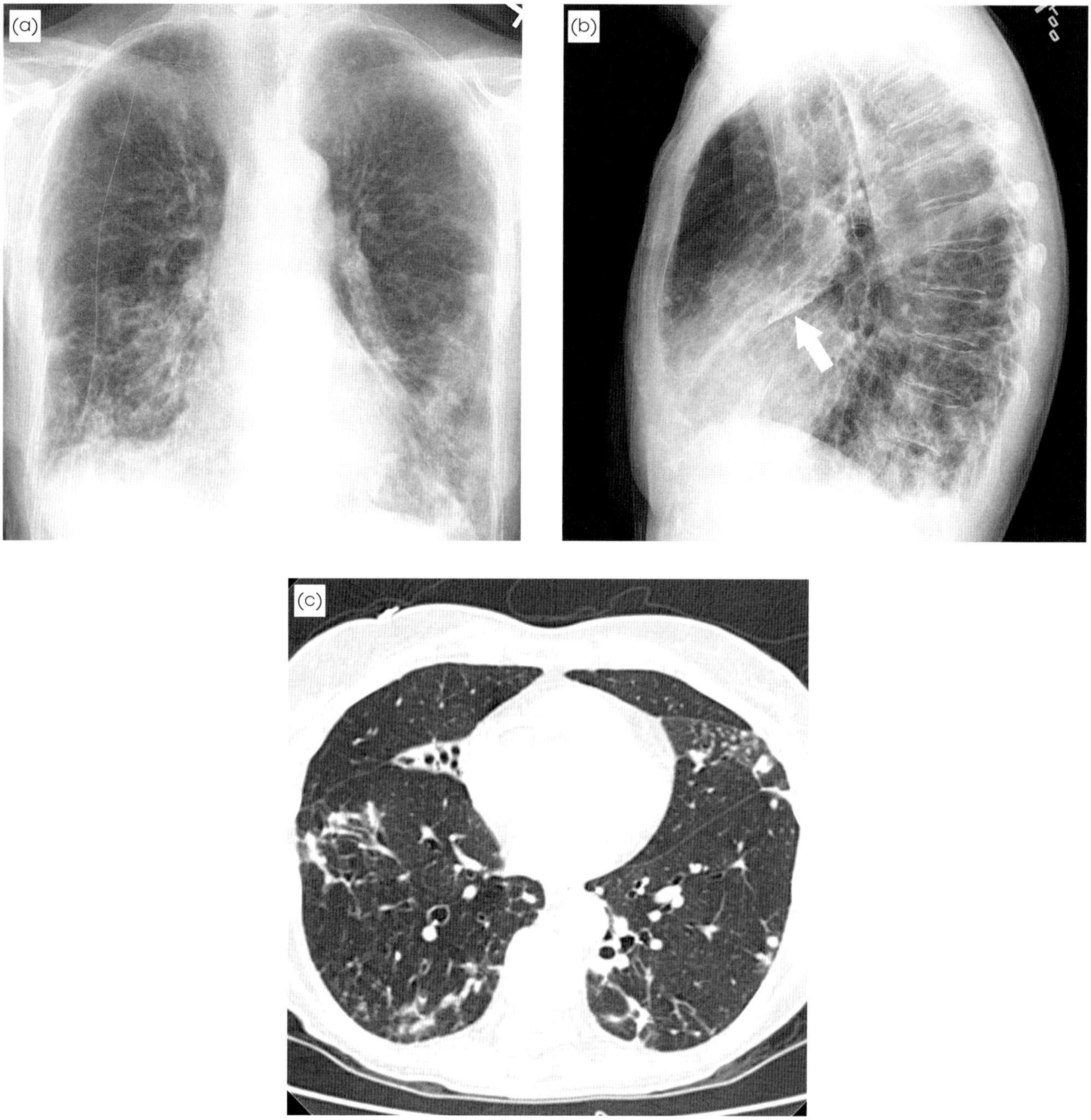

Figure 39.2 Bronchiectatic NTMI. (a) Posteroanterior and (b) lateral chest radiographs of a 72-year-old woman with chronic cough show lower lung zone reticular and heterogeneous opacities and obscuration of the cardiac borders consistent with middle lobe and lingular involvement. Middle lobe bronchiectasis is also seen. Lateral radiograph shows extensive heterogeneous opacities in the lower lobes and volume loss in the right middle lobe and lingula (arrow). (c) Unenhanced chest CT shows characteristic findings of bronchiectatic NTMI, including middle lobe and lingular volume loss, bronchiectasis, tree-in-bud opacities, discrete nodules, and mosaic attenuation.

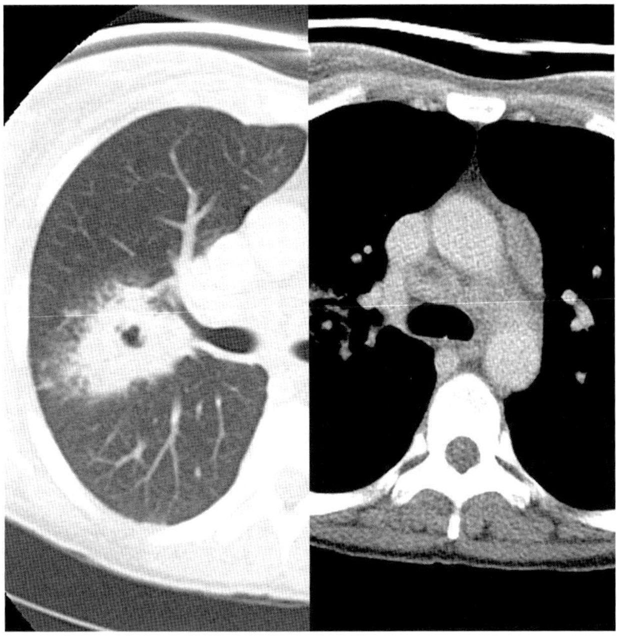

Figure 39.3 NTM infection in HIV. Composite image with contrast-enhanced chest CT of a 35-year-old HIV-positive man with fever and malaise shows right upper lobe consolidation with intrinsic cavitation (left) and mediastinal lymphadenopathy (right).

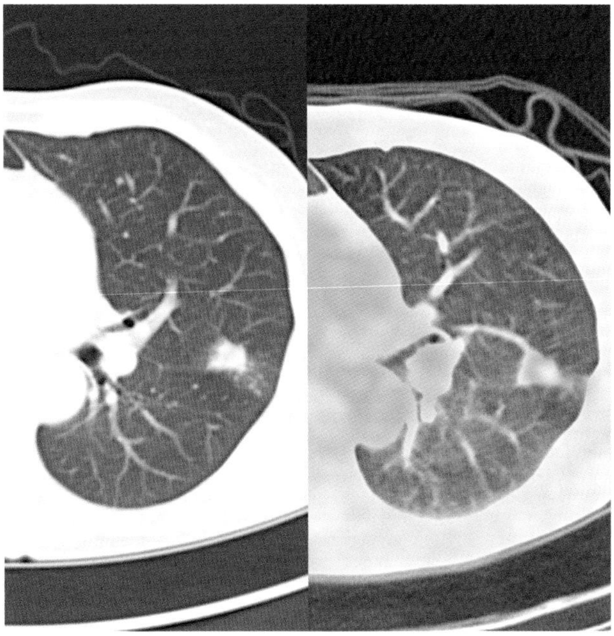

Figure 39.5 Asymptomatic NTMI with discrete nodule. Composite image with unenhanced chest CT (left) and FDG PET/CT (right) of an asymptomatic 72-year-old woman with MAC shows a 2-cm left upper lobe spiculated solitary nodule that exhibits increased FDG uptake on PET/CT.

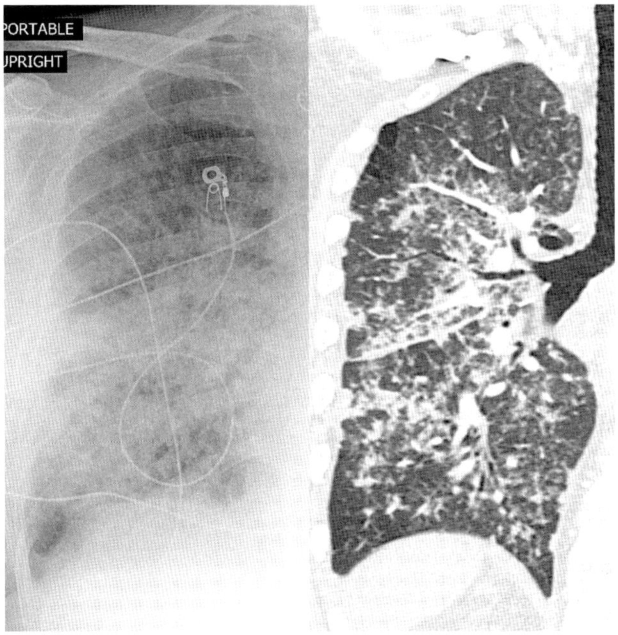

Figure 39.4 NTMI in immune compromise. Composite image with anteroposterior chest radiograph (left) and unenhanced coronal chest CT of a 61-year-old man with a history of orthotopic heart transplantation, progressive dyspnea, and fever shows diffuse reticulonodular opacities (left) and extensive coalescent peribronchovascular nodules (right).

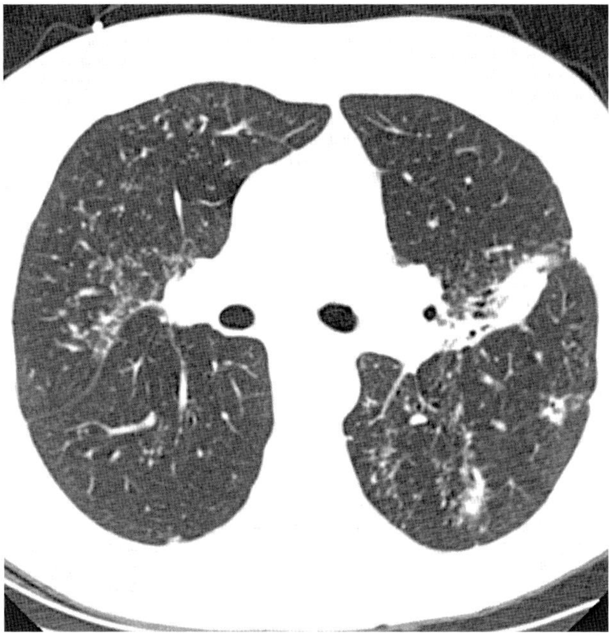

Figure 39.6 NTMI in a patient with impaired deglutition. Unenhanced chest CT of a 67-year-old man with achalasia, chronic cough, and MAC related to aspiration shows scattered centrilobular nodules, tree-in-bud opacities, and left upper lobe focal scarring and traction bronchiectasis.

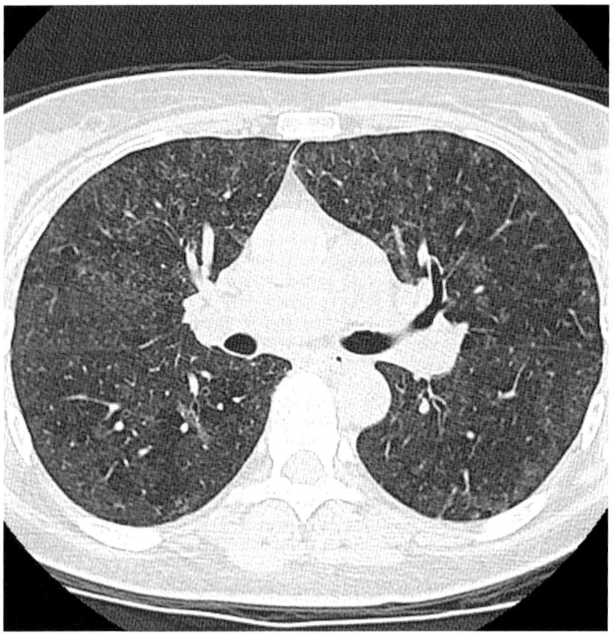

Figure 39.7 Hypersensitivity pneumonitis (hot tub lung). Thin-section chest CT of a 42-year-old man with chronic dyspnea and cough shows diffuse ill-defined ground-glass opacities and mosaic attenuation. Both the patient's indoor pool water and the bronchoalveolar lavage cultures grew MAC.

Suggested Reading

Fritscher LG, Marras TK, Bradi AC, Fritscher CC, Balter MS, Chapman KR. Nontuberculous mycobacterial infection as a cause of difficult-to-control asthma: A case–control study. *Chest*. 2011 Jan;139(1):23–27.

Griffith DE, Aksamit T, Brown-Elliott BA, Catanzaro A, Daley C, Gordin F, et al.; ATS Mycobacterial Diseases Subcommittee; American Thoracic Society; Infectious Disease Society of America. An official ATS/IDSA statement: Diagnosis, treatment, and prevention of nontuberculous mycobacterial diseases. *Am J Respir Crit Care Med*. 2007 Feb 15;175(4):367–416.

Martinez S, McAdams HP, Batchu CS. The many faces of pulmonary nontuberculous mycobacterial infection. *AJR Am J Roentgenol*. 2007 Jul;189(1):177–186.

CHAPTER 40

Mycoplasma and Viral Pneumonia

Diana Palacio

Definition

Mycoplasma pneumoniae and viruses remain among the most common causes of community-acquired pneumonia and account for approximately 30% or more of all cases. *Mycoplasma pneumoniae* is a bacterium that lacks a cell wall, which results in certain microbiologic features absent in other bacteria. A wide variety of viruses may infect the lungs, commonly influenza, parainfluenza, adenovirus, and cytomegalovirus (CMV).

Clinical Features

Viral and mycoplasma pneumonia is transmitted from person to person through respiratory droplets. Infections by these organisms should be considered in epidemics affecting confined populations, such as military recruits, prisoners, boarding school students, patients at both extremes of age, patients with chronic illnesses, and patients with a history of smoking and/or previous mechanical ventilation. Lower respiratory tract symptoms are not common; they are found in 10–30% of patients with viral pneumonia and in 3–5% of those with mycoplasma pulmonary infection. Symptoms of viral and *M. pneumoniae* pneumonia often exhibit a slow onset and are not initially severe. Cough, shaking chills, shortness of breath, wheezing, dyspnea on exertion, and pleuritic chest pain may be seen.

Mycoplasma pneumoniae pneumonia usually affects individuals younger than age 40 years and healthy immune-competent individuals, but it may be associated with comorbidities including diabetes, cardiovascular disease, chronic liver disease, and cerebrovascular accident. Infected older patients may present with altered mental status. The term "walking pneumonia" refers to clinically mild pulmonary infection for which patients may not seek medical attention and is common in *M. pneumoniae* pneumonia. *Mycoplasma pneumoniae* pneumonia tends to be severe in children with sickle cell anemia.

Viral pneumonias may affect immunocompetent and immunocompromised hosts. Patients with a high risk for viral pneumonia include the elderly and patients with chronic cardiopulmonary disease, patients who are status post bone marrow transplant, and those with hematologic malignancies. Immunocompetent patients typically have self-limited infections that are frequently not severe enough for them to seek medical attention. However, severe pulmonary disease may be seen in clinical practice (e.g., influenza H1N1). Swyer–James syndrome is defined as constrictive bronchiolitis that may complicate childhood adenovirus pulmonary infection. Immunocompromised patients may have severe life-threatening viral infections (e.g., CMV, parainfluenza, respiratory syncytial virus, and adenovirus).

Viral pneumonia is typically accompanied by classic influenza symptoms, including mild or high fever, headache, myalgias, malaise, and loss of appetite. Leukocytosis may be present but is typically less severe that that associated with bacterial pneumonia. Appropriately treated adults typically experience a full recovery.

Anatomy and Physiology

Mycoplasma pneumoniae pneumonia may manifest as cellular bronchiolitis, bronchopneumonia, or frank pneumonic consolidation. Cellular bronchiolitis and edematous and ulcerative lesions of the bronchial walls are common pathologic findings.

Overall, viruses preferentially target the epithelial cells, in which they replicate and eventually disseminate through the adjacent interstitium.

Diffuse alveolar damage, alveolar hemorrhage, edema, fibrin deposition, type II cell hyperplasia, and hyaline membrane formation may occur in severe cases of viral pneumonia and, less frequently, in *M. pneumoniae* pneumonia.

How to Approach the Image

In clinical practice, *M. pneumoniae* and viral pneumonias are characterized as either community-acquired pneumonia or pneumonia in the immunocompromised patient; however, they are discussed separately in this chapter. As with other pneumonias, *M. pneumoniae* and viral pneumonias are often initially assessed with chest radiography, with CT reserved for cases in which chest radiography is inconclusive or when complications are suspected clinically.

What Not to Miss

A normal chest radiograph does not exclude the possibility of *M. pneumoniae* or viral pneumonias.

Early in the disease, the presence of bronchial wall thickening and centrilobular nodules on chest CT is a

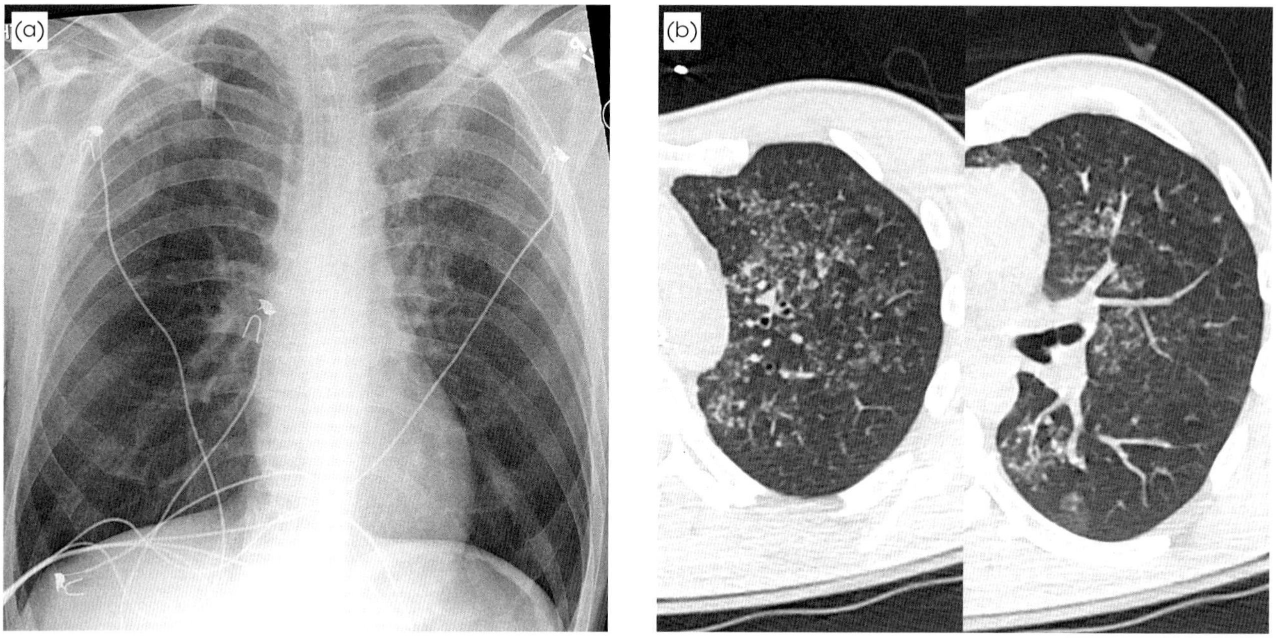

Figure 40.1 *Mycoplasma pneumoniae* bronchiolitis. (a) Anteroposterior chest radiograph of a 32-year-old man with fever and shortness of breath shows subtle hazy opacities in the left upper lobe. (b) Composite image with unenhanced chest CT of the same patient shows profuse centrilobular micronodules and ground-glass opacities consistent with infectious bronchiolitis.

helpful feature of *M. pneumoniae* pneumonia that allows differentiation from *Streptococcus pneumonia*, which often manifests with consolidation. In later disease, both exhibit consolidation.

Differential Diagnosis

Viral bronchiolitis manifesting with centrilobular micronodules and "tree-in-bud" opacities must be differentiated from other causes of noninfectious cellular bronchiolitis, such as aspiration and follicular bronchiolitis. Other etiologies of cellular bronchiolitis, such as respiratory and hypersensitivity pneumonitis, are commonly associated with centrilobular ground-glass nodules on thin-section chest CT, a feature that is not common in infection.

The imaging findings of endobronchial spread of viral or *M. pneumoniae* pneumonia (i.e., centrilobular nodules and/or tree-in-bud opacities) are indistinguishable from those of tuberculosis, nontuberculous mycobacterial infection, and bacterial bronchopneumonia. As a result, affected patients may require isolation until *M. tuberculosis* is excluded.

In severe cases of viral and mycoplasma pneumonia with extensive airspace disease, findings are often indistinguishable from those of pulmonary edema or pulmonary hemorrhage.

Imaging Findings

Chest Radiography

- Chest radiography may be normal in both viral and *M. pneumoniae* pneumonia.
- Poorly defined nodular opacities, patchy consolidation (bronchopneumonia), and segmental consolidation are common findings in viral and *M. pneumoniae* pneumonia (Figs. 40.1 and 40.2).
- Unilateral or patchy bilateral consolidations are common in cases of rapid disease progression (Fig. 40.3).
- Pleural effusions, when present, tend to be small.

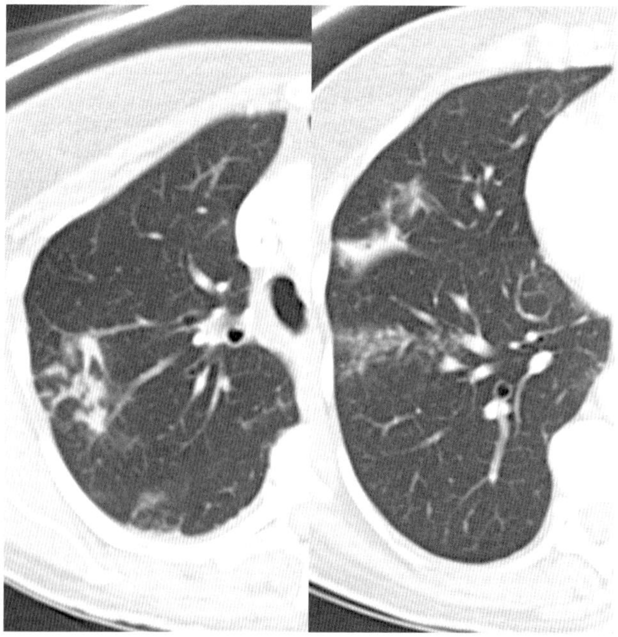

Figure 40.2 *Mycoplasma pneumoniae* bronchopneumonia. Composite image with contrast-enhanced chest CT of a 37-year-old man with dyspnea and fever shows multifocal lobular airspace disease characteristic of bronchopneumonia.

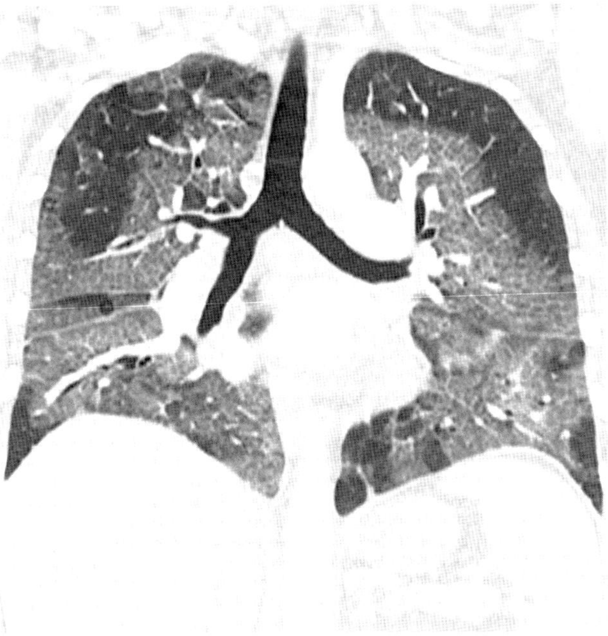

Figure 40.3 Influenza (H1N1) pneumonia. Composite image with posteroanterior (PA) chest radiograph (left) and unenhanced chest CT (right) of an 18-year-old man with rapidly progressive dyspnea and fever shows heterogeneous right basilar and perihilar opacities (left). CT shows confluent subpleural right lower lobe consolidation and scattered lobular opacities in the right lower and middle lobes.

CT

- CT is helpful in demonstrating abnormalities that may be subtle or not apparent on radiography (Figs. 40.3–40.6).

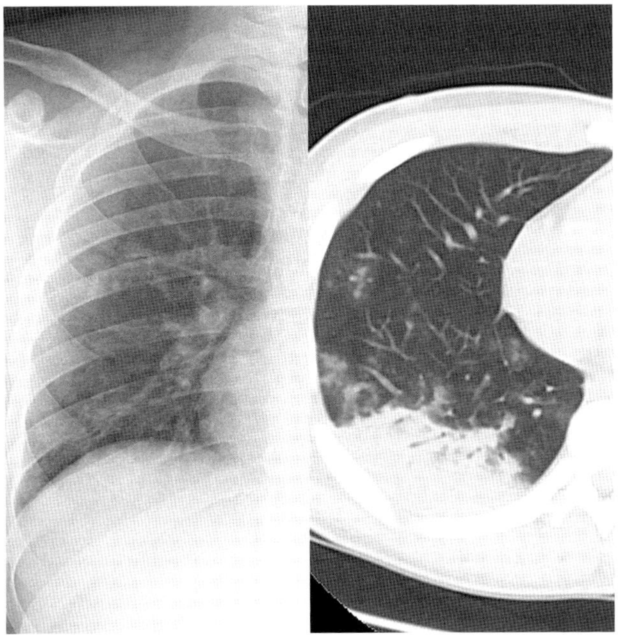

Figure 40.4 Influenza pneumonia. Composite image with chest CT of two different patients with influenza pneumonia shows multifocal peripheral ground-glass opacities (left) and profuse centrilobular micronodules and tree-in-bud opacities (right). Both are common findings of pulmonary viral infection.

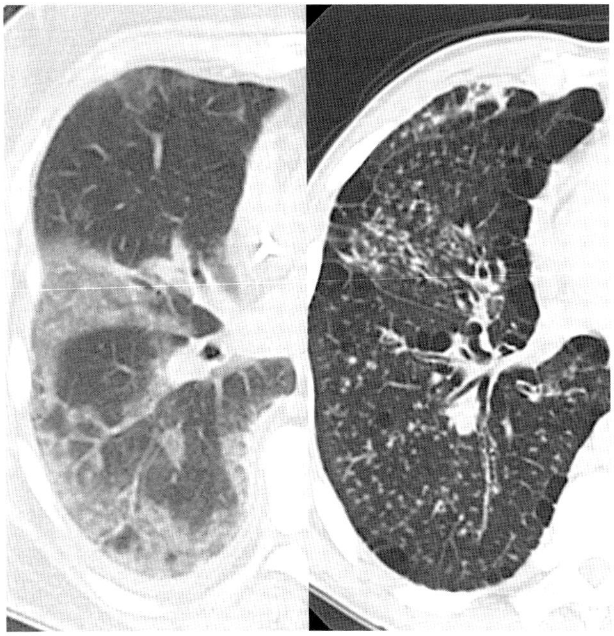

Figure 40.5 CMV pneumonia. Composite image with chest CT of two different patients with CMV pneumonia following bone marrow transplantation (left) and associated with chronic lymphocytic leukemia (right) shows left upper lobe subsegmental ground-glass opacities (left) and nodular consolidation in the left upper lobe and heterogeneous airspace disease in the left lower lobe (right).

- Characteristic pattern: Infectious bronchiolitis manifesting as centrilobular nodules often with tree-in-bud appearance and peribronchial thickening (Fig. 40.1).

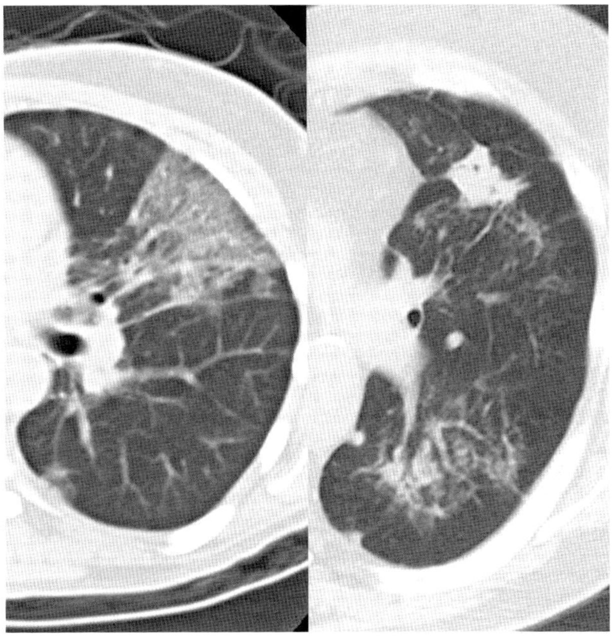

Figure 40.6 Adenovirus pneumonia. Composite image with chest CT of two different patients with adenovirus pneumonia shows multiple small discrete pulmonary nodules (left) and extensive pulmonary ground-glass opacities (right).

Source: Fig. 40.6, left, courtesy Tomas Franquet, MD.

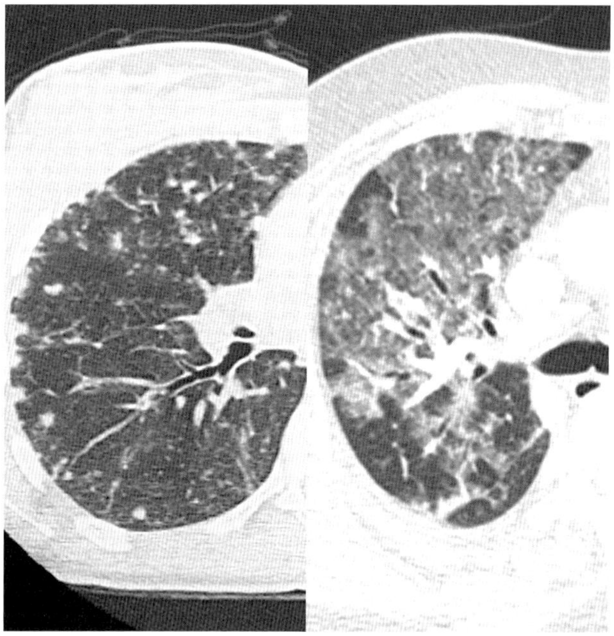

Figure 40.7 *Mycoplasma pneumoniae* pneumonia and acute respiratory distress syndrome. Coronal contrast-enhanced chest CT of a 27-year-old woman with acute shortness of breath and fever shows extensive bilateral ground-glass opacities superimposed on reticular opacities, the so-called "crazy-paving" pattern.

- The bronchopneumonia pattern is characterized by lobular airspace opacities that affect some secondary pulmonary lobules and spare others, and bronchial wall thickening is frequent in *M. pneumoniae* pneumonia.
- Discrete pulmonary nodules with or without surrounding ground-glass opacities have been described in a variety of viral infections.
- The "crazy paving" pattern consisting of interstitial thickening with superimposed ground-glass opacities may be seen in *M. pneumoniae* and viral pneumonias (Fig. 40.7).
- Pleural effusions are uncommon in viral and *M. pneumoniae* pneumonias.
- Swyer–James syndrome is a chronic sequela related to viral infection that manifests with bilateral mosaic attenuation, expiratory air trapping, bronchial wall thickening, and bronchiectasis (Fig. 40.8).

Clinical Issues

- The appropriate timing and indication of imaging in the evaluation of atypical pneumonia remains controversial.
- Pneumonia caused by atypical pathogens such as viruses and *M. pneumoniae* tends to clear more quickly than classic lobar pneumonia caused by bacterial pathogens.
- The radiologic resolution of viral and *M. pneumoniae* pneumonias is slower in elderly patients and in those with multilobar involvement. Follow-up imaging for 12–14 weeks may be appropriate before classifying the pneumonia as nonresolving.

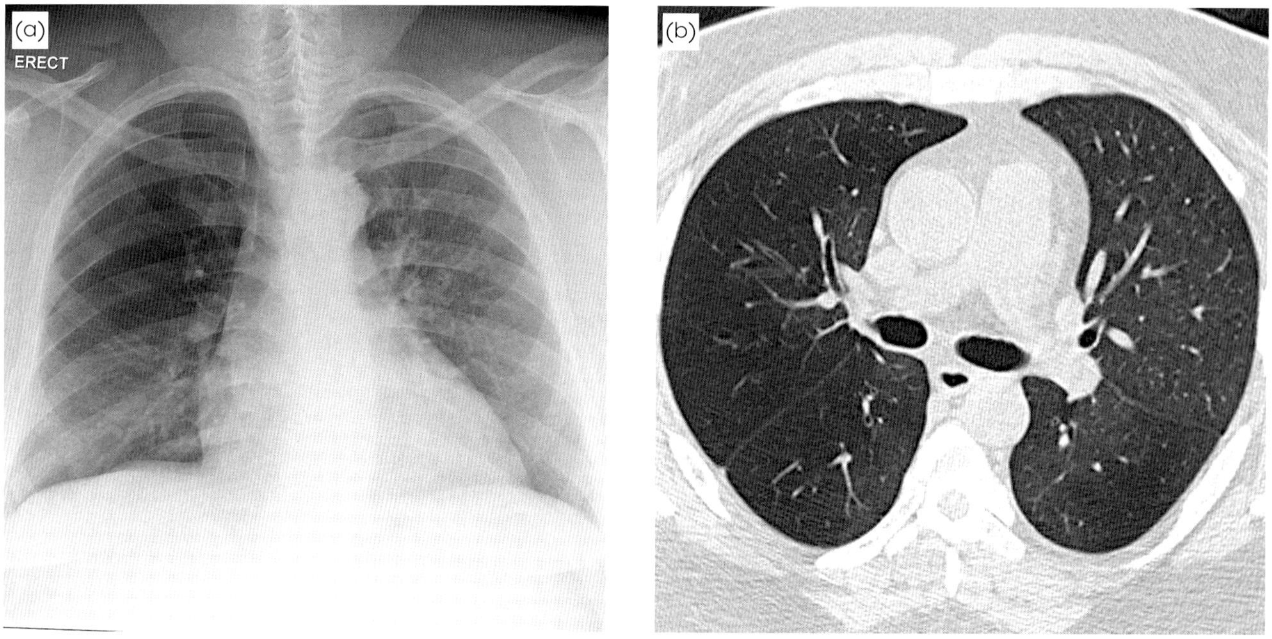

Figure 40.8 Swyer–James syndrome from remote adenovirus infection. (a) PA chest radiograph of a 28-year-old man with documented severe childhood adenovirus pneumonia shows lucency and paucity of vascular markings in the right mid and upper lung zones

Key Points

- The combination of centrilobular nodules, peribronchial thickening, and lobular ground-glass attenuation on CT is the most suggestive pattern identified in patients with *M. pneumoniae* pneumonia.
- Although cellular bronchiolitis is a nonspecific finding, a patchy or clustered distribution should raise the possibility of infectious etiology, with the most likely causative agents being *M. pneumoniae*, tuberculosis, and viral bronchiolitis.
- The radiologic findings of adult viral and *M. pneumoniae* pneumonias are variable and depend on the host and the virulence of the pathogen. The imaging findings overlap with those found in pneumonias caused by atypical microorganisms (virus, *Pneumocystis jirovecii* pneumonia, etc.).
- CT imaging of immunocompetent patients with suspected viral or mycoplasma pneumonia is not indicated unless there is suspicion of complications. CT may be performed in patients with normal, equivocal, or nonspecific radiographic findings. Conversely, CT is often indicated in immunocompromised patients with a normal chest radiograph and suspected pulmonary infection.

Suggested Reading

Franquet T. Imaging of pulmonary viral pneumonia. *Radiology.* 2011;260:18–39.

Kim EA, Lee KS, Primack SL, et al. Viral pneumonias in adults: Radiologic and pathologic findings. *RadioGraphics.* 2002;22:S13.

Miyashita N, Sugiu T, Kawai Y, et al. Radiographic features of *Mycoplasma pneumoniae* pneumonia: Differential diagnosis and performance timing. *BMC Med Imaging.* 2009;9:7.

Nei T, Yamano Y, Sakai F, et al. *Mycoplasma pneumoniae* pneumonia: Differential diagnosis by computerized tomography. *Intern Med.* 2007;46:1083–1087.

Reittner P, Muller NL, Heyneman L, et al. *Mycoplasma pneumoniae* pneumonia: Radiographic and high-resolution CT features in 28 patients. *AJR Am J Roentgenol.* 2000;174:37–40.

Reynolds JH, McDonald G, Alton H, et al. Pneumonia in the immunocompetent patient. *Br J Radiol.* 2010;83:998–1009.

Ruuskanen O, Lahti E, Jennings LC, et al. Viral pneumonia. *Lancet.* 2011;377:1264–1275.

Section VIII

The Immunocompromised Patient

CHAPTER 41

Introduction to the Immunocompromised Patient

Santiago Martínez-Jiménez

Introduction

The imaging findings of various complications of immunosuppression have been described. Although such complications are often of infectious etiology, neoplastic processes are also common.

An important group of immunocompromised patients are those infected with HIV. Patients with AIDS are known to develop specific infections and malignancies that often correlate with the level of $CD4^+$ lymphocytes. Certain diseases typically occur at low levels of $CD4^+$, and others are more common at higher levels. Chapter 42 provides updated information on the epidemiology of HIV infection and particularly AIDS, with emphasis on the imaging abnormalities that occur as manifestations of pulmonary diseases in this patient population.

Certain diseases associated with immunocompromise other than AIDS (e.g., congenital immunodeficiencies or patients under treatment with immunomodulant medications) are relatively well understood by clinicians and radiologists. However, the role of immune compromise in other disorders is less well recognized, including immune compromise in patients with respiratory conditions associated with increased susceptibility to infection such as asthma and chronic obstructive pulmonary disease. These patients are often treated with immune suppressors such as corticosteroids, which may further compromise their immune status. Similarly, in patients with autoimmune conditions there is increased risk of pulmonary infection due to both the disease and the treatment with immune modulators. In addition, patients with malignancy and those with diabetes may be at risk for opportunistic infection due to immunosuppression related to the disease and its treatment.

The list of nonsteroidal immunomodulators is large and beyond the scope of this work. However, radiologists must become familiar with common drug treatments that produce immunosuppression, including tumor necrosis factor inhibitors (e.g., infliximab and etanercept) and T-cell suppressors (e.g., cyclosporine, tacrolimus, and sirolimus).

AIDS

During the past few decades, as a result of medical research on HIV, the epidemiology of AIDS has significantly changed from a highly lethal disease in the 1980s to a chronic illness with significantly better overall life expectancy.

In clinical practice, patients with HIV infection may present with clinical patterns that, if recognized, can help make the diagnosis (Figs. 41.1 and 41.2). The first and most problematic group of patients are those with an unknown HIV status. In this group of patients, it is difficult to consider the possibility of an HIV-related complication. However, the clinical history may offer clues to the patient's HIV status. Knowledge of risk factors is critical in these cases: sexual intercourse among men, promiscuity,

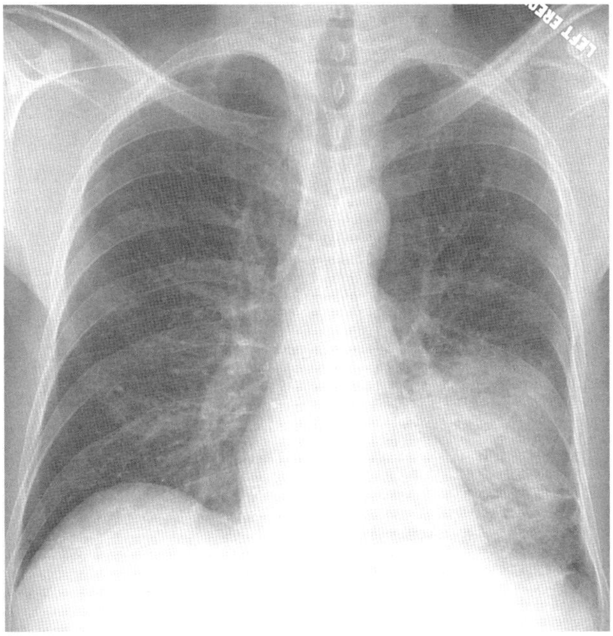

Figure 41.1. *Rhodococcus equi* pneumonia in HIV. Posteroanterior chest radiograph of a 47-year-old man shows a left lower lobe consolidation secondary to rhodococcal pneumonia, an opportunistic infection occasionally seen in immunocompromised patients.

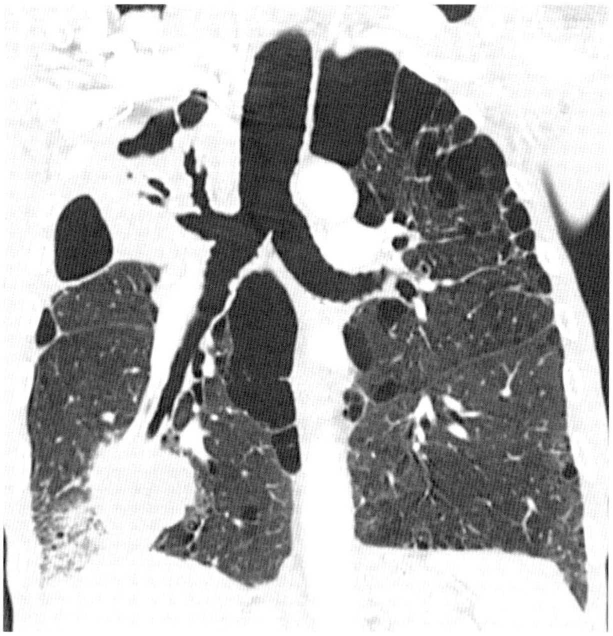

Figure 41.2. Lung cancer, atypical mycobacterial infection, and emphysema in HIV. Coronal unenhanced chest CT shows right upper lobe cavitary disease from atypical mycobacterial infection, extensive centrilobular and paraseptal emphysema, and a lobulated right lower lobe mass proven to represent primary lung cancer.

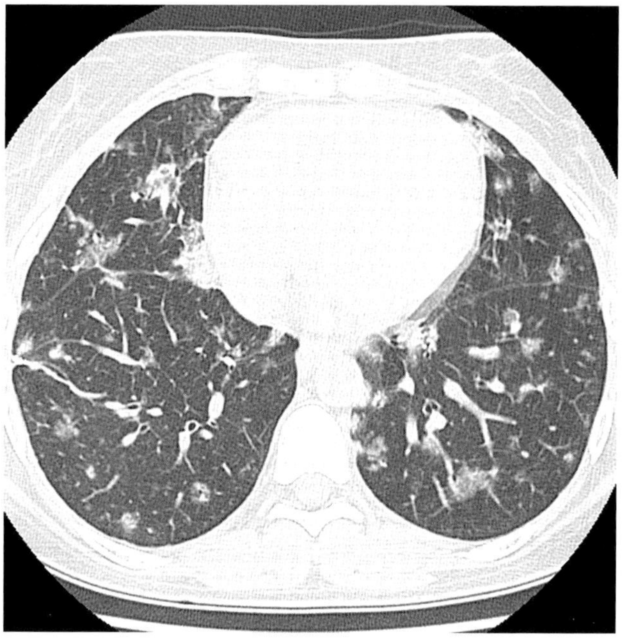

Figure 41.3. Lymphocytic interstitial pneumonia (LIP) in common variable immunodeficiency. Unenhanced chest CT of a 41-year-old woman shows scattered bilateral ill-defined ground-glass nodules. Open lung biopsy revealed LIP.

sex worker, transgender, intravenous drug use, prisoners, alcoholics, people with disabilities, and immigrants. In the United States, the African American population is at significantly higher risk compared to Latinos, and the latter have a higher risk compared to White individuals. Radiologists may be the first to suspect HIV-related disease, even in the absence of a known HIV status. For example, a young individual with risk factors for HIV infection and no history of cardiac disease who presents with an abnormal chest radiograph concerning for with pulmonary edema (i.e., perihilar opacities, thickened septal lines, and pleural effusions) may be suspected of Kaposi sarcoma, particularly if the patient does not have a history consistent with heart failure.

In patients with known HIV-positive status and pulmonary abnormalities, knowledge of the CD4 lymphocyte count is critical. Patients with near normal CD4 counts are more likely to have bacterial pneumonia or tuberculosis, whereas patients with low CD4 counts are more likely to have Kaposi sarcoma, cytomegalovirus pneumonia, atypical mycobacterial infection, or disseminated fungal infection.

Other Causes of Immunosuppression

As previously mentioned, there are many other causes of immunocompromise besides AIDS. Knowledge of specific risk factors is important in the interpretation of abnormal chest imaging studies in affected patients (Figs. 41.3 and 41.4). Correlation with the clinical presentation and the past medical history is crucial for accurate radiologic interpretation. For example, a patient with diffuse bilateral mosaic attenuation on thin-section chest CT may be suspected of having one of several small airways diseases. However, if the patient is known to have congenital immunodeficiency, the finding is likely small airways disease as

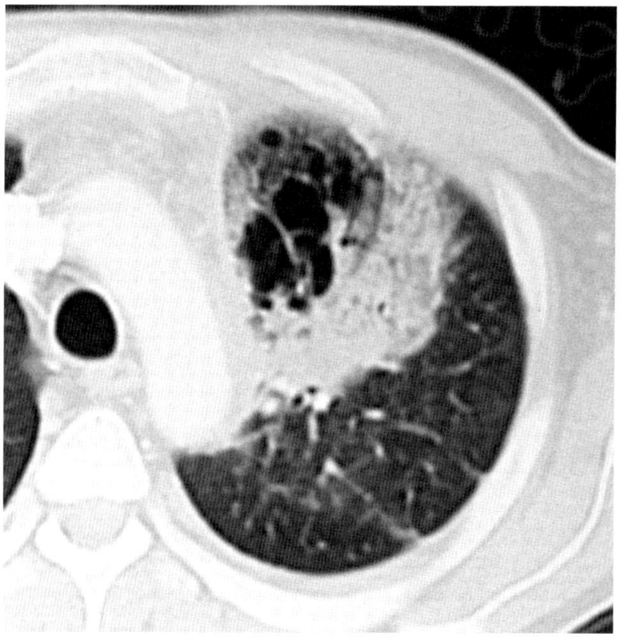

Figure 41.4. Mucormycosis in diabetes mellitus type 2. Contrast-enhanced chest CT shows a cavitary mass-like left upper lobe consolidation proven to represent mucormycosis on open lung biopsy.

the sequela of recurrent infections rather than idiopathic constrictive bronchiolitis.

Suggested Reading

Benito N, Moreno A, Miro JM, Torres A. Pulmonary infections in HIV-infected patients: An update in the 21st century. *Eur Respir J.* 2012 Mar;39(3):730–745.

Hampson FA, Chandra A, Screaton NJ, Condliffe A, Kumararatne DS, Exley AR, et al. Respiratory disease in common variable immunodeficiency and other primary immunodeficiency disorders. *Clin Radiol.* 2012 Jun;67(6):587–595.

Klein NC, Go CH, Cunha BA. Infections associated with steroid use. *Infect Dis Clin North Am.* 2001 Jun;15(2):423–432.

Lichtenberger JP 3rd, Sharma A, Zachary KC, Krishnam MS, Greene RE, Shepard JA, et al. What a differential a virus makes: A practical approach to thoracic imaging findings in the context of HIV infection: Part 2. Extrapulmonary findings, chronic lung disease, and immune reconstitution syndrome. *AJR Am J Roentgenol.* 2012;198(6):1305–1312.

CHAPTER 42

The Immunocompromised Patient: AIDS

Juliana Bueno

Definition

AIDS is caused by infection with HIV that results in decreased immunity and favors infectious or neoplastic conditions.

The onset of clinical AIDS is defined by a CD4 count of less than 200 cells/mm^3 or CD4 cells less than 14% of all leukocytes in an HIV-positive patient, even in the absence of opportunistic infections. As CD4 count decreases, the likelihood of developing infections and malignancies increases. Prolonged life expectancy after introduction of highly active antiretroviral therapy (HAART) has allowed HIV infection and AIDS to be regarded as a chronic disease.

Clinical Features

CD4 count correlates with degree of immunosuppression and is used as a marker of variety of pulmonary manifestations (i.e., at certain levels, some diseases are more common). Figure 42.1 shows the distribution of infections according to the CD4 count. Neoplastic disorders (e.g., lymphoma and Kaposi sarcoma) and opportunistic infections due to bacteria, fungi, and virus are more common when CD4 levels are less than 200 cells/mm^3.

Bacterial pneumonia is now the most common pulmonary infection in patients with AIDS. Although it can occur at any level of immunosuppression (including >400 cells/mm^3), it is more common at severe immunosuppression. *Streptococcus pneumoniae, Haemophilus influenzae*, and *Staphylococcus aureus* are the most common causative microorganisms. Common symptoms include fever, dyspnea, cough, and pleuritic pain. Bacterial pulmonary infections are more common among intravenous drug abusers and smokers.

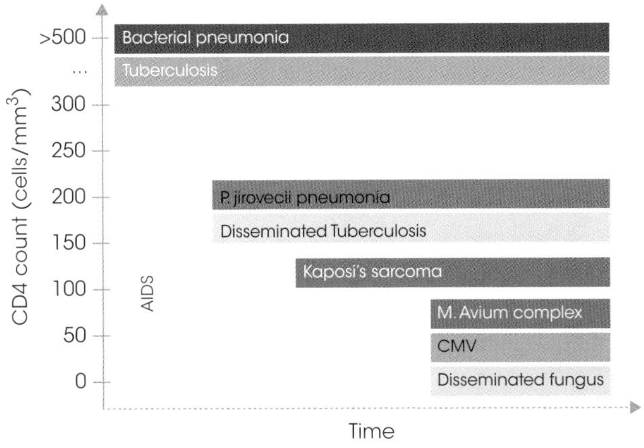

Figure 42.1. Frequency of opportunistic diseases according to CD4 count. As immunosuppression progresses, the incidence of infection and malignancy increases.

Although the incidence of *Pneumocystis jirovecii* pneumonia (or *Pneumocystis* pneumonia (PCP)) has decreased since the introduction of HAART and prophylaxis, it continues to be the most common fungal infection in AIDS, especially in individuals with CD4 counts less than 200 cells/mm^3. The most common presentation includes fever, cough, and dyspnea over days or weeks. Patients present with hypoxia and elevated lactate dehydrogenase level. *Pneumocystis jirovecii* can be detected on bronchoalveolar lavage with high sensitivity. Other mycoses, such as histoplasmosis and cryptococcosis, are often disseminated infections and remain common in patients with AIDS and CD4 levels less than 100 cells/mm^3. Cryptococcal pneumonia is often associated with meningitis.

Although *Mycobacterium tuberculosis* is common in AIDS, its incidence has significantly decreased in the HAART era. Intravenous drug users are at a higher risk of developing tuberculosis (TB). At relative high CD4 counts (>350 cells/mm^3), symptoms are similar to those of affected immunocompetent patients and include low-grade fever, cough, weight loss, night sweats, and malaise. Among nontuberculous mycobacteria, *Mycobacterium avium-intracellulare* (MAC) is the most common isolated pathogen, often with CD4 counts less than 50 cells/mm^3. Symptoms are often nonspecific and include fever, weight loss, and fatigue.

Lung cancer, lymphoma, and Kaposi sarcoma (KS) have an increased incidence among patients with AIDS. Lung cancer is more common at CD4 counts greater than 400 cells/mm^3, whereas lymphoma and KS are more likely to occur at CD4 counts less than 200 cells/mm^3. In the era of HAART, diffuse large B-cell lymphoma and Burkitt lymphoma are the most common HIV-associated lymphomas. KS is more common among homosexual and bisexual men. Epstein–Barr virus and human herpesvirus-8 are strongly associated with lymphoma and KS, respectively.

Immune reconstitution syndrome is a paradoxical clinical deterioration after initiation of HAART more likely to occur in the setting of low CD4 counts (<50 cells/mm^3). As immune response improves, indolent infections or neoplastic disorders appear to worsen clinically and on imaging. This is especially common in patients with partially treated or untreated TB or MAC infection.

Anatomy and Physiology

HIV affects primarily the immune system and affects a variety of cells, including lymphocytes, T helper (CD4$^+$) macrophages, and dendritic cells. This significantly compromises cell-mediated immunity, leading to opportunistic infections and malignancies.

How to Approach the Image

Awareness of HIV status is critical when interpreting imaging studies in affected patients. However, patients and physicians may be unaware of HIV infection. Thus, knowledge of populations at risk of HIV infection is valuable. The likelihood of HIV infection is higher in homosexual men, intravenous drug users, and promiscuous individuals. Imaging features of infection and malignancy in patients with AIDS are not significantly different from those in patients without AIDS. However, certain imaging findings in patients with AIDS may suggest a specific diagnosis (e.g., diffuse ground-glass opacities often correlate with PCP). *Pneumocystis jirovecii* pneumonia and Kaposi sarcoma are less likely in compliant patients on PCP prophylaxis and/or HAART.

What Not to Miss

- A normal chest radiograph does not exclude an opportunistic infection; chest CT is often indicated in patients with respiratory symptoms. Approximately 40% of patients with PCP may have a normal chest radiograph at presentation.
- Consider PCP in patients with AIDS, a CD4 count less than 200 cells/mm^3, and diffuse ground-glass opacities on chest CT.
- KS should be considered in patients with AIDS, a CD4 count less than 150 cells/mm^3, and imaging features of pulmonary edema without supporting clinical evidence.
- Spontaneous pneumothorax in an HIV-positive patient should raise concern for PCP.

Differential Diagnosis

- Diffuse ground-glass opacities (GGO): PCP is the most common infection with diffuse GGO and should be suspected in HIV-positive patients with hypoxemia. Cytomegalovirus infection is less frequent, occurs in severe immunosuppression, and manifests with scattered GGO.
- Consolidation: Regardless of CD4 count, focal or multifocal consolidations usually represent bacterial pneumonia.
- Nodules: Single or multiple nodules occur in multiple opportunistic infections, including *Nocardia* spp., *Cryptococcus* spp., and *Aspergillus* spp.
- Cavitary nodules: Septic embolism should be considered in patients with intravenous drug use or an extrapulmonary source of sepsis. Other atypical infections may also cavitate.
- Nodule/mass with lymphadenopathy: Consider TB, MAC, and lymphoma in patients with a low CD4 count. Consider AIDS-associated lymphoma with poor response to antibiotics.
- Miliary pattern: Consider disseminated tuberculosis but also disseminated MAC, toxoplasmosis, and fungi.

Imaging Findings

- Bacterial bronchiolitis (pyogenic airways disease) and pneumonia (Figs. 42.2 and 42.3): Chest radiography is insensitive and often normal. Thin-section CT often demonstrates centrilobular and tree-in-bud nodular opacities. Pneumonia manifests as airspace disease and is often multifocal. Abscess formation manifesting as cavitary mass or consolidation is more frequent than in the general population.
- TB (Fig. 42.4): Radiographic manifestations correlate with level of immunosuppression. Patients with CD4

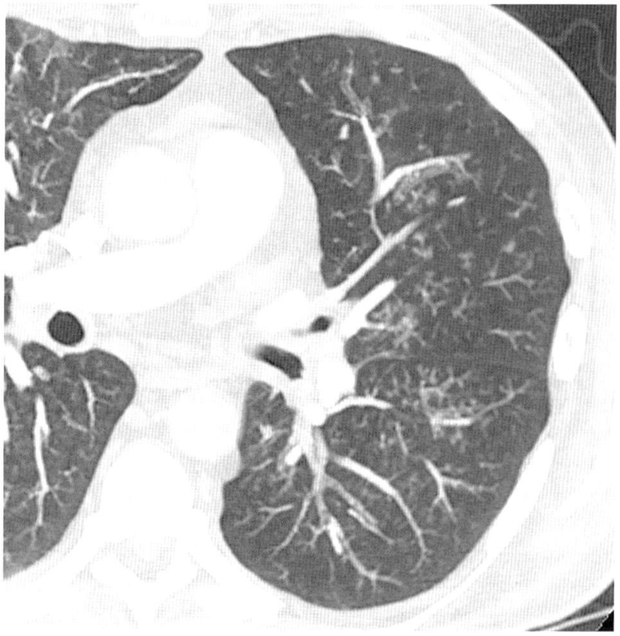

Figure 42.2. Pyogenic airways disease. Maximum intensity projection (MIP) reformation contrast-enhanced chest CT of a 55-year-old HIV-positive man with fever and dyspnea shows scattered centrilobular and tree-in-bud nodules.

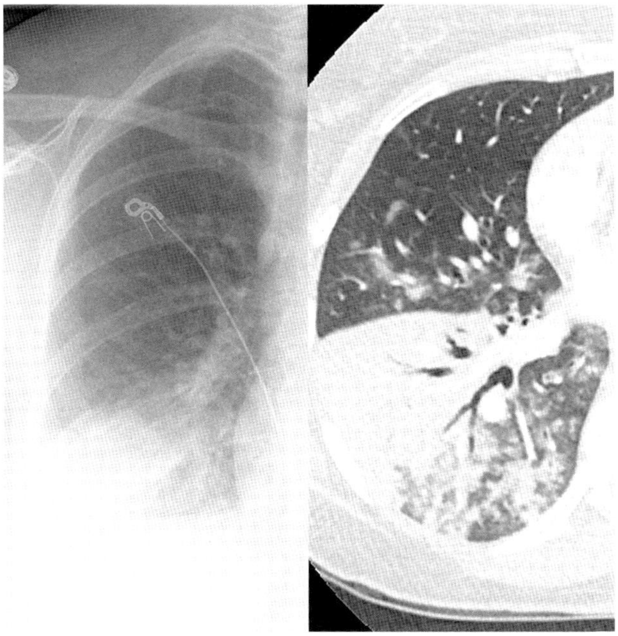

Figure 42.3. Bacterial pneumonia. Composite image with anteroposterior (AP) chest radiograph (left) and contrast-enhanced chest CT (right) of a 46-year-old HIV-positive man with dyspnea and fever shows a right lower lobe consolidation with surrounding centrilobular nodules and tree-in-bud opacities and less severe right middle lobe involvement.

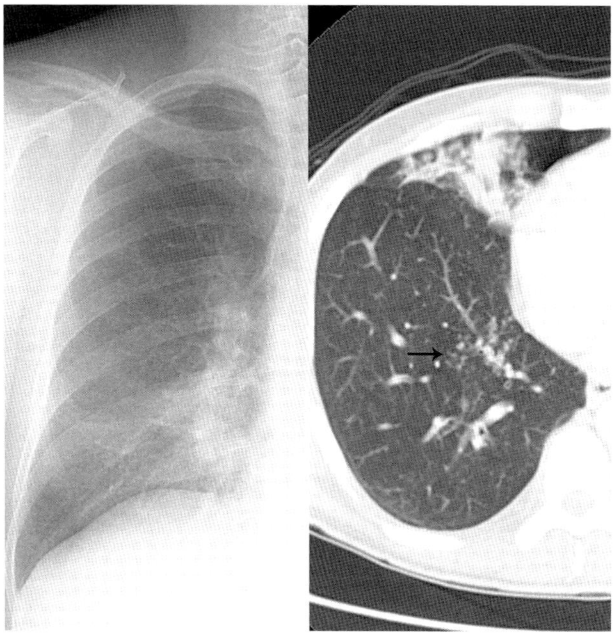

Figure 42.5. Atypical mycobacterial infection due to MAC. Composite image with PA chest radiograph (left) and unenhanced chest CT (right) of a 42-year-old HIV-positive man with nonspecific constitutional symptoms shows a right middle lobe consolidation and right lower lobe bronchial wall thickening and centrilobular nodules (arrow) due to multilobar involvement.

count greater than 200 cells/mm^3 exhibit the postprimary pattern of disease, with upper lobe cavitary disease and endobronchial spread manifesting as centrilobular nodules and tree-in-bud opacities. Patients

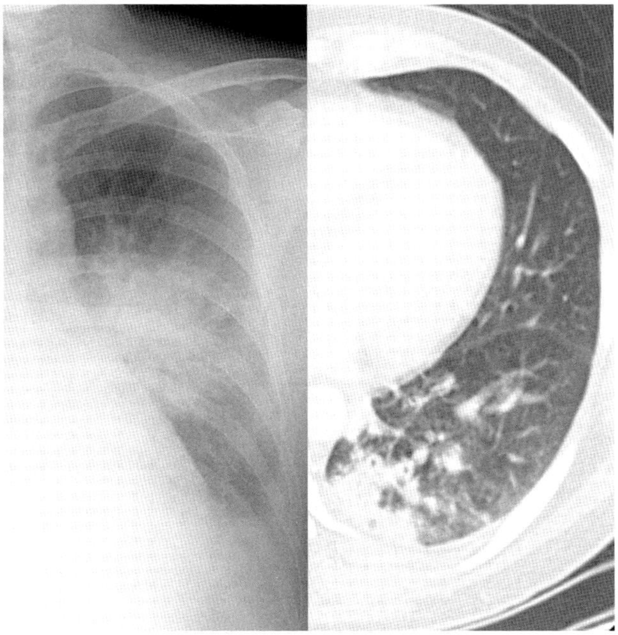

Figure 42.4. Multidrug-resistant tuberculosis. Composite image with posteroanterior (PA) chest radiograph (left) and contrast-enhanced chest CT (right) of a 37-year-old HIV-positive man with cough and constitutional symptoms shows a left perihilar consolidation and left lower lobe subsegmental consolidation on CT.

with CD4 count less than 200 cells/mm^3 exhibit the primary pattern of disease characterized by consolidation and lymphadenopathy and may have miliary disease. Disseminated TB with extrapulmonary involvement is more common in advanced immunosuppression and frequently manifests with extensive multifocal lymphadenopathy (tuberculous lymphadenitis) and pleural involvement (tuberculous empyema) that may progress to empyema necessitatis.

- MAC (Fig. 42.5): Radiographic findings resemble those of TB, including multifocal consolidation and lymphadenopathy. Cavitation is not uncommon.
- PCP (Fig. 42.6): Chest radiography may be normal or demonstrate mild diffuse hazy opacities. CT typically shows diffuse GGO, often with perihilar predominance and sparing of scattered secondary pulmonary lobules. Associated smooth interlobular thickening, the so-called "crazy paving" pattern, is not uncommon. Pneumatoceles may occur as disease evolves and may produce secondary spontaneous pneumothorax. Absence of CT abnormalities is very sensitive for exclusion of PCP.
- Fungal infections other than PCP (Fig. 42.7): Chest radiographs are often normal or show reticular or reticulonodular opacities. CT may show a miliary pattern or diffuse airspace disease.
- KS (Fig. 42.8): KS often mimics pulmonary edema on chest radiography, manifesting with diffuse peribronchovascular opacities, peribronchial cuffing, septal lines, and pleural effusions. CT findings include hilar,

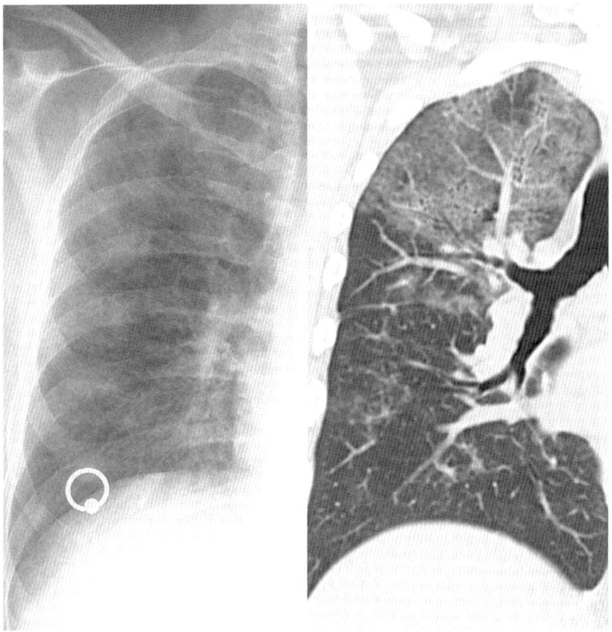

Figure 42.6. PCP. Composite image with PA chest radiograph (left) and coronal contrast-enhanced chest CT (right) of an HIV-positive 22-year-old man with with dyspnea and fever shows upper lobe predominant hazy opacities that manifest as GGO on CT.

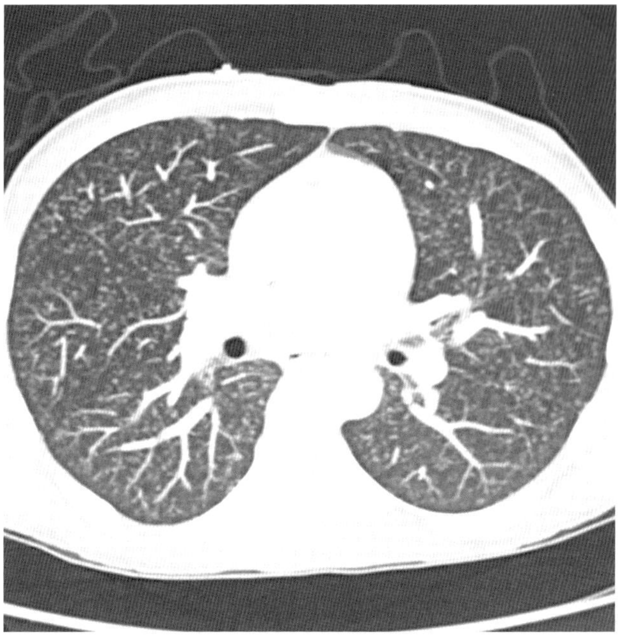

Figure 42.7. Miliary histoplasmosis. MIP reformatted unenhanced chest CT of a 33-year-old man with dyspnea and fever shows randomly distributed (or miliary) micronodules.

mediastinal, and axillary lymphadenopathy. "Flame-shaped" nodules or peribronchovascular nodules with ill-defined or spiculated margins and surrounding GGO are characteristic findings on CT.

- Non-Hodgkin lymphoma (Fig. 42.9): Common manifestations include hilar/mediastinal lymphadenopathy; pulmonary nodules, masses, and airspace disease; and pleural effusions.
- Immune reconstitution syndrome: Development or worsening of parenchymal opacities or lymphadenopathy. Lymphadenopathy may demonstrate hypodense centers from necrosis on CT.

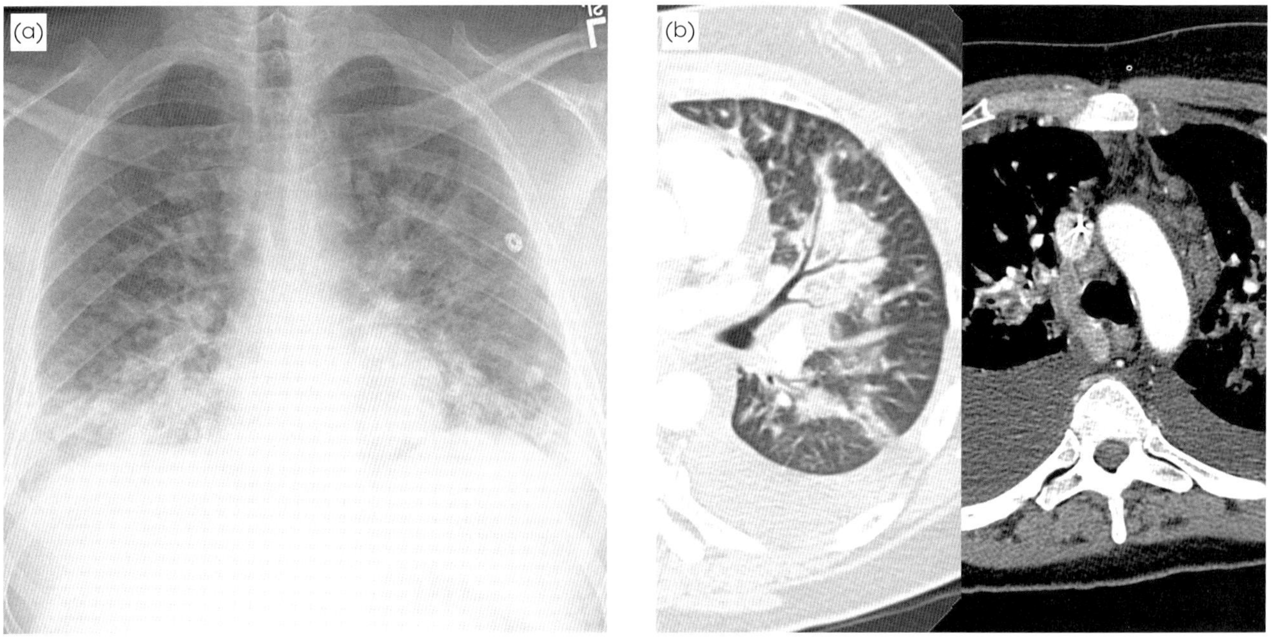

Figure 42.8. Kaposi sarcoma. (a) AP chest radiograph of a 55-year-old HIV-positive man with chronic cough and dyspnea shows bilateral basilar predominant heterogeneous opacities with associated septal lines and small pleural effusions. (b) Composite image with contrast-enhanced chest CT of the same patient shows ill-defined peribronchovascular airspace disease, mediastinal lymphadenopathy, and bilateral pleural effusions.

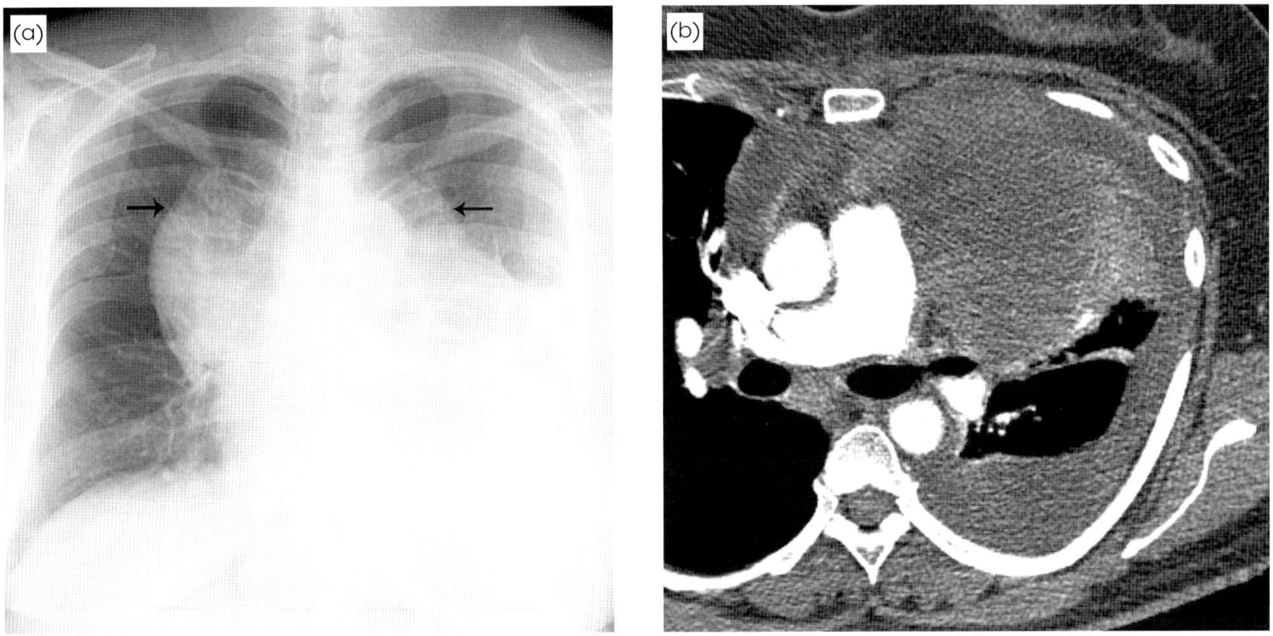

Figure 42.9. Diffuse large B-cell non-Hodgkin lymphoma. (a) AP chest radiograph of an HIV-positive 45-year-old woman with low-grade fever, weight loss, and fatigue shows marked mediastinal widening (arrows) and a left pleural effusion. (b) Contrast-enhanced chest CT of the same patient shows loss of a large heterogeneous anterior mediastinal mass, subcarinal and left hilar lymphadenopathy, and a left pleural effusion.

Source: Fig. 42.9b courtesy Carlos S. Restrepo, MD.

Clinical Issues

With the advent of HAART in the late 1990s, the epidemiology of AIDS complications has changed. Previously common diseases have decreased in incidence (e.g., PCP, KS, and non-Hodgkin lymphoma), whereas some may remain prevalent (e.g., bacterial pneumonia). In addition, new diseases have emerged (lung cancer, leukemia, hepatocellular carcinoma, skin cancers, etc.). Constant update by clinicians and radiologists is required.

Key Points

- Imaging abnormalities in HIV-positive patients should be correlated with the CD4 count to narrow the differential diagnosis.
- Diffuse GGO on CT in a patient with AIDS and hypoxemia is virtually diagnostic of PCP.
- CT is indicated in HIV-positive patients with respiratory symptoms and normal chest radiographs.
- Suspect TB in patients with advanced AIDS and low CD4 counts presenting with consolidation and lymphadenopathy.
- KS may simulate cardiogenic pulmonary edema on imaging and should be suspected in patients without clinical evidence of edema.

Suggested Reading

Benito N, Moreno A, Miro JM, Torres A. Pulmonary infections in HIV-infected patients: An update in the 21st century. *Eur Respir J.* 2012 Mar;39(3):730–745.

Castañer E, Gallardo X, Mata JM, Esteba L. Radiologic approach to the diagnosis of infectious pulmonary diseases in patients infected with the human immunodeficiency virus. *Eur J Radiol.* 2004;51:114–112.

Chong S, Lee KS, Yi CA, Chung MJ, Kim TS, Han J. Pulmonary fungal infection: Imaging findings in immunocompetent and immunocompromised patients. *Eur J Radiol.* 2006;59: 371–383.

Eisner MD, Kaplan LD, Herndier B, Stulbarg MS. The pulmonary manifestations of AIDS-related non-Hodgkin's lymphoma. *Chest.* 1996 Sep;110(3):729–736.

Jeong YJ, Lee KS. Pulmonary tuberculosis: Up-to-date imaging and management. *AJR Am J Roentgenol.* 2008;191:834–884.

Lichtenberger JP 3rd, Sharma A, Zachary KC, Krishnam MS, Greene RE, Shepard JA, et al. What a differential a virus makes: A practical approach to thoracic imaging findings in the context of HIV infection: Part 2. Extrapulmonary findings, chronic lung disease, and immune reconstitution syndrome. *AJR Am J Roentgenol.* 2012;198(6):1305–1312.

Restrepo CS, Martínez S, Lemos JA, Carrillo JA, Lemos DF, Ojeda P, et al. Imaging manifestations of Kaposi sarcoma. *RadioGraphics.* 2006 Jul–Aug;26(4):1169–1185.

CHAPTER 43

The Immunocompromised Patient: Non-AIDS

Juliana Bueno

Definition

Immunosuppression is a state in which the immune system is compromised to a level at which there is an increased risk of infections and certain malignancies. This may be related to humoral deficiency (i.e., antibodies), cellular deficiency (e.g., lymphocytes and neutrophils), complement deficiency, etc.

Immunodeficiencies may be primary (i.e., congenital) or secondary (i.e., acquired). Although more than 100 well-recognized immunodeficiencies have been described, this chapter focuses on common immunodeficiencies seen in clinical practice. Primary immunodeficiencies discussed in this chapter include immunoglobulin A (IgA) deficiency, common variable immunodeficiency, X-linked agammaglobulinemia, and chronic granulomatous disease. Secondary immunodeficiencies include those occurring in bone marrow (BMT) and solid organ transplant recipients and chronic corticosteroid therapy. Complementary information on opportunistic fungal infections can be found in Chapter 37.

Clinical Features

IgA deficiency is the most common immune deficiency (1 in 700 White individuals of European origin) and is thought to be inherited. Common variable immunodeficiency (CVID) is a humoral immunodeficiency manifesting after 24 months of age or in early adulthood (1 in 10,000 individuals). X-linked agammaglobulinemia (Bruton agammaglobulinemia) is a humoral immunodeficiency manifesting after 2 months of age (1 in 200,000 individuals). Chronic granulomatous disease consists of failure of phagocytes to kill engulfed microorganisms (1 in 200,000 individuals). These entities manifest with recurrent infections such as pneumonia and subsequent bronchiectasis. CVID may also be associated with an increased incidence of lymphoma.

Patients on chronic corticosteroid therapy are at increased risk of infection due to immunosuppression. Bacterial infection is the most common complication, often due to *Staphylococcus aureus, Streptococcus pneumoniae*, and enterobacteria. Other common bacteria include *Listeria monocytogenes, Salmonella* spp., *Brucella* spp., *Legionella* spp., and *Nocardia* spp. There is also an increased incidence of tuberculosis, which is more likely to be disseminated (miliary). The most common fungus remains *Pneumocystis jirovecii. Strongyloides stercoralis* infection is a relatively common life-threatening parasitic infection.

Diabetes, hematologic malignancies, renal insufficiency, solid organ transplantation, and metabolic acidosis are debilitating conditions that lead to immunosuppression. Fungal infections such as mucormycosis and candidiasis are not infrequent in these patients.

Malnutrition from alcoholism, diabetes, chronic granulomatous disease, or connective tissue disorders is associated with mild to moderate degrees of immunosuppression, and affected patients are prone to infections such as semi-invasive aspergillosis.

Patients who undergo splenectomy or have conditions that cause splenic dysfunction, such as sickle cell disease, are prone to develop infections by encapsulated bacteria such as *Streptococcus pneumoniae, Salmonella* spp., *Neisseria meningitidis, Escherichia coli, Klebsiella pneumoniae*, and *Haemophilus influenzae*.

Familiarity with the time course of immune dysfunction following BMT is essential for imaging interpretation and formulation of a narrow differential diagnosis in cases of opportunistic infection. Table 43.1 illustrates the different stages of immunosuppression related to therapy, after transplantation, as well as the most frequent infections in each stage. Important noninfectious entities should be taken into account in these patients because they frequently exhibit similar imaging manifestations.

Anatomy and Physiology

Humoral immunodeficiency is characterized by impaired production of antibodies with compromised phagocytosis and opsonization and resultant predisposition to infections by encapsulated bacteria. The severity of the infection and imaging manifestations vary according to the degree of immunosuppression. Cellular immunodeficiency is characterized by impaired T-cell function and may be primary or secondary. Common causes of secondary cellular immunodeficiency are chemotherapy, BMT, lymphoma, and corticosteroid therapy. Infection by

Table 43.1 - Infection at different stages after transplanatation

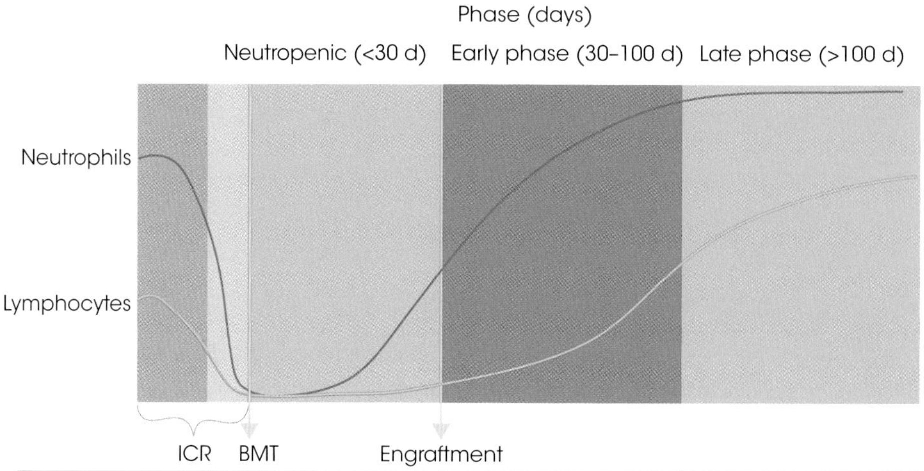

	Neutropenic (<30 d)	Early phase (30–100 d)	Late phase (>100 d)
Infectious causes	Invasive aspergillosis Candidiasis Bacterial pneumonia	CMV PCP	Uncommon
Non-Infectious causes	Pulmonary edema Drug reactions DAH	Engraftment syndrome	OB COP GVHD

intracellular pathogens such as viruses (herpes simplex virus), *Mycobacterium* spp., *Listeria* spp., and other opportunistic microorganisms, such as *P. jirovecii, Toxoplasma gondii*, and *Mycobacterium avium-intracellulare*, is common. More frequently, systemic debilitating diseases lead to combined immunosuppression.

In patients undergoing BMT, immunosuppression starts with the conditioning regimen of chemotherapy and total body irradiation, usually 1 week before the transplant. Profound neutropenia occurs in all patients during the first month after the transplant (neutropenic phase). Neutrophils slowly start to recover within the first 2–4 weeks, although recovery of lymphocytes may take months. Recovery of both humoral and cell-mediated immune functions may take up to 6–12 months, and affected patients remain at risk for opportunistic infections for a relatively long period of time.

How to Approach the Image

Because immunodeficiencies constitute an extensive and highly heterogeneous group of diseases, imaging interpretation must be performed with knowledge of the underlying condition and/or treatment time line whenever possible.

What Not to Miss

A normal chest radiograph does not exclude infection in immunocompromised patients with respiratory symptoms; further assessment with chest CT should always be considered.

Differential Diagnosis

- Diffuse ground-glass opacities (GGO): Opportunistic infection, pulmonary edema (cardiogenic and noncardiogenic), drug toxicity, and diffuse alveolar hemorrhage. Differentiation of these conditions on imaging is not possible, and further evaluation is required.
- Pulmonary nodules/masses with the CT halo sign: Typically opportunistic fungal infections, but other infections may produce this finding. Pulmonary infarction, septic embolism, and vasculitis should also be considered.
- Centrilobular nodules and/or tree-in-bud opacities: Bacterial, mycobacterial, fungal, and viral infection. Aspiration bronchiolitis should also be considered.
- Diffuse bronchiectasis: Immunodeficiency should always be considered in young individuals with diffuse bronchiectasis. Other etiologies include post-infectious bronchiestasis, cystic fibrosis, and inhalational injury.

Imaging Findings

- Imaging abnormalities in primary immunodeficiencies are nonspecific.
- Recurrent infections: Infection often manifests as cellular bronchiolitis (i.e., centrilobular nodules and/or tree-in-bud opacities) or frank airspace disease. Diffuse bronchiectasis results from recurrent infection. Additional findings include mosaic attenuation or expiratory air trapping, bronchial wall thickening, and bronchiectasis. Follicular bronchiolitis may

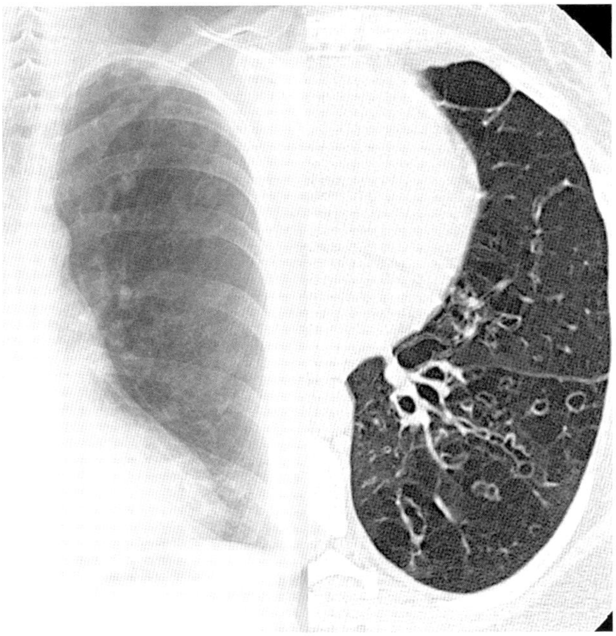

Figure 43.1. IgA deficiency. Composite image of a 41-year-old man with a history of recurrent infections. (Left) Chest radiograph shows some linear opacities and tram tracking in the lower lobes suggesting bronchiectasis. (Right) Chest CT shows extensive cylindrical bronchiectasis in a background of mosaic attenuation from associated small airways disease.

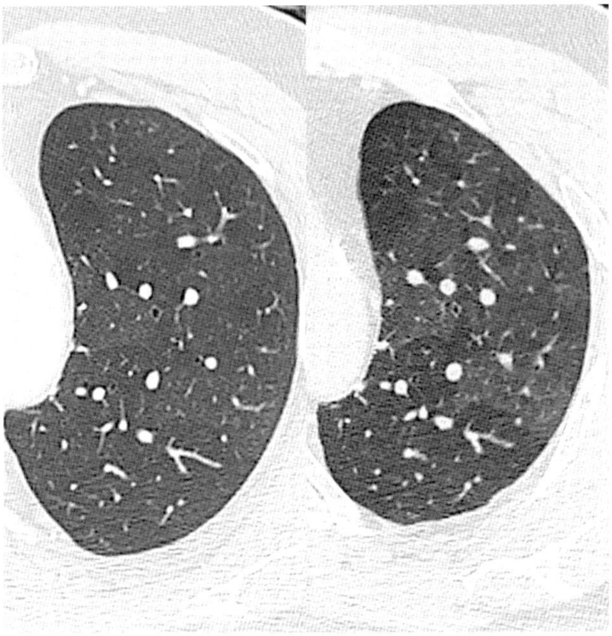

Figure 43.3. X-linked agammaglobulinemia (Bruton agammaglobulinemia). Composite image of a 37-year-old man with chronic cough. (Left) Inspiration chest CT shows very subtle mosaic attenuation. (Right) Expiration chest CT demonstrates marked air trapping consistent with small airways disease.

mimic infection and may be associated with nodules, bronchial wall thickening, and bronchiectasis (Figs. 43.1–43.3).

- *Pneumocystis jirovecii* pneumonia (PCP) (Fig. 43.4): Chest radiography may be normal or show subtle bilateral opacities. CT shows diffuse bilateral GGO.
- Opportunistic infections in BMT recipients can be categorized based on the post-transplant phase:
- Neutropenic phase (<30 days, before engraftment): Profound neutropenia predisposes to aggressive infections, including angioinvasive aspergillosis (Fig. 43.5). Radiography may be normal, but CT often demonstrates nodules or masses surrounded by

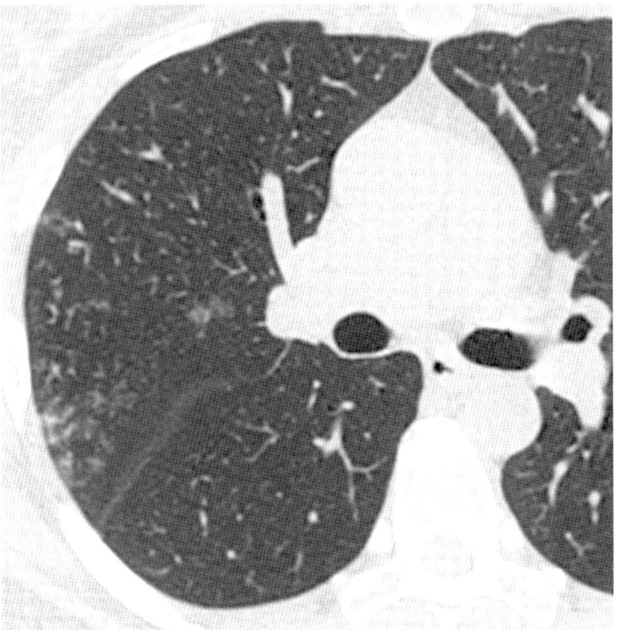

Figure 43.2. Common variable immunodeficiency. Composite image of a 53-year-old man with fever and dyspnea. Chest CT shows clustering of nodules in the right upper lobe consistent with infectious bronchiolitis.

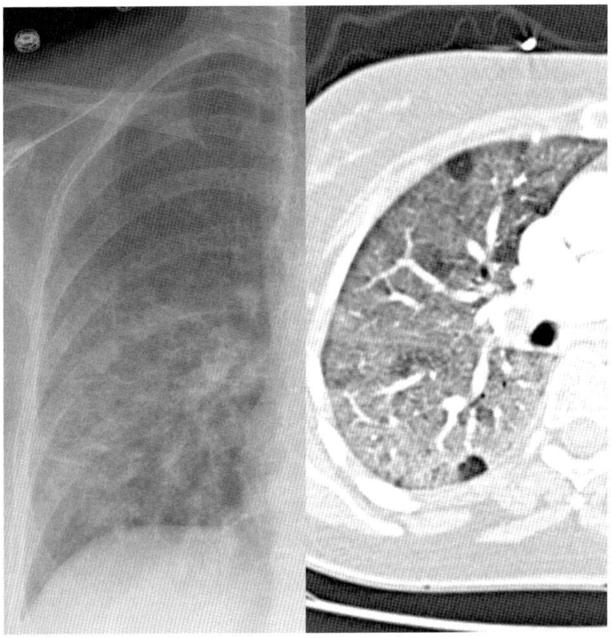

Figure 43.4. PCP pneumonia. Composite image of a 37-year-old woman with Crohn disease on chronic corticosteroid therapy. (Left) Chest radiograph shows diffuse hazy opacities. (Right) Chest CT demonstrates diffuse ground-glass opacities.

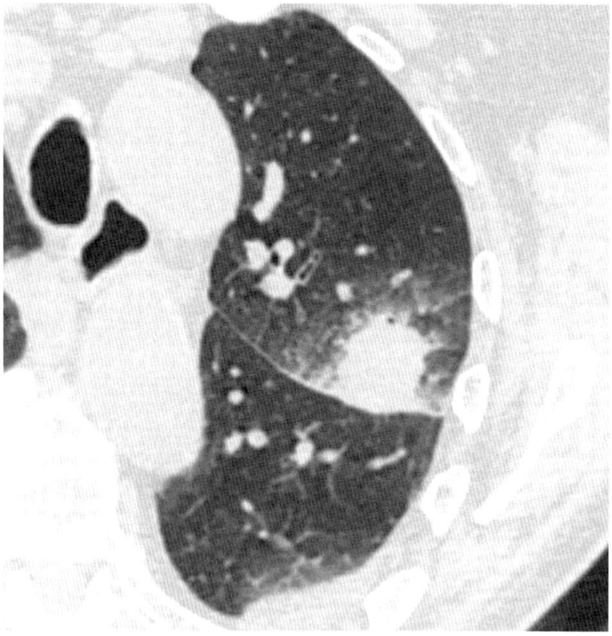

Figure 43.5. Angioinvasive aspergillosis. A 62-year-old woman 20 days after BMT. Chest CT shows a left upper lobe nodule with surrounding ground-glass opacities.

GGO (CT halo sign), which represents hemorrhagic infarction.

- Early phase (30–100 days, after engraftment): Gradual recovery of neutrophil function leads to decreased risk of fungal infection but increased risk of viral infections such as cytomegalovirus (CMV) pneumonitis (Fig. 43.6). Chest radiography may show mid and lower lung diffuse hazy opacities and nodules. CT shows multiple micronodules associated with consolidations and GGO.
- Late phase (>100 days): With continued recovery of immunity, most pulmonary complications are noninfectious.

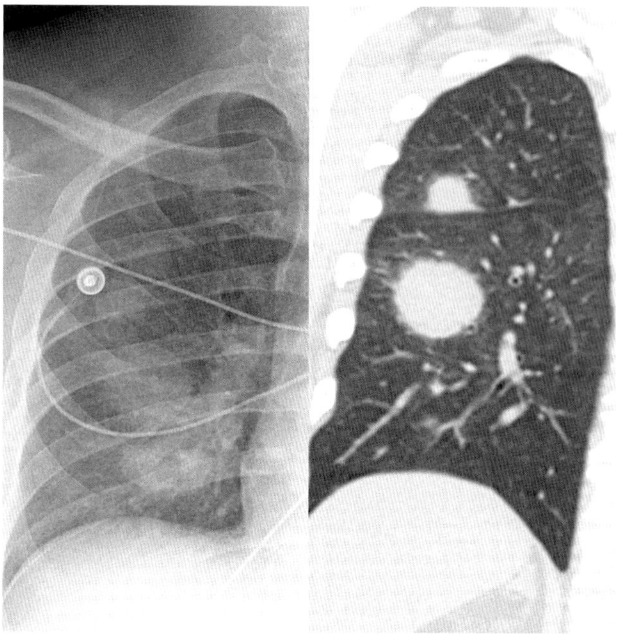

Figure 43.7. *Nocardia* pneumonia. Composite image of a 37-year-old man with a history of renal transplant presenting with dyspnea and fever. (Left) Chest radiograph shows an ill-defined right lower lobe mass. (Right) Chest CT demonstrates several soft tissue nodules.

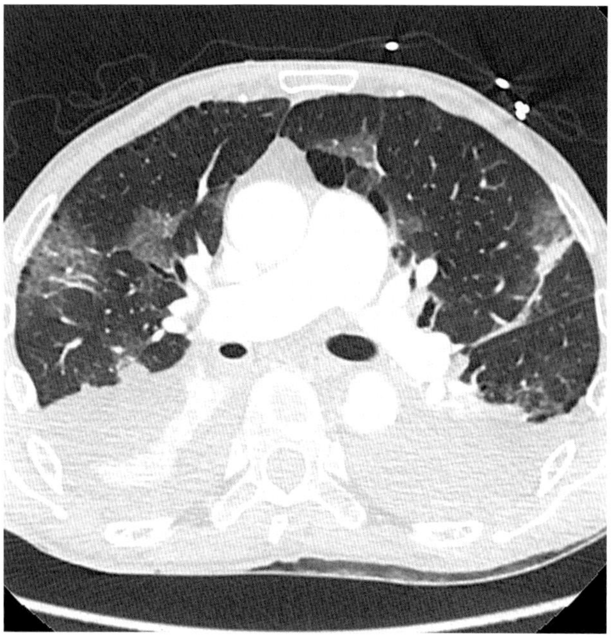

Figure 43.6. CMV pneumonia. A 43-year-old man with history of renal transplant presenting with shortness of breath and fever. Chest CT shows scattered ground-glass opacities and bilateral pleural effusions.

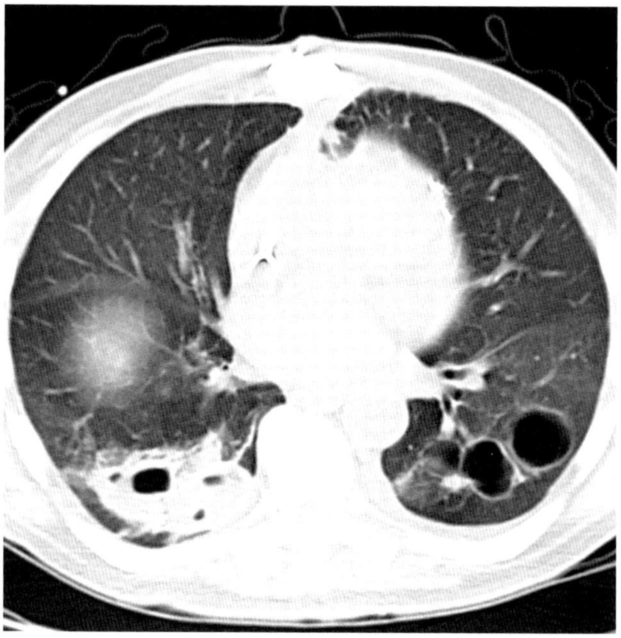

Figure 43.8. *Serratia* pneumonia. A 68-year-old man with a history of heart transplant presenting with dyspnea and fever. Chest CT demonstrates several lower lobe cavitary nodules consistent with pulmonary abscesses.

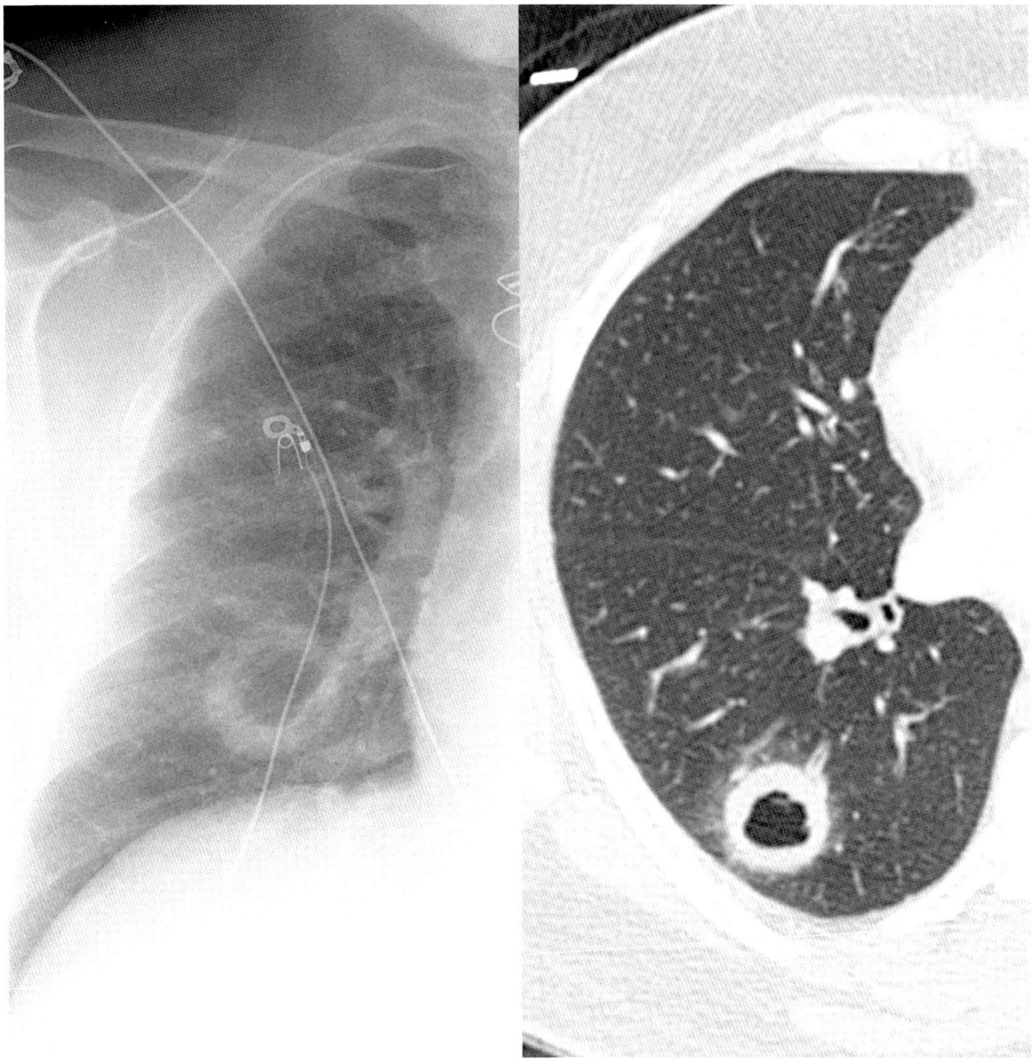

Figure 43.9. Mucormycosis. Composite image of a 42-year-old man with a history of heart transplant presenting with fever and cough. (Left) Chest radiograph shows a cavitary nodule in the right lower lobe. (Right) Chest CT demonstrates a thick-wall cavitary nodule.

- Infection due to atypical organisms is common in solid organ transplant and often manifests as pulmonary nodules that may be cavitated and exhibit surrounding GGO (Figs. 43.7–43.10).
- Strongyloidiasis: Diffuse airspace disease in radiography and CT; focal consolidations should suggest superimposed bacterial pneumonia.

Clinical Issues

- *Pneumocystis jirovecii* pneumonia is often associated with AIDS, but it is also common in other immunosuppressive states, including chronic corticosteroid therapy.
- Strongyloidiasis is rarely diagnosed prospectively unless there is a high index of suspicion. The disease is more prevalent among patients on chronic steroids therapy and/or after transplantation.

Key Points

- Clinical and imaging evaluation of infection in immunocompromised patients with diseases other than AIDS is challenging given the varied types of immunosuppression.
- Familiarity with typical complications of common immunosuppression states (congenital immunodeficiencies, chronic corticosteroid treatment, transplant recipients, etc.) and their corresponding imaging manifestations may help suggest the correct diagnosis.
- Chest radiography is typically the first imaging study performed, but it is often normal or shows nonspecific abnormalities. Thin-section CT is indicated when the chest radiograph is normal and allows identification of subtle imaging abnormalities and the formulation of a narrow differential diagnosis, thus

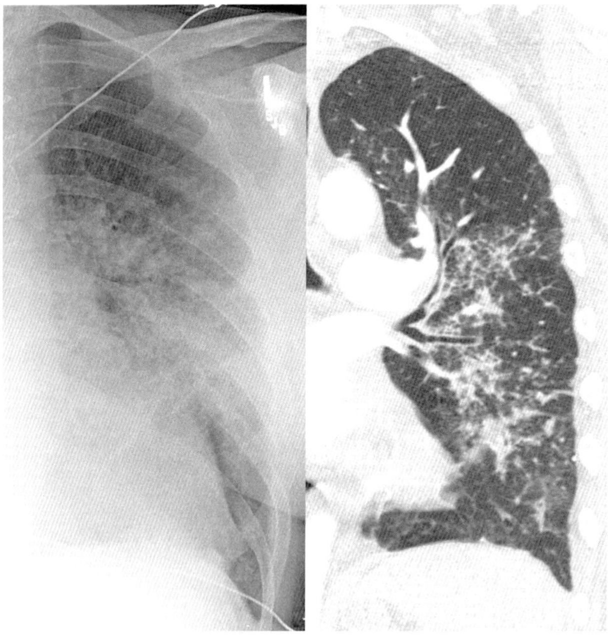

Figure 43.10. Atypical mycobacterial infection. Composite image of a 38-year-old man with a history of heart transplant presenting with dyspnea and cough. (Left) Chest radiograph shows perihilar heterogeneous opacities. (Right) Chest CT demonstrates perihilar reticular and ground-glass opacities.

helping guide management and evaluate response to treatment.

- Close correlation with the timing after BMT allows radiologists to formulate a differential diagnosis and clinicians to determine the most appropriate empiric therapy.
- Although the CT halo sign is not specific, clinicians should always consider angioinvasive fungal infection in patients with neutropenia.
- Consider the primary immunodeficiency in young individuals with diffuse bronchiectasis and recurrent infections.

Suggested Reading

Al-Herz W, Bousfiha A, Casanova JL, Chapel H, Conley ME, Cunningham-Rundles C, et al. Primary immunodeficiency diseases: An update on the classification from the International Union of Immunological Societies Expert Committee for Primary Immunodeficiency. *Front Immunol.* 2011 Nov 8;2:54.

Chong S, Lee KS, Yi CA, Chung MJ, Kim TS, Han J. Pulmonary fungal infection: Imaging findings in immunocompetent and immunocompromised patients. *Eur J Radiol.* 2006;59:371–383.

Coy D, Ormazabal A, Godwin JD, Lalani T. Imaging evaluation of pulmonary and abdominal complications following hematopoietic stem cell transplant. *RadioGraphics.* 2005;25:305–318.

Hampson FA, Chandra A, Screaton NJ, Condliffe A, Kumararatne DS, Exley AR, et al. Respiratory disease in common variable immunodeficiency and other primary immunodeficiency disorders. *Clin Radiol.* 2012 Jun;67(6):587–595.

Klein NC, Go CH, Cunha BA. Infections associated with steroid use. *Infect Dis Clin North Am.* 2001 Jun;15(2):423–432

Wah T, Moss HA, Robertson RJH, Barnard DL. Pulmonary complications following bone marrow transplantation. *Br J Radiol.* 2003;76:373–379.

Section IX

Neoplasms of the Lung and Tracheobronchial Tree

CHAPTER 44

Introduction to Neoplasms of the Lung and Tracheobronchial Tree

Melissa L. Rosado-de-Christenson

Introduction

Cancer is second only to cardiovascular disease as a leading cause of death in the United States and in many Western countries, and it constitutes a major source of morbidity for affected patients. Although the most common cancers in men and women (excluding basal and squamous cell skin cancers) are prostate and breast cancers, respectively, lung cancer is the leading cause of cancer mortality for North American men and women. Although numerous primary neoplasms affect the lung and tracheobronchial tree, lung cancer accounts for the vast majority—approximately 95%. The most common cell type of lung cancer is adenocarcinoma, followed by squamous cell, small cell, and large cell carcinomas in decreasing order of frequency. Other primary lung malignancies are uncommon and include carcinoid tumor and primary pulmonary lymphoma (both Hodgkin and non-Hodgkin), pulmonary blastoma, carcinosarcoma, and, rare primary pulmonary sarcomas. Airway malignancies include squamous cell, adenoid cystic, and mucoepidermoid carcinomas. Benign neoplasms of the lung and airways are rare. They include hamartoma, papilloma, and mesenchymal neoplasms such as lipoma, leiomyoma, and neurogenic neoplasm. Pulmonary metastases are common and probably represent the most common pulmonary malignancies. Frequent extrapulmonary primary sources include primary malignancies of the breast, colon, kidney, gynecologic organs, prostate, and head and neck. Radiologists play an important role in patient management through accurate diagnosis, staging, and imaging follow-up for restaging following treatment, and surveillance for disease recurrence.

Clinical Presentation

Patients with neoplasms of the lung and airways exhibit a wide variety of clinical presentations. Because of the highly aggressive behavior of most lung cancers, affected patients often present with advanced disease (Figs. 44.1 and 44.2). Local effects of the tumor may produce cough, wheezing, dyspnea, or hemoptysis (Fig. 44.3). Symptoms may relate to locally invasive behavior by the tumor and vary depending on whether the mediastinal vessels, the aerodigestive track, or the chest wall is involved. In addition, symptoms may result from the presence of distant metastases or from systemic effects of the neoplasm such as paraneoplastic syndromes. Advanced lung cancer may also produce constitutional symptoms, including malaise and weight loss. A small percentage of patients are asymptomatic and are diagnosed incidentally. Benign lesions of the lung may be entirely asymptomatic or may produce airway-related symptoms due to involvement of the tracheobronchial tree.

Approach to Neoplasms of the Lung and Tracheobronchial Tree

Malignant neoplasms of the lung and airways are common. Therefore, radiologists must have a very high index of suspicion when detecting thoracic abnormalities on radiography because both malignant and benign neoplasms exhibit protean imaging manifestations. Because lung cancer is often advanced at presentation, lymphatic and hematogenous metastases may be the principal radiographic manifestations of malignancy.

Nodules and Masses

Identification of pulmonary nodules on radiography is important because these may be the initial manifestation of primary lung cancer (Fig. 44.1). However, only a small percentage of pulmonary nodules are malignant. Thus, many nodules discovered and evaluated on imaging turn out to be benign lesions, often related to remote fungal infection. Pulmonary masses have a higher likelihood of representing pulmonary malignancy. Thus, lung masses should undergo further assessment with chest CT for the purposes of initial staging.

Atelectasis and Consolidation

Lung malignancies located in the central tracheobronchial tree may be inconspicuous on radiography or may be obscured by secondary effects from the centrally obstructing neoplasm. These lesions may initially manifest with the sequelae of central airway obstruction, including atelectasis

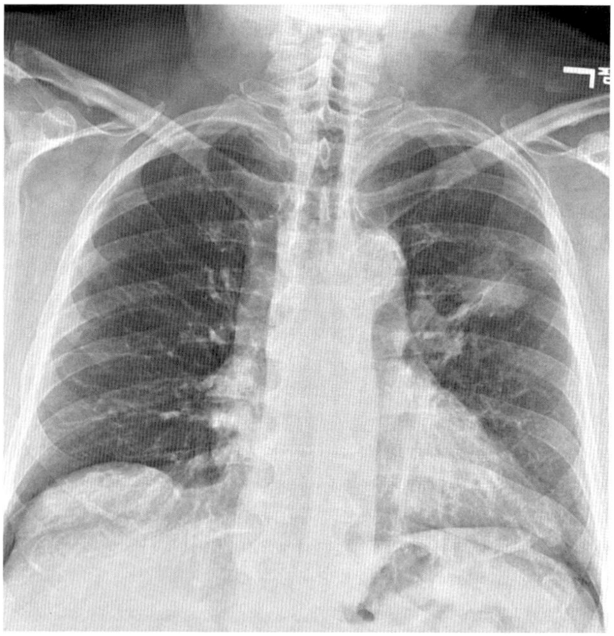

Figure 44.1. Advanced lung cancer. PA chest radiograph of a 62-year-old man with right lower extremity pain shows a left upper lobe lung cancer that manifested as a polylobular lung mass without evidence of intrathoracic lymphadenopathy. The lower extremity pain was secondary to lytic femoral metastases (not shown).

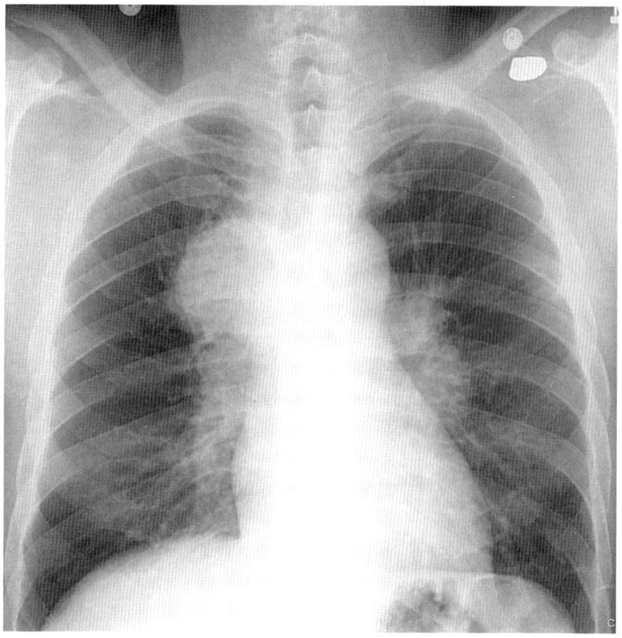

Figure 44.2. Advanced lung cancer. PA chest radiograph of a 54-year-old man with advanced lung cancer shows a dominant right upper lobe lung cancer manifesting as a large paramediastinal mass. Note contralateral left hilar and mediastinal lymphadenopathy consistent with lymph node metastases.

and post-obstructive pneumonia. For this reason, consolidations and atelectasis should always be viewed with suspicion. Follow-up imaging is helpful in documenting complete resolution. In cases in which the abnormalities persist, it is important to further assess the central airways with bronchoscopy or CT (Fig. 44.3).

Lymphadenopathy

Highly aggressive primary lung cancers such as small cell carcinoma are usually metastatic at the time of presentation (Fig. 44.2). In these cases, the principal chest radiographic abnormality may be hilar and/or mediastinal lymphadenopathy. Although such findings usually suggest the possibility of malignant lymphoma or metastatic disease, advanced lung cancer should always be a consideration. Tissue sampling allows determination of cell type and formulation and implementation of an appropriate treatment regimen.

Extrapulmonary Involvement

Lung cancer is often locally invasive and may grow into mediastinal vascular structures, the aerodigestive tract or the pleura, chest wall, or diaphragm. Cross-sectional imaging is important in the assessment of the extent of pulmonary involvement in order to determine potential resectability. Although chest CT is often employed for this purpose, MRI is helpful in cases in which patients cannot tolerate intravenous contrast and in the evaluation of chest wall invasion.

Airway Involvement

Pulmonary neoplasms such as carcinoid tumors, bronchial gland carcinomas, hamartomas, and benign mesenchymal neoplasms may predominantly involve the central airways (Fig. 44.3). Careful analysis of the tracheobronchial tree

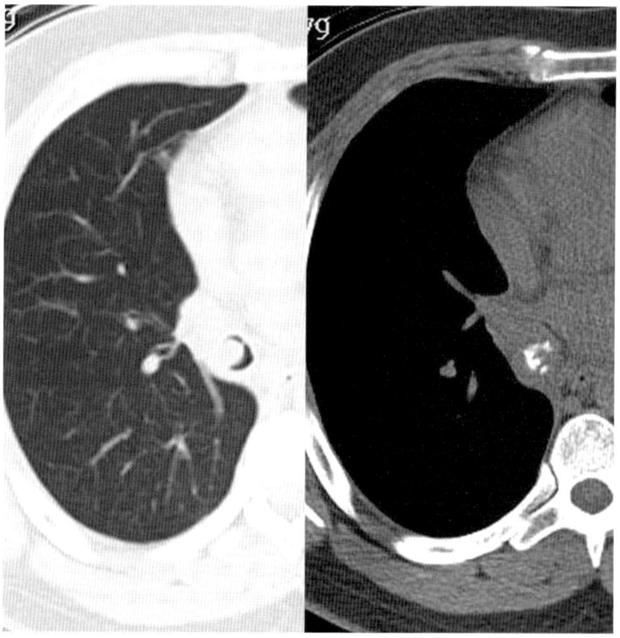

Figure 44.3. Carcinoid. Composite image with unenhanced chest CT in lung (left) and soft tissue (right) window of a 30-year-old man with hemoptysis shows a bronchial carcinoid manifesting as an endoluminal nodule with intrinsic calcification in the bronchus intermedius.

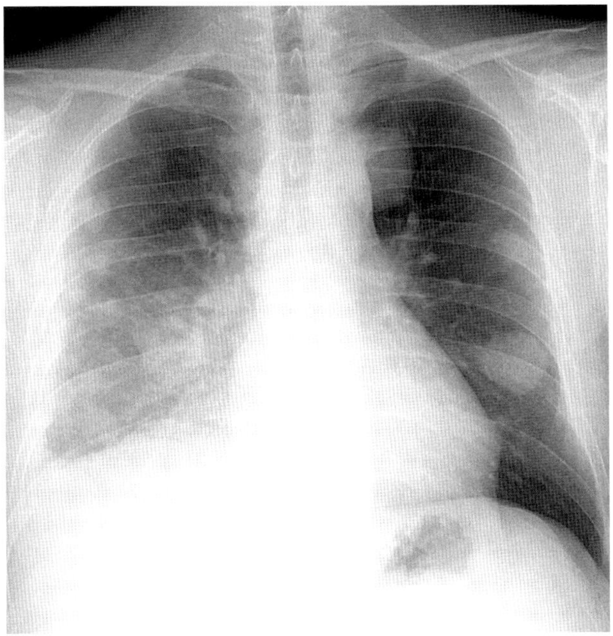

Figure 44.4. Metastases. PA chest radiograph of a 45-year-old man with metastatic renal cell carcinoma shows extensive thoracic metastases including multiple pulmonary metastases, mediastinal lymphadenopathy, and a right malignant pleural effusion with circumferential solid pleural metastases.

allows visualization of an endoluminal component of the neoplasm. These lesions are generally readily accessible to bronchoscopic biopsy. Multiplanar cross-sectional imaging allows determination of length of airway involvement for surgical planning.

Metastatic Disease

Pulmonary metastases are common and typically manifest as multifocal pulmonary nodules or masses in a patient with a known primary malignancy (Fig. 44.4). In the absence of a known primary malignancy, metastases should still be considered, but a differential diagnosis for multifocal lung disease should also be provided. Radiologists should also become familiar with atypical manifestations of pulmonary metastases, including solitary lesion, cavitation, calcification, lymphangitic carcinomatosis, and endovascular tumor growth.

Suggested Reading

Aquino SL. Imaging of metastatic disease to the thorax. *Radiol Clin North Am.* 2005;43:481–495.

Centers for Disease Control and Prevention, National Center for Health Statistics. Leading causes of death. http://www.cdc.gov/nchs/fastats/leading-causes-of-death.htm.

Hoyert DL. 75 years of mortality in the United States, 1935–2010. *NCHS Data Brief*, No. 88, March 2012.

Siegel RL, Miller KD, Jemal A. Cancer statistics, 2015. *CA Cancer J Clin.* 2015;65:5–29.

CHAPTER 45

Lung Cancer

Melissa L. Rosado-de-Christenson

Definition

Lung cancer is the most common primary lung malignancy and the most common fatal malignancy of men and women in the United States. It is estimated that there will be more than 220,000 new cases of lung cancer and more than 150,000 deaths related to lung cancer in the United States in 2018. Lung cancer typically affects patients older than age 60 years, and risk is highest among those in this age group. Approximately 70% of patients with lung cancer present with advanced stage disease. The overall 5-year survival for patients with lung cancer is 17.7%, and it is better for patients with localized early stage disease. Small cell lung cancer has a very poor prognosis, with 5-year survival of only 6%. The National Lung Screening Trial demonstrated a 20% reduction in lung cancer mortality for patients screened with low-dose chest CT compared to those screened with chest radiography. The wide availability of multidetector CT has resulted in increased detection of indolent lung cancers in asymptomatic patients.

Clinical Features

The most important risk factor for lung cancer is cigarette smoking. Other risk factors are radon exposure, secondhand smoke, occupational and environmental exposure to carcinogens such as asbestos, various toxins, and therapeutic radiation. Note that asbestos exposure and cigarette smoking have a synergistic effect that increases risk up to 100 times compared to that of nonsmokers who are not exposed to asbestos. Additional risk factors include chronic obstructive pulmonary disease, pulmonary fibrosis, tuberculosis, and increasing age. Genetic predisposition may also play a role in lung cancer development. All cell types of lung cancer are strongly associated with cigarette smoking, but adenocarcinomas may affect nonsmokers.

Patients with lung cancer are typically older adults with a significant smoking history. A variety of constitutional symptoms may be present, including weight loss, loss of appetite, and respiratory symptoms such as cough, hemoptysis, dyspnea, wheezing, and recurrent pneumonia. Affected patients may present with symptoms related to locally invasive disease, including facial swelling from superior vena cava (SVC) obstruction (SVC syndrome), hoarseness from recurrent laryngeal nerve involvement, chest wall pain and Horner syndrome from invasion of the sympathetic chain and stellate ganglion. In addition, patients may present with bone pain, headache, or seizures related to metastatic disease. Patients with lung cancer may also present with paraneoplastic syndromes, including Cushing syndrome, syndrome of inappropriate antidiuretic hormone secretion, autoimmune neuropathy (e.g., Lambert–Eaton myasthenic syndrome), hypercalcemia, and hypertrophic osteoarthropathy.

Anatomy and Physiology

The principal cell types of lung cancer are adenocarcinoma (40%), squamous cell (25%), small cell (15%), and large cell (10%) carcinomas.

Adenocarcinoma is the most common cell type of lung cancer and typically manifests as a peripheral solitary lung nodule or mass (Figs. 45.1 and 45.2), but it may also manifest as multifocal nodules, masses, and/or consolidations. Although adenocarcinomas may grow slowly, they metastasize early, often to the brain and adrenal gland. Indolent adenocarcinomas typically manifest as subsolid peripheral lung nodules that exhibit slow growth and often increase in CT attenuation over time.

Squamous cell carcinoma (SCC) tends to be a central tumor arising in mainstem, lobar, and segmental bronchi. It may manifest as a hilar mass that may be associated with bronchial obstruction, bronchiectasis, mucoid impaction, or post-obstructive atelectasis. They are rapidly growing, locally invasive tumors that metastasize late. Approximately 30% of SCCs are peripheral and may exhibit necrosis or cavitation.

Small cell lung cancer (SCLC) is an aggressive malignant neuroendocrine carcinoma, is strongly associated with smoking, and affects older smokers. SCLC typically manifests as a large central mass with frequent mediastinal and hilar lymphadenopathy (Fig. 45.3), and most affected patients have metastases at presentation.

Large cell carcinoma is a diagnosis of exclusion. There are multiple subtypes, some of which demonstrate neuroendocrine features. These tend to be large peripheral masses that typically affect older male smokers.

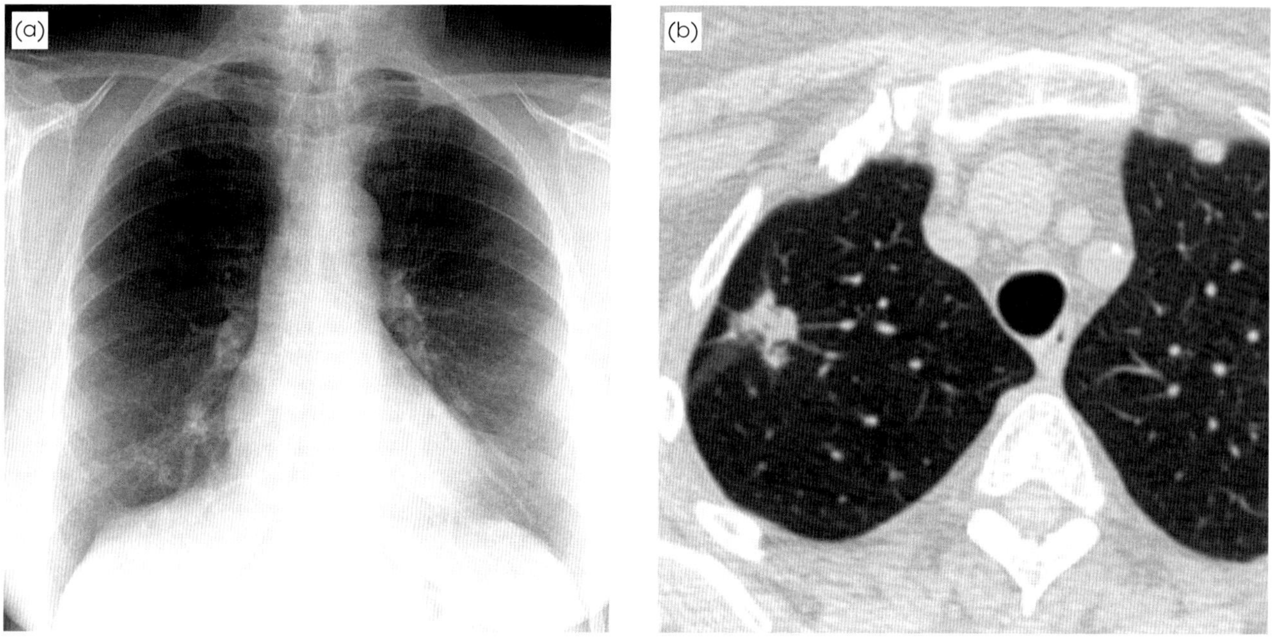

Figure 45.1. Lung cancer: lung nodule. (a) Posteroanterior (PA) chest radiograph of a 72-year-old woman smoker with dyspnea and cough shows a small right upper lobe indeterminate lung nodule. (b) Unenhanced chest CT of the same patient shows a polylobular right upper lobe nodule with spiculated margins and pleural tags. A moderately differentiated adenocarcinoma with visceral pleural involvement was diagnosed at surgery.

How to Approach the Image

All chest radiographs should be carefully scrutinized for lung nodules, masses, or airway abnormalities. Because early lung cancer may be difficult to perceive on radiography, comparison to prior studies is very important for the detection of new subtle abnormalities. The hila must be assessed for lymphadenopathy. The pulmonary lobes and fissures must be evaluated for findings of volume loss. The lines, stripes, and interfaces of the mediastinum must be assessed for contour abnormalities that may relate to lymphadenopathy. Because many patients with lung cancer present with advanced disease, the chest wall soft tissues and skeletal structures must be assessed to exclude local invasion or metastatic disease.

What Not to Miss

- Lung nodules: Early lung cancer can be subtle; careful image analysis includes comparison to prior studies to detect subtle changes and identify small nodules.
- Consolidation or atelectasis may obscure an underlying neoplasm; post-treatment follow-up chest radiography should be performed to document resolution and detect persistent abnormalities. The latter should be further evaluated with chest CT or bronchoscopy to exclude underlying malignancy.
- Lymphadenopathy in association with a lung nodule or mass should raise suspicion for malignancy and may indicate advanced disease.
- Extrapulmonary involvement may occur via direct invasion of adjacent thoracic structures or via lymphatic or hematogenous metastases.

Differential Diagnosis

Other Pulmonary Neoplasm

- Carcinoid tumor, hamartoma, and solitary metastasis can manifest as pulmonary nodules or masses indistinguishable from lung cancer.
- Hamartoma and lymphoma may manifest as pulmonary masses.
- Lymphoma may manifest as solitary or multiple pulmonary nodules and/or consolidations.

Pulmonary Infection

- Granulomas are often calcified, but they may also manifest as indeterminate lung nodules.
- Round pneumonia and lung abscess may manifest as pulmonary masses with or without cavitation.
- Fungal pneumonias may manifest with nodules, masses, or consolidations and may exhibit associated lymphadenopathy.

Atelectasis

- Atelectasis should always be evaluated to exclude a centrally obstructing lesion that is not always neoplastic and may include mucus plug, granulomatous disease, and extrinsic compression from reactive lymphadenopathy.
- Rounded atelectasis may manifest as a mass that may mimic lung cancer; it results from in-folding of subpleural lung adjacent to pleural thickening from prior asbestos exposure or following surgery (particularly sternotomy and cardiothoracic surgery).

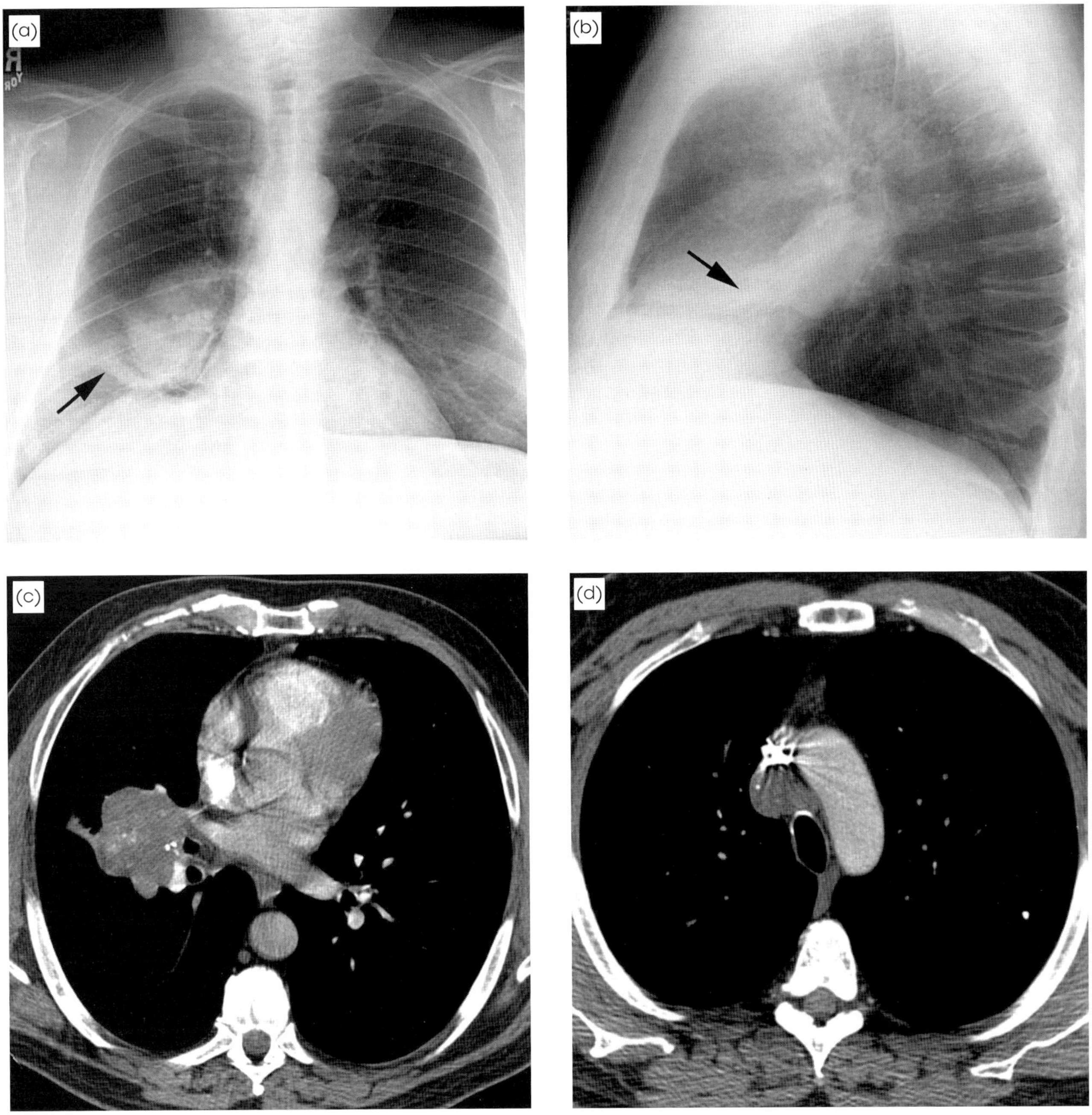

Figure 45.2. Lung cancer: lung mass. (a, b) PA and lateral chest radiographs of a 58-year-old man with a 90 pack-year history of smoking and recent hemoptysis show a large polylobular right hilar mass with associated middle lobe subsegmental atelectasis (arrows). Right paratracheal fullness is suspicious for lymphadenopathy. (c, d) Contrast-enhanced chest CT of the same patient shows a large heterogeneous right hilar mass with intrinsic punctate calcifications. The lesion completely obstructs the middle lobe bronchus and encases or invades the right lower lobe pulmonary arteries. Note right paratracheal lymphadenopathy (d) that is highly suspicious for metastatic disease.

- Inflammatory process
  - Organizing and lipoid pneumonias and sarcoidosis may manifest with solitary or multiple mass-like consolidations.
  - Vasculitis may manifest with solitary or multiple pulmonary nodules, masses, or consolidations that may exhibit cavitation.

Imaging Findings

Lung cancer has a wide variety of imaging manifestations:

- Pulmonary nodule (Fig. 45.1) with variable border characteristics and attenuation patterns; may exhibit calcification.
- Pulmonary mass (Fig. 45.2) with variable border characteristics; may exhibit cavitation.

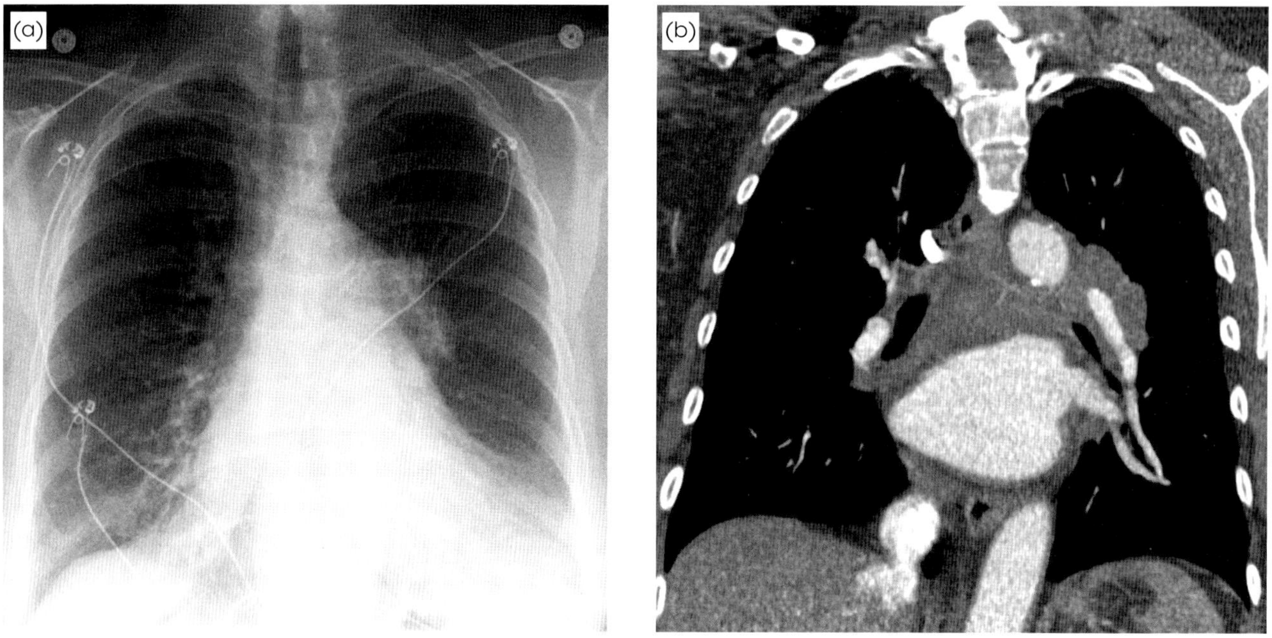

Figure 45.3. Lung cancer: lymphadenopathy. (a) PA chest radiograph of a 63-year-old woman with a 150 pack-year smoking history and chest pain shows a left hilar mass with associated aortopulmonary window lymphadenopathy. (b) Coronal contrast-enhanced chest CT of the same patient confirms extensive left hilar and mediastinal coalescent lymphadenopathy encasing the left pulmonary artery and proximal descending aorta. Biopsy demonstrated small cell lung cancer.

- Pulmonary consolidation (Fig. 45.4) may be a manifestation of lung cancer either as a result of a centrally obstructing lesion or from lepidic (respecting the underlying interstitium) growth of the neoplasm.
- Atelectasis may result from centrally obstructing neoplasms; large central neoplasms with resultant atelectasis may exhibit the S sign of Golden, in which a convex contour produced by the mass accompanies the lobar collapse.

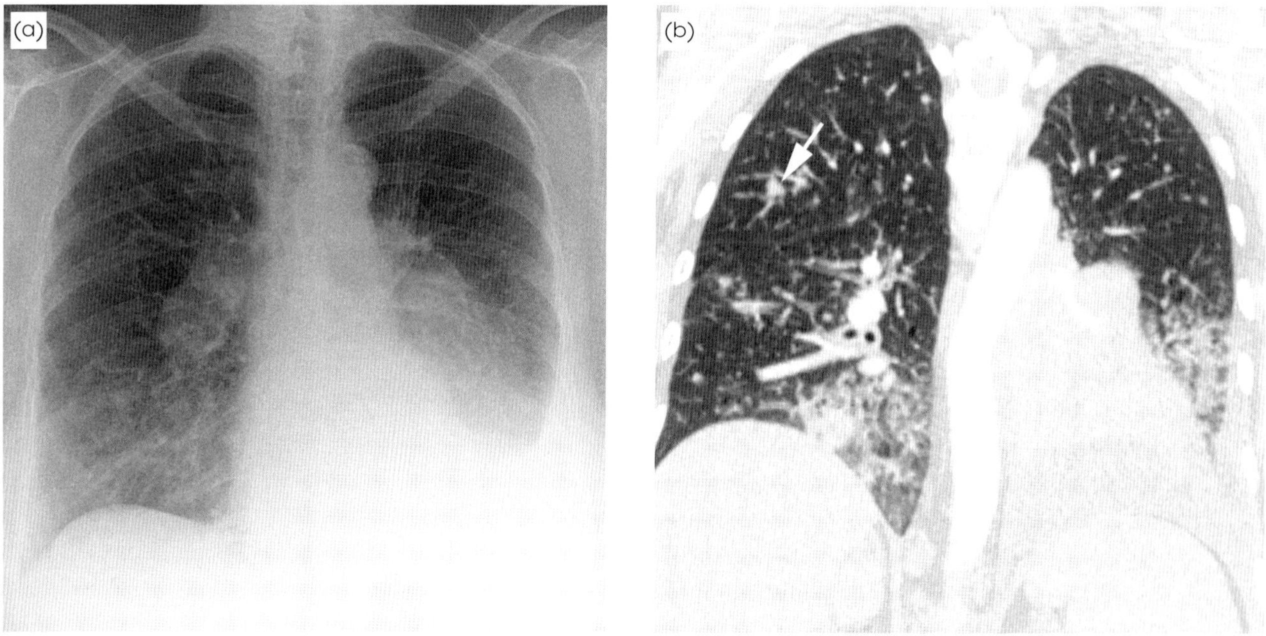

Figure 45.4. Lung cancer: lymphadenopathy, consolidation, and metastases. (a) PA chest radiograph of a 70-year-old woman with advanced lung cancer shows left lower lobe mass-like consolidation, moderate left pleural effusion, bilateral hilar lymphadenopathy, and multifocal small pulmonary nodules. (b) Coronal contrast-enhanced chest CT of the same patient confirms a left hilar mass, left lower lobe consolidation, and multifocal pulmonary nodules (arrow) representing hematogenous metastases. Biopsy confirmed adenocarcinoma.

- Lymphadenopathy (Fig. 45.3) may be the only manifestation of aggressive undifferentiated lung cancers such as SCLC and may involve the hilum/hila and/or mediastinum.
- Multifocal lung nodules (Fig. 45.4), masses, and consolidations may occur in the setting of multifocal or metastatic lung cancer.
- Extrapulmonary involvement may occur adjacent to a lung mass such as in Pancoast tumors, in which the tumor may invade the adjacent chest wall. Direct mediastinal involvement by the lesion may also occur. Hematogenous distant metastases may affect the chest wall skeleton and soft tissues.

All pulmonary masses should be regarded as suspicious for primary lung cancer, particularly those with spiculated or lobular borders, cavitation, heterogeneous attenuation, associated intrathoracic lymphadenopathy, and/or local invasion.

Clinical Issues

- Lung cancer is a common malignancy of older adults, particularly long-term smokers.
- Affected patients may have a variety of presenting symptoms or may be entirely asymptomatic.
- Solid lung cancers have mean doubling times ranging from 30 to 400 days (mean, 150 days).
- Rapidly growing lesions (doubling time < 30 days) are more likely related to infection, inflammation, or hemorrhage.
- Asymptomatic patients at high risk for lung cancer should be considered for low-dose chest CT screening, provided a multidisciplinary team is available to manage positive screening studies.

Key Points

- Chest radiographs should always be compared to prior studies (when available) to detect new subtle abnormalities.
- Indeterminate nodules found on radiography (particularly if new) should be further evaluated with chest CT.
- Unexplained atelectasis, persistent consolidation, and recurrent respiratory complaints in a high-risk patient should warrant further evaluation with chest CT and/or bronchoscopy to exclude underlying lung cancer.
- Suspicious lesions should undergo tissue sampling to exclude malignancy.

Suggested Reading

Aberle DR, Adams AM, Berg CD, et al. Reduced lung-cancer mortality with low-dose computed tomographic screening. *N Engl J Med.* 2011;365:395–409.

Siegel RL, Miller KD, Jemal A. Cancer statistics 2018. *CA Cancer J Clin.* 2018;68:7–30.

Travis WD, Brambilla E, Riely GJ. New pathologic classification of lung cancer: Relevance for clinical practice and clinical trials. *J Clin Oncol.* 2013;31:992–1001.

CHAPTER 46

Lung Cancer: Nodules and Masses

Ryo E. C. Benson

Definition

Lung cancer may manifest as a pulmonary nodule or mass. A lung nodule is a roughly spherical pulmonary density measuring 3 cm or less. A small nodule measures less than 1 cm. A mass is a roughly spherical pulmonary lesion that measures greater than 3 cm. Solid pulmonary lesions exhibit soft tissue attenuation and completely obscure or replace the underlying pulmonary architecture. Subsolid lesions may exhibit homogeneous ground-glass attenuation (nonsolid lesions) or a mixture of soft tissue and ground-glass opacity. Ground-glass opacity lesions allow visualization of the underlying pulmonary architecture.

Clinical Features

The likelihood that a lung nodule represents a lung cancer relates to patient demographics and increases in patients older than 40 years (particularly those older than 60 years), patients with a history of smoking, and patients who have a first-degree relative with a history of cancer or lung cancer. Patients with pulmonary fibrosis, chronic obstructive pulmonary disease, asbestos exposure, and/or thoracic therapeutic irradiation are more likely to develop lung cancer.

A pulmonary mass is very likely to be malignant and will typically represent a primary lung cancer, regardless of the presence or absence of risk factors for lung cancer.

Anatomy and Physiology

Lung cancer often affects the upper lobes and is more frequent in the right lung. Lung cancers that manifest as a pulmonary nodule or mass may be peripheral or central; may transgress interlobar fissures; and may invade adjacent structures, including the pleura, the mediastinum and its structures, and the chest wall.

How to Approach the Image

Detection and assessment of indeterminate lung nodules (Fig. 46.1) is critical for the early diagnosis of lung cancer. The smallest detectable nodule on chest radiography measures approximately 4 mm. The detection rate of a 1-cm

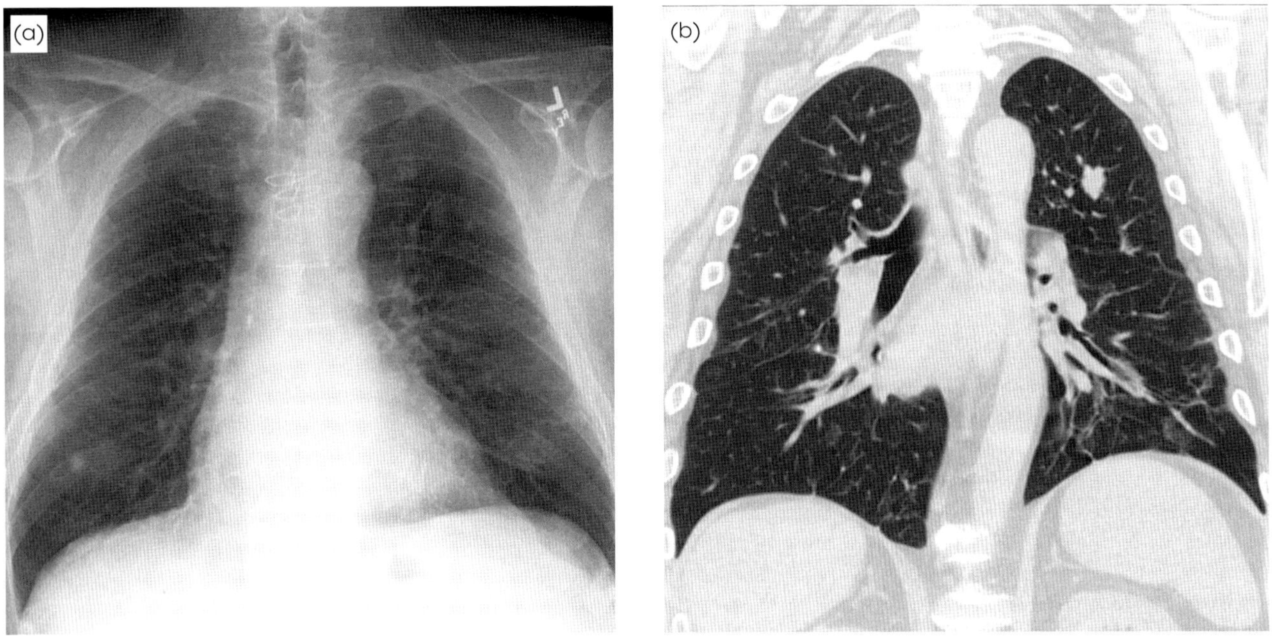

Figure 46.1. Solid lung nodule: adenocarcinoma. (a) Posteroanterior chest radiograph of an asymptomatic patient shows a right basilar granuloma and a subtle solitary left upper lung zone indeterminate lung nodule with ill-defined borders. (b) Coronal unenhanced chest CT of the same patient shows a polylobular slightly spiculated left upper lobe nodule surgically proven to represent an adenocarcinoma.

nodule ranges from 40% to 87%. Once a nodule is detected on radiography, pseudonodules (nonpulmonary lesions that may mimic a lung nodule) such as nipple shadows, skin lesions, bone islands, pleural plaques, and rib fracture callus must be excluded. The average size of a missed lung cancer is 1.6 cm, indicating that larger lesions are also missed. Note that the vast majority of noncalcified lung nodules are benign, with proven lung cancer ranging from 0.3% to 2.7% of all surgically resected lesions (the percentage would be even lower in unresected image-detected nodules).

Comparison to prior chest radiographs for documentation of stability or assessment of interval change is critical for determining the probability of malignancy. Further characterization of lung nodules detected on radiography is accomplished with chest CT. Although not routinely utilized currently, computer-aided detection (CAD) may become an important adjunct tool for nodule detection, characterization, and growth assessment in the future. Careful assessment of such nodules often allows the radiologist to decide whether the lesion is benign, possibly malignant, or indeterminate. Possibly malignant lung nodules require further assessment with PET/CT to assess metabolic activity and/or tissue sampling. Indeterminate lung nodules require imaging follow-up to assess growth and determine malignant potential.

Recorded measurement of solid nodules is the average of the nodule length and width. CT imaging of subsolid nodules is optimally performed with contiguous 1–1.5 mm thin sections. Measurement of both solid and ground-glass components is required. Comparison to remote CT studies is helpful in determining slow nodule growth.

What Not to Miss

- Comparison to old studies is critical in the detection of subtle new pulmonary nodules. In addition, stable nodules are often benign or indolent lesions.
- Thin-section CT imaging is important in the detection and characterization of intrinsic calcification and/or fat in lung nodules, which may allow the prospective diagnosis of benignity.
- Nodules (Fig. 46.2) or masses with spiculated or lobular contours are suspicious for malignancy.
- Thin-section CT imaging is critical in the assessment of subsolid nodules for determination of extent of solid component and detection of cystic changes and intrinsic air bronchograms (Figs. 46.3 and 46.4).
- Perifissural and juxtapleural nodules with a flat morphology on multiplanar imaging often represent intrapulmonary lymphoid tissue, and may exhibit changes in size and morphology on follow-up imaging.

Differential Diagnosis

Solitary Pulmonary Nodule

Primary Lung Cancer

- 20–30% of patients with lung cancer have a solitary pulmonary nodule (SPN) on radiography at presentation.

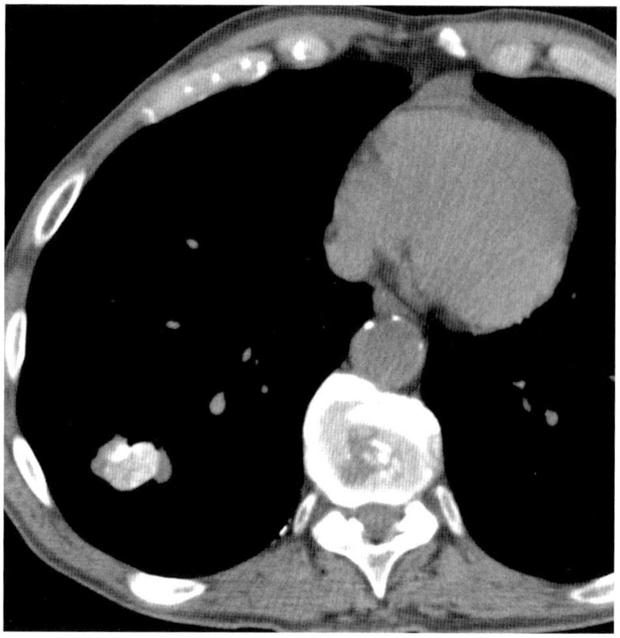

Figure 46.2. Solid lung nodule: squamous cell carcinoma. Unenhanced chest CT of an asymptomatic patient shows a polylobular right lower lobe pulmonary nodule with cloud-like calcification. Biopsy demonstrated squamous cell carcinoma.

- Polylobular and spiculated lung nodules are highly suspicious for primary lung cancer.

Granuloma

- Most common SPN.
- Generally exhibits central, laminar, or diffuse calcification.

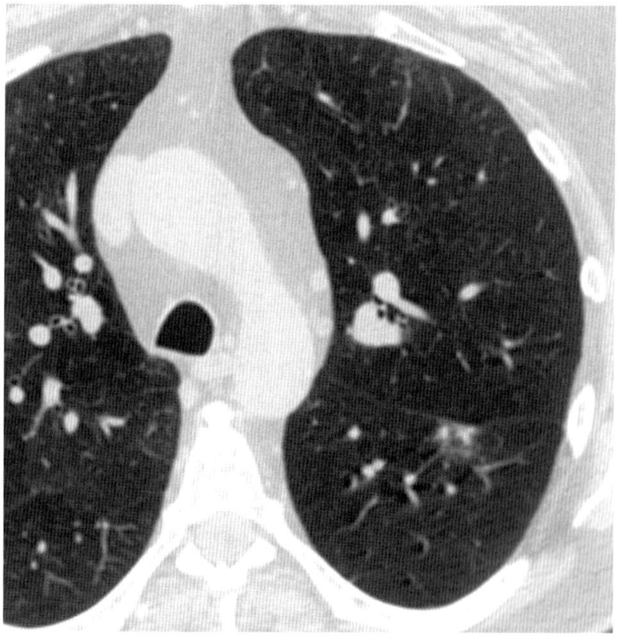

Figure 46.3. Part-solid lung nodule. Unenhanced chest CT of an asymptomatic patient shows a left lower lobe superior segment part-solid nodule with predominant ground-glass attenuation and two solid components, the larger measuring more than 5 mm, concerning for indolent lung cancer. Stability or growth at 3–6 month follow-up CT may require surgical resection/biopsy.

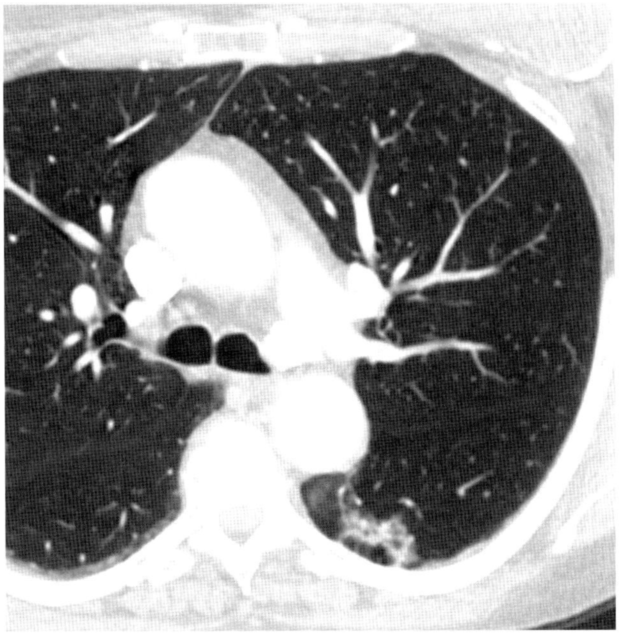

Figure 46.4. Part-solid lung nodule. Unenhanced chest CT of an asymptomatic 63-year-old former smoker shows a 2.4-cm left lower lobe part-solid nodule with pleural tags and predominant solid components. Lepidic predominant well-differentiated adenocarcinoma was diagnosed at surgery.

- May exhibit satellite micronodules.
- Granulomas exhibit increased FDG uptake on FDG PET/CT and may be indistinguishable from lung cancer in the absence of calcification (Fig. 46.5).

Intrapulmonary Lymph Node

- One-third of noncalcified solid small nodules seen on screening CT.

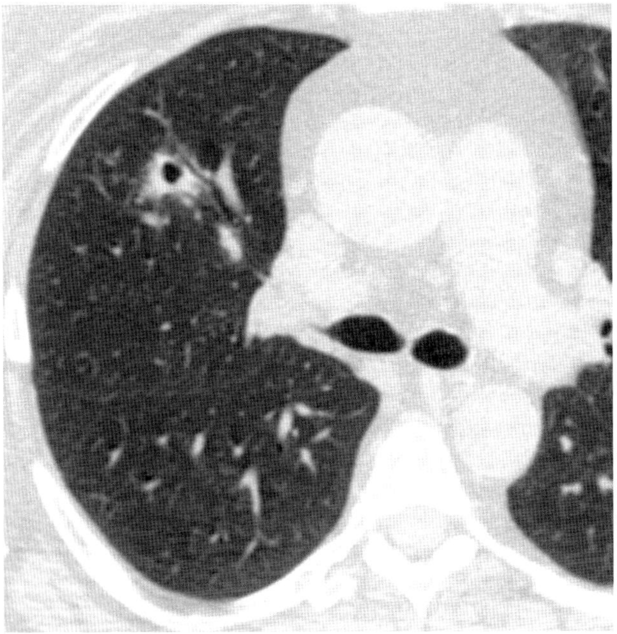

Figure 46.5. Cavitary lung nodule. Unenhanced chest CT of an asymptomatic smoker shows a right upper lobe spiculated nodule with intrinsic cavitation that did not resolve on follow-up imaging. Surgical excision revealed a cavitary granuloma.

- Most are less than 1 cm, juxtapleural, perifissural or septal, and located caudal to the carina; often exhibit ovoid, lentiform, or triangular morphology.

Hamartoma

- Rare benign primary lung neoplasm.
- Identification of intrinsic macroscopic fat and/or typical "popcorn" calcification may be diagnostic.

Solitary Metastasis

- Rare; primary lung cancer should always be considered, even in patients with documented extrapulmonary primary malignancy.

Carcinoid

- Younger age group. May exhibit a bronchial relationship, calcification, and contrast enhancement

Pulmonary Mass

Primary Lung Cancer

- High likelihood of malignancy with increasing size
- May exhibit spiculated or lobular borders, cavitation, and amorphous, often eccentric calcification

Other Pulmonary Neoplasms

- Hamartoma, carcinoid, lymphoma, sarcoma, and metastasis

Infectious Process

- Lung abscess, round pneumonia
- Signs and symptoms of infection; response to antimicrobial treatment
- May exhibit cavitation (with or without air–fluid levels), necrosis

Inflammatory Process

- Lipoid pneumonia, organizing pneumonia
- Consolidation, may be mass-like and exhibit spiculated borders

Other

- Rounded atelectasis; may manifest as subpleural pulmonary mass, associated with adjacent pleural thickening and the comet tail sign (curvilinear morphology of bronchovascular structures coursing toward the lesion)

Imaging Findings

Most SPNs are benign. Most solitary lung masses are malignant. Imaging assessment relies on evaluation of the following:

Size

- More than 90% of nodules less than 2 cm are benign.
- Most SPNs less than 9 mm detected on chest radiography are calcified granulomas (Fig. 46.1).

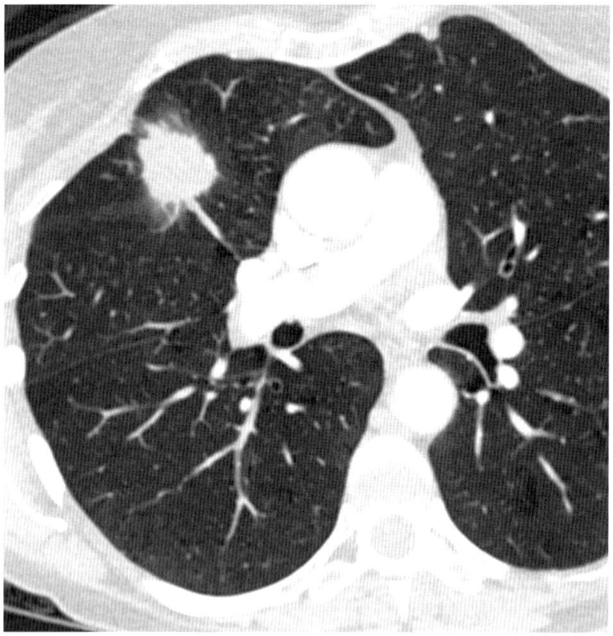

Figure 46.6. Lung mass. Contrast-enhanced chest CT of an asymptomatic patient shows a right upper lobe spiculated mass with surrounding ground-glass opacity and retraction of the adjacent visceral pleura. The findings are highly suspicious for primary lung cancer, and further assessment with tissue sampling is indicated.

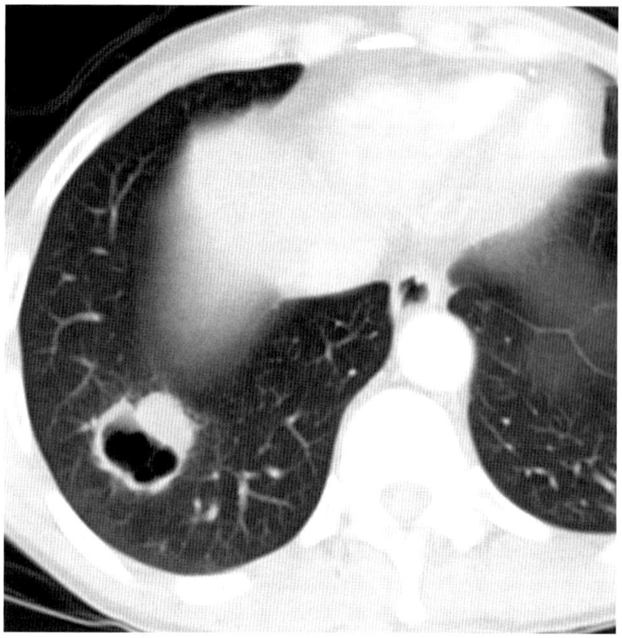

Figure 46.7. Cavitary lung mass. Contrast-enhanced chest CT of a patient with a past history of treated head and neck cancer shows a right lower lobe mass with irregular borders, intrinsic cavitation, and a nodular cavity wall measuring up to 1.5 cm anteriorly. Primary squamous cell carcinoma was diagnosed by image-guided biopsy.

- Lesions measuring 3 cm or more are highly suspicious for malignancy (Fig. 46.6).

Morphology
- Well-circumscribed spherical lesions are more likely to be benign.
- Lesions with irregular, spiculated, and/or lobular borders or with pleural tags are suspicious for malignancy.

CT Attenuation
- Heterogeneity or subsolid attenuation is suspicious for malignancy; half of part-solid nodules smaller than 1.5 cm and one-third of nonsolid or ground-glass nodules larger than 1.5 cm are malignant.
- Ground-glass opacity components of malignant subsolid nodules correlate with lepidic tumor growth, and solid components correlate with invasive behavior.
- Cavitary nodules or masses with thick nodular walls greater than 16 mm in thickness are suspicious for malignancy (Fig. 46.7).

Metabolic Activity
- Increased metabolic activity on FDG PET/CT suggests malignancy (Fig. 46.8); infectious/inflammatory processes may produce false-positive findings; indolent and small malignancies may produce false-negative findings.

CT Enhancement
- Nodule enhancement of greater than 20 Hounsfield units (HU) suggests malignancy.
- Nodule enhancement of less than 15 HU usually denotes benignity.

Growth
- Lung cancers typically exhibit tumor doubling times ranging from 100 to 400 days.
- Indolent lung cancers may manifest as subsolid lesions that exhibit doubling times of more than 400 days. Average doubling times may be on the order of 3–5 years.

Associated Findings
- Other pulmonary nodules or masses in the same lobe, other ipsilateral lobes, or contralateral lung
- Local invasion of pleura, mediastinum, and chest wall
- Lymphadenopathy
- Pleural effusion with or without associated solid pleural nodules or masses
- Lytic or sclerotic skeletal lesions indicating metastases
- Upper abdominal lesions involving abdominal lymph nodes, liver, and/or adrenal glands representing metastatic disease

Clinical Issues
- Tissue diagnosis should be strongly considered in all pulmonary masses.
- Imaging follow-up of solid nodules requires stratification of affected patients into low-risk and high-risk categories. High-risk patients are those with a history of smoking, exposure to carcinogens, or

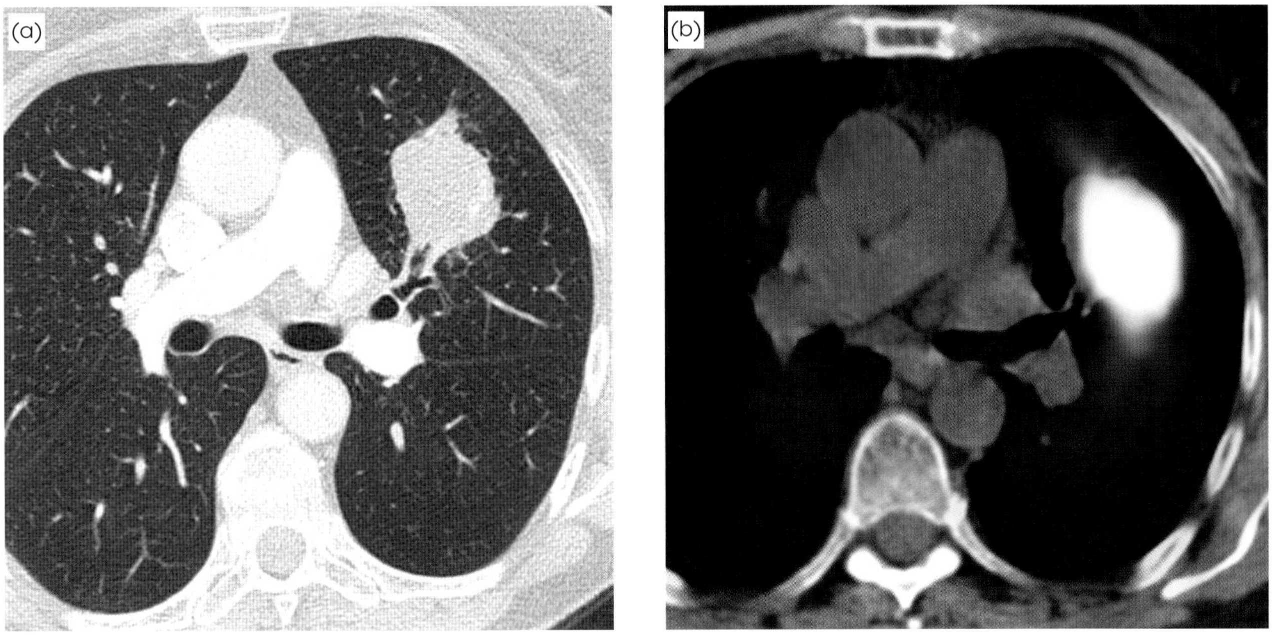

Figure 46.8. Lung mass. (a) Contrast-enhanced chest CT of a 54-year-old woman smoker with cough and dyspnea shows a left upper lobe mass with irregular borders that obliterates the left upper lobe anterior segmental bronchus. (b) Fused FDG PET/CT of the same patient shows marked increased FDG uptake in the mass (maximum standardized uptake value = 12), indicating intense metabolic activity and no metastatic disease. Image-guided biopsy revealed squamous cell carcinoma.

Table 46.1 - Fleischner Society Guidelines for Management of Incidentally Detected Solid Pulmonary Nodules in Adults

SOLID NODULES	< 6 mm (< 100 mm³)	6–8 mm (100–250 mm³)	> 8 mm (> 250 mm³)
Single			
Low-risk patient	No routine follow-up	CT at 6–12 months, then consider CT at 18–24 months	Consider CT at 3 months, PET/CT, or tissue sampling
High-risk patient	Optional CT at 12 months	CT at 6–12 months, then CT at 18–24 months	Consider CT at 3 months, PET/CT or tissue sampling
Multiple			
Low-risk patient	No routine follow-up	CT at 3–6 months, then CT at 18–24 months	CT at 3–6 months, then consider CT at 18–24 months
High-risk patient	Optional CT at 12 months	CT at 3–6 months, then consider CT at 18–24 months	CT at 3–6 months, then consider CT at 18–24 months

Notes:
1. In general, nodules < 6 mm usually require no follow up unless there are growth, upper lobe location, or suspicious features

history of lung cancer in a first-degree relative. The Fleischner guidelines for management of solid nodules apply to patients who are age 35 years or older (Table 46.1).

- Imaging follow-up of subsolid nodules does not rely on risk factors for malignancy (Table 46.2). The solid component of a primary lung adenocarcinoma usually correlates with invasive behavior on histology.
- Indeterminate nodules greater than 1 cm should be evaluated with PET/CT, tissue sampling, or close follow-up after therapy.

Key Points

- Lung cancers often manifest as pulmonary nodules or masses. Lobulation and spiculation are features of malignancy.
- Lung cancers may exhibit intrinsic calcifications that are often eccentric, cloud-like, or amorphous.
- Cavitation in a nodule or mass, particularly when eccentric, irregular, or nodular, should suggest malignancy.
- Imaging follow-up of well-defined solid nodules with benign morphology may be discontinued at 12–18

Table 46.2 - Fleischner Society Guidelines for Management of Incidentally Detected Subsolid Pulmonary Nodules in Adults

SUBSOLID NODULES	< 6 mm (< 100 mm³)	≥ 6 mm (> 100 mm³)
Single		
Ground-glass	No routine follow-up	CT at 6–12 months to confirm persistence, then CT every 2 years until 5 years
Part-solid	No routine follow-up	CT at 3–6 m. If unchanged and solid component remains <6mm, annual CT should be performed for 5 years
Multiple	CT at 3–6 months; if stable, consider CT at 2 and 4 years	CT at 3–6 months. Subsequent management based on the most suspicious nodule(s).

Notes:
1. Part-solid nodule cannot be defined as such unless it is > 6 mm
2. In general nodules < 6 mm require no follow-up unless suspicious or if growing or with developing solid components

months provided that the nodule is accurately measured and definitely stable.

- Indolent lung cancers manifesting as subsolid nodules may exhibit stability over years and may be followed with CT for up to 5 years.
- Subsolid nodules and nodules with air bronchograms or cystic changes likely represent indolent malignancies and may not demonstrate FDG uptake on PET/CT. Because persistent subsolid nodules have a high incidence of malignancy, surgical biopsy is often preferred over image-guided needle biopsy.
- Detection of nodule growth requires careful comparison with the earliest available imaging study in order to identify subtle changes in size.

Suggested Reading

De Hoop B, Van Ginneken B, Gietema H, Prokop M. Pulmonary perifissural nodules on CT scans: Rapid growth is not a predictor of malignancy. *Radiology*. 2012;265:611–616.

MacMahon H, Naidich DP, Goo JM, et al. Guidelines for management of incidental pulmonary nodules detected on CT images: From the Fleischner Society 2017. *Radiology*. 2017; 237: 395–400.

Winer-Muram HT. The solitary pulmonary nodule. *Radiology*. 2006;239:34–49.

CHAPTER 47

Lung Cancer: Atelectasis and Consolidation

Ryo E. C. Benson

Definition

Atelectasis (or collapse) is defined as reduced lung inflation and volume that may be complete or partial with resultant reduction or absence of alveolar gas and impairment of gas exchange. It may result from resorption of alveolar gas distal to central airway obstruction resulting in increased opacity or attenuation of the affected lung.

Consolidation refers to replacement of alveolar gas typically by exudative fluid (in cases of pneumonia) or other material and results in increased lung density or attenuation and obscuration of underlying normal anatomic landmarks.

Airspace disease in the form of atelectasis and consolidation may obscure an associated central neoplasm. Neoplastic cells may also replace the gas in the alveolar airspaces manifesting as airspace opacity or consolidation.

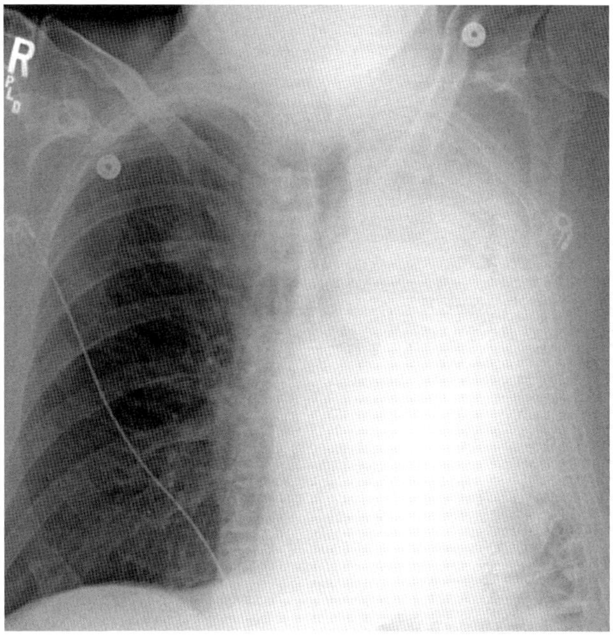

Figure 47.1. Left lung atelectasis. Anteroposterior (AP) chest radiograph of an elderly man with severe dyspnea shows an opaque left hemithorax from left lung atelectasis. Note left mediastinal and tracheal shift, left hemidiaphragm elevation, and abrupt cutoff of the left mainstem bronchus consistent with centrally obstructing lung cancer diagnosed on bronchoscopy.

Clinical Features

Patients with centrally obstructing lung cancers may present with symptoms including chest pain, cough, and hemoptysis. Partially obstructing neoplasms may produce recurrent pulmonary infection or wheezing. Completely obstructing neoplasms may result in complete or partial atelectasis of a lobe or lung, depending on collateral circulation (Figs. 47.1 and 47.2). Consolidated lung distal to a centrally obstructing lung cancer is often not infected but, rather, involved by endogenous lipoid pneumonia—so-called "golden" or "cholesterol" pneumonia.

Recurrent or persistent pulmonary opacities should raise concern for underlying tumor. Unexplained atelectasis or volume loss should raise concern for centrally obstructing lesion (Fig. 47.3). The most common histologic types of lung cancer to produce these findings are squamous cell and small cell carcinomas (Fig. 47.4). These histologic cell types are intimately related to cigarette smoking. Adults who present with pneumonia or atelectasis must be followed to complete resolution. Pneumonia that persists after 6 weeks or recurs in the same lobe must be further evaluated with chest CT or bronchoscopy (Fig. 47.5).

Anatomy and Physiology

Any neoplasm or tumor obstructing a bronchus, whether by endoluminal growth, extrinsic compression, or airway invasion, may produce post-obstructive atelectasis or consolidation. Thus, recurrent or persistent pneumonia and unexplained atelectasis (particularly when lobar or larger) should always raise concern for underlying lung cancer.

Squamous cell lung carcinoma is characterized by endoluminal tumor growth in a central airway. Small cell carcinomas are central locally invasive neoplasms that rarely exhibit endoluminal growth but may produce bronchial obstruction often associated with hilar and mediastinal lymphadenopathy.

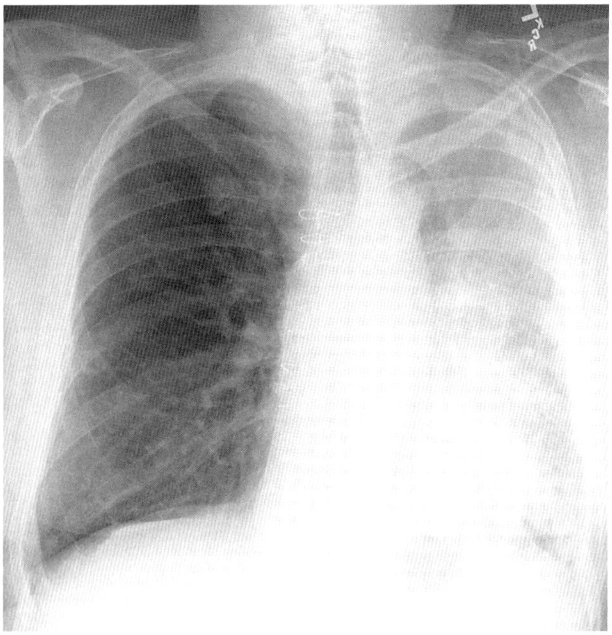

Figure 47.2. Luftsichel sign. Posteroanterior (PA) chest radiograph of an elderly smoker with cough and weight loss shows complete left upper lobe atelectasis manifesting with the luftsichel sign, an arcuate lucency surrounding the aortic arch and produced by adjacent compensatory hyperinflation of the left lower lobe. A centrally obstructing squamous cell carcinoma was confirmed on endoscopic biopsy.

How to Approach the Image

Atelectasis and consolidation are often initially diagnosed on radiography and manifest with increased pulmonary opacity that may be subtle (Fig. 47.3). Visualization of an endoluminal or centrally located mass associated with atelectasis or pneumonia allows the radiologist to suggest malignancy as the most likely etiology and recommend further imaging with chest CT or direct visualization of the airway obstruction with bronchoscopy.

Although atelectasis may be caused by benign conditions such as mucus plugging and granulomatous disease, malignancy must always be considered. Atelectasis may be subtle on radiography, and direct and indirect signs of volume loss must be recognized. The absence of air bronchograms within an opaque atelectatic lung indicates a centrally obstructing lesion as the etiology of atelectasis (Fig. 47.1). Atelectasis of a lobe or combined lobes supplied by a single bronchus should raise concern of an endobronchial tumor.

A central convexity associated with the atelectasis is a feature of malignancy that indicates the presence of an underlying mass and is the basis for the S sign of Golden. The luftsichel sign of left upper lobe atelectasis is a crescentic air lucency about the aortic arch produced by compensatory hyperinflation of the left lower lobe superior segment interposed between the aorta and the atelectatic left upper lobe (Fig. 47.2). Unexplained or persistent atelectasis should prompt further evaluation with follow-up chest radiographs, bronchoscopy, or a chest CT.

Most consolidations in symptomatic patients represent pneumonia. However, post-obstructive consolidation may occur in the absence of volume loss and occasionally exhibits bulging fissures in cases of "drowned lung" due to central obstruction. In addition, lepidic and invasive mucinous adenocarcinomas may manifest with consolidation (Fig. 47.6).

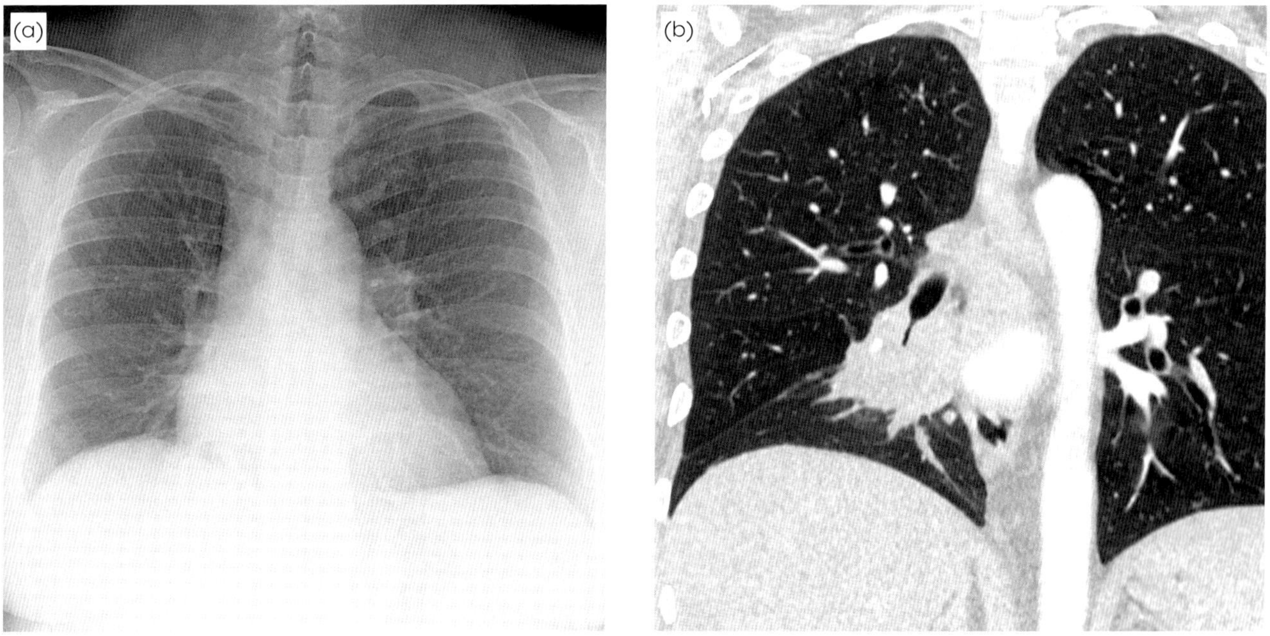

Figure 47.3. Volume loss from central mass. (a) PA chest radiograph of a 52-year-old woman with persistent cough and dyspnea shows subtle right lung volume loss and a right retrocardiac opacity. (b) Coronal contrast-enhanced chest CT of the same patient shows a central lung cancer encasing and obstructing the right lower lobe bronchus with resultant right lower lobe volume loss.

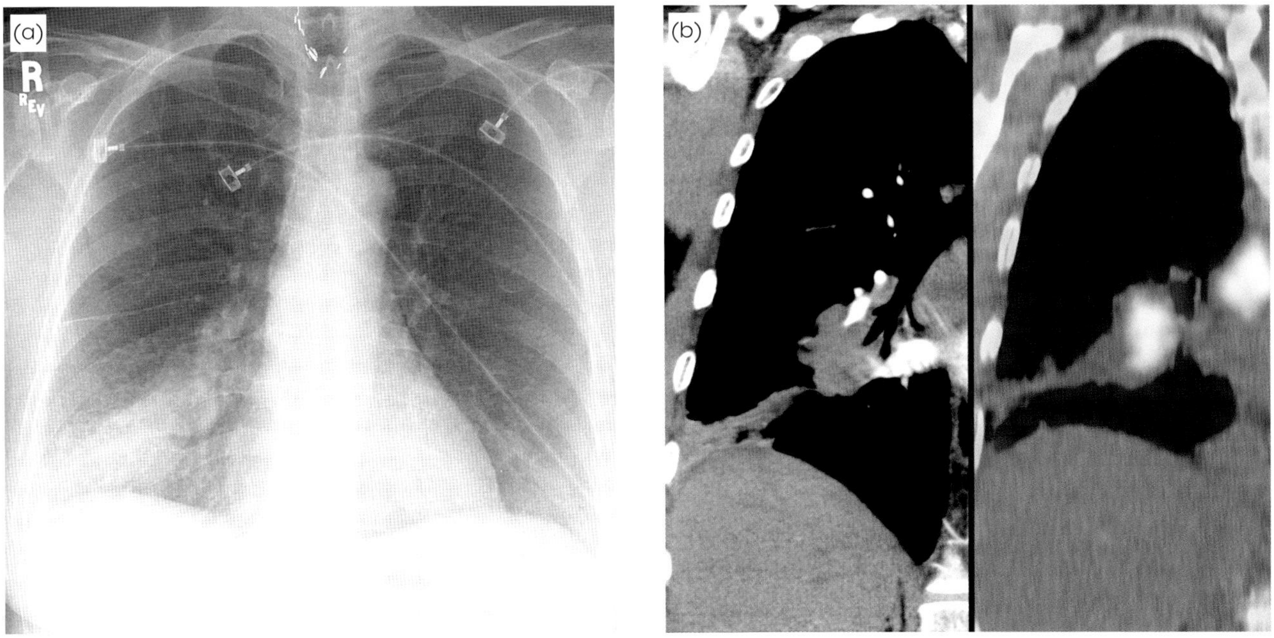

Figure 47.4. Subsegmental atelectasis from central mass. (a) AP chest radiograph of a 56-year-old woman with dyspnea shows right lower lobe subsegmental atelectasis and an associated central mass. (b) Composite image with coronal contrast-enhanced chest CT (left) and coronal FDG PET/CT (right) of the same patient shows right lower lobe subsegmental atelectasis distal to a central mass. FDG uptake in the mass allows differentiation of tumor from adjacent airspace disease and shows hypermetabolic subcarinal lymph node metastases. Biopsy showed small cell lung cancer.

Careful analysis of the tracheobronchial tree should be part of the systematic assessment of every chest radiograph, particularly in symptomatic smokers, for recognition of endoluminal densities or airway narrowing.

Differential Diagnosis

Neoplasm

- Carcinoid: Indolent malignancy with typical central location; may completely or partially obstruct airway.

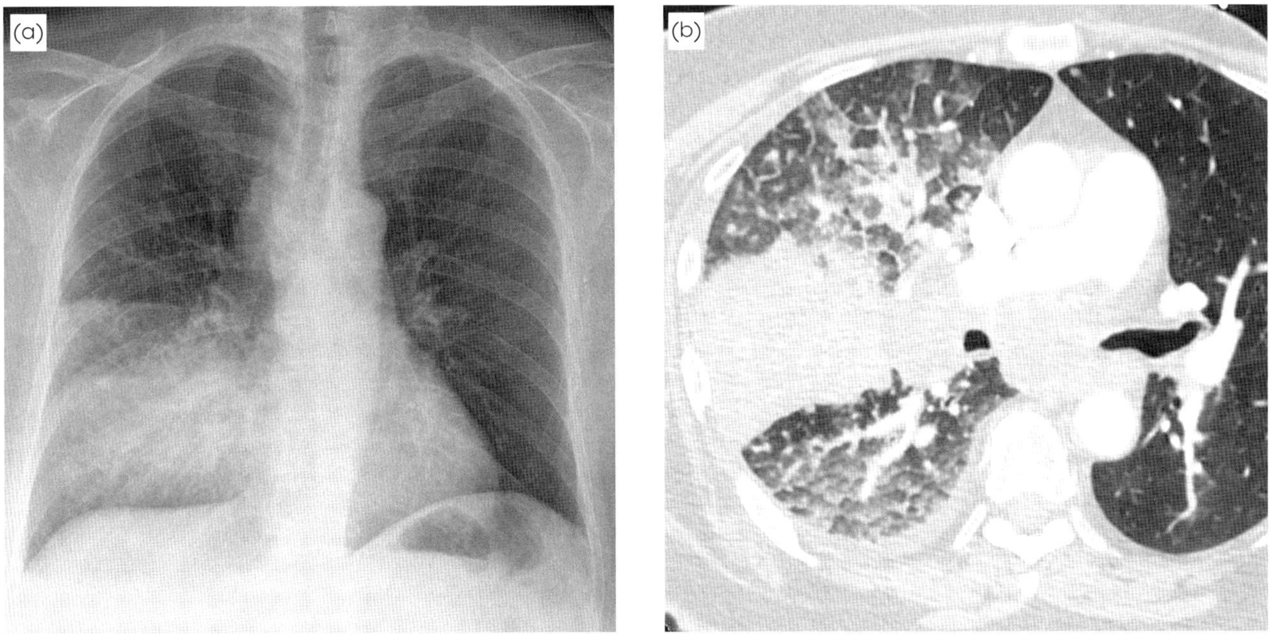

Figure 47.5. Postobstructive consolidation from advanced lung cancer. (a) PA chest radiograph of a 60-year-old woman with persistent pneumonia shows dense middle lobe consolidation. Right paratracheal lymphadenopathy should raise suspicion for malignancy. (b) Contrast-enhanced chest CT of the same patient shows mediastinal and hilar lymphadenopathy encasing the bronchus intermedius and obliteration of the middle lobe bronchus. Note dense consolidation in the right lung with surrounding interlobular septal thickening from lymphangitic carcinomatosis and a small right pleural effusion.

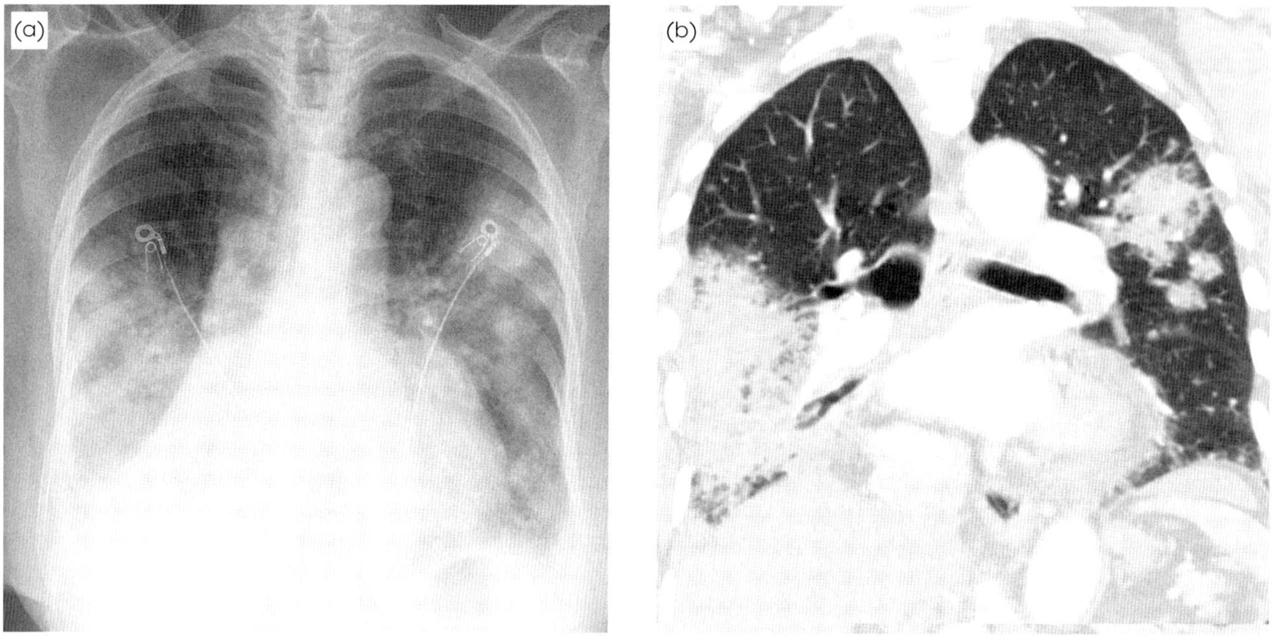

Figure 47.6. Multifocal consolidation. (a) AP chest radiograph of a 94-year-old woman with advanced invasive mucinous pulmonary adenocarcinoma shows multifocal bilateral consolidations. (b) Contrast-enhanced chest CT of the same patient shows bilateral nodular and mass-like consolidations that represented advanced multifocal invasive mucinous adenocarcinoma initially thought to represent multifocal pulmonary infection.

Affected patients are younger than those with lung cancer. Association with cigarette smoking is not strong.

- Mucoepidermoid carcinoma: Rare malignancy that primarily affects segmental airways. Affected patients are younger than those with lung cancer.
- Lymphoma: Primary pulmonary lymphoma is rare, but it may manifest as a pulmonary consolidation with air bronchograms.

Inflammatory Process

- Infection/inflammation: Pulmonary infection typically manifests with consolidation, which can be correlated with history and sputum analysis.
- Broncholith: Calcified lymph node; typically adjacent to an airway; may produce extrinsic airway stenosis or become endoluminal due to erosion through the airway wall and may result in post-obstructive atelectasis/consolidation.
- Bronchial stenosis: Acquired process due to infection (including fibrosing mediastinitis) or trauma; may result in post-obstructive volume loss or pneumonitis.

Other

- Foreign body: History of aspirated foreign body; most are not radiopaque but may be visible on CT. Bronchoscopy may be required for visualization.
- Mucous plug: May produce acute airway obstruction, typically in intubated patients. May resolve spontaneously or require removal with bronchoscopy-guided therapy/suction.

What Not to Miss

- Complete atelectasis and early consolidation may be subtle. Careful radiographic analysis allows identification of early abnormalities that may produce obscuration of normal anatomic landmarks.
- Recurrent or persistent atelectasis or pneumonia may be the only imaging abnormality in patients with central lung cancers and should prompt further investigation with chest CT and/or bronchoscopy.
- Radiographic visualization of a central mass with peripheral volume loss or consolidation (S sign of Golden), the luftsichel sign of left upper lobe atelectasis, or the bronchus cutoff sign should raise concern for lung cancer.
- The central airways must be carefully assessed on every chest radiograph or CT but particularly in the setting of wheezing, dyspnea, cough, or other recurrent/persistent respiratory complaints.

Imaging Findings

Radiography

- Atelectasis or volume loss of a lobe, lobes, or lung with absence of air bronchograms (Figs. 47.1–47.3)
  - Direct signs: Increased opacity associated with bronchovascular crowding (incomplete atelectasis), displacement of interlobar fissures, and location shift of preexistent granulomas (shifting granuloma sign)
  - Indirect signs: Mediastinal shift, hemidiaphragm elevation, juxtaphrenic peak, hilar displacement,

rib crowding, and compensatory hyperinflation of adjacent or contralateral uninvolved lung
- Assessment of interlobar fissures adjacent to atelectasis for identification of central mass
- Identification of S sign of Golden or luftsichel sign
- Direct visualization of obstructing endoluminal nodule or mass (Fig. 47.1)
- Consolidation
  - Post-obstructive pneumonia
  - Manifestation of lepidic growth and invasive mucinous lung adenocarcinomas (Fig. 47.6)
- Associated abnormalities: Lymphadenopathy, pleural effusion, and chest wall involvement

CT

- Assessment of extent of involvement by atelectasis or consolidation
- Evaluation of atelectatic or consolidated lung for underlying nodules and/or masses
- Differentiation of central neoplasm from atelectatic or consolidated lung based on differences in contrast enhancement; tumor typically enhances to a lesser degree than atelectatic lung
- Assessment of central airways
  - Direct visualization of endoluminal tumor and assessment of extent of airway involvement: Abrupt cutoff of airway, airway stenosis, and endoluminal nodule or mass (Figs 47-3 and 47-4)
  - Differentiation of central tumor from distal mucus plugs
  - Assessment of fissure margins for central nodules or masses (S sign of Golden)
  - Assessment of proximal extent of lesion
- Identification of associated abnormalities: Lymphadenopathy, pleural effusion, skeletal metastases, soft tissue metastases, and metastatic disease in upper abdominal organs

PET/CT

- FDG uptake by tumor and other areas of involvement (metastases to lymph nodes and other organs)
- Differentiation of central tumor from surrounding atelectasis (accurate size determination may be difficult due to nondiagnostic CT component) (Fig. 47.4)

Clinical Issues

- Centrally obstructing pulmonary neoplasms are readily accessible via bronchoscopy for tissue diagnosis.
- The more centrally located the lung cancer, the higher the T designation, and therefore the higher the tumor stage. Central neoplasms have a propensity for hilar and mediastinal lymph node metastases.
  - Central tumor obstructing an entire lung or less, extending to the hilum is designated T2.
- Small cell lung carcinomas are centrally located and are typically advanced at presentation. Surgical excision is advocated only for a select group of patients with limited disease. Most small cell lung cancers are treated with chemoradiation or chemotherapy, generally with a poor prognosis.

Key Points

- Consolidations in adults should be followed to radiographic resolution in order to exclude underlying malignancy.
- Persistent airspace disease not responding to therapy for more than 6 weeks and recurrent airspace disease in the same lung/lobe should prompt further evaluation with chest CT or bronchoscopy.
- The absence of an air bronchogram in consolidated or atelectatic lung indicates a centrally obstructing lesion.

Suggested Reading

Gelbman BD, Cham MD, Kim W, et al. Radiographic and clinical characterization of the false negative results from CT-guided needle biopsies of lung nodules. *J Thorac Oncol.* 2012;7:815–820.

Onitsuka H, Tsukuda M, Araki A, Murakami J, Torii Y, Masuda K. Differentiation of central lung tumor from postobstructive lobar collapse by rapid sequence computed tomography. *J Thorac Imaging.* 1991;6:28–31.

Yang RM, Li L, Wei XH, et al. Differentiation of central lung cancer from atelectasis: Comparison of diffusion-weighted MRI with PET/CT. *PLoS One.* 2013;8:e60279.

CHAPTER 48

Lung Cancer: Lymphadenopathy and Extrapulmonary Involvement

Ryo E. C. Benson

Definition

Lymphadenopathy refers to pathologic enlargement of lymph nodes and is a common manifestation of metastatic lung cancer. However, lymph node enlargement does not always signify malignancy, and normal-sized lymph nodes may contain neoplastic cells.

Extrapulmonary involvement by lung cancer may occur via direct extension (local invasion), lymphatic or hematogenous spread, or seeding of body cavities (pleura and pericardium). Lung cancer may invade or involve the mediastinum and its organs and structures, the pleura, the diaphragm, and the chest wall. It may also metastasize to involve extrathoracic sites, including the brain, liver, adrenal gland, and skeleton.

Clinical Features

Patients with lung cancer metastatic to lymph nodes may be relatively asymptomatic and may be diagnosed incidentally. Enlarged lymph nodes may also produce symptoms by compressing or invading airways, and affected patients may present with cough, chest pain, hemoptysis, or dyspnea. Invasion of vascular structures may produce upper extremity swelling and/or superior vena cava syndrome. Patients with central lymphadenopathy associated with lymphatic congestion and those with lymphangitic carcinomatosis (spread of cancer involving the lymphatics) may present with dyspnea and, occasionally, nonproductive cough or hemoptysis. Lymphadenopathy in the setting of lung cancer portends a worse prognosis, with hilar, ipsilateral mediastinal, and contralateral thoracic or extrathoracic lymphadenopathy denoting increasing degrees of disease progression.

Approximately 5–15% of patients with lung cancer have pleural effusions and may present with dyspnea or nonspecific chest pain. Malignant pleural effusion is characterized by malignant cells in the pleural fluid. Patients with lung cancer and pleural effusion have a poorer prognosis, regardless of whether or not neoplastic cells are identified in the pleural fluid.

Patients with extrapulmonary involvement by lung cancer may present with a variety of respiratory and nonrespiratory complaints. Superior vena cava syndrome is characterized by facial and upper extremity edema, venous distention in the neck and chest wall, and sometimes mental status changes, plethora, papilledema, or cyanosis. Although it may occur with any lung cancer cell type, it is typical of small cell carcinoma. Pancoast tumors cause chest wall pain, and Pancoast syndrome with brachial plexus and sympathetic ganglia involvement characteristically produces ipsilateral radicular pain, shoulder pain, and Horner's syndrome (miosis, ptosis, and anhidrosis). Direct or hematogenous involvement of the spine may result in acute compression fractures or intraspinal involvement, and affected patients may present with back pain, neurologic deficits, weakness, pain, or even loss of bowel/bladder function.

Patients may also present with metastases to the brain, adrenal glands, liver, and bones. Some of these lesions may produce seizures, mental status changes, pain, and/or pathologic fractures.

Anatomy and Physiology

Lung cancer commonly metastasizes to intrathoracic lymph nodes generally depending on the location of the primary tumor. It typically spreads sequentially to intrapulmonary, hilar, and ipsilateral mediastinal lymph nodes. However, skip metastases to mediastinal lymph nodes and metastases to contralateral lymph nodes may also occur.

Adenocarcinoma is the cell type most commonly associated with pleural effusion. The pleura may be involved by direct invasion, lymphatic permeation, drop metastases, or hematogenous tumor emboli. Given its innervation, patients with parietal pleural invasion often present with local pain.

Some lung cancers have a propensity to invade adjacent structures. For example, small cell carcinoma is often locally invasive with frequent mediastinal vascular and airway encasement and/or obstruction. Some peripheral lung cancers may grow through the pleura to directly invade the adjacent chest wall osseous and soft tissue structures.

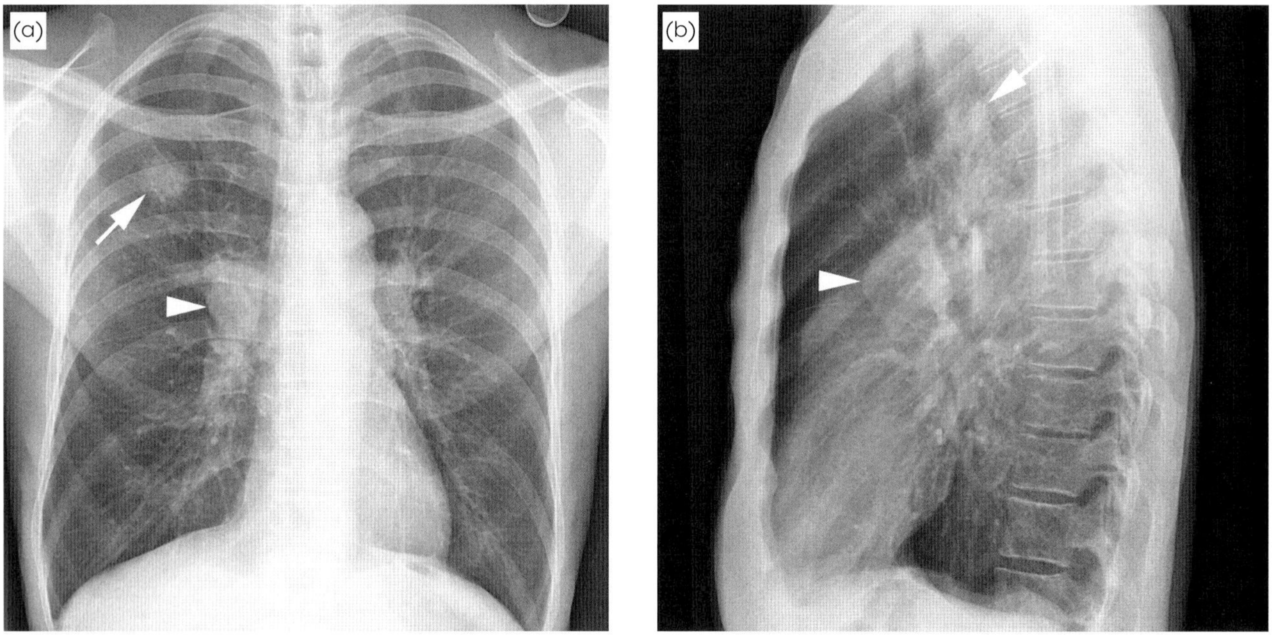

Figure 48.1. Hilar lymphadenopathy. (a, b) Posteroanterior (PA) and lateral chest radiographs of a 47-year-old man show a right upper lobe nodule (arrow) with associated right hilar enlargement (arrowhead) from metastatic lymphadenopathy.

How to Approach the Image

Chest radiographs must be carefully evaluated for hilar and/or mediastinal contour abnormalities that may represent lymphadenopathy (Figs. 48.1 and 48.2). Comparison to prior studies is of paramount importance for detection of subtle abnormalities. Chest CT studies must be systematically scrutinized with attention to all intrathoracic lymph node stations as well as supraclavicular, cervical, axillary, and upper abdominal lymph nodes. Mediastinal lymphadenopathy is readily identified with or without contrast, but contrast administration facilitates distinction of hilar lymph nodes from adjacent vascular structures (Fig. 48.3). Careful scrutiny of the skeleton is important because osseous involvement may be subtle.

The adrenal glands and visualized portions of the liver should be evaluated on every chest CT. Abnormal

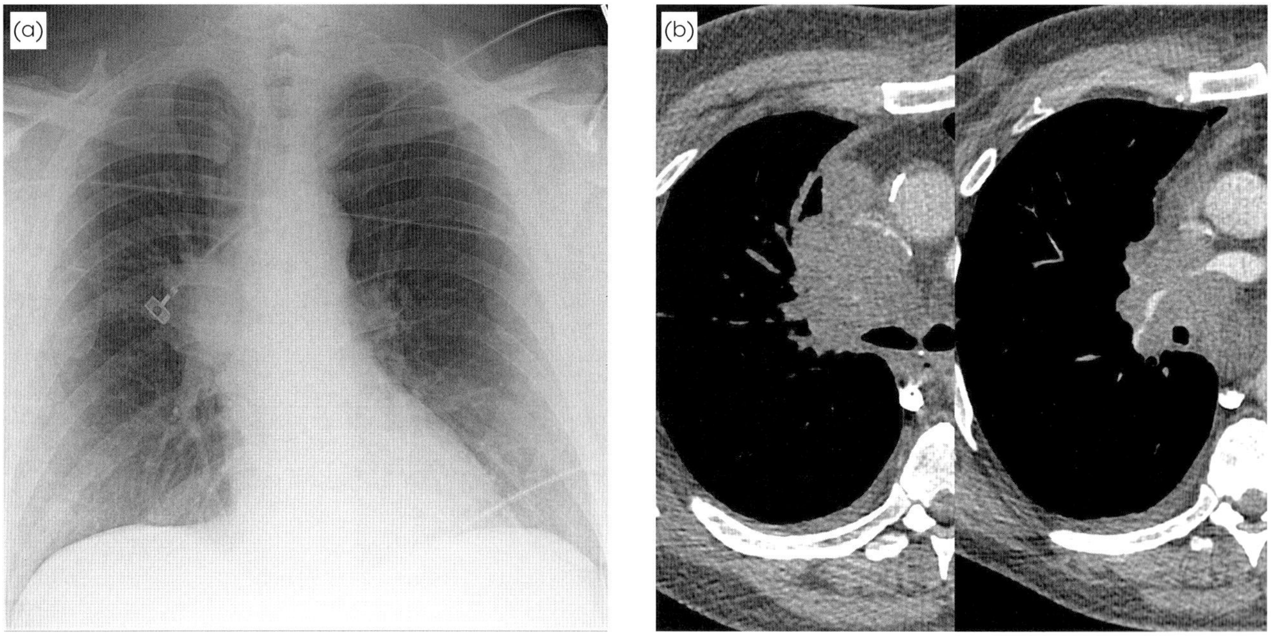

Figure 48.2. Lymphadenopathy and local vascular and airway invasion. (a) Anteroposterior (AP) chest radiograph of a 72-year-old man with small cell lung cancer and severe dyspnea shows right hilar and mediastinal enlargement. (b) Composite image with contrast-enhanced chest CT of the same patient shows locally invasive conglomerate right hilar and mediastinal lymphadenopathy nearly obliterating the superior vena cava (left) and encasing and narrowing the right pulmonary artery and bronchus intermedius (right).

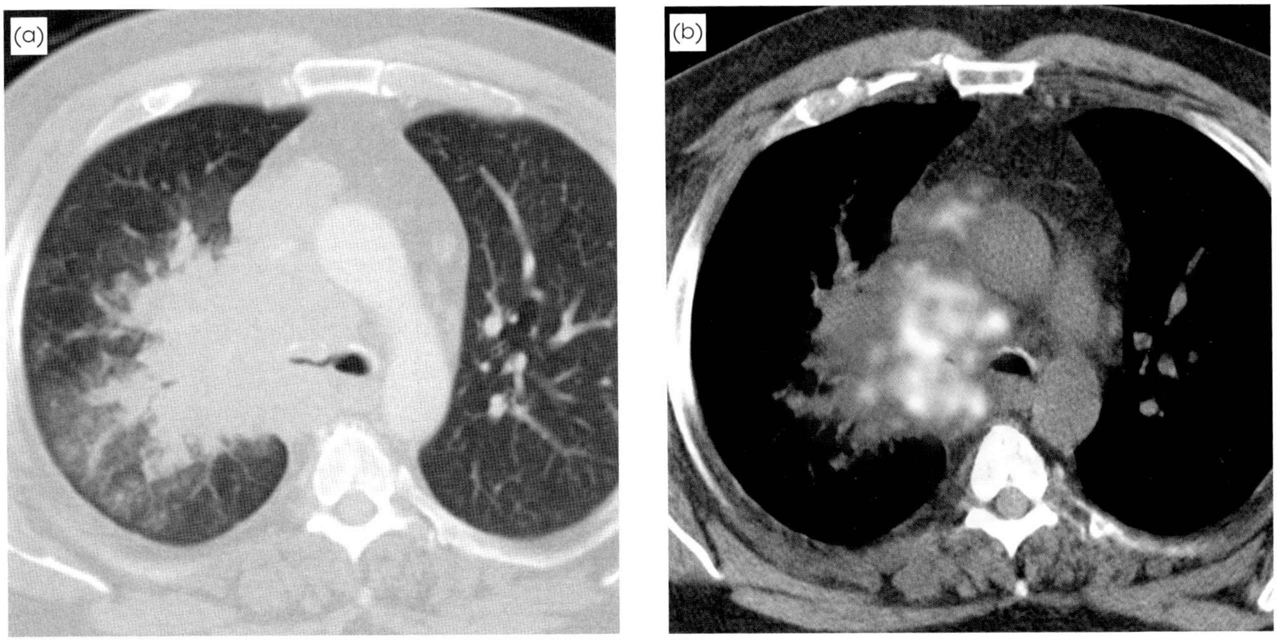

Figure 48.3. Mediastinal lymphadenopathy and local airway invasion. (a) Contrast-enhanced chest CT of a 64-year-old man with severe dyspnea shows a large irregular right upper lobe mass that invades the mediastinum encasing and narrowing the right mainstem bronchus and superior vena cava. (b) FDG PET/CT of the same patient shows intense FDG uptake in the central mass and adjacent hilar and mediastinal metastatic lymphadenopathy.

abdominal findings may require further assessment with dedicated abdominal imaging, including MRI. CT is superior to radiography for the detection of bone erosions, as manifestations of metastatic disease, and MRI is superior to CT in the evaluation of the chest wall bones and soft tissues. Brain MRI is often used for tumor detection and is more sensitive than brain CT.

Bone scintigraphy is useful in detecting skeletal metastases but is not specific. FDG PET/CT is the study of choice for identifying distant metastases, except in the brain and kidney due to normal FDG uptake in these areas.

What Not to Miss

Lymphadenopathy

- Hilar lymphadenopathy may manifest as a minor change in contour from a prior normal appearance or as increased hilar density (Figs. 48.1 and 48.2).
- Enlarged hila from lymphadenopathy must be differentiated from enlarged pulmonary arteries in pulmonary hypertension.
- Knowledge of normal radiographic anatomy allows detection of subtle abnormalities of mediastinal lines, stripes, and interfaces to identify lymphadenopathy.
- Extrathoracic lymph nodes visible on chest CT must be assessed for asymmetry or enlargement.

Extrapulmonary Involvement

- Pleural effusions must be evaluated for associated pleural thickening and/or solid nodules, which are virtually diagnostic of malignant pleural effusion (Fig. 48.4).
- Lesions abutting the mediastinum, chest wall, or diaphragm must be assessed for evidence of local invasion.

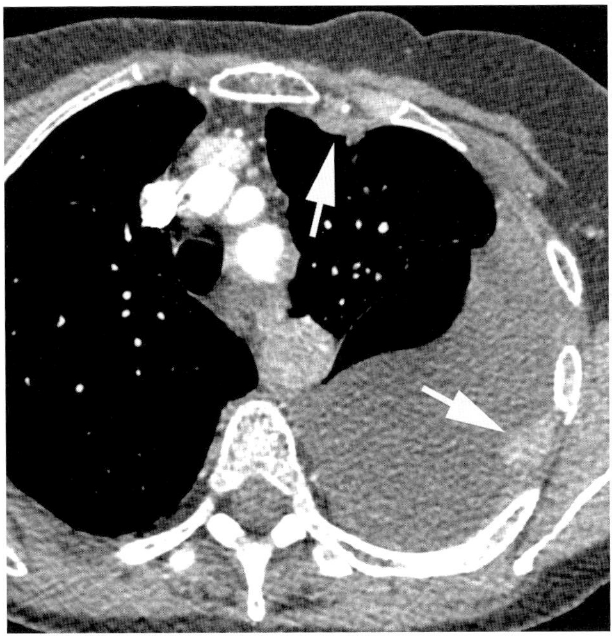

Figure 48.4. Malignant pleural effusion. Contrast-enhanced chest CT of a 58-year-old woman with advanced adenocarcinoma shows a large left pleural effusion with enhancing pleural nodules (arrows) consistent with malignant pleural effusion.

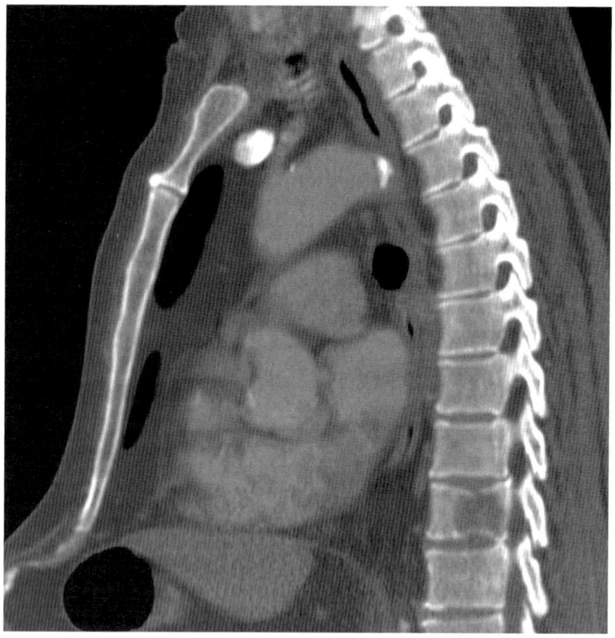

Figure 48.5. Skeletal metastases. Sagittal contrast-enhanced chest CT of an elderly man with small cell lung cancer shows a lytic metastasis of the T10 vertebral body with a pathologic fracture of the superior endplate.

- Chest wall osseous structures, especially the ribs and sternum, must be evaluated for subtle erosion or pathologic fracture, particularly in patients with chest wall pain (Fig. 48.5).

Differential Diagnosis

Lymphadenopathy

- Sarcoidosis
  - Affected patients are typically younger than those with lung cancer.
  - Lymphadenopathy is typically bilateral and symmetric with frequent hilar involvement.
  - Perilymphatic pulmonary micronodules support the diagnosis.
  - Sarcoidosis is a diagnosis of exclusion based on correlation of imaging, laboratory, physical exam, and histologic findings.
- Granulomatous infection (tuberculosis, histoplasmosis, and coccidiomycosis)
  - May produce asymmetric hilar and/or mediastinal lymphadenopathy and mimic lung cancer.
  - Fungal infection may be confirmed with fungal titers and occurs in endemic areas.
  - Tuberculosis may be diagnosed on sputum analysis, particularly in patients with cavitary lesions.
  - Histoplasmosis may be complicated by mediastinal fibrosis.
- Metastases
  - Head and neck cancers, genitourinary malignancies, thyroid cancer, breast cancer, and melanoma frequently involve mediastinal lymph nodes.
  - Breast cancer may involve intrathoracic lymph nodes, particularly internal thoracic/mammary lymph nodes.
- Lymphoma/leukemia
  - May exhibit intra- and extrathoracic lymphadenopathy.
  - Hodgkin lymphoma may contiguously affect upper mediastinal lymph nodes (paratracheal, prevascular).
  - Non-Hodgkin lymphoma may affect intrathoracic lymph nodes and often exhibits abdominal lymphadenopathy and splenomegaly.

Extrapulmonary Involvement

- Vascular invasion
  - Lymphadenopathy from extrapulmonary malignancy
  - Invasive thymic epithelial neoplasm
  - Mediastinal fibrosis
- Chest wall involvement
  - Infection: Tuberculosis, actinomycosis, fungal infection
  - Primary chest wall neoplasm: Chondrosarcoma, myeloma
  - Extrapulmonary chest wall metastases

Imaging Findings

Lymphadenopathy

Radiography

- Hilar enlargement and/or increased density, typically asymmetric
- Focal or diffuse mediastinal and/or hilar enlargement
- Associated findings
  - Central or peripheral pulmonary nodule, mass, or consolidation (Figs 48.1)
  - Multifocal nodules, masses, or consolidations in advanced disease
  - Pleural effusion, may be massive
  - Lytic or sclerotic skeletal metastases
  - Upper abdominal lymphadenopathy and/or solid organ metastases

CT/MRI

- Optimal evaluation of lymphadenopathy; intravenous contrast for evaluation of hilar lymphadenopathy and differentiation from adjacent vascular structures
- Size criteria for enlargement: Short axis larger than 1 cm for most intrathoracic lymph nodes, subcarinal lymph node enlargement greater than 1.3–1.5 cm.
- Lymph node metastases may exhibit contrast enhancement or intrinsic low attenuation from necrosis.

- Associated findings
  - Peripheral nodule, mass, or consolidation in adenocarcinoma
  - Central endoluminal nodule or mass in squamous cell carcinoma
- Coalescent mass-like hilar/mediastinal lymphadenopathy is frequent in small cell lung cancer.

PET/CT

- High negative predictive value
- FDG uptake in lymph node metastases (Fig 48.3); false positive in infectious/inflammatory lymphadenopathy
- Staging of lung cancer

Extrapulmonary Involvement

Radiography

- Tumor mass abutting mediastinum with focal or diffuse mediastinal enlargement
- Pleural effusion, may be massive
- Direct chest wall invasion with or without skeletal erosion/destruction (Fig 48.6)

CT/MRI

- Limited contact with mediastinum or preservation of tissue planes may indicate tumor resectability.
- Direct mediastinal invasion by adjacent tumor; confidently identified in cases of encasement/ invasion of mediastinal structures (Figs. 48.2 and 48.3)
  - Invasion of central tracheobronchial tree (trachea, carina)
  - Vascular encasement/invasion of aorta, pulmonary arteries, pulmonary veins, superior vena cava
    - Greater than 90° contact with aorta suggests invasion/unresectability
    - Brachiocephalic vein and superior vena cava invasion/obstruction usually with associated vascular collaterals
  - Esophageal invasion: Tumor abutting esophagus, mural esophageal thickening, endoluminal lesion
  - Pericardial invasion: Pericardial effusion, pericardial thickening or nodules
  - Cardiac invasion: Left atrial invasion via pulmonary veins
- Pleural thickening, nodules, masses
- Pleural effusion: May be small, moderate, large, or massive; associated solid pleural nodules or masses virtually diagnostic of malignant pleural effusion (Fig 48.4)
- Brain, adrenal, liver, soft tissue, or skeletal metastases may be identified on CT or MR prior to diagnosis of the primary lung cancer (Fig 48.5).
- Direct chest wall invasion (Fig 48.6)
  - Loss of extrapleural fat
  - Rib erosion/invasion and/or pathologic fracture
  - Intercostal muscle involvement
  - Pancoast tumor: Apical tumor with local invasion of adjacent ribs, vertebral bodies, subclavian vessels, brachial plexus, and/or cervical sympathetic nerves, and stellate ganglion

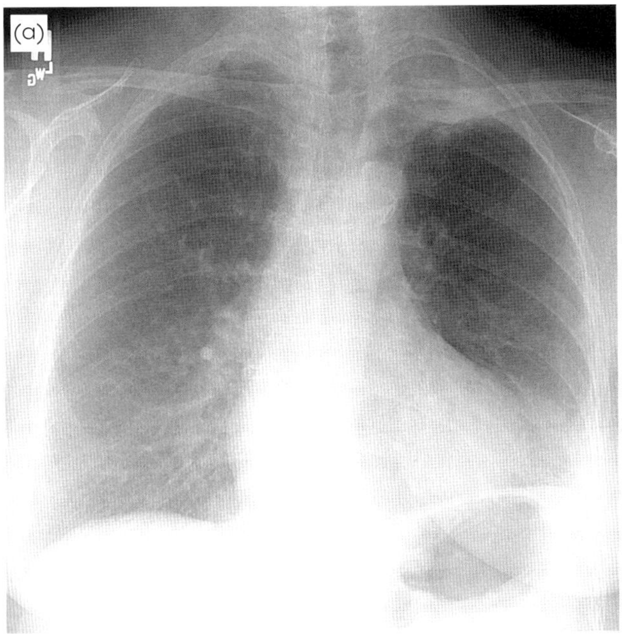

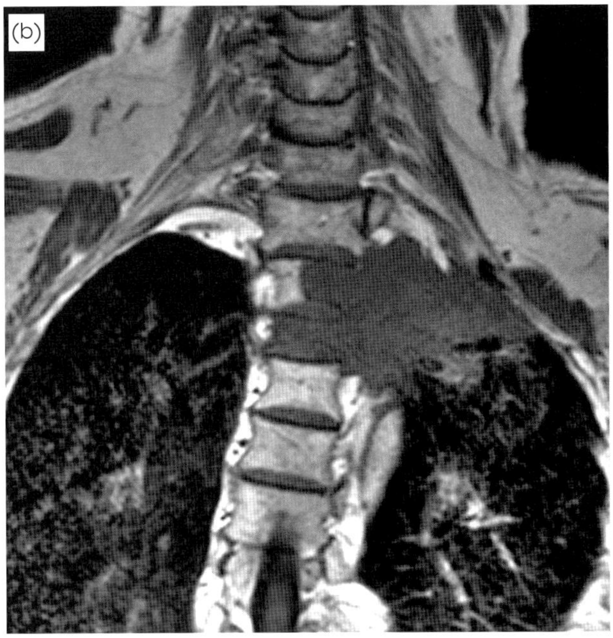

Figure 48.6. Pancoast tumor. (a) PA chest radiograph of a 79-year-old woman with a 50 pack-year smoking history shows a Pancoast tumor manifesting as asymmetric left apical opacity and subtle elevation of the left hemidiaphragm. (b) Coronal T1-weighted MR of the same patient shows a left apical mass directly invading at least two upper thoracic vertebral bodies with obliteration of the left apical extrapleural fat. Biopsy showed moderately differentiated squamous cell carcinoma.

FDG PET/CT

- Staging of lung cancer
- FDG uptake by intra- and extrathoracic metastases

Clinical Issues

- Extensive lymphadenopathy, especially when contralateral or supraclavicular, precludes surgical resection.
- Involvement of the aerodigestive tract implies unresectable tumor.
- Malignant pleural and/or pericardial effusion considered nonsurgical stage IV disease.

Key Points

- Lung cancer may initially manifest with hilar and/or mediastinal lymphadenopathy from metastatic disease.
- Normal-sized lymph nodes may contain micrometastases.
- Lung cancer may initially manifest with extrapulmonary involvement and/or metastatic disease.
- PET/CT upstages many lung cancers through detection of unsuspected distant metastases.

Suggested Reading

Almeida FA, Uzbeck M, Ost D. Initial evaluation of the nonsmall cell lung cancer patient: Diagnosis and staging. *Curr Opin Pulm Med.* 2010:16;307–314.

Detterbeck FC, Boffa DJ, Kim AW, et al. The eighth edition lung cancer stage classification. *Chest* 2017;151:193–203.

UyBico SJ, Wu CC, Suh RD, Le NH, Brown N, Krishnam MS. Lung cancer staging essentials: The new TNM staging system and potential imaging pitfalls. *RadioGraphics.* 2010 Sep;30(5): 1163–1181.

CHAPTER 49

Lung Cancer: Staging

Ryo E. C. Benson

Definition

Cancer staging is a process used to evaluate the extent of spread of malignancy in order to determine the most appropriate treatment and predict prognosis. Clinical staging is an estimate of the extent of disease prior to surgery based on imaging, bronchoscopy, biopsy, and mediastinoscopy. Surgical–pathologic staging is performed when the tumor and associated lymph nodes are resected, based on histologic analysis. Restaging is used to determine the extent of disease after treatment based on a combination of imaging and histologic analysis of suspicious lesions.

Clinical Features

Patients with lung cancer present with a variety of symptoms and signs. However, affected patients may be entirely asymptomatic, particularly those with localized peripheral lung cancers. As lung cancer becomes more advanced, affected patients may present with thoracic complaints including cough, dyspnea, chest pain, and hemoptysis. Extrathoracic clinical manifestations of lung cancer may occur with metastatic disease and may include bone pain related to pathologic fractures, constitutional symptoms of malaise, weight loss and anorexia, or symptoms related to paraneoplastic syndromes.

Table 49.1 - TNM Classification System

	N0	N1	N2	N3
T1a (≤ 1 cm)	IA1	IIB	IIIA	IIIB
T1b (> 1–2 cm)	IA2	IIB	IIIA	IIIB
T1c (> 2–3 cm)	IA3	IIB	IIIA	IIIB
T2a Central tumor, Visceral pleural invasion	IB	IIB	IIIA	IIIB
T2a (> 3–4 cm)	IB	IIB	IIIA	IIIB
T2b (> 4–5 cm)	IIA	IIB	IIIA	IIIB
T3 (> 5–7 cm)	IIB	IIIA	IIIB	IIIC
T3 Invasion	IIB	IIIA	IIIB	IIIC
T3 (Satellite nodule)	IIB	IIIA	IIIB	IIIC
T4 (> 7 cm)	IIIA	IIIA	IIIB	IIIC
T4 Invasion	IIIA	IIIA	IIIB	IIIC
T4 Ipsilateral nodule	IIIA	IIIA	IIIB	IIIC
M1a Contralateral nodule	IVA	IVA	IVA	IVA
M1a Pleural/Pericardial disseminaion	IVA	IVA	IVA	IVA
M1b Single metastasis	IVA	IVA	IVA	IVA
M1c Muliple metastases	IVB	IVB	IVB	IVB

Anatomy and Physiology

Lung cancer staging uses the TNM classification system. The T designation refers to the primary tumor, N to thoracic lymph node involvement, and M to metastases to lung, other organs, or distant lymph nodes (Table 49.1).

T Designation

Tx—Primary tumor cannot be assessed or tumor proven by malignant cells in sputum or bronchial washings, but not visible on imaging or bronchoscopy.

T0—No evidence of primary tumor

TIS—Carcinoma in situ (squamous cell carcinoma or adenocarcinoma)

T1—Nodule ≤ 3 cm surrounded by lung or endoluminal lesion located at or peripheral to a lobar bronchus
- T1a (mi)—Minimally invasive adenocarcinoma
- T1a (ss)—Superficial spreading tumor
- T1a—Nodule ≤1 cm
- T1b—Nodule >1 cm and ≤2 cm (Fig. 49.1)
- T1c—Nodule > 2 cm and ≤3 cm (Fig. 49.2)

T2—Mass >3 cm and ≤5 cm; visceral pleural involvement or endoluminal lesion in the mainstem bronchus without carinal involvement or with post-obstructive atelectasis involving part of or an entire lung

T2a—Mass >3 cm and ≤4 cm

T2b—Mass >4 cm and ≤5 cm

T3—Mass >5 cm and ≤7 cm; tumor of any size involving chest wall, parietal pleura, phrenic nerve, and parietal pericardium; and metastatic lung nodule within ipsilateral tumor lobe (Fig. 49.3)

T4—Mass >7 cm; involvement of trachea or carina, diaphragm, mediastinum, aorta, heart, vertebral body, recurrent laryngeal nerve, pulmonary trunk,

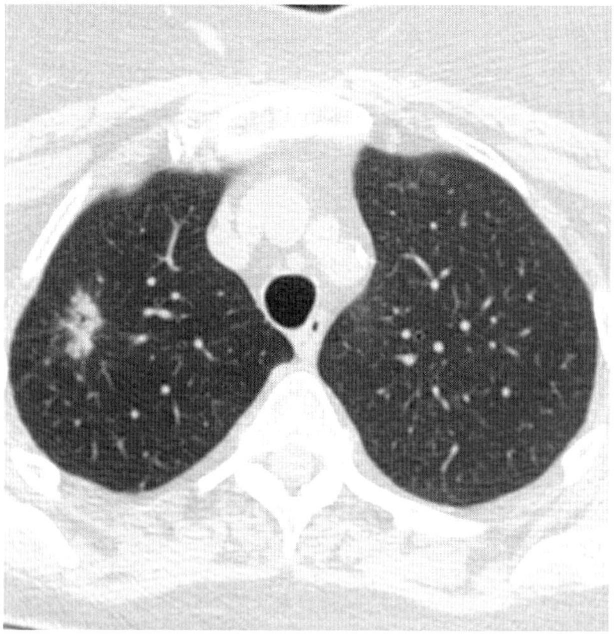

Figure 49.1. Stage I lung cancer. Unenhanced chest CT shows a right upper lobe adenocarcinoma manifesting as a spiculated nodule that measures 1.8 cm in longest dimension. In the absence of lymphadenopathy or metastases, this is a stage IA2 lesion: T1b, N0, M0.

and metastatic nodule in ipsilateral lung but in a different lobe from the primary tumor (Fig. 49.4)

N Designation

Nx—Regional lymph nodes cannot be assessed. (Note: Designation to be incorporated in future staging classifications)

N0—No regional lymph node involvement

N1—Metastases to ipsilateral hilar or intrapulmonary lymph nodes (Fig. 49.2)

- N1a—Single lymph node station N1 involvement
- N1b—Multiple lymph node station N1 involvement

N2—Metastases to ipsilateral mediastinal lymph nodes, including subcarinal (Fig. 49.5)

- N2a1—Single station N2 lymph node involvement without N1 involvement (skip lymph node metastasis)
- N2a2—Single station N2 lymph node involvement with N1 lymph node involvement
- N2b—Multiple station N2 involvement

N3—Metastases to contralateral hilar or mediastinal lymph nodes and/or metastases to ipsilateral or contralateral supraclavicular or scalene lymph nodes (Fig. 49.6)

Lymph Node Stations

Station 1: Supraclavicular lymph nodes, midline demarcates right and left sides

Station 2: Right and left upper paratracheal lymph nodes, left tracheal wall demarcates right and left sides

Station 3: Prevascular (3a) and posterior retrotracheal (3p) lymph nodes from thoracic inlet to carina

Station 4: Right and left lower paratracheal lymph nodes, left tracheal wall demarcates right and left sides

Station 5: Aortopulmonary window (subaortic) lymph nodes

Station 6: Para-aortic lymph nodes adjacent to ascending aorta and aortic arch

Station 7: Subcarinal lymph nodes

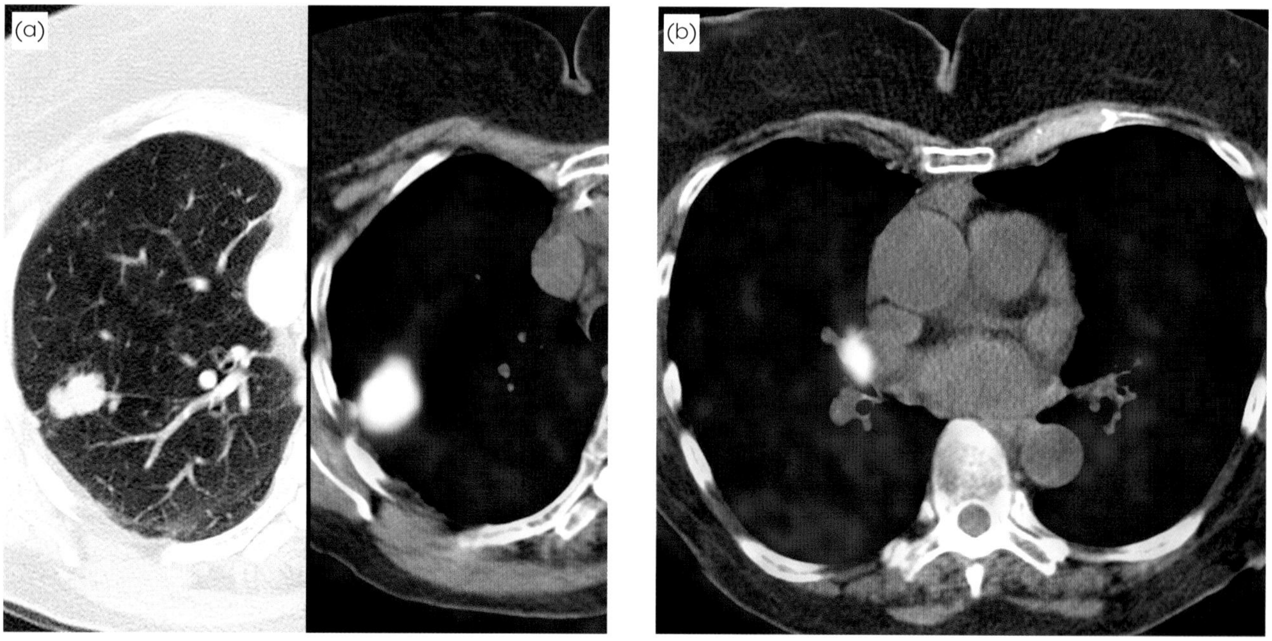

Figure 49.2. Stage II lung cancer. (a) Composite image with contrast-enhanced chest CT (left) and FDG PET/CT (right) shows a polylobular 2.8-cm adenocarcinoma with intense FDG uptake. (b) FDG PET/CT of the same patient shows intense FDG uptake in an ipsilateral right hilar lymph node not evident on chest CT. In the absence of metastases, this is a stage IIB lesion: T1c, N1, M0.

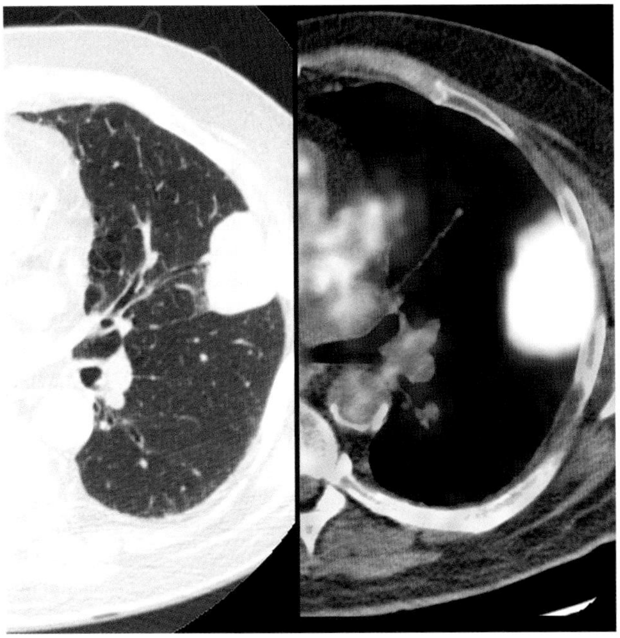

Figure 49.3. Stage II lung cancer. Composite image with unenhanced chest CT (left) and FDG PET/CT (right) shows a left upper lobe peripheral large cell lung cancer that measures 5.3 cm with a maximum standardized uptake value of 10.5, without parietal pleural invasion at surgery. In the absence of lymphadenopathy or metastases, this is a stage IIB lesion: T3, N0, M0.

Station 8: Paraesophageal lymph nodes adjacent to the esophagus from lower border of bronchus intermedius on the right and upper border of the left lower lobe bronchus on the left to the diaphragm

Station 9: Pulmonary ligament lymph nodes

Station 10: Main hilar lymph nodes

Stations 11–14: Interlobar, lobar, segmental, and subsegmental lymph nodes, respectively

Note that the following intrathoracic lymph nodes do not have designated stations: axillary, internal thoracic/mammary, diaphragmatic, and juxtacardiac lymph nodes.

M Designation

M0—No distant metastases

M1—Distant metastases

M1a—Metastases to pleura and pericardium, including malignant pleural or pericardial effusion and contralateral metastatic lung nodule (Fig. 49.7)

M1b—Single extrathoracic metastasis to distant organ or lymph node

M1c—Multiple extrathoracic metastases to one or more organs

Note that although lymphangitic carcinomatosis indicates advanced disease, it is not included in the TNM definition/designation.

The TNM staging system is recommended for the staging of small cell lung cancer (especially very limited disease). However, the Veterans Administration Lung Cancer Study Group staging system distinguishes limited-stage disease (LD) from extensive-stage disease (ED). LD is disease confined to one hemithorax and therefore treatable within a single radiation port. ED is cancer spread beyond LD.

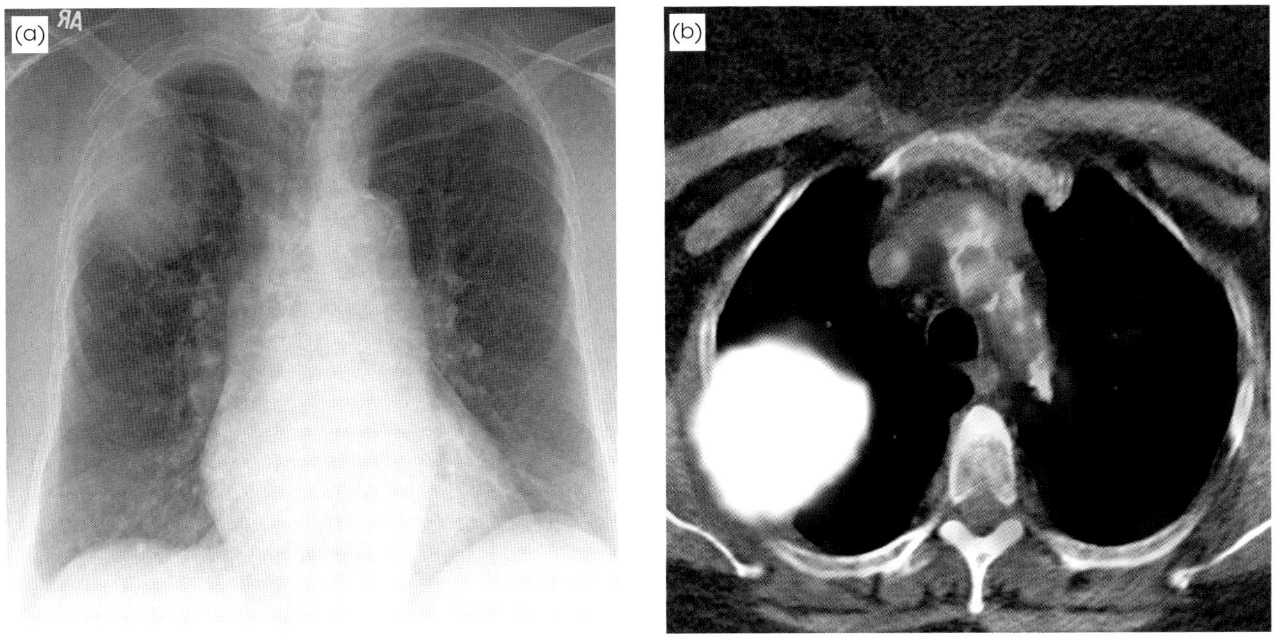

Figure 49.4. Stage III lung cancer. (a) Posteroanterior chest radiograph of a 76-year-old woman smoker with right chest wall pain shows a 7.5-cm peripheral right upper lobe adenocarcinoma with chest wall invasion and rib destruction. (b) FDG PET/CT of the same patient shows intense FDG uptake in the mass and chest wall invasion but no evidence of lymphadenopathy or metastases. This is a stage IIIA lesion: T4, N0, M0.

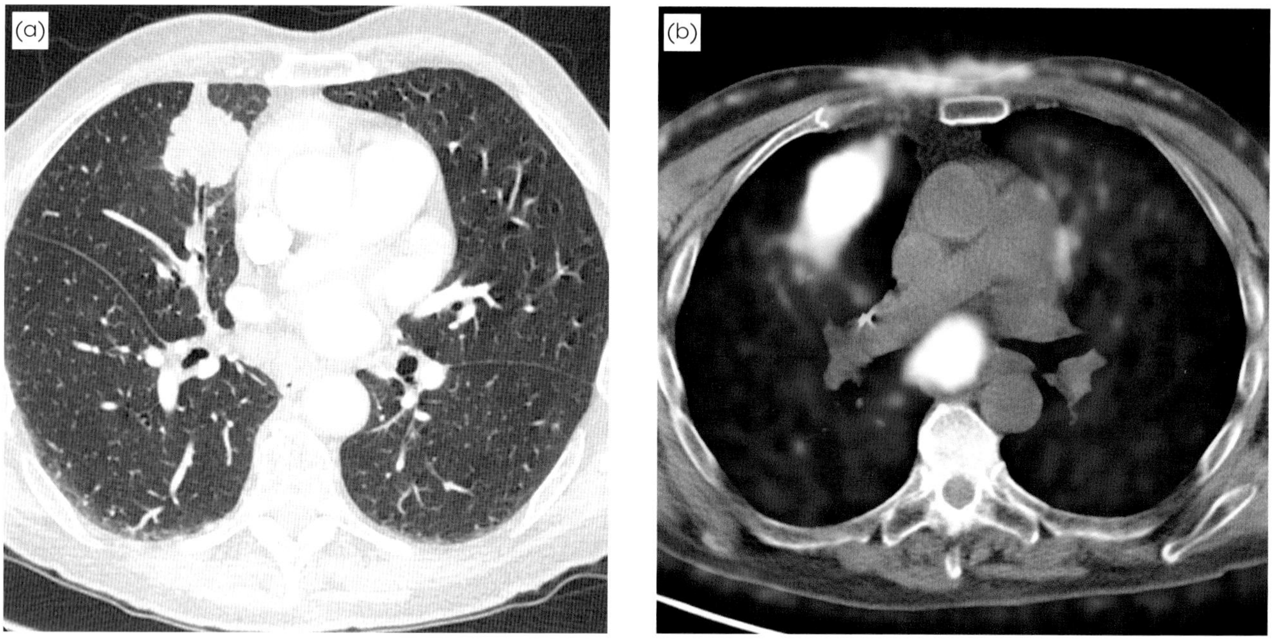

Figure 49.5. Stage III lung cancer. (a) Contrast-enhanced chest CT shows a middle lobe polylobular 3.5-cm adenocarcinoma and conspicuous subcarinal soft tissue suspicious for lymphadenopathy. (b) FDG PET/CT of the same patient shows intense FDG uptake in the mass and subcarinal lymph node metastases. In the absence of distant metastases, this is a stage IIIA lesion: T2a, N2, M0.

Important notes regarding TNM staging:

T designation

Highest T designation should be chosen if tumor demonstrates multiple T descriptors

For subsolid tumors, maximum dimension of the solid component is used to assign the T category, but maximum dimension of ground-glass component should also be recorded

Tumor extension from lymph node metastasis does not count as T involvement

Involvement of hilar fat is T2a

Involvement of mediastinal fat is T4

Involvement of parietal pericardium is T3

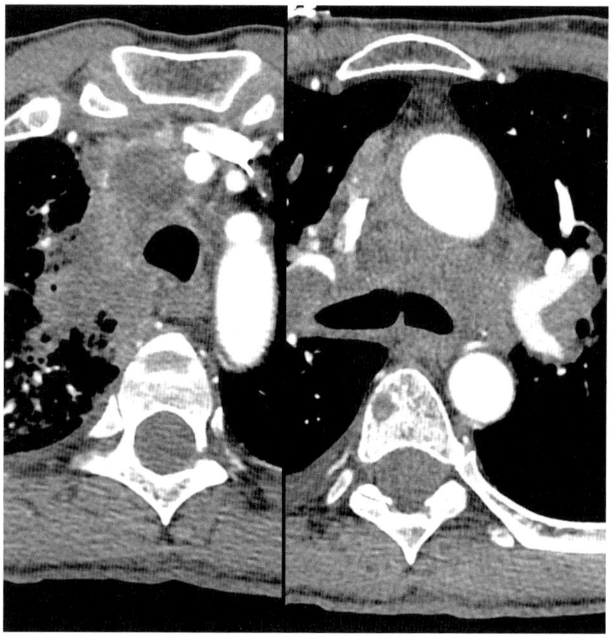

Figure 49.6. Stage III lung cancer. Composite image with contrast-enhanced chest CT shows an advanced right upper lobe adenocarcinoma with local mediastinal invasion and superior vena cava obstruction (left). Note contralateral left paratracheal and left hilar metastatic lymphadenopathy (right). In the absence of distant metastases, this is a stage IIIC lesion: T4, N3, M0.

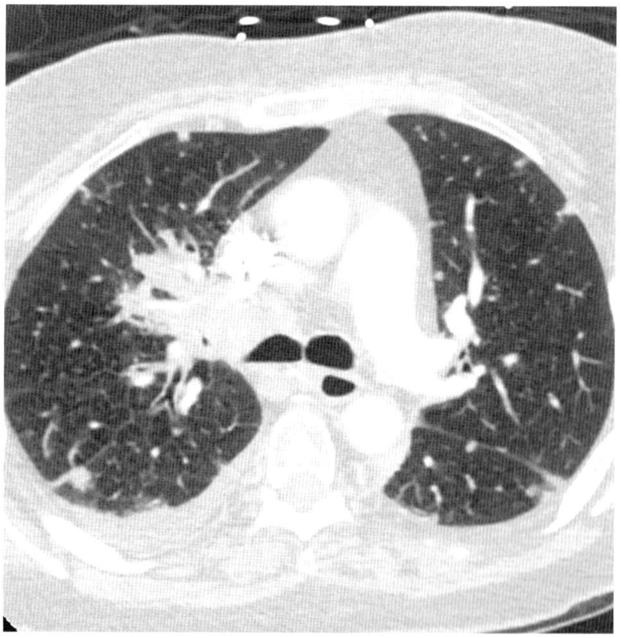

Figure 49.7. Stage IV lung cancer. Contrast-enhanced chest CT shows a right upper lobe adenocarcinoma with mediastinal invasion, small bilateral pleural effusions, and multifocal bilateral pulmonary metastases. This is a stage IVA lesion: T4, N2, M1a.

Involvement of visceral pericardium is T4
Pancoast tumor is T3 if only thoracic nerve roots are involved
Pancoast tumor is T4 with involvement of C8 or more cephalad nerve roots, brachial plexus cords, or spinal canal

N designation

Direct extension of primary tumor into adjacent lymph node counts as lymph node involvement

How to Approach the Image

Evaluation of chest radiographs of patients with suspected lung cancer should include clinical staging (Fig. 49.4). Multifocal pulmonary involvement, lymphadenopathy, pleural effusion, and suspicious skeletal lesions should be noted as suspicious and further evaluated with chest CT.

CT is usually employed in the initial staging of lung cancer (Fig. 49.5). Evaluation should include assessment for intra- and/or extrathoracic lymphadenopathy, evaluation of pleural effusions for pleural nodules that may indicate malignancy, and examination of the chest wall for lytic or sclerotic skeletal lesions and soft tissue metastases. The upper abdomen should be scrutinized for hepatic lesions, lymphadenopathy, and adrenal enlargement. Abdominal abnormalities suspicious for malignancy should be further evaluated with dedicated abdominal imaging.

MRI is usually employed as a problem-solving tool in cases in which CT is equivocal. It is particularly useful for assessment of vascular invasion in patients in whom intravenous contrast is contraindicated and in selected cases of suspected chest wall involvement, including patients with Pancoast tumor, for assessment of vascular and brachial plexus involvement.

FDG PET/CT is the imaging modality of choice for staging lung cancer and is based on the metabolic activity of malignant neoplasms.

What Not to Miss

- All radiographs of patients with lung cancer should be assessed for subtle lymphadenopathy and chest wall involvement.
- Large and massive pleural effusions are highly suspicious for malignancy and should be thoroughly assessed for pleural thickening, nodules, or masses.
- Contrast-enhanced CT is the optimal modality for assessment of hilar lymphadenopathy and differentiation of abnormal lymph nodes from adjacent vessels (Fig. 49.6).
- Enlarged lymph nodes are not necessarily neoplastic, and normal lymph nodes may contain micrometastases.
- Indolent lung cancers may produce false-negative findings on FDG PET/CT, and infectious/inflammatory processes may produce false-positive findings.

Differential Diagnosis

T Designation

- Nodule: Granuloma, carcinoid, hamartoma, solitary metastasis, arteriovenous malformation
- Mass: Metastasis, lymphoma, lung abscess, intralobar sequestration
- Endoluminal lesion: Carcinoid, adenoid cystic carcinoma, mucoepidermoid carcinoma, hamartoma, lipoma, neurogenic neoplasm

N Designation

- Neoplastic lymphadenopathy: Metastases, lymphoma
- Non-neoplastic lymphadenopathy: Infection (fungal, mycobacterial), sarcoidosis, pneumoconiosis, Castleman disease

M Designation

- Pleura: Metastases, mesothelioma, lymphoma
- Chest wall: Metastases, myeloma, chondrosarcoma

How to Approach the Image

Evaluation of chest radiographs of patients with suspected lung cancer should include clinical staging (Fig. 49.4). Multifocal pulmonary involvement, lymphadenopathy, pleural effusion, and suspicious skeletal lesions should be noted as suspicious and further evaluated with chest CT.

CT is usually employed in the initial staging of lung cancer (Fig. 49.5). Evaluation should include assessment for intra- and/or extrathoracic lymphadenopathy, evaluation of pleural effusions for pleural nodules that may indicate malignancy, and examination of the chest wall for lytic or sclerotic skeletal lesions and soft tissue metastases. The upper abdomen should be scrutinized for hepatic lesions, lymphadenopathy, and adrenal enlargement. Abdominal abnormalities suspicious for malignancy should be further evaluated with dedicated abdominal imaging.

MRI is usually employed as a problem-solving tool in cases in which CT is equivocal. It is particularly useful for assessment of vascular invasion in patients in whom intravenous contrast is contraindicated and in selected cases of suspected chest wall involvement, including patients with Pancoast tumor, for assessment of vascular and brachial plexus involvement.

FDG PET/CT is the imaging modality of choice for staging lung cancer and is based on the metabolic activity of malignant neoplasms.

What Not to Miss

- All radiographs of patients with lung cancer should be assessed for subtle lymphadenopathy and chest wall involvement.
- Large and massive pleural effusions are highly suspicious for malignancy and should be thoroughly assessed for pleural thickening, nodules, or masses.

- Contrast-enhanced CT is the optimal modality for assessment of hilar lymphadenopathy and differentiation of abnormal lymph nodes from adjacent vessels (Fig. 49.6).
- Enlarged lymph nodes are not necessarily neoplastic, and normal lymph nodes may contain micrometastases.
- Indolent lung cancers may produce false-negative findings on FDG PET/CT, and infectious/inflammatory processes may produce false-positive findings.

Differential Diagnosis

T Designation
- Nodule: Granuloma, carcinoid, hamartoma, solitary metastasis, arteriovenous malformation
- Mass: Metastasis, lymphoma, lung abscess, intralobar sequestration
- Endoluminal lesion: Carcinoid, adenoid cystic carcinoma, mucoepidermoid carcinoma, hamartoma, lipoma, neurogenic neoplasm

N Designation
- Neoplastic lymphadenopathy: Metastases, lymphoma
- Non-neoplastic lymphadenopathy: Infection (fungal, mycobacterial), sarcoidosis, pneumoconiosis, Castleman disease

M Designation
- Pleura: Metastases, mesothelioma, lymphoma
- Chest wall: Metastases, myeloma, chondrosarcoma

Imaging Findings

T Designation
- Nodule: Size (largest dimension), relationship to pleura, location within airway
- Mass: Size (largest dimension), relationship to pleura, location of airway involvement, features of local invasion (mediastinum and its structures, chest wall)
- Assessment of extent of atelectasis associated with centrally obstructing lesions
- Identification and assessment of additional ipsilateral and/or contralateral lung nodules
- Contrast-enhanced CT for distinction of neoplasm from surrounding or adjacent atelectasis or consolidation
- MRI used for problem solving, particularly to determine locally invasive behavior. Whole body MR/PET may be comparable to FDG PET/CT for lung cancer staging.

N Designation
- Identification of hilar, mediastinal, supraclavicular, and scalene lymph nodes; short axis measurement
- Assessment of affected lymph node stations
- Identification of coalescent lymphadenopathy and locally invasive behavior
- Contrast-enhanced chest CT allows distinction of hilar lymph nodes from adjacent structures
- PET-CT for assessment of metabolic activity of suspicious lymph nodes

M Designation
- Assessment of pleura and pericardium for thickening, nodules, masses
- Assessment of skeleton for lytic or blastic metastases
- CT and FDG PET/CT for initial staging and post-treatment restaging

Clinical Issues

- Stage I and stage II lung cancers are resectable.
- Stage IIIA lung cancers are potentially resectable.
- Stage IIIB and stage IV lung cancers are unresectable, although stage IIIB may be "downstaged" with preoperative neoadjuvant chemotherapy.
- Stage IV lesions are treated with radiation and/or chemotherapy; select stage IV lung cancers with solitary adrenal or brain metastasis may be surgically treated (Fig. 49.7).
- CT better predicts resectability than unresectability because of limited ability to accurately determine mediastinal invasion and microscopic lymph node involvement. Surgical resection should be considered for limited mediastinal contact or preserved mediastinal fat plane on CT.
- Mediastinoscopy: Access to paratracheal and upper subcarinal lymph nodes.
- Chamberlain procedure or left parasternal mediastinotomy: Access to aortopulmonary and subaortic lymph nodes.
- Mediastinal lymph node spread of lung cancer is the most important determinant of surgical resectability.
- Small cell lung cancer is almost always treated medically. Limited disease may be treated with surgery and chemoradiation, whereas extensive disease is treated primarily with chemotherapy. Some patients in either group are treated with thoracic radiation therapy. Prophylactic cranial radiation may be beneficial in all patients.
- Most lung cancers metastasize to brain, bone, liver, and adrenal gland.

Key Points

- CT has limited accuracy for lung cancer staging (sensitivity and specificity of approximately 65%).
- Malignant pleural effusion is considered stage IVA disease as are contralateral metastatic lung nodules and single distant metastases. Multiple distant metastases are considered stage IVB disease.

- The TNM staging system does not fully address all thoracic lymph nodes (e.g., internal thoracic/mammary, diaphragmatic, and axillary), lymphangitic carcinomatosis, or concurrent pulmonary nodules (pathologically unconfirmed as malignant or benign).
- PET/CT has improved sensitivity and specificity to greater than 90% for detection of mediastinal lymph node involvement and has been shown to reduce futile thoracotomies.
- Because false-positive PET/CT occur, mediastinoscopy or endoscopic bronchial ultrasound biopsy should be performed prior to surgical resection to accurately assess mediastinal lymph node involvement.

Suggested Reading

Asamura H, Chansky K. Crowley J, et al. The International Association for the Study of Lung Cancer lung cancer staging project. Proposals for the revision for the N descriptors in the forthcoming 8th edition of the TNM classification for lung cancer. *J Thorac Oncol.* 2015;10:1675–1684.

Colt HG, Murgu SD, Korst RJ, Slatore CG, Unger M, Quadrelli S. Follow-up and surveillance of the patient with lung cancer after curative-intent therapy: Diagnosis and management of lung cancer, 3rd ed.: American College of Chest Physicians evidence-based clinical practice guidelines. *Chest.* 2013;143 (5 Suppl):e437S–e454S.

Detterbeck FC, Boffa DJ, Kim AW, et al. The eighth edition lung cancer stage classification. *Chest.* 2017;151(1):193–203.

Goldstraw P, Chansky K, Crowley J, The IASCL lung cancer staging project: Proposals for revision of the TNM stage groupings in the forthcoming (eighth) edition of the TNM classification for lung cancer. *J Thorac Oncol.* 2016;11(1):39–51.

CHAPTER 50

Bronchial Carcinoids and Bronchial Gland Carcinomas

Ryo E. C. Benson

Definition

Bronchial carcinoid is a rare low-grade malignant neuroendocrine neoplasm comprising 1%–2% of primary lung malignancies. Most carcinoids occur in the abdomen, and the lung is the second most common location. Pulmonary carcinoids are thought to originate from Kulchitsky (neuroendocrine) cells in the bronchial mucosa. The majority are typical carcinoids (TCs) characterized by the absence of necrosis and less than 2 mitoses per 10 high power fields (HPF). Atypical carcinoids (ACs) account for 10–16% of cases, may exhibit necrosis, and/or have 2–10 mitoses/HPF. Carcinoids exhibit reactivity to immunohistochemical markers. Pulmonary carcinoids are rarely associated with tumorlets and diffuse idiopathic pulmonary neuroendocrine cell hyperplasia (DIPNECH). Tumorlets invade the bronchial basement membrane and measure less than 5 mm. DIPNECH is a neuroendocrine cell proliferation confined to the bronchial epithelium and measures less than 5 mm.

Bronchial gland carcinomas include adenoid cystic carcinoma (ACC) and mucoepidermoid carcinoma (MEC). These malignancies arise in the submucosal regions of the central airways and preferentially affect the trachea and central bronchi, respectively.

Clinical Features

Bronchial carcinoids affect patients of any age with equal gender distribution. Patients with TCs are usually in their mid-40s and are a decade younger than those with ACs. Carcinoid is the most common primary lung malignancy of childhood and may affect adolescents. Presenting symptoms include recurrent infection, cough, hemoptysis, wheezing, chest pain, dyspnea, and constitutional symptoms. Patients with peripheral tumors are often asymptomatic. Pulmonary carcinoids are rarely associated with paraneoplastic syndromes, carcinoid syndrome, or carcinoid heart disease. Patients with DIPNECH are usually elderly women with chronic cough or dyspnea, but they may also be asymptomatic.

ACC is the second most common primary tracheal malignancy (after squamous cell carcinoma). Affected patients exhibit a wide age range at presentation but are typically 30–50 years of age. Patients with tracheobronchial ACC may present with cough, stridor, wheezing, hemoptysis, and/or chest pain.

MEC is a rare primary lung neoplasm that characteristically involves the segmental bronchi. Affected patients are typically younger than age 40 years.

The intimate association with cigarette smoking seen in cases of lung cancer is not documented with carcinoids or bronchial gland carcinomas. Treatment is complete surgical resection. Patient prognosis varies with tumor histology, tumor grade, and the feasibility of complete excision.

Anatomy and Physiology

Grossly, carcinoid tumors and bronchial gland carcinomas are well-defined central lesions with an airway relationship and frequent airway wall invasion. ACCs preferentially affect the trachea. Because these lesions arise deep in the bronchial mucosa, they often exhibit well-defined borders on imaging. The central location of these neoplasms explains the frequency of atelectasis and post-obstructive pneumonitis caused by increasing degrees of airway obstruction.

How to Approach the Image

- Carcinoid may be missed on radiography when manifesting as an endoluminal nodule (Fig. 50.1).
- Carcinoid may exhibit indirect findings of obstruction, including recurrent consolidation or atelectasis (Fig. 50.2).
- Contrast-enhanced chest CT allows differentiation of enhancing central tumor from adjacent atelectasis/consolidation.
- ACCs typically affect the trachea and may be missed on radiography.
- MEC may also affect the trachea but typically affects segmental bronchi and may be indistinguishable from carcinoid.
- Careful analysis of the central airways on radiography and CT is mandatory for detecting airway-associated lesions.

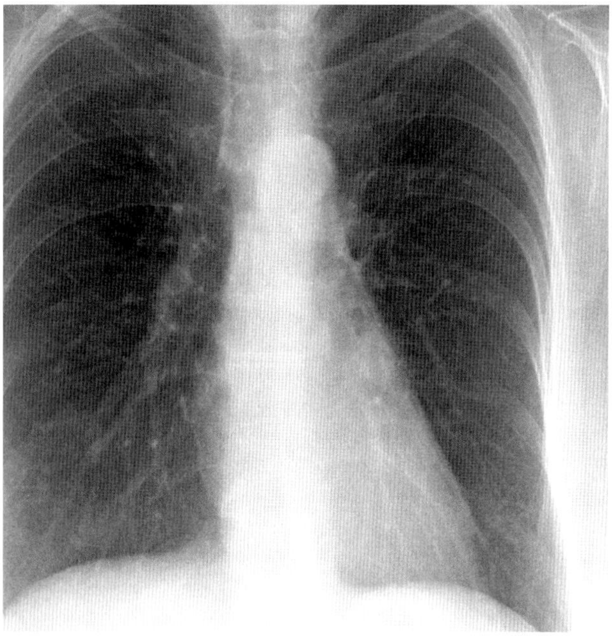

Figure 50.1. Central carcinoid. Posteroanterior (PA) chest radiograph shows a carcinoid tumor manifesting as an endoluminal nodule that obliterates the left lower lobe bronchus lumen. Prospective diagnosis of such cases requires careful evaluation of the airways on radiography.

What Not to Miss

- Recurrent infection or atelectasis in the same pulmonary lobe should suggest an endoluminal obstructing lesion.

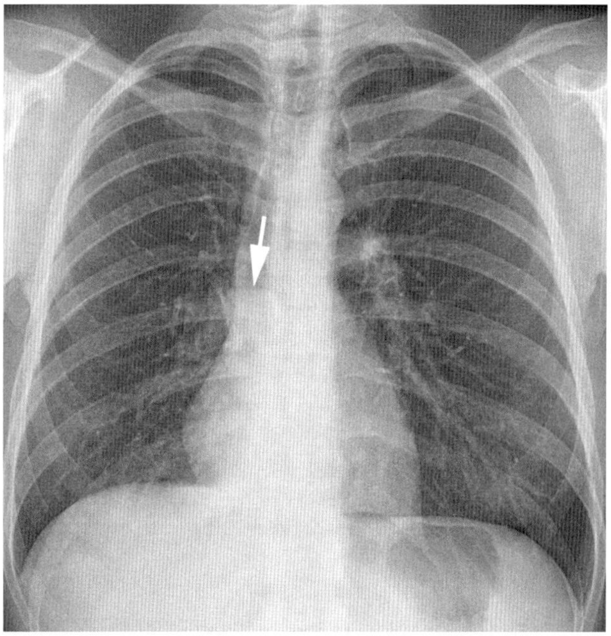

Figure 50.2. Central carcinoid. PA chest radiograph shows subtle right lower lobe opacity related to volume loss secondary to a centrally obstructing carcinoid. The superior aspect of the tumor is visible within the bronchus intermedius (arrow).
Source: Courtesy C. W. Walker, MD.

- In such cases, contrast-enhanced CT will allow optimal evaluation of the central airways and identification of endoluminal nodules or partially endoluminal masses.
- Patients with upper airway complaints or stridor should be evaluated for tracheal abnormalities including neoplasms. The tracheal lumen may be reduced by 75% before upper airway symptoms occur.

Differential Diagnosis

Endobronchial Lesion

- Mucous plug: Most common airway pseudotumor; exhibits low attenuation and no enhancement on CT
- Broncholith: Completely calcified; remote granulomatous disease (calcified granulomas) elsewhere
- Hamartoma: Rare benign neoplasm; may exhibit fat and/or calcification
- Other mesenchymal neoplasm: Lipoma and neurogenic neoplasm

Tracheal Lesion

- Squamous cell carcinoma (SCC): Most common primary malignant tracheal neoplasm; patients older at presentation (50–60 years) than those with ACC, almost all are smokers; male-to-female ratio of 4:1
- Squamous cell papilloma: Common benign central airway tumor; typically affects male smokers
- Laryngotracheal papillomatosis: Solitary or multiple endoluminal tracheobronchial tumors; may exhibit nodular surface irregularity and thin-walled cavities when involving the lung

Solitary Pulmonary Nodule

- Granuloma: May exhibit central, laminar, or complete calcification; often associated with calcified hilar/mediastinal lymph nodes
- Lung cancer: May manifest as solitary nodule; may exhibit airway relationship; may exhibit calcification
- Solitary metastasis: Rare; metastases typically multifocal angiocentric pulmonary nodules
- Hamartoma: Rare; may exhibit fat and/or calcification; popcorn calcification may be diagnostic
- Arteriovenous malformation: Feeding and draining vessel(s); contrast enhancement equal to that of other pulmonary vessels

Imaging Findings

Carcinoid

Radiography

- Indirect features of central obstruction: Chronic or recurrent atelectasis/pneumonia
- Endoluminal nodule/mass, central nodule/mass

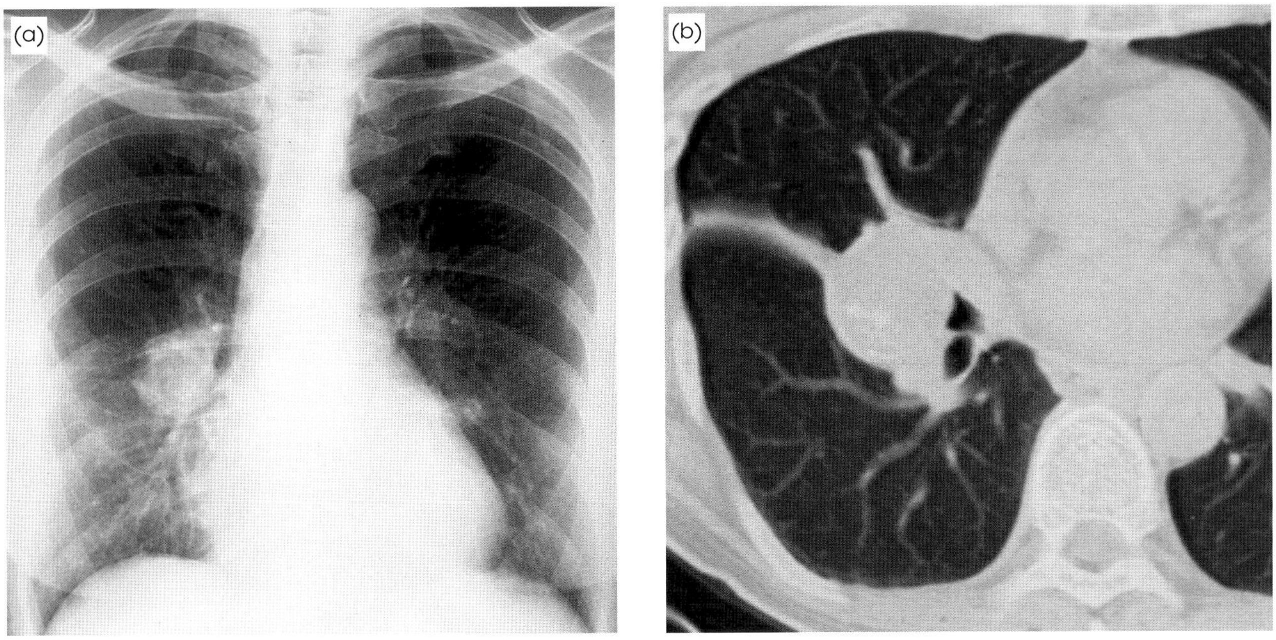

Figure 50.3. Central carcinoid. (a) PA chest radiograph demonstrates a well-circumscribed polylobular right hilar mass. (b) Unenhanced chest CT (lung window) of the same patient shows a well-defined spherical tumor with an endoluminal component in the middle lobe bronchus. The lesion exhibits intrinsic punctate calcification seen in approximately 30% of bronchial carcinoids.

CT

- Well-defined, smooth or lobular nodule or mass; size range of 2–5 cm (average size, 3 cm)
- Central location: Completely endoluminal, partially endoluminal ("tip of the iceberg"), or abutting airway (Fig. 50.3)
- Central nodule/mass with post-obstructive atelectasis, consolidation, mucoid impaction, or bronchiectasis
- Bronchus sign: Bronchus leading to tumor (Fig. 50.4)
- Contrast enhancement: Allows distinction of neoplasm from surrounding atelectasis or consolidation (Fig. 50.5)

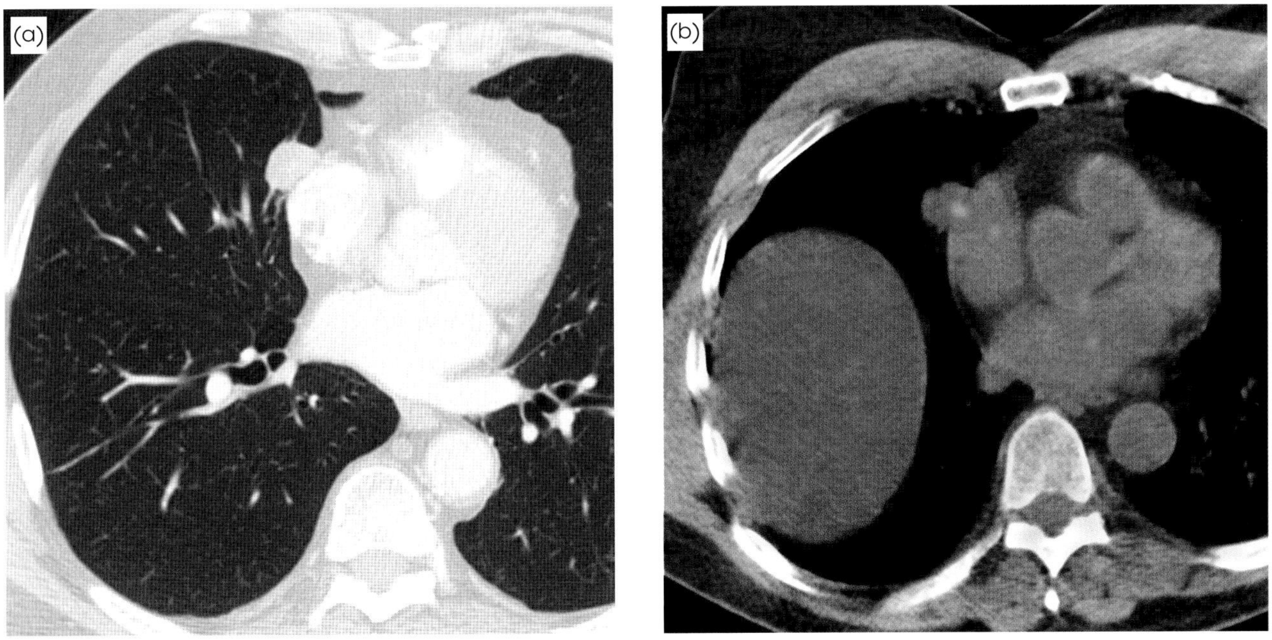

Figure 50.4. Typical carcinoid. Bronchus sign. (a) Contrast-enhanced chest CT shows a carcinoid manifesting as a middle lobe nodule. A branch of the middle lobe medial segmental bronchus courses into the lesion—the so-called bronchus sign. (b) Fused FDG PET/CT of the same patient demonstrates mildly increased FDG uptake in the nodule, with maximum standardized uptake value = 3.4.

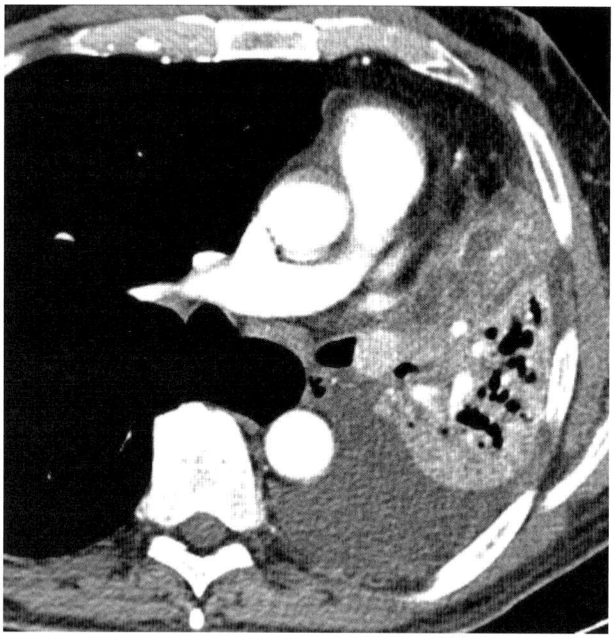

Figure 50.5. Central carcinoid. Contrast-enhanced chest CT shows a homogeneously and intensely enhancing endobronchial carcinoid in the left mainstem bronchus with associated left lung post-obstructive atelectasis and bronchiectasis and a moderate left pleural effusion.

- Calcification in approximately 30%; more common in larger and central tumors (Fig. 50.6)
- TC and AC often indistinguishable: AC more common in the periphery, larger in size, and more likely to be associated with lymphadenopathy

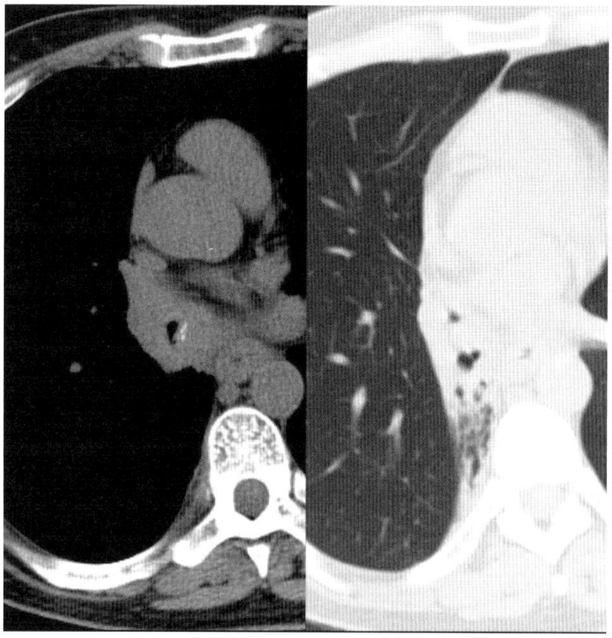

Figure 50.6. Central carcinoid. Composite image with unenhanced chest CT in soft tissue (left) and lung (right) window shows a carcinoid tumor with intrinsic calcifications that narrows the bronchus intermedius and produces severe right lower lobe atelectasis.

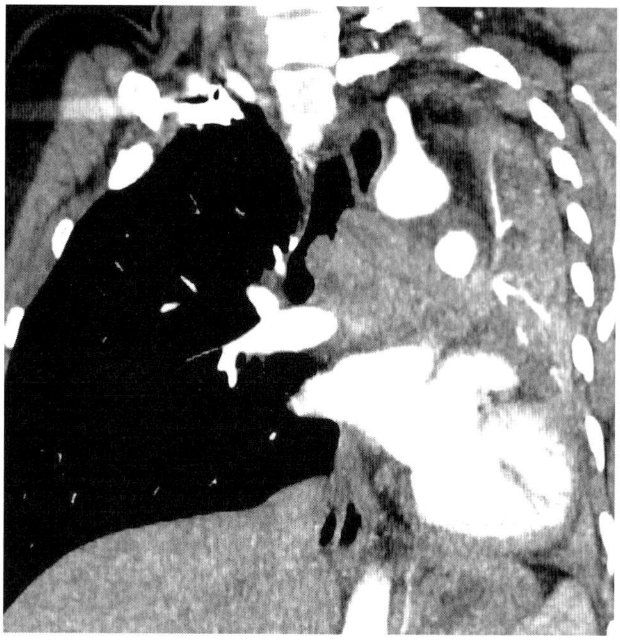

Figure 50.7. Adenoid cystic carcinoma. Coronal contrast-enhanced chest CT of a patient with adenoid cystic carcinoma shows a large polylobular tumor of the distal trachea, which produces complete obstruction of the left mainstem bronchus and complete left lung atelectasis.

- With widespread utilization of multidetector CT, incidental detection of greater numbers of peripheral carcinoids reported

Nuclear Scintigraphy

- FDG PET/CT: Variable FDG uptake; often insignificant uptake

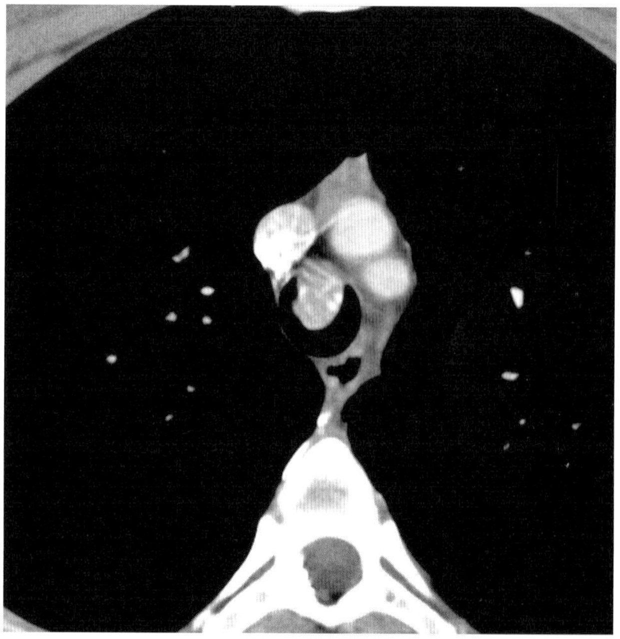

Figure 50.8. Mucoepidermoid carcinoma. Contrast-enhanced chest CT demonstrates an enhancing nodule arising from the anterior tracheal wall with intrinsic punctate calcifications. Although mucoepidermoid carcinoma often affects the bronchi, it may also arise in the trachea.

- Octreotide (somatostatin analog) scintigraphy for carcinoids with somatostatin receptors

ACC

- Smooth, lobular, or irregular endoluminal nodule versus circumferential tracheal narrowing (Fig. 50.7)
- More readily detected on CT than radiography. Multiplanar reformations demonstrate airway narrowing, mural and mediastinal fat infiltration, circumferential airway wall thickening, or stenosis.
- Multiplanar imaging allows determination of length of airway involvement.

MEC

- Similar imaging characteristics as carcinoid (Fig. 50.8)
- Frequent (50%) punctate calcifications
- Ovoid, smooth, or lobulated endobronchial lesion paralleling airways with preferential involvement of segmental airways

Clinical Issues

- Good prognosis for completely resected TCs, with 5-year survival of 87–100%.
- Five-year survival of patients with ACs of 44–88% due to lymph node metastases. Long-term follow-up is recommended.
- Good prognosis for patients with DIPNECH, with 5-year survival of 83%. Many patients do not require treatment. A minority of patients progress to respiratory failure and death.
- Long-term survival for patients with ACC is 40% at 15 years due to slow growth and propensity for local recurrence.
- Five-year survival of patients with completely resected MEC is 92–100%, especially for low-grade lesions.

Key Points

- A well-defined central neoplasm in a young patient should suggest the diagnosis of carcinoid tumor.
- Carcinoid manifests as a well-defined lesion on CT that may exhibit an airway relationship and typically enhances with contrast, allowing distinction from adjacent atelectasis or consolidation.
- SCC is the most common primary tracheal malignancy, followed by ACC. The latter affects patients who are younger than those with SCC.
- MEC is a rare malignancy that predominantly affects segmental airways and may be indistinguishable from carcinoid.

Suggested Reading

Benson RE, Rosado-de-Christenson ML, Martínez-Jiménez S, Kunin JR, Pettavel PP. Spectrum of pulmonary neuroendocrine proliferation and neoplasms. *RadioGraphics*. 2013;33:1631–1649.

Ferretti GR, Bithigoffer C, Righini CA, Arbib F, Lantuejoul S, Jankowski A. Imaging of tumors of the trachea and central bronchi. *Radiol Clin North Am*. 2009;47:227–241.

Jeung MY, Gasser B, Gangi A, et al. Bronchial carcinoid tumors of the thorax: Spectrum of radiologic findings. *RadioGraphics*. 2002;22:351–365.

CHAPTER 51

Pulmonary Metastases

Tyler H. Ternes

Definition

Pulmonary metastases represent spread of malignancy to the lung parenchyma.

Clinical Features

The clinical presentation of patients with pulmonary metastases is highly variable. Many patients with a few small pulmonary metastases are asymptomatic. However, with increased number and size of metastatic foci, affected patients may develop dyspnea, cough, and/or hemoptysis. Some patients may present with chest pain, particularly in the setting of tumor emboli and associated pulmonary infarcts.

Metastatic disease to the lungs may be the initial manifestation of disease in a patient not previously known to have cancer. Alternatively, metastases may be found as part of the evaluation of a newly diagnosed extrathoracic malignancy. The lungs are a common site for metastatic disease. Breast, colon, lung, and kidney cancers are the most common causes of pulmonary metastases because they represent some of the most common primary malignancies. However, some less prevalent neoplasms have a high likelihood to produce lung metastases, including choriocarcinoma, testicular tumors, melanoma, osteosarcoma, and Ewing sarcoma. Due to the greatly increased rates of cancer in adults, metastatic disease is inherently much more common in older populations.

Anatomy and Physiology

Aside from lymphadenopathy and pleural metastases (which are discussed elsewhere), there are three main routes by which neoplasm spreads within the chest: the airways, the bloodstream, and the lymphatics. The vast majority of pulmonary metastases disseminate to the lungs via the bloodstream (hematogenously), typically a basilar predominant process, given the dominant pulmonary blood flow to the lower lung zones (Fig. 51.1). Endobronchial spread of tumor also occurs, but it is relatively uncommon. It may result from hematogenous seeding of the airway, direct airway invasion by an adjacent neoplasm, and, much less commonly, via tracheobronchial dissemination from other airway tumors. Lymphangitic carcinomatosis represents tumor invasion of the pulmonary lymphatics. This can result from hematogenous metastatic disease and subsequent involvement of lymphatics by tumor in adjacent pulmonary arteries, retrograde lymphatic invasion from affected hilar lymph nodes, or direct lymphatic invasion by an adjacent malignancy (e.g., lung cancer).

How to Approach the Image

- Any pulmonary nodule in a patient with known malignancy should be carefully evaluated, with comparison to previous examinations if available.
- CT has been shown to have higher sensitivity for nodule detection than radiography; therefore, it should be the modality of choice for patients undergoing workup for metastatic disease.
- The most sensitive imaging study for complete evaluation of the extent of metastatic disease is FDG PET/CT due to the fact that most malignant neoplasms are FDG avid. However, PET/CT is approved only for selected clinical scenarios, currently including assessment of solitary pulmonary nodules, lymphoma, melanoma, and cancers of the lung, esophagus, colon, breast, and head and neck.

What Not to Miss

The radiologist should carefully look for findings that may suggest metastatic disease on chest imaging studies of patients with known malignancy:

- Any suspicious pulmonary nodule (Fig. 51.1).
- Irregular interlobular septal thickening, representing lymphangitic carcinomatosis (Fig. 51.2).
- Pulmonary artery filling defects typically represent bland thrombus but may rarely represent endovascular metastases and should prompt careful evaluation for other signs of metastatic disease.

Differential Diagnosis

Infection

- Clinical signs of infection are typically present.
- Several infections may manifest with pulmonary nodules.

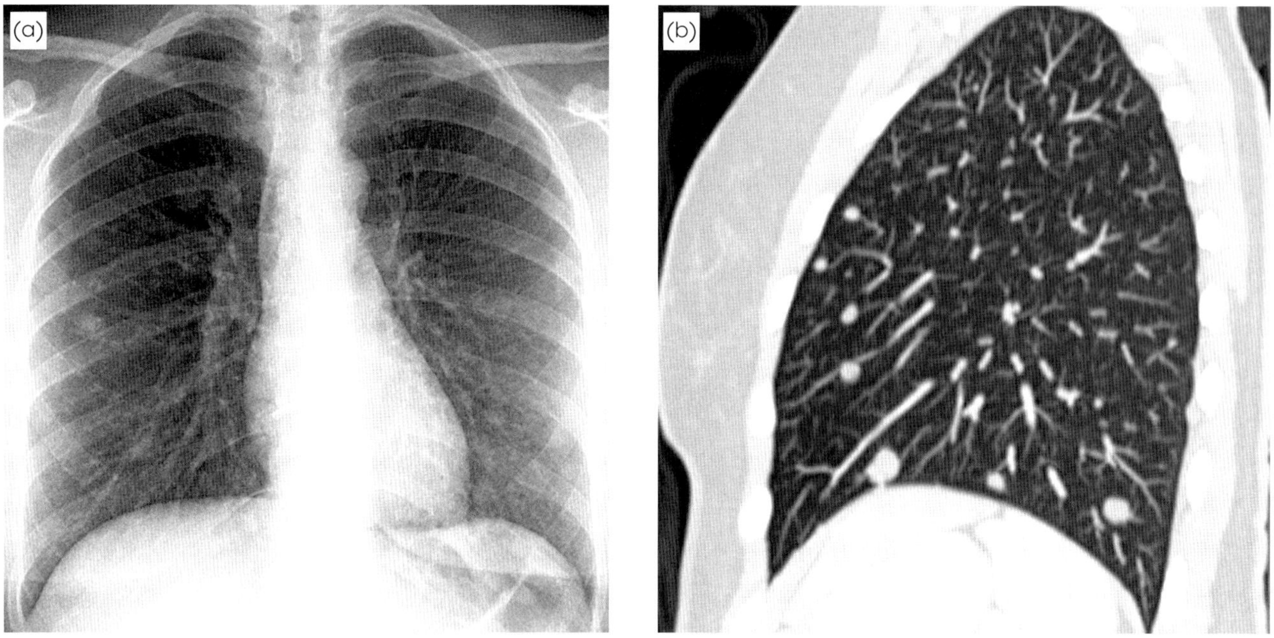

Figure 51.1. Hematogenous metastases. (a) Posteroanterior (PA) chest radiograph of a 62-year-old woman with progressive cough and small cell lung cancer shows multiple bilateral lower lung zone predominant rounded indeterminate pulmonary nodules. (b) Sagittal contrast-enhanced chest CT maximum intensity projection image of the same patient shows multiple basilar predominant pulmonary nodules that represented hematogenous metastases. Basilar predominance of hematogenous metastases is common due to preferential pulmonary blood flow to the lung bases.

- Remote infection may manifest as granulomas, which are often calcified.

Septic Emboli

- Signs and symptoms of systemic infection are typically present.
- There may be a history of illicit drug use, and sources may include poor dentition and infected heart valves.
- These are typically multiple peripheral lung nodules, often demonstrating cavitation.

Primary Lung Cancer

- Single pulmonary nodule/mass
- May exhibit associated hilar or mediastinal lymphadenopathy
- Mimics a solitary pulmonary metastasis

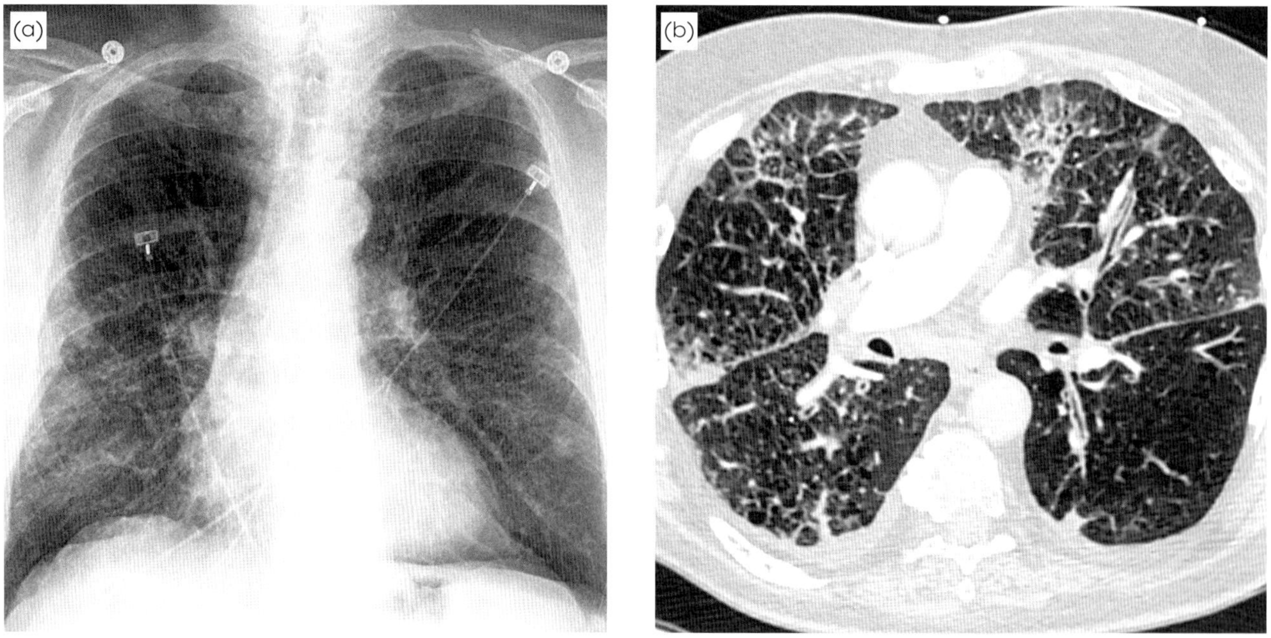

Figure 51.2. Lymphangitic carcinomatosis. (a) PA chest radiograph of a 79-year-old man with prostate cancer and progressive dyspnea shows bilateral asymmetric reticular opacities. (b) Contrast-enhanced chest CT of the same patient shows asymmetric interlobular septal thickening, bronchial wall thickening, and trace bilateral pleural fluid.

Granulomatosis with Polyangiitis

- Multiple bilateral pulmonary nodules, masses, or consolidations, often cavitary
- Pulmonary hemorrhage manifesting as ground-glass opacity surrounding pulmonary nodules (CT halo sign)

Pulmonary Edema

- Interlobular septal thickening, typically smooth and diffuse; lymphangitic carcinomatosis often exhibits asymmetric nodular interlobular septal thickening
- Bronchial wall thickening
- Pleural effusions are very common
- May exhibit reactive lymph node enlargement

Sarcoidosis

- Perilymphatic nodules/micronodules and frequent symmetric lymphadenopathy
- Typically spares lung bases, whereas hematogenous metastases do not

Imaging Findings

Hematogenous Metastases

- Lung metastases are typically hematogenous and often manifest as peripheral basilar predominant lung nodules given the dominant blood flow of the lung (Fig. 51.1). Several imaging patterns are described.

Miliary Nodules

- Very small nodules (< 3 mm), usually innumerable (Fig. 51.3)

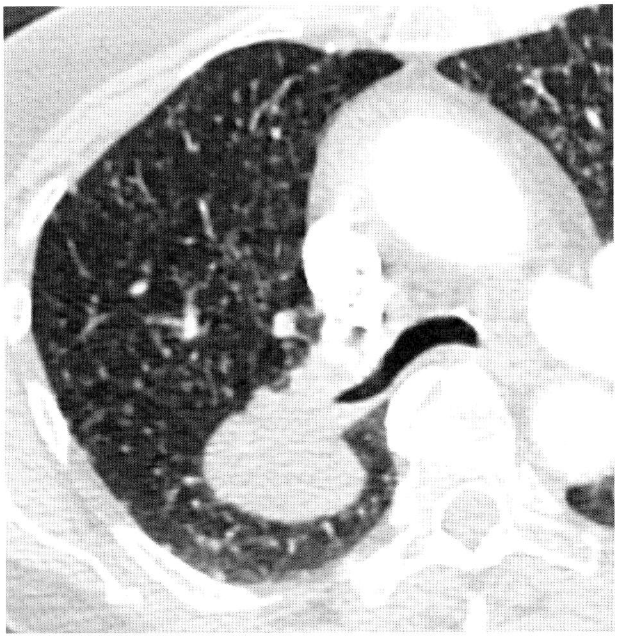

Figure 51.3. Miliary metastases. Contrast-enhanced chest CT of a 60-year-old man with right upper lobe lung cancer shows innumerable miliary lung nodules representing hematogenous pulmonary metastases.

- Medullary thyroid carcinoma, renal cell carcinoma, and melanoma

"Cannonball" Metastases

- Implies multiple large spherical lesions
- Sarcoma, colorectal carcinoma, testicular carcinoma, and renal cell carcinoma

Solitary Pulmonary Nodule

- Rare manifestation of metastatic disease
- Melanoma, sarcoma, colorectal carcinoma, and renal cell carcinoma

CT Halo Sign

- Ground-glass opacity surrounding a solid nodule or mass (Fig. 51.4)
- Indicates surrounding hemorrhage
- Medullary thyroid carcinoma, renal cell carcinoma, choriocarcinoma, or melanoma

Airspace Opacities

- Appearance of consolidation or airspace disease that mimics pneumonia
- Lepidic growth (preserved alveolar walls)
- Adenocarcinoma

Cavitary Nodules or Masses

- Nodules with central lucency (Fig. 51.5)
- Squamous cell carcinoma, adenocarcinoma, and sarcoma

Calcified Nodules or Masses

- Various patterns of calcification
- Osteosarcoma, chondrosarcoma, papillary thyroid carcinoma, and mucinous adenocarcinoma
- Some neoplasms will also calcify following treatment.

Tumor Emboli

- May manifest as filling defects in small or medium-sized arteries similar to pulmonary thromboemboli
- Beading of subsegmental vessels, tree-in-bud opacities: mosaic attenuation due to areas of decreased blood flow
- Sarcoma, renal cell carcinoma, hepatocellular carcinoma, and melanoma

Lymphangitic Carcinomatosis

- Interlobular septal thickening and thickening of the axial interstitium that may be smooth or nodular and is often asymmetric (Fig. 51.2)
- Lung cancer, breast cancer, and several gastrointestinal/genitourinary adenocarcinomas

Endobronchial Metastases

- Lobar or segmental atelectasis
- Endobronchial lesion(s) (Fig. 51.6)

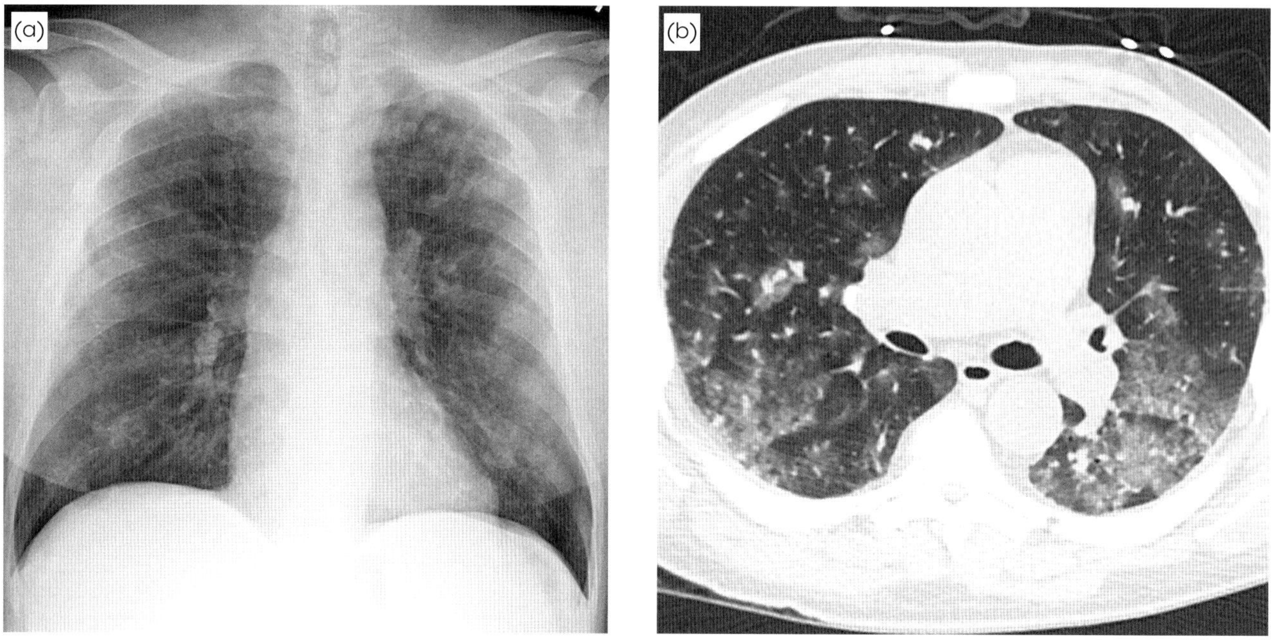

Figure 51.4. Hemorrhagic metastases. (a) PA chest radiograph of a 58-year-old man with prostate cancer and progressive dyspnea and hemoptysis shows multifocal heterogeneous airspace opacities, for which there is a broad differential diagnosis not limited to infection and metastatic disease. (b) Unenhanced chest CT of the same patient shows bilateral multifocal solid nodules and ground-glass opacities. Biopsy confirmed metastatic prostate cancer. The ground-glass opacities represented pulmonary hemorrhage surrounding metastatic foci.

- Mimic primary lung cancer
- Lung cancer, renal cell carcinoma, melanoma, breast cancer, head and neck cancer, and several adenocarcinomas

Clinical Issues

- The presence of pulmonary metastases is in general regarded as stage IV disease and therefore represents unresectable disease.

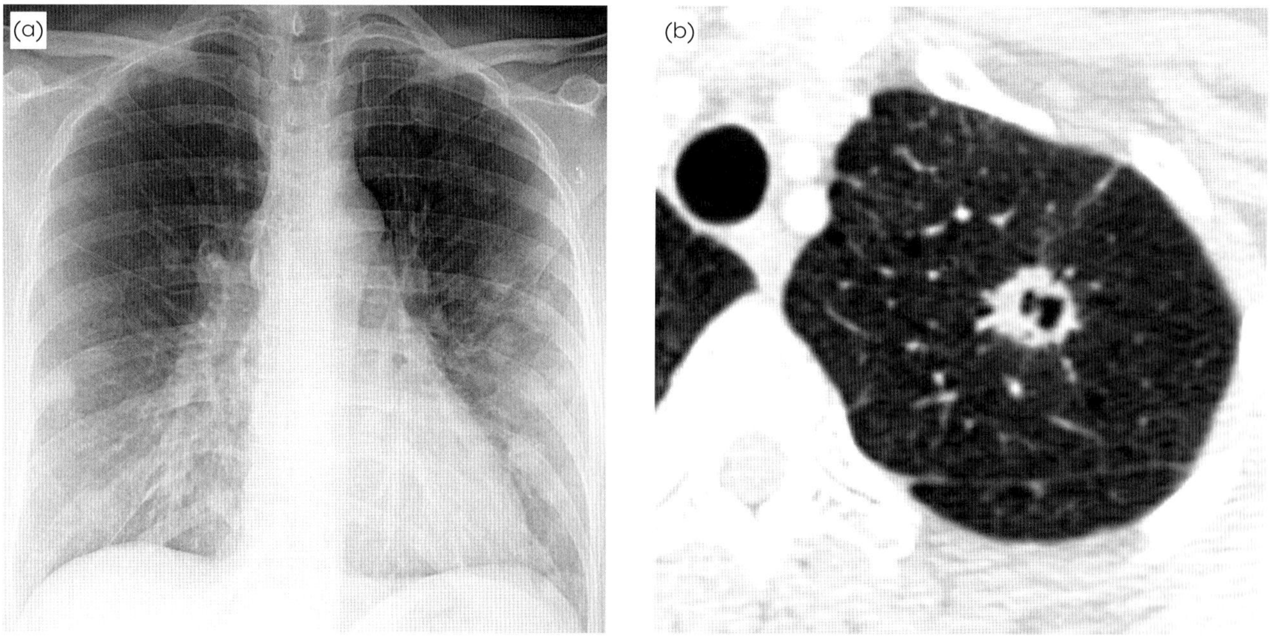

Figure 51.5. Cavitary metastases. (a) PA chest radiograph of a 57-year-old woman with cough and a history of breast cancer shows numerous bilateral pulmonary nodules that represented pulmonary metastases. (b) Contrast-enhanced chest CT of the same patient demonstrates one of many pulmonary nodules in the left upper lobe that exhibits spiculation and central cavitation. Lung biopsy confirmed metastatic disease.

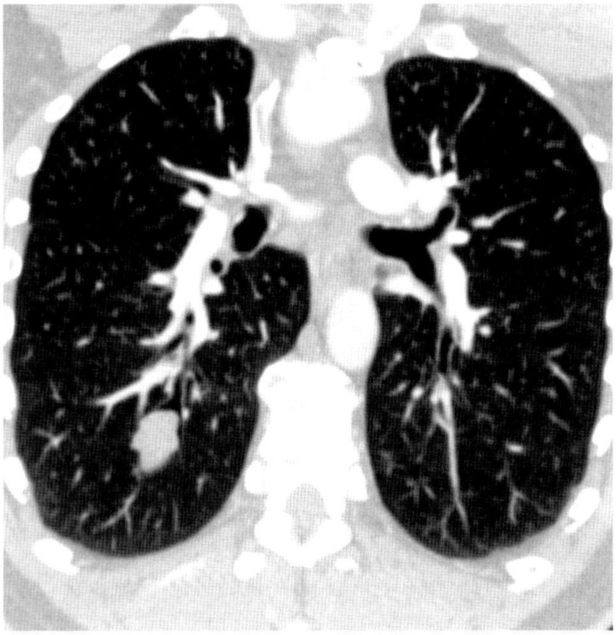

Figure 51.6. Endobronchial metastasis. Oblique axial contrast-enhanced chest CT of a patient with metastatic sarcoma shows a polyobular nodule within the right lower lobe posterior basilar segmental bronchus diagnosed as an endobronchial metastasis on biopsy.

- Prognosis is dependent on the cell type of the primary malignancy because some have better chemotherapeutic responses.
- In the setting of metastatic disease isolated to the lungs, with one or very few lesions, a metastasectomy may be considered.

Key Points

- Pulmonary metastatic disease most often manifests as numerous pulmonary nodules with basilar and peripheral predominance.
- The majority of pulmonary metastases are due to hematogenous spread of malignancy.
- Asymmetric interlobular septal and thickening of the axial interstitium are concerning for lymphangitic carcinomatosis.
- CT is superior to chest radiography for detection and evaluation of metastatic disease. FDG PET/CT has increased sensitivity in the evaluation of extent of disease progression.

Suggested Reading

Aquino SL. Imaging of metastatic disease to the thorax. *Radiol Clin North Am.* 2005;43(3):481–495.

Seo JB, Im JG, Goo JM, Chung MJ, Kim MY. Atypical pulmonary metastases: Spectrum of radiologic findings. *RadioGraphics.* 2001;21(2):403–417.

CHAPTER 52

Hamartoma and Benign Tumor-like Lesions

Tyler H. Ternes

Definition

Pulmonary hamartoma is a benign pulmonary neoplasm that contains various mesenchymal components, including cartilage, calcium, fat, epithelial cells, and smooth muscle. Hamartoma accounts for the majority of benign lung tumors, and although it was previously thought to represent a congenital lesion, it is now classified as a benign true neoplasm of mesenchymal origin.

Other rare benign lesions may arise in the airways or lung parenchyma. Pulmonary chondromas are considered a distinct type of mesenchymal neoplasm and differ from hamartoma in that they are composed almost entirely of cartilage, whereas hamartoma contains a greater variety of tissues.

Lipomas are rare, typically occur in the central airways, and are composed entirely of fat. Leiomyomas are rare benign neoplasms believed to arise from the smooth muscle of the bronchial walls or blood vessels. Neurogenic neoplasms are rare and may arise in the lung or in the airways.

Clinical Features

Hamartomas most frequently affect patients in the sixth decade of life, and men have a two- or threefold increased incidence compared to women. Most hamartomas are discovered incidentally on chest imaging. Symptoms are rare, typically occur with central lesions, and include cough, hemoptysis, and recurrent pneumonia. Hamartomas demonstrate a very slow growth rate. The potential for malignant transformation is exceptionally low.

Patients with the Carney triad may develop pulmonary chondromas in addition to gastric leiomyosarcomas and extra-adrenal paragangliomas.

Anatomy and Physiology

Pulmonary hamartomas are well-encapsulated lesions and are easily "shelled out" from the surrounding normal lung parenchyma. Histologic analysis reveals a variety of tissue components including cartilage, which may exhibit chondroid calcification, fat, epithelial tissues, and smooth muscle. Most hamartomas are located in the lung periphery. However, up to 20% occur centrally within a bronchus. Most hamartomas are less than 4 cm in size. Hamartomas and other benign pulmonary neoplasms may arise within the airway lumen and may produce airway obstruction, which may lead to atelectasis and consolidation.

How to Approach the Image

The vast majority of pulmonary hamartomas are incidentally discovered on imaging studies obtained for other reasons. A careful inspection of the chest radiograph is mandatory for the detection of small, often subtle indeterminate pulmonary nodules. Each nodule should be evaluated for the presence or absence of calcification and, when present, the pattern of calcification must be analyzed. A minority of hamartomas (15%) demonstrate radiographic evidence of calcification. A classic pattern is "popcorn" calcification.

The majority of lung nodules found on radiography will require further evaluation with chest CT. Use of thin-section CT (1 mm) is imperative to identify subtle calcifications and avoid errors in attenuation values attributable to volume averaging. Approximately 60% of hamartomas exhibit macroscopic fat (−40 to −120 HU). Up to 15% of hamartomas demonstrate classic popcorn calcification on CT. Although nodules are often identified on "lung window," "soft tissue" window settings allow easier identification of calcium or fat (Figs. 52.1–52.4).

What Not to Miss

When evaluating pulmonary nodules with CT, the radiologist must determine the presence or absence of the following:

- *Fat* helps confirm a benign etiology and may be diagnostic of hamartoma.
- *Calcification* must be further characterized as benign or malignant (Fig. 52.5); popcorn calcification suggests a hamartoma.

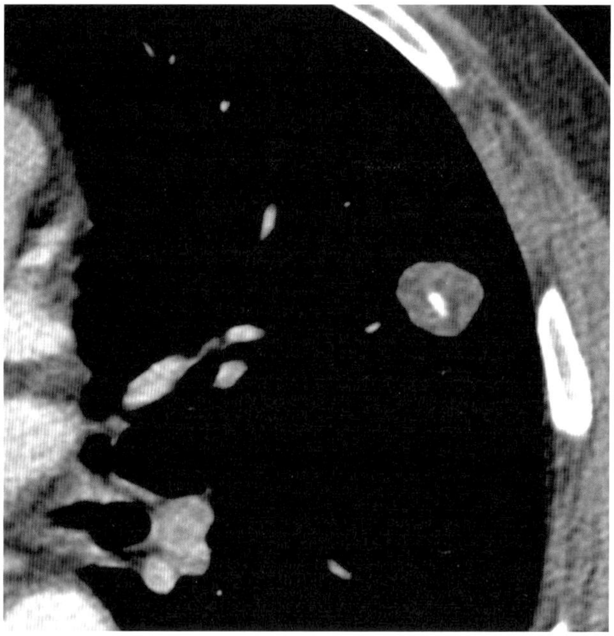

Figure 52.1. Hamartoma. Contrast-enhanced chest CT of an asymptomatic 57-year-old man shows a left upper lobe hamartoma manifesting as a lung nodule with central calcification and subtle fat attenuation foci. In cases with subtle or equivocal fat attenuation, tissue diagnosis may be required to exclude malignancy.

- *Sequela of endobronchial obstruction* by hamartoma, including post-obstructive atelectasis, pulmonary hemorrhage, and infection.
- *Other neoplasms* to suggest Carney triad in the setting of newly diagnosed pulmonary chondroma: gastric leiomyosarcoma and extra-adrenal paraganglioma.

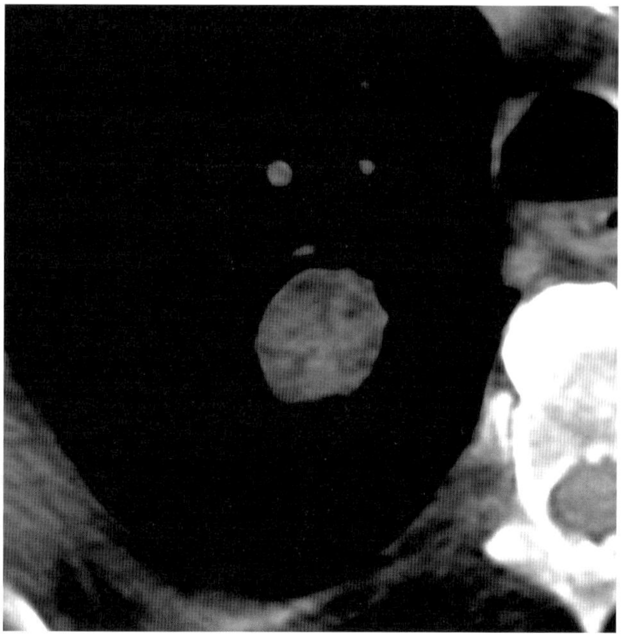

Figure 52.2. Hamartoma. Unenhanced chest CT of an asymptomatic 81-year-old man shows a right upper lobe nodule with intrinsic low-attenuation foci due to macroscopic fat, highly suggestive of hamartoma.

Differential Diagnosis

The differential diagnosis of a solitary pulmonary nodule includes common benign conditions, malignant lung neoplasms, and pulmonary hamartomas.

Primary Lung Cancer

- Often manifests as a solitary pulmonary nodule or mass

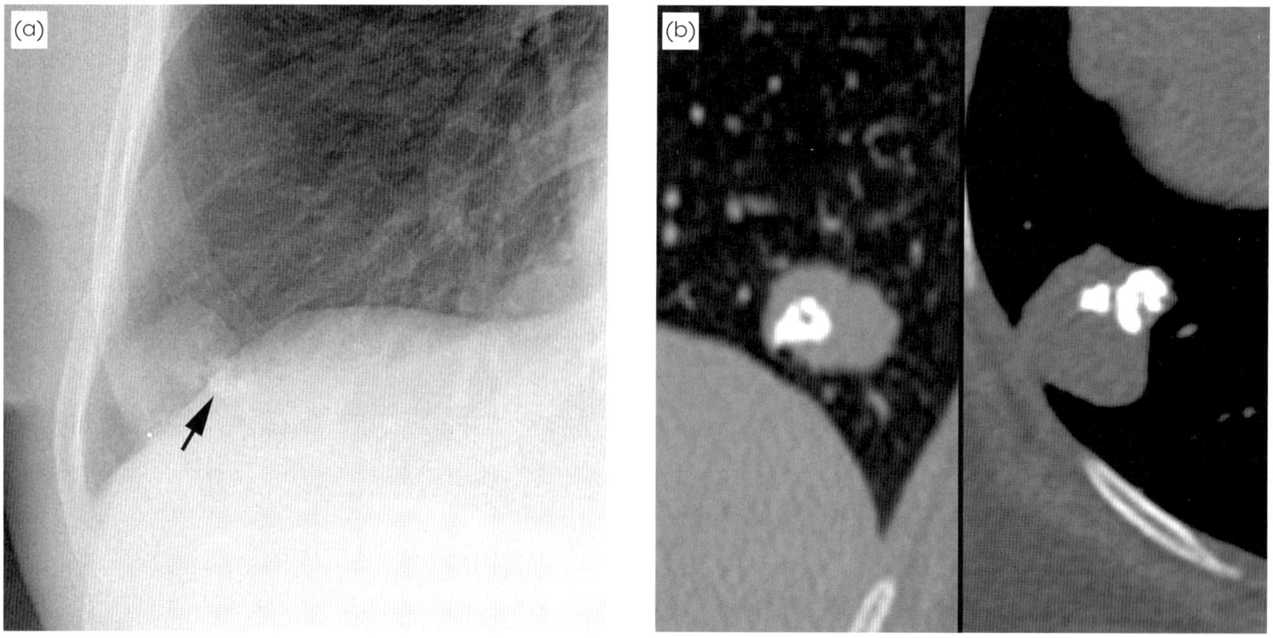

Figure 52.3. Hamartoma with popcorn calcification. (a) Coned-down posteroanterior (PA) chest radiograph of an asymptomatic 66-year-old woman shows an ill-defined right lower lobe nodule with intrinsic "popcorn"-like calcification (arrow). (b) Composite image with sagittal (left) and axial (right) unenhanced chest CT of the same patient shows a polylobular right lower lobe soft tissue nodule with intrinsic eccentric "rings and arcs" cartilage-like calcification consistent with pulmonary hamartoma.

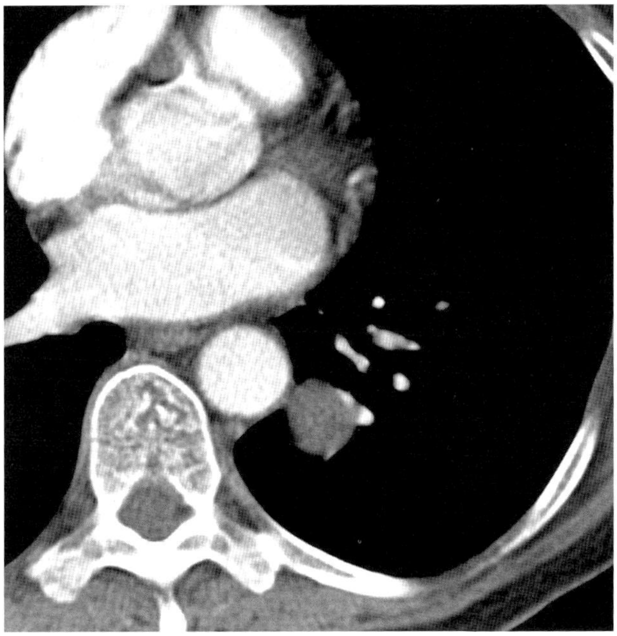

Figure 52.4. Hamartoma. Contrast-enhanced chest CT of a 61-year-old man with cough shows an indeterminate left lower lobe nodule diagnosed as a hamartoma after surgical excision. Fat and cartilaginous calcification are not always present, and further workup is warranted to exclude malignancy.

- Does not exhibit intrinsic fat but may demonstrate calcification (Fig. 52.5)
- May exhibit aggressive morphologic features, including lobular or spiculated margins and pleural tags

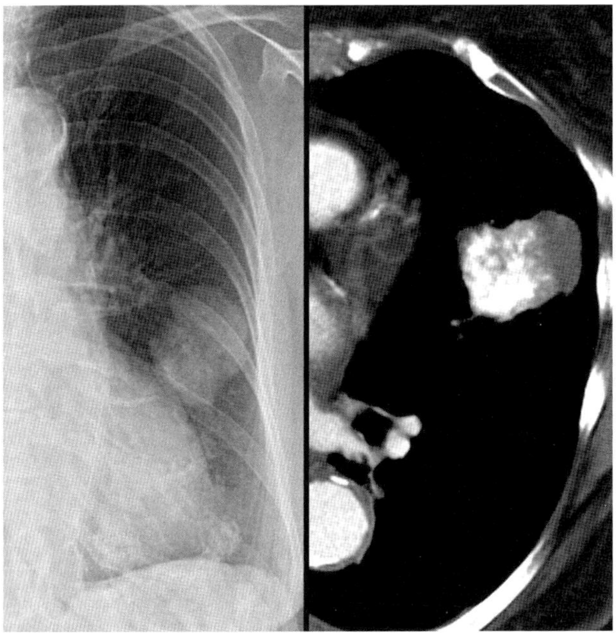

Figure 52.5. Lung cancer with calcification. Composite image of an 84-year-old woman with progressive cough with coned-down PA chest radiograph (left) and contrast-enhanced chest CT (right) shows a left upper lobe mass with extensive eccentric amorphous calcification. Biopsy confirmed non-small cell lung cancer.

- Often is FDG avid on PET/CT, whereas hamartoma is typically not; small lung cancers (< 7 mm) may not exhibit metabolic activity on PET/CT

Solitary Pulmonary Metastasis

- Pulmonary metastases rarely manifest as solitary pulmonary nodules; primary lung cancer should always be considered despite a history of primary malignancy.
- Most metastases do not exhibit calcification. Exceptions include osteosarcoma, chondrosarcoma, synovial sarcoma, thyroid carcinoma, and some mucinous neoplasms.

Carcinoid

- Approximately 80% are small central nodules that often exhibit an endobronchial component or abut a central airway; 20% are peripheral.
- All carcinoid tumors are malignant and should be resected.
- Tumors may exhibit calcification (38%) and contrast enhancement.

Granuloma

- May exhibit varying amounts of calcification with central, diffuse, and concentric or target-like morphology (Fig. 52.6)
- Does not exhibit intrinsic fat
- Typically results from prior histoplasmosis or tuberculosis

Lipoid Pneumonia

- Results from repeated inhalation of mineral oil (Fig. 52.7)
- Typically manifests as consolidation with fat attenuation

Imaging Findings

Hamartoma

- Most are incidentally discovered on chest radiography
- Typically a solitary pulmonary nodule or mass with smooth or lobular margins
- Calcification in up to 15% on radiography; classically "popcorn" (Fig. 52.3)
- Solitary nodule with intrinsic fat and calcification on CT considered diagnostic of hamartoma (Fig. 52.2)

Lipoma

- Rare neoplasm that typically affects adult males
- Characteristically occurs within central airways
- Exhibits diffuse fat attenuation on CT mimicking hamartoma
- May produce endoluminal obstruction

Chondroma

- Exceedingly rare neoplasm composed of cartilage

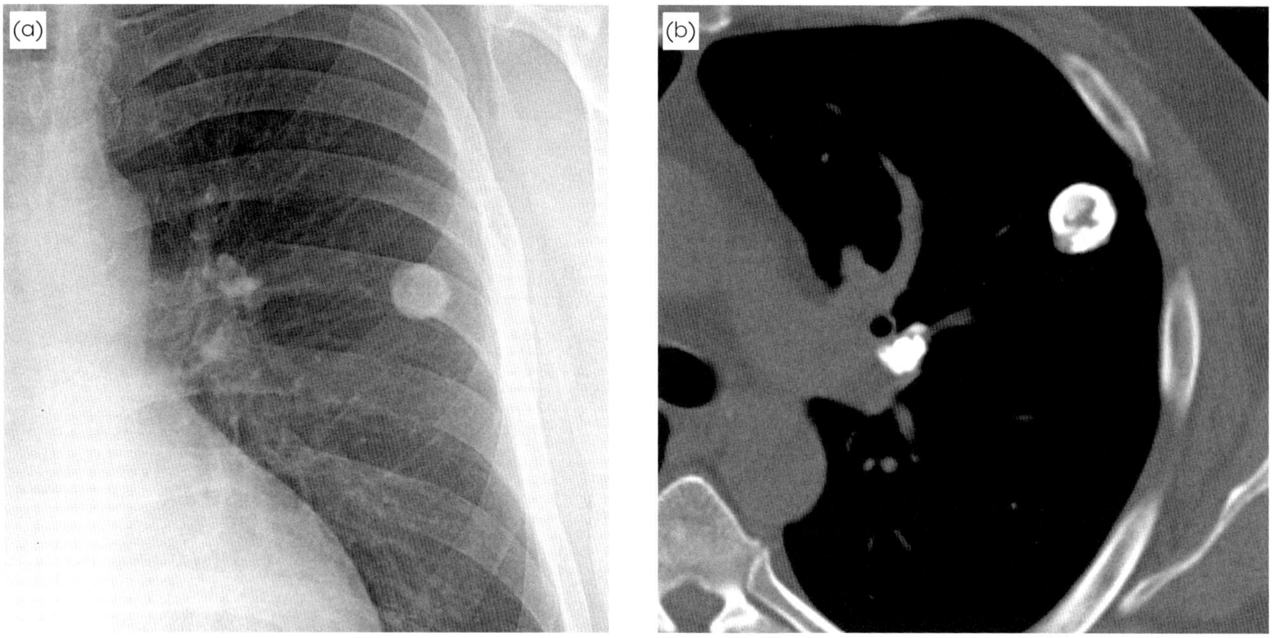

Figure 52.6. Granuloma. (a) PA chest radiograph of an asymptomatic 54-year-old man demonstrates a round, densely calcified left upper lobe nodule. (b) Unenhanced CT chest of the same patient shows the densely calcified left upper lobe nodule consistent with a granuloma (likely from histoplasmosis). Peripheral curvilinear (lamellar) calcification should not be confused with the cartilaginous calcification seen in hamartomas.

- Frequently exhibits calcification (30%), which may demonstrate typical morphologic features of chondroid tissue (rings and arcs)

Leiomyoma

- Rare neoplasm that typically affects women
- May manifest as a peripheral lung nodule or endoluminal lesion that may produce bronchial obstruction
- Well-defined lobular margins

Neurogenic Neoplasms

- May manifest as solitary nodules or endoluminal lesions (Fig. 52.8)

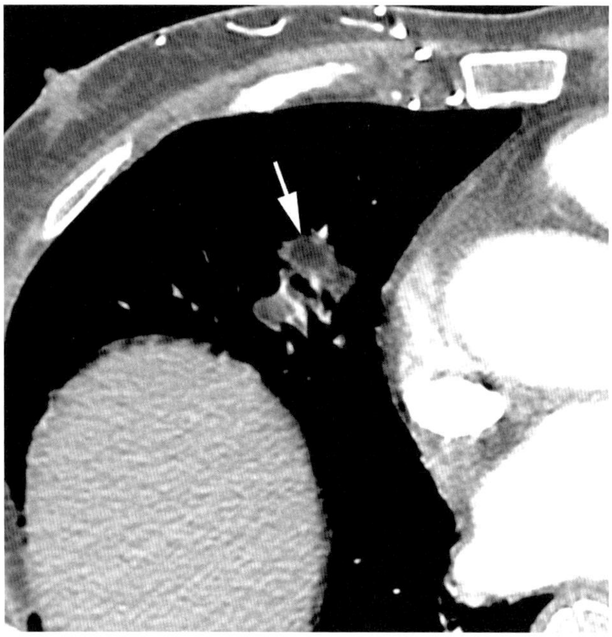

Figure 52.7. Lipoid pneumonia. Contrast-enhanced chest CT of a 74-year-old man with chronic cough shows a middle lobe heterogeneous consolidation with fat attenuation (arrow) representing lipoid pneumonia, secondary to aspiration of mineral oil.

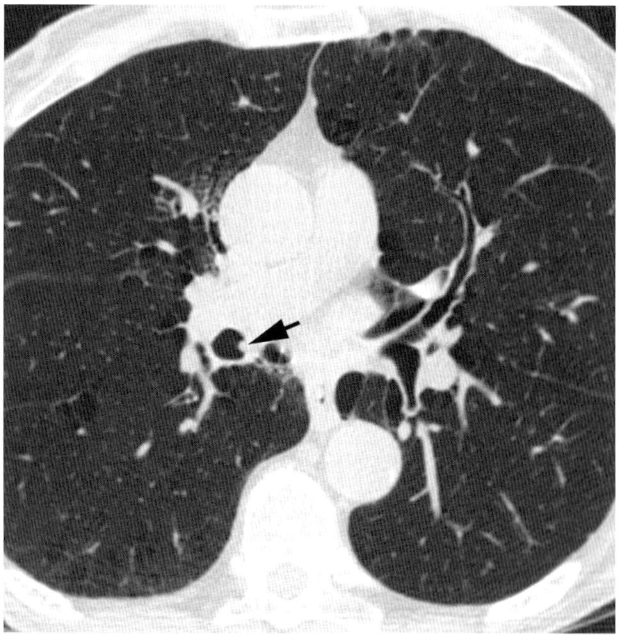

Figure 52.8. Neurofibroma. Axial unenhanced chest CT of a 62-year-old man shows a small endoluminal nodule (arrow) in the bronchus intermedius. Biopsy confirmed endobronchial neurofibroma.

Clinical Issues

- Pulmonary hamartomas may require tissue diagnosis particularly if fat attenuation is subtle or not present on CT.
- Pulmonary hamartomas may exhibit FDG avidity on PET/CT and may mimic pulmonary malignancies.
- Surgical resection is usually not necessary for lesions with characteristic CT findings, unless the patient is symptomatic due to a central lesion or if the nodule is rapidly enlarging.
- Endobronchial hamartomas may be resected bronchoscopically.
- Surgery should also be considered in patients with central lesions and post-obstructive atelectasis or infection.
- Hamartomas account for the majority of benign lung neoplasms. Other benign neoplasms occurring in the lungs and airways include lipoma, chondroma, and leiomyoma, but these are very rare.
- If a pulmonary chondroma is diagnosed, additional investigation should be considered to exclude concurrent leiomyosarcoma and extra-adrenal paraganglioma (Carney triad).

Key Points

- Pulmonary hamartomas are benign neoplasms composed of various mesenchymal components.
- The presence of chondroid calcification (popcorn pattern) and/or macroscopic fat can be diagnostic of hamartoma.
- Very slow growth is an expected finding.
- Treatment of pulmonary hamartoma is usually conservative. Surgical resection can be considered if the CT findings are nondiagnostic, if biopsy is inconclusive, or if the lesion demonstrates rapid growth.

Suggested Reading

Meyer CA, White CS. Cartilaginous disorders of the chest. *RadioGraphics*. 1998;18(5):1109–1123.

Siegelman SS, Khouri NF, Scott WWJr, et al. Pulmonary hamartoma: CT findings. *Radiology*. 1986 Aug;160(2):313–317.

Section X

Airways Disease

CHAPTER 53

Airways Disease

Brent P. Little

Introduction

A variety of neoplastic, infectious, inflammatory, iatrogenic, inhalational, and congenital disorders may affect the airways. Large airway diseases involve the trachea and bronchi, whereas small airway diseases involve the bronchioles. Familiarity with the normal radiographic and CT appearances of the airways and the imaging features of airway diseases enables the radiologist to provide the most accurate and helpful interpretation of imaging studies.

Anatomy

The large airways include the trachea; the mainstem, lobar, and segmental bronchi; and several generations of subsegmental bronchi. The trachea is 6–9 cm in length and its 18–22 C-shaped incomplete rings of cartilage maintain its normal ovoid cross-sectional shape and support its posterior membranous wall which is devoid of cartilage. Bronchi have a similar structure, but their walls contain cartilaginous plates rather than rings. The small airways measure less than 1 or 2 mm in diameter and include the distal smallest subsegmental bronchi and the bronchioles. Unlike the large airways, bronchiolar walls have a thin layer of smooth muscle without cartilage and measure approximately 0.15 mm. The small airways are not visible on imaging studies, including thin-section CT, unless they become abnormally thickened or dilated or become filled with exudative material.

A distal bronchiole, accompanied by an arteriole and lymphatics, supplies the center of each secondary pulmonary lobule, a polyhedral unit of lung measuring 1–2.5 cm in diameter. From the center of each lobule, the terminal bronchioles branch into one to three respiratory bronchioles, which open into alveolar ducts and terminate in the alveolar sacs. The pulmonary acinus is a functional unit of gas exchange that includes respiratory bronchioles and all supplied alveoli; 3–12 acini are found within each secondary lobule. The airways and alveoli within the acinus are not normally visible on thin-section CT, but their structures may become manifest in some small airway diseases.

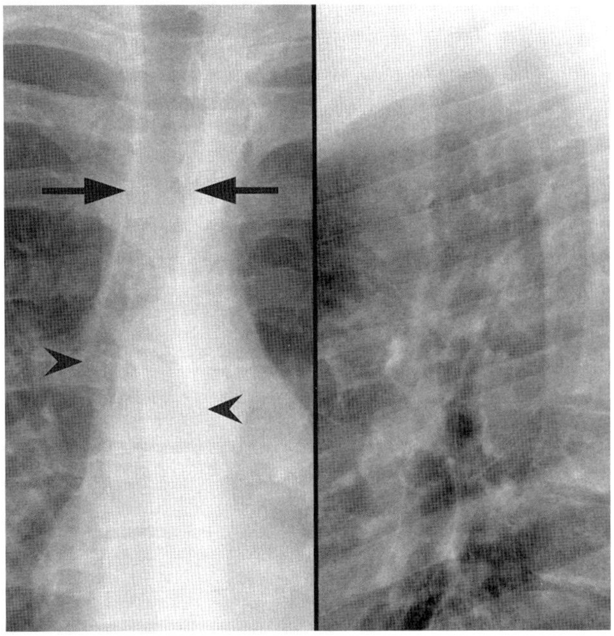

Figure 53.1. Radiography of the normal trachea. Composite image of coned-down posteroanterior (left) and lateral (right) radiographs shows the normal thin-walled, tubular appearance of the air-filled trachea (arrows) with parallel walls. The right and left mainstem bronchi are also visualized (arrowheads).

Normal Appearance at Radiography and CT

The normal trachea is visible on frontal and lateral radiographs as a smooth, lucent, thin-walled column of air (Fig. 53.1). On CT, the normal trachea has a thin, 1-to 3-mm wall and a round or ovoid shape when imaged axially during inspiration. On expiratory CT imaging, the noncartilaginous posterior tracheal wall flattens or bows inward (Fig. 53.2). Mainstem and lobar bronchi have thin walls and are visualized on both radiography and CT. Normal bronchi are smooth and approximately the same size as their accompanying pulmonary artery. Proximal subsegmental bronchi may be identified at CT, but airways in the outer one-third of the lung (including bronchioles) cannot be resolved unless abnormally thickened or dilated.

Differential Diagnosis and Imaging Findings of Airways Diseases

- Neoplasms: Primary malignancies of the large airways are more common than benign lesions. Squamous cell carcinoma is the most common tracheal malignancy

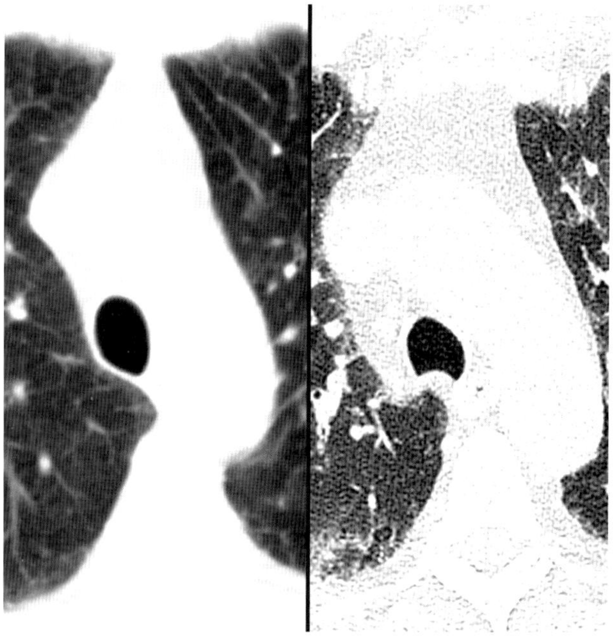

Figure 53.2. CT of the normal trachea. Composite image of axial CT of the trachea during inspiration (left) and expiration (right) shows its typical ovoid appearance in inspiration, with a thin smooth posterior wall. In expiration (right), the posterior wall of the trachea appears thickened and bows inward.

(Fig. 53.3), followed by other tumors, including adenoid cystic and mucoepidermoid carcinoma.
- Tracheal or bronchial nodule or mass
- Focal/segmental tracheal/bronchial wall thickening, often irregular or nodular

- Inflammatory/noninfectious conditions of the large airways: Amyloidosis, granulomatous polyangiitis, and relapsing polychondritis
  - Smooth or nodular thickening of trachea/bronchi, either focal, multifocal, or diffuse
  - Nodular calcification of trachea/bronchi
- Infection: Tuberculosis, bacterial, viral, and invasive fungal infections can involve the large or small airways. Infections involving the small airways may cause impaction of the bronchioles and alveoli by mucous and cellular debris, manifesting as clusters of small centrilobular airway nodules.
  - Smooth, often circumferential thickening of trachea and/or bronchi
  - "Tree-in-bud" nodules—small centrilobular nodules in clusters, extending from a short linear opacity, representing impacted bronchioles and alveolar ducts/sacs; resemble a budding tree in the spring season (Fig. 53.4)
- Iatrogenic/post-traumatic conditions: Trauma, radiation, surgery, or endotracheal tube placement may result in injury to the trachea or bronchi.
  - Focal, usually smooth, narrowing of the trachea at the site of a prior endotracheal tube balloon, trauma, radiation, or surgery
  - Bronchial or tracheal stenosis or malacia at an anastomotic site
- Congenital diseases of the airways: Cystic fibrosis, primary ciliary dyskinesia, and congenital immunodeficiency. A destructive cycle of repeated infection

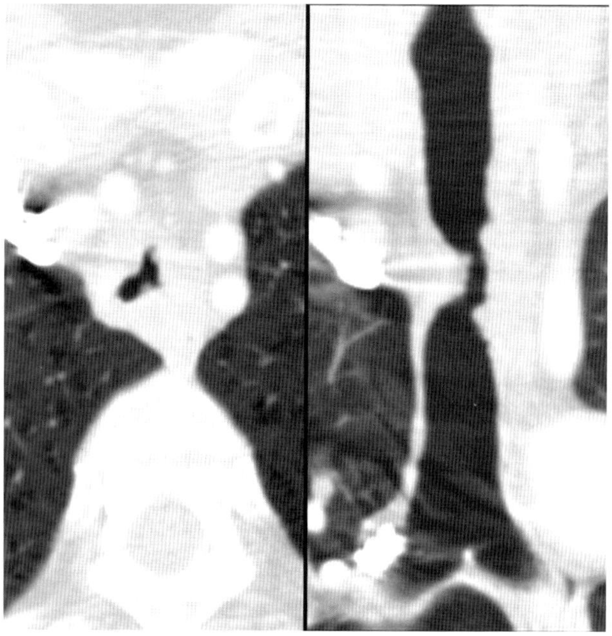

Figure 53.3. Tracheal squamous cell carcinoma. Composite image of axial CT (left) and coronal CT (right) shows irregular circumferential thickening of the trachea with severe narrowing of the tracheal lumen. The coronal CT (right) shows the luminal mass extending over a short segment of the tracheal wall.

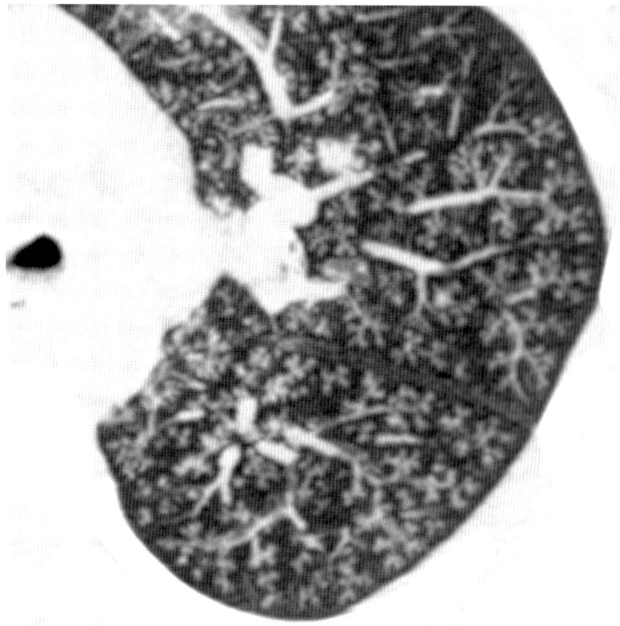

Figure 53.4. Viral bronchiolitis with tree-in-bud pattern (parainfluenza pneumonia). Chest CT maximum intensity projection image shows innumerable centrilobular tree-in-bud nodules that involved both lungs.

and airway dysfunction leads to chronic airway damage, usually resulting in bronchiectasis.
  - Tracheal dilatation and/or bronchiectasis
  - Small airway thickening and tree-in-bud nodules (chronic bronchiolar impaction from dysfunction/infection)
- Inhalational or idiopathic small airways disease: Constrictive bronchiolitis, respiratory bronchiolitis, hypersensitivity pneumonitis, allergic bronchopulmonary aspergillosis, and asthma. Primarily affect bronchioles and may have characteristic imaging appearances. Hazy (ground-glass) centrilobular nodules are a manifestation of many of these diseases, representing bronchiolar and peribronchiolar inflammation.
  - Centrilobular ground-glass nodules (often upper and mid-lung predominant)
  - Tree-in-bud nodules (less common than in airways infection)
  - Bronchial wall thickening
  - Air trapping
  - Bronchiectasis may occur.
- Emphysema: Although it results in lung parenchymal destruction, emphysema may be classified as an airways-related inhalational disease, typically caused by cigarette smoking.
  - Hyperlucent lungs on chest radiography
  - Centrilobular areas of low attenuation on CT with ill-defined, imperceptible walls
  - Bronchial wall thickening and centrilobular ground-glass nodules possible as manifestations of respiratory bronchiolitis
- Tracheomalacia/bronchomalacia: Weakness or deficiency of cartilage may cause collapse of the trachea and/or bronchi during expiration; may result in stridor and obstructive symptoms.
  - Abnormal tracheal or bronchial collapse on expiratory imaging
  - Marked thin crescent-shaped tracheal lumen ("frown sign")

Conclusion: General Approach to Imaging of Airways Diseases

Causes of airways diseases are diverse, but many have similar imaging findings. Diseases of the large airways can manifest as masses, thickening, stenosis, or airway collapse on expiration. Imaging clues to small airway diseases include air trapping and centrilobular nodules/tree-in-bud opacities. Bronchiectasis/bronchioloectasis may be a sign of chronic airway damage. Knowledge of normal anatomy and common imaging patterns of disease is essential for accurate radiologic diagnosis of airway diseases.

Suggested Reading

Gosset N, Bankier AA, Eisenberg RL. Tree-in-bud pattern. *Am J Roentgenol.* 2009;193(6):W472–W477.

Gotway MB, Reddy GP, Webb WR, Elicker BM, Leung JWT. High-resolution CT of the lung: Patterns of disease and differential diagnoses. *Radiol Clin North Am.* 2005;43(3):513–542.

Webb EM, Elicker BM, Webb WR. Using CT to diagnose nonneoplastic tracheal abnormalities. *Am J Roentgenol.* 2000;174(5):1315–1321.

CHAPTER 54

Tracheal Narrowing and Tracheomalacia

Aalok Turakhia, Brent P. Little, and Travis S. Henry

Definition

The etiologies of tracheal narrowing and stenosis are myriad. An important first step in formulating an imaging differential diagnosis is to classify tracheal narrowing into the following categories: neoplastic (benign and malignant), idiopathic, traumatic, inflammatory/infiltrative, and that caused by underlying pulmonary disease.

Clinical Features

In patients with tracheal narrowing, the most common symptoms are related to airway compromise. Symptoms of airway obstruction commonly occur if the airway lumen has narrowed to one-third or less of its normal luminal diameter. Primary symptoms include persistent cough, dyspnea, and respiratory stridor—nonspecific symptoms that are often overlooked or misdiagnosed as acute bronchitis or reactive airway disease, thus delaying appropriate therapy. Mucosal inflammation and ulceration may lead to hemoptysis. If distal tracheal or bronchial narrowing becomes severe, post-obstructive changes including pneumonia, segmental or lobar atelectasis, and mucous plugging may occur.

Anatomy and Physiology

The trachea is a fibroelastic structure extending inferiorly from the cricoid cartilage in the larynx to the carina, where it divides into the right and left mainstem bronchi. Typically, the length of the trachea ranges from 6 to 9 cm. For women, the upper limits of the coronal and sagittal diameters are 21 and 23 mm, respectively. Men, on average, have a slightly larger trachea, with the upper limits of normal for coronal and sagittal tracheal diameters being 25 and 27 mm, respectively. The trachea is lined by a pseudostratified ciliary columnar mucosa; the submucosa consists of loose connective tissue with serous and mucus glands. Arterial blood supply is from branches of the inferior thyroid and bronchial arteries. Approximately 18–22 U-shaped cartilage rings provide rigidity to the anterior trachea. The posterior wall of the trachea is membranous and more flexible, comprised in part by the trachealis muscle. This distinction between the anterior and the posterior tracheal composition is important in developing a differential diagnosis for tracheal pathology.

How to Approach the Image

On chest radiography, the overlap of mediastinal structures and osseous elements of the thorax can significantly limit visualization of tracheal pathology. Helical CT performed with thin, 3-mm collimation and 1- to 1.5-mm interval reconstructions is adequate to demonstrate tracheal abnormalities. When evaluating a tracheal lesion, it is important to first determine whether the process is focal (short segment) or diffuse (long segment). Next, one must determine its location along the tracheobronchial wall and look for signs of wall invasion or direct extension into adjacent structures to further refine the differential diagnosis. The presence of fat or calcium is also useful in narrowing the list of diagnostic considerations.

What Not to Miss

Careful inspection of the trachea must be included in every radiologist's search pattern when interpreting chest radiographs and CT studies. Utilization of axial, coronal, and sagittal images will optimize detection of tracheal abnormalities.

Differential Diagnosis

The differential diagnosis of airway narrowing can be classified into broad categories: iatrogenic/traumatic, neoplastic (benign and malignant), idiopathic, inflammatory/infiltrative, and those caused by underlying pulmonary disease. The length of involvement (i.e., short or long segment) and location (e.g., at the thoracic inlet) can also help narrow the differential.

Neoplastic—Malignant

- Squamous cell carcinoma: Most common primary malignant lesion of the trachea. Smokers are at increased risk; affects men more often than women by a ratio of 4:1 (Fig. 54.1).
- Adenoid cystic carcinoma: Tumor of the minor salivary glands in the tracheal submucosa, with a better prognosis than squamous cell carcinoma. Accounts for one-third of primary malignant tracheal lesions, with no gender predilection and no association with smoking (Figs. 54.2).

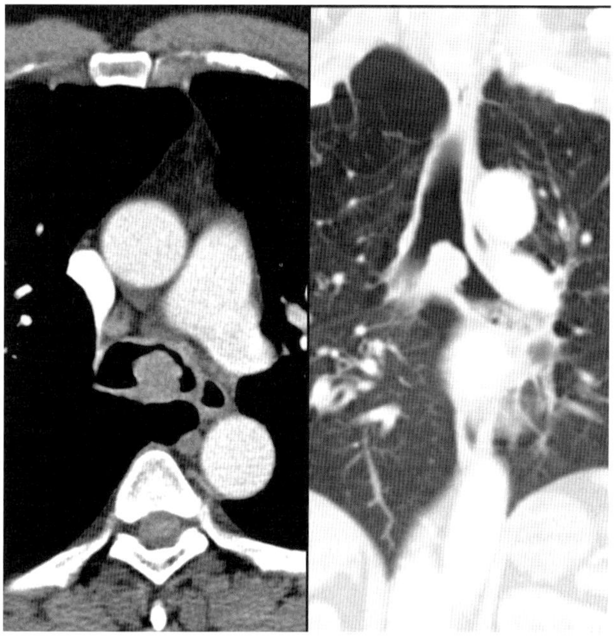

Figure 54.1. Squamous cell carcinoma. Composite image of axial (left) and coronal (right) contrast-enhanced chest CT shows an irregular, polypoid mass arising from the posterior wall of the trachea at the level of the carina (left) that causes severe narrowing of the left main bronchial lumen (right). Squamous cell carcinoma is the most common primary malignant tumor of the trachea.

- Mucoepidermoid carcinoma: Arises from the minor salivary glands of the tracheobronchial tree; however, it is exceedingly rare, accounting for only 0.1–0.2% of thoracic malignancies.

Neoplastic—Benign

- Tracheobronchial papillomatosis: Benign neoplasm resulting from infection by human papilloma virus, acquired either during transit through the birth canal or later in life from oral–genital contact. It is the most common laryngeal tumor in pediatric population and is often seen in the trachea or proximal bronchi (Fig. 54.3).
- Lipoma: Most common in late middle-aged men, this mass originates from submucosal fat in the tracheobronchial tree. It may produce symptoms of airway compromise, including cough, wheezing, or post-obstructive pneumonia.
- Other benign neoplasms: Solitary papillomas, hamartomas, and other benign tumors may also occur as focal endoluminal airway nodules or masses.

Traumatic/Iatrogenic

- Post-intubation stenosis: Tracheal stenosis from prolonged intubation typically develops 4–6 weeks or later following extubation. Overinflation of the endotracheal tube cuff results in vascular compromise and ischemic necrosis of the trachea (Fig. 54.4).
- Post-tracheostomy stenosis: Usually occurs from damage to the cricoid cartilage and first tracheal ring, resulting in focal collapse of the airway.
- Post-transplant stenosis: Usually occurs at a bronchial anastomosis due to ischemia; less commonly occurs distal to the site.
- Trauma: Deposition of granulation tissue or fibrin at the site of blunt or penetrating trauma may cause focal stenosis.

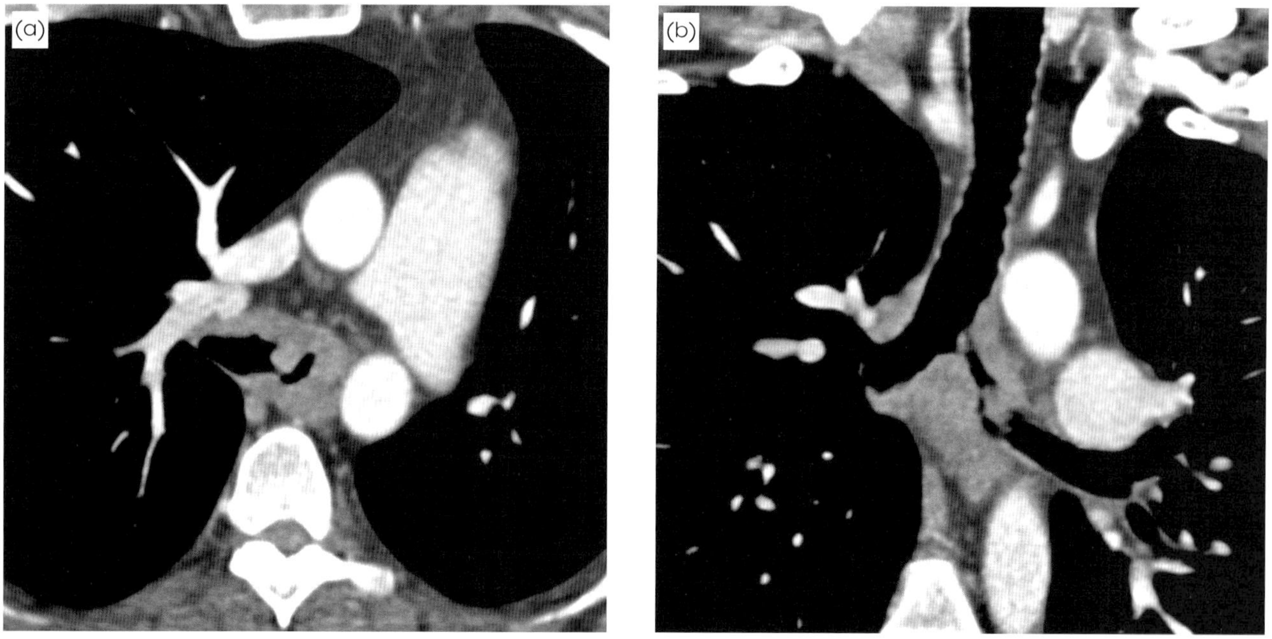

Figure 54.2. Adenoidcystic carcinoma. (a) Axial contrast-enhanced CT shows a lobulated and circumferential tumor involving the distal trachea and proximal aspects of the left and right main bronchi. (b) Coronal CT shows the submucosal and longitudinal tumor growth pattern that is characteristic of adenoidcystic carcinoma, the second most common primary tracheal malignant tumor. Subcarinal lymphadenopathy represents metastatic tumor, which typically involves regional lymph nodes.

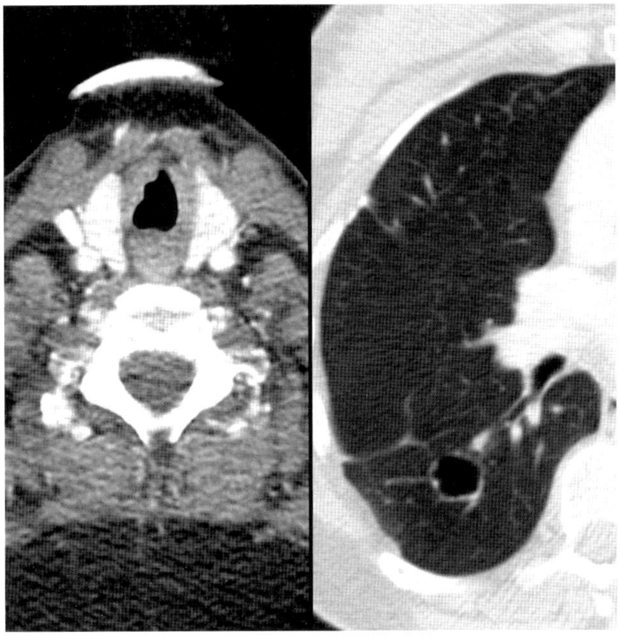

Figure 54.3. Tracheobronchial papillomatosis. Composite image of cervical (left) and chest CT (right) shows endoluminal mucosal nodules along the right lateral tracheal wall (left) and a thin-walled cyst in the right lower lobe (right). Additional findings of solid and cavitating pulmonary nodules (not shown) involved the posterior-dependent aspects of both lungs.

- Post-radiation stenosis: Although less radiosensitive than lung parenchyma, the trachea may become stenotic following radiation therapy, particularly in patients receiving doses greater than 73.6 Gy.

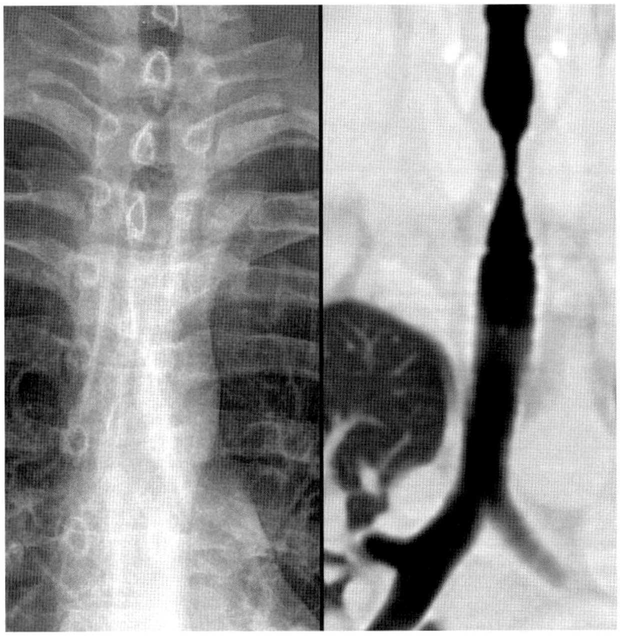

Figure 54.4. Tracheal stenosis. Composite image of coned-down posteroanterior (PA) chest radiograph (left) and coronal CT (right) shows a focal area of tracheal stenosis at the level of the thoracic inlet that developed 6 months after prolonged tracheal intubation.

Infection

Infectious tracheitis may be caused by a variety of bacterial, fungal, and viral etiologies and by tuberculosis (TB). Postinfectious stenosis is most commonly a sequela of endobronchial TB, and despite appropriate therapy, some degree of airway stenosis is seen in up to 90% of patients.

Infiltration/Inflammatory

- Amyloidosis: Heterogeneous group of disorders characterized by deposition of abnormal extracellular deposition of insoluble proteinaceous material.
- Granulomatosis with polyangiitis (formerly Wegener granulomatosis): A c-ANCA-positive, necrotizing granulomatous vasculitis that classically involves the upper airways and kidneys but can also involve the lower respiratory tract and other organs; increased prevalence in middle-aged men (Fig. 54.5).
- Relapsing polychondritis: A very rare autoimmune disorder characterized by recurrent episodes of cartilaginous inflammation and fibrosis. Typically involved sites include the ear, nose, and tracheobronchial tree.
- Tracheobronchopathia osteochondroplastica (TBO): TBO is an idiopathic condition characterized by deposition of multiple submucosal osteocartilagenous nodules. It is seen in men with a 3:1 predilection over women, and it typically affects patients older than age 50 years.

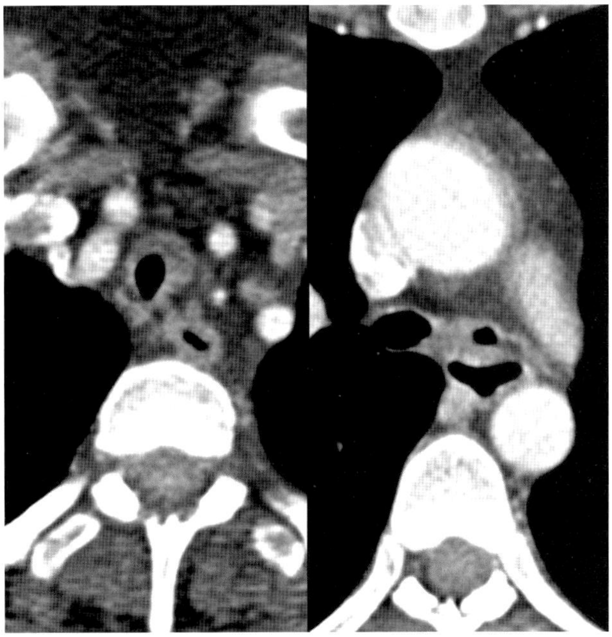

Figure 54.5. Granulomatosis with polyangiitis. Composite image of contrast-enhanced chest CT at the level of the trachea (left) and carina (right) shows multisegmental circumferential soft tissue thickening and narrowing of the trachea and mainstem bronchi. The abnormality does not spare the posterior trachea, as would be expected in relapsing polychondritis and tracheobronchopathia osteochondroplastica. Tracheal amyloid may have a similar appearance.

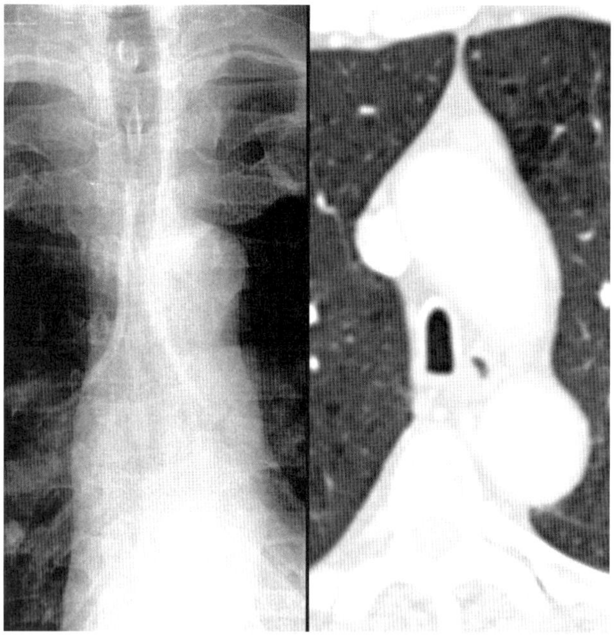

Figure 54.6. Saber sheath trachea. Composite image of coned-down PA chest radiograph (left) and contrast-enhanced chest CT (right) shows saber sheath deformity of the trachea in a patient with emphysema and a long history of COPD. The smooth, symmetric tracheal narrowing begins at the level of the thoracic inlet, with narrowing of the coronal diameter of the trachea.

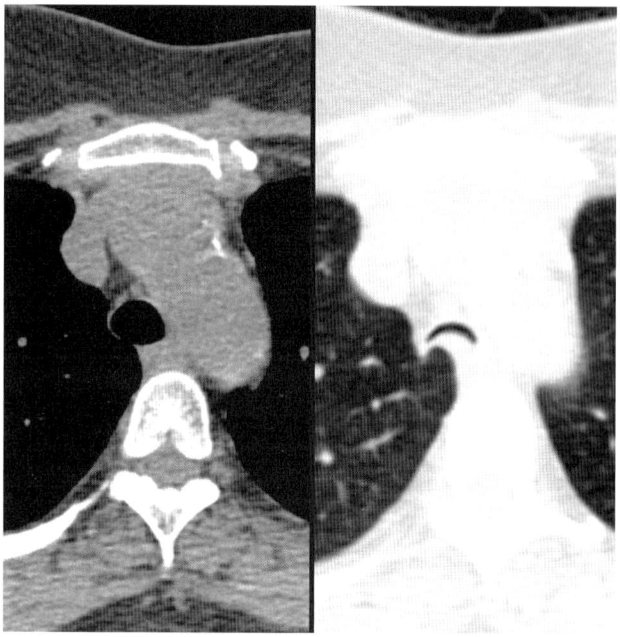

Figure 54.7. Tracheomalacia. Composite image of chest CT images obtained during inspiration (left) and expiration (right) shows a normal tracheal configuration during inspiration, with severe collapse deformity on expiration that shows a narrow crescent-shaped tracheal lumen that has been likened to a downturned mouth ("frown sign").

Underlying Pulmonary Disease

- Saber-sheath trachea: Common abnormality of the intrathoracic trachea that typically affects men with underlying chronic obstructive pulmonary disease (COPD). Smooth narrowing in the coronal plane that begins at the level of the thoracic inlet; likely due to chronically elevated intrathoracic pressure (Fig. 54.6).

Tracheomalacia/Tracheobronchomalacia

- Results from weakness and/or redundancy in the tracheal or bronchial walls, and it is characterized by airway collapse during the expiratory phase of respiration (Fig. 54.7). Although the precise etiology is unknown, histologic studies have demonstrated decreased cartilage-to-muscle ratios and increased diameter of the membranous tracheal wall. The prevalence of tracheomalacia ranges from 4.1% to 23% in symptomatic populations.

Imaging Findings

Neoplastic—Malignant

- Squamous cell carcinoma: Large, irregular, polypoid mass arising from the posterior wall of the trachea (Fig. 54.1). Rarely, squamous cell carcinoma may manifest as a sessile lesion or with circumferential nodular thickening on CT. Invasion of the adjacent mediastinal fat or vessels is readily detected on CT.
- Adenoid cystic carcinoma: As this lesion infiltrates along submucosal planes, adenoid cystic carcinoma can be detected on CT as a homogeneous soft tissue mass circumferentially narrowing the tracheal wall or as a soft tissue mass extending through the tracheal wall (Fig. 54.2a); a longitudinal growth pattern may be apparent on coronal or sagittal reformatted images (Fig. 54.2b). Calcification within the tumor is rare.
- Mucoepidermoid carcinoma: Smooth or ovoid endoluminal soft tissue nodule or mass in the tracheobronchial tree, conforming to the branching features of the airways. Calcification/ossification have been reported in 50% of cases.

Neoplastic—Benign

- Tracheobronchial papillomatosis: Endoluminal focal or multifocal mucosal nodules resulting in airway narrowing. Pulmonary nodules/masses with or without cavitation and thin-walled cysts occur. Findings predominantly involve the posterior-dependent portion of the lungs (Fig. 54.3).
- Lipoma: Circumscribed lesion with macroscopic fat.
- Other lesions: Other benign lesions, such as adenomas and hemangiomas, can manifest as endoluminal soft tissue masses.

Infection

- Usually smooth thickening of the trachea and/or bronchi.
- Can be focal or diffuse.
- Ancillary findings may include tree-in-bud nodules or cavities in tuberculosis.

Traumatic/Iatrogenic

- Post-intubation stenosis: Most often seen in the subglottic airway, these stenoses are focal, rarely extending more than 2 cm, and are generally smooth and symmetric, attaining an "hourglass" configuration (Fig. 54.4). Mild irregularity can be seen if nodular granulation tissue is present.
- Post-tracheostomy stenosis: Damage to cricoid cartilage or tracheal ring results in collapse and narrowing in transverse plane.
- Trauma: Similar "hourglass" focal stenosis as with post-intubation stenosis.

Infiltration/Inflammatory
Circumferential, Not Sparing Posterior Trachea

- Amyloidosis: Diffuse nodular mucosal thickening with irregular narrowing. Calcification and ossification is sometimes seen.
- Granulomatosis with polyangiitis (formerly Wegener granulomatosis): Circumferential thickening and irregularity of the tracheal wall (Fig. 54.5) with ulceration that may be focal or diffuse.

Sparing the Posterior Tracheal Wall

- Relapsing polychondritis: Thickened tracheal wall with destruction of the tracheal cartilage, sparing the posterior (noncartilaginous) membranous trachea.
- TBO: TBO exhibits thickened tracheal cartilage with deposition of multifocal nodules ± calcifications, sparing the posterior trachea.

Underlying Pulmonary Disease

- Saber-sheath trachea: Marked decrease in coronal diameter that begins at the level of the thoracic inlet, with increased sagittal diameter (Fig. 54.6). Inward displacement of the lateral tracheal walls may be seen.

Tracheomalacia

On inspiratory CT images, the trachea may have a normal round or ovoid shape, with anteroposterior (AP) larger than transverse diameter; however, a lunate (crescent-shaped) trachea, with a larger transverse than AP diameter, is thought to occur more frequently in patients with tracheomalacia (Fig. 54.7).

- CT at end-forced expiration demonstrates collapse of the trachea along its AP dimension. Whereas older studies suggested using a diagnostic threshold of a minimum of 50% collapse relative to the tracheal diameter at inspiration, recent evidence suggests using a threshold of 70%, increasing the specificity for tracheomalacia. Many asymptomatic patients have a mild degree of tracheal collapse at expiration.
- Airway collapse in tracheomalacia can be segmental or diffuse.
- Bronchial collapse at expiration is often also present, correlating with tracheobronchomalacia.
- Isolated collapse of the bronchus intermedius on expiratory CT imaging is often a normal finding, especially in elderly patients.

Clinical Issues

- Findings that suggest impending airway collapse and/or obstruction must be communicated to the clinician.
- In cases of suspected malignant airway lesions, careful attention should be paid to signs of adjacent mediastinal fat invasion and identification of intrathoracic lymphadenopathy.
- Post-intubation or post-traumatic tracheal stenosis is often treated by serial balloon dilatation, stenting, or segmental resection with re-anastamosis. Evaluation of both the length and the degree of stenosis is important.
- Tracheomalacia is a dynamic process that is best evaluated with inspiratory and forced expiratory CT images to demonstrate tracheal collapse.
- Like other tracheal diseases, tracheomalacia may mimic asthma, or affected patients may present with nonspecific symptoms. Significant respiratory dysfunction may result if tracheomalacia goes untreated.

Key Points

- A wide variety of etiologies may cause tracheal narrowing.
- Determining whether a process is focal or diffuse is an important first step in formulating a focused differential diagnosis.
- Lesion location along the tracheobronchial wall, the presence or absence of calcifications, and evidence of extension through the tracheal wall are important characteristics that may help to further narrow the differential diagnosis.
- In the adult population, most tracheal tumors are malignant, and squamous cell carcinoma is the most common tumor detected.

Suggested Reading

Chung JH, Kanne JP, Gilman MD. CT of diffuse tracheal diseases. *AJR Am J Roentgenol.* 2011;196(3):W240–246.

Park CM, Goo JM, Lee HJ, et al. Tumors in the tracheobronchial tree: CT and FDG-PET features. *RadioGraphics.* 2009;29(1):55–71.

Prince JS, Duhamel DR, Levin DL, Harrell JH, Friedman PJ. Nonneoplastic lesions of the tracheobronchial wall: Radiologic findings with bronchoscopic correlation. *RadioGraphics.* 2002;22(Special Issue):S215–S230.

Ridge CA, O'Donnell CR, Yee EL, Majid A, Boiselle PM. Tracheobronchomalacia: Current concepts and controversies. *J Thorac Imaging.* 2001;26:278–289.

Webb EM, Elicker BM, Webb WR. Using CT to diagnose nonneoplastic tracheal abnormalities: Appearance of the tracheal wall. *AJR Am J Roentgenol.* 2000;174:1315–1321.

CHAPTER 55

Bronchiectasis

Bethany Milliron, Brent P. Little, and Travis S. Henry

Definition

Bronchiectasis represents irreversible bronchial dilatation. It can be focal or diffuse, and it usually results from chronic infection, proximal airway obstruction, or a congenital bronchial abnormality. *Traction bronchiectasis* refers to irregular bronchial dilatation in the setting of surrounding pulmonary fibrosis.

Clinical Features

Patients with bronchiectasis may present with chronic cough, hemoptysis, recurrent pneumonia, or general malaise. Spirometry often demonstrates an obstructive physiology, and some patients may have bronchial reactivity, frequently resulting in diagnostic confusion with chronic obstructive pulmonary disease and asthma. Treatment is usually directed at symptoms or treatment of the underlying etiology. In cases of severe bronchiectasis within a pulmonary lobe or segment, surgical resection is sometimes performed.

Cystic fibrosis (CF), a disorder of abnormal chloride transport, remains the most devastating congenital cause of bronchiectasis, with an average life span of 37 years for affected patients. Routine newborn serum screening is now performed in the United States; a positive immunoreactive trypsinogen (IRT) serum result is suggestive and is confirmed by a second IRT test or by DNA testing for a mutation in the CFTR transporter. A sweat test showing increased chloride levels remains the gold standard for establishing the diagnosis of CF. Treatment of frequent pulmonary infections is supportive, and the only definitive therapy for CF is lung transplantation.

Patients affected by other congenital causes of bronchiectasis, such as bronchial atresia, tracheobronchomegaly, or primary ciliary dyskinesia, may present in childhood or later in life with recurrent infections, intractable cough, or other respiratory symptoms.

Anatomy and Physiology

Bronchial and bronchiolar dilation due to increased intraluminal airway pressures (due to coughing or barotrauma) may be reversible in the acute setting (sometimes seen in pneumonia and acute respiratory distress syndrome (ARDS)). True bronchiectasis is irreversible, explained by Cole's "vicious cycle hypothesis." Airway infection leads to inflammation and obstruction due to bronchial impaction with fluid and inflammatory/immune cells. The obstructed airway is thus subjected to both the primary effects of the infectious pathogen and host-mediated inflammatory tissue damage. Tissue damage impairs mucociliary clearance, predisposing to further infection and inflammation and further damage to the airways. Ultimately, the architecture of the airway is permanently altered. As bronchiectasis becomes more severe, the normal ciliated epithelium is replaced by squamous or columnar epithelium with eventual loss of the elastin layer of the bronchial wall and destruction of the bronchial muscle and cartilage.

How to Approach the Image

The imaging findings of bronchiectasis may be subtle on chest radiography. Common findings include a "tram track" appearance with parallel lines corresponding to ectatic bronchi with thickened walls; mucous plugging may manifest as nodules. Thin-section CT is the imaging method of choice for diagnosing bronchiectasis because it allows accurate assessment of the severity and distribution of bronchiectasis.

Is Bronchiectasis Present?

The morphologic criteria for diagnosing bronchiectasis include bronchial dilatation compared to its paired bronchial artery (signet ring sign), lack of tapering of the bronchi, and identification of bronchi in the peripheral lung, within 1 cm of the pleural surface.

What Is the Morphology/Grade of Severity?

- Cylindrical—Smooth and tubular, with parallel walls (mild)
- Varicoid—Alternating dilatation and constriction, irregular/corrugated walls (moderate)
- Cystic—Saccular dilatation, often clustered (severe) (Fig. 55.1)

What Is the Distribution?

Craniocaudal (upper or lower lung zones) and axial (central or peripheral) distributions are important to note because they help narrow the differential diagnostic considerations.

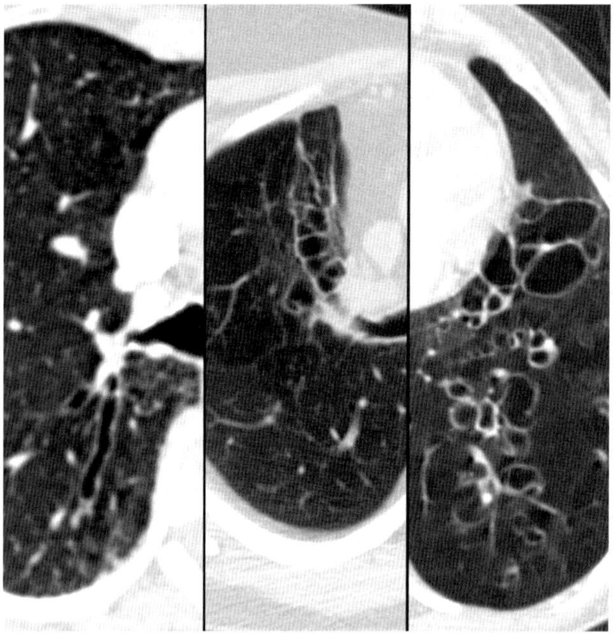

Figure 55.1. Grades of severity of bronchiectasis. Composite image of chest CT of three patients with increasing grades of bronchiectasis shows cylindrical (mild) bronchiectasis (left), varicose (moderate) bronchiectasis (middle), and cystic (severe) bronchiectasis (right). Cylindrical bronchiectasis is characterized by parallel airway walls (tram track sign), varicose bronchiectasis manifests as alternating areas of bronchial dilatation and constriction, and cystic bronchiectasis is characterized by clustered areas of cyst-like bronchial dilatation.

What Is the Clinical History?

The patient's clinical history is of paramount importance. Did the patient have a recent stroke and is therefore at risk for recurrent aspiration? Is there a history of multiple pneumonias at a young age? If the time course is rapid, findings may represent a reversible form of bronchial dilatation (e.g., pneumonia or ARDS) rather than permanent bronchiectasis.

Other Findings?

- Centrilobular or tree-in-bud nodules may represent mucous impaction or infection/inflammation of distal bronchioles and alveolar ducts.
- Perilymphatic nodules are a common imaging manifestation of sarcoidosis (especially in the upper and mid lung zones).
- High-attenuation mucous in bronchiectatic airways is a frequent CT manifestation of allergic bronchopulmonary aspergillosis (ABPA), caused by the accumulation of fungal debris with metal salts (magnesium).

Volume Loss and Architectural Distortion

Sarcoidosis may result in upper lobe scarring and volume loss with elevation of the pulmonary hila.

Pulmonary fibrosis causes architectural distortion, manifesting as peripheral and basilar predominant reticulation, traction bronchiectasis, and eventually honeycombing. Tuberculosis (TB) may cause asymmetric upper lobe volume loss, focal architectural distortion, and regional bronchiectasis.

What Not to Miss

- On chest radiography, bronchiectasis may be confused with other conditions, such as pulmonary fibrosis or edema. Bronchiectasis manifests as parallel linear (tram track) and/or ring-like opacities. Chest CT may be used for confirmation of cases suspected on radiography.
- On CT, findings of bronchiectasis include bronchi that are larger than their accompanying pulmonary artery and a lack of smooth tapering as bronchi course to the lung periphery. Bronchial wall thickening and irregularity is often present.
- Focal, asymmetric bronchiectasis in the presence of cavities and/or a tree-in-bud pattern of nodules can be seen in infections such as TB and nontuberculous mycobacterial disease.
- Bronchiectasis limited to contiguous bronchi should prompt a search for an obstructing endobronchial or peribronchial lesion. For example, endobronchial carcinoid tumors typically grow slowly and may cause bronchiectasis of distal bronchi due to a "ball valve" mechanism.

Differential Diagnosis

The predominant distribution of findings of bronchiectasis may help to narrow the differential diagnosis as follows.

Upper and Mid Lung Zones

- Sarcoidosis/silicosis/other pneumoconioses
- CF (Fig. 55.2)
- ABPA
- TB (Fig. 55.3)

Lower Zone

- Recurrent aspiration/infection
- Pulmonary fibrosis with traction bronchiectasis (Fig. 55.4)
- Congenital immunodeficiencies

Middle Lobe/Lingula

- Chronic atypical mycobacterial infection (Fig. 55.5)
- Primary ciliary dyskinesia (Kartagener syndrome)
- Post-ARDS fibrosis

Central Distribution

- Sarcoidosis (Fig. 55.6)
- ABPA (Fig. 55.7)
- CF

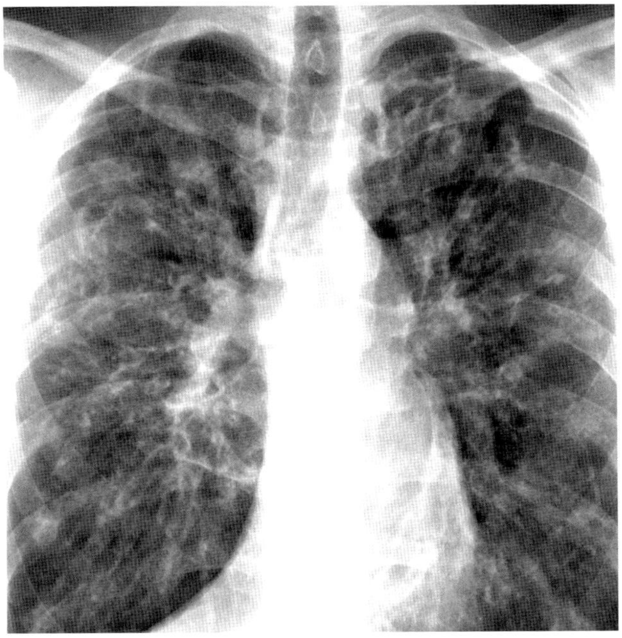

Figure 55.2. Cystic fibrosis. Coned-down posteroanterior (PA) chest radiograph shows bilateral upper lobe predominant findings of bronchiectasis, with overlapping areas of parallel linear opacities (tram tracking) and ring-like opacities representing underlying cylindrical and cystic bronchiectasis. Small areas of nodularity in the left upper lobe represent mucoid impaction in bronchiectatic airways.

- Tracheobronchomegaly (Mournier–Kuhn syndrome) (Fig. 55.8)

Mid-Order Bronchi

- Williams–Campbell syndrome

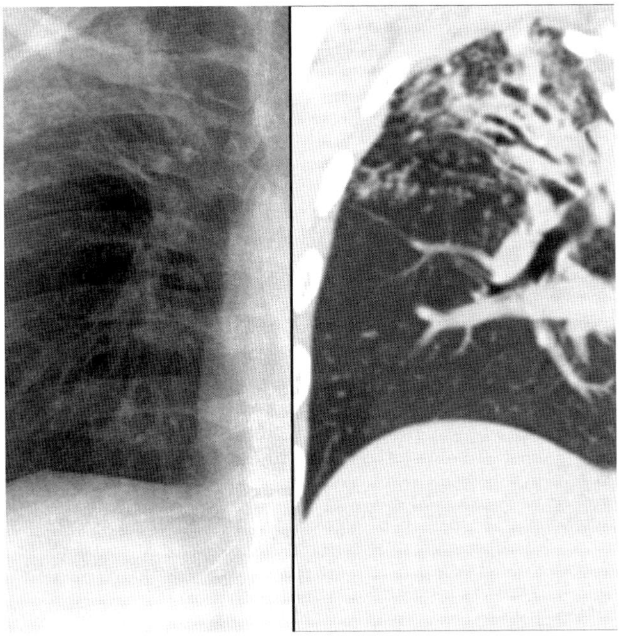

Figure 55.3. Tuberculosis. Composite image of coned-down PA chest radiograph (left) and coronal CT (right) shows loss of volume in the right upper lobe with airway wall thickening, bronchiectasis, and centrilobular nodules and tree-in-bud opacities (right). Sputum culture revealed mycobacterium tuberculosis.

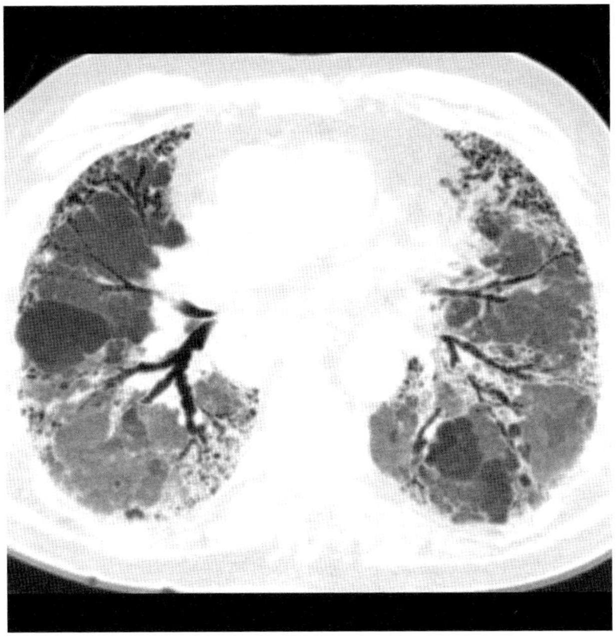

Figure 55.4. Pulmonary fibrosis (scleroderma). Axial CT (MinIP image) of a 69-year-old man with pulmonary fibrosis and scleroderma shows peripheral findings of interstitial fibrosis with fine honeycombing and extensive traction bronchiectasis likely due to a combination of chronic aspiration and fibrotic NSIP.

Peripheral Distribution

- Aspiration/recurrent infection
- Pulmonary fibrosis

Focal Bronchiectasis

- Bronchial obstruction due to tumor or foreign body

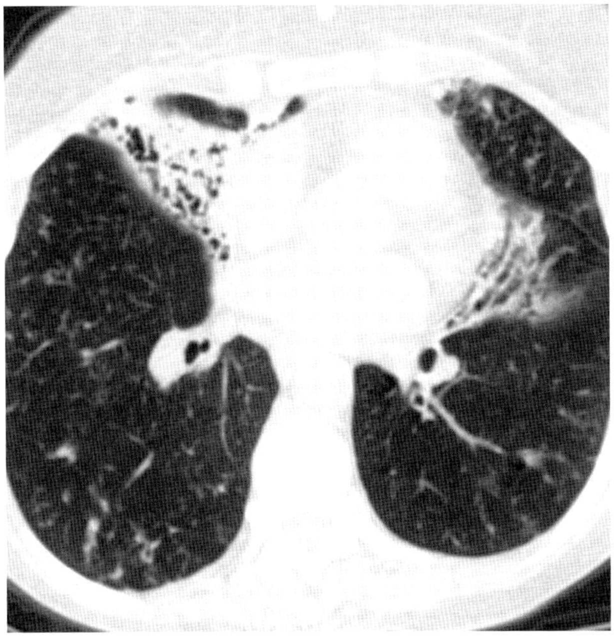

Figure 55.5. Chronic MAI infection. Chest CT of a 76-year-old woman with chronic MAI infection shows atelectasis and bronchiectasis in the middle lobe and lingula and also areas of bronchiectasis and centrilobular nodules in both lower lobes.

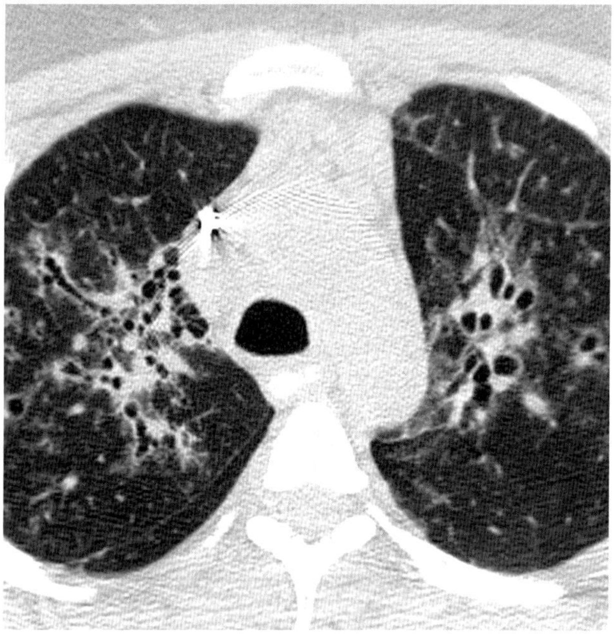

Figure 55.6. Sarcoidosis. Chest CT of a 43-year-old woman with sarcoidosis shows central symmetric upper lobe predominant bronchiectasis and peribronchovascular architectural distortion that is characteristic of sarcoidosis. The imaging findings of sarcoidosis tend to be more symmetric and peribronchovascular in distribution than those of tuberculosis.

Imaging Findings

Recurrent Aspiration or Infection

- Bronchiectasis most prominent in the dependent lung zones, usually bilateral with a peripheral distribution

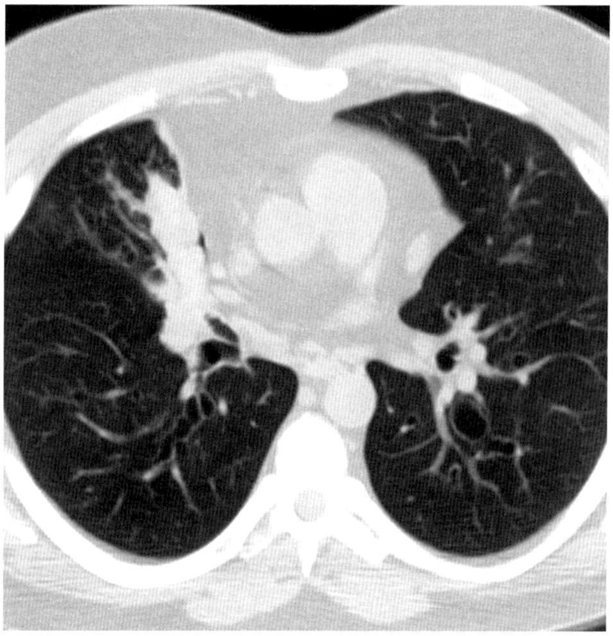

Figure 55.7. ABPA. Chest CT of a 46-year-old man with ABPA shows central bronchiectasis in both lower lobes and in the middle lobe, where mucoid impaction manifests as a dense tubular opacity. CT with mediastinal window (not shown) revealed high-attenuation bronchial impaction, representing fungal debris containing high concentrations of iron and manganese.

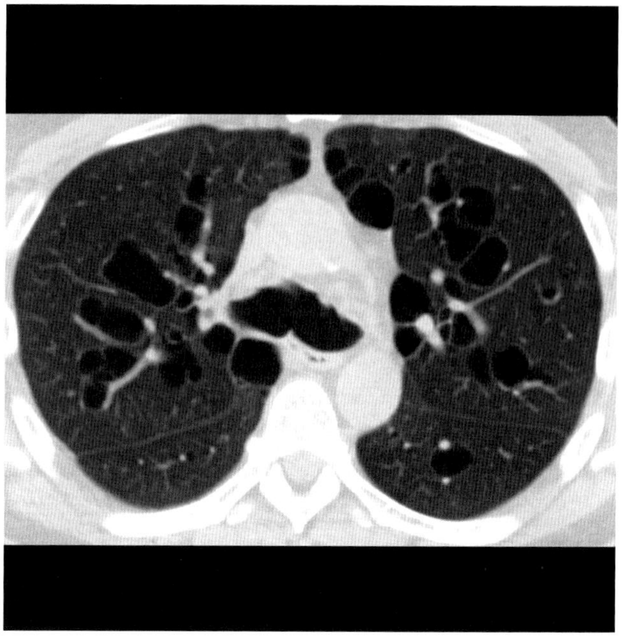

Figure 55.8. Tracheobronchomegaly (Mournier–Kuhn syndrome). Axial chest CT of a 55-year-old man with tracheobronchomegaly shows dilatation of the trachea, main, segmental, and proximal subsegmental bronchi. Images of the upper trachea revealed a corrugated appearance (not shown), and tracheobronchomegaly is characterized by bronchiectasis with a central distribution.

- Concurrent mucous plugging or obstruction with debris in bronchiectatic airways

Mycobacterial Infection

Tuberculosis

- Bronchiectasis is usually asymmetric, upper lobe predominant; may occur in patients with active post-primary TB and in those with scarring from healed TB (Fig 55.3).
- Tree-in-bud nodules and cavities are common in active TB infection.

Atypical Mycobacterial Infection (*Mycobacterium avium-intracellulare* and Others)

- *Mycobacterium avium-intracellulare* (MAI) is most common; 80% of patients are female, most in their seventh or eighth decade of life, and 86% are Caucasian (Fig. 55.5).
- Bronchiectasis and tree-in-bud nodules characteristically involve the lingula and middle lobe.
- Bronchiectasis is typically more symmetric and extensive than in patients with TB.

Sarcoidosis

- 25% of patients with pulmonary sarcoidosis may develop progressive pulmonary fibrosis with traction bronchiectasis, typically manifesting with upper lobe volume loss and elevation of the hila (Fig 55.7).

- Sarcoidosis tends to be more symmetric and peribronchovascular than TB.

Congenital Causes

Cystic Fibrosis

- Upper lobe predominant but relatively diffuse cystic and cylindrical bronchiectasis
- Nodules/tubular opacities representing mucoid impaction
- Tree-in-bud nodules and mosaic attenuation/air trapping
- Bronchial wall and peribronchial interstitial thickening (Fig. 55.2)

Hypogammaglobulinemia

- Lower and middle lobe predominant cylindrical bronchiectasis with marked bronchial wall thickening
- Scattered mucoid impaction and tree-in-bud nodules representing small airways impaction/bronchiolitis

Immotile Cilia Syndrome

- Usually mid and lower lung predominant
- Tree-in-bud nodules and mucous plugging common
- 50% of affected patients have dextrocardia or complete situs inversus (Kartagener syndrome)

Tracheobronchomegaly (Mournier–Kuhn Syndrome)

- Affected patients present in third or fourth decade of life with cough and recurrent infection
- Enlarged trachea and central bronchi
- Trachea often has "corrugated" appearance, with or without diverticula (Fig. 55.8)

Williams–Campbell Syndrome

- Rare cartilage deficiency of mid-order subsegmental bronchi, sparing the trachea and the distal airways
- Cystic bronchiectasis limited to subsegmental bronchi

Allergic Bronchopulmonary Aspergillosis

- Hypersensitivity reaction and inflammation from immune reaction to the presence of endobronchial *Aspergillis*
- Central/proximal bronchiectasis seen in nearly 100% of cases, usually cystic or varicoid
- High-attenuation mucus impaction on CT due to fungal debris with metal salts (magnesium) (Fig. 55.8)

Interstitial Lung Disease

- Traction bronchiectasis, an associated finding of fibrosis, may be seen in usual interstitial pneumonia and fibrotic nonspecific interstitial pneumonitis (NSIP).
- Peripheral bronchi and bronchioles (bronchiolectasis) are commonly involved.
- Fibrotic NSIP may manifest with central lower zone bronchiectasis.

Tumor or Foreign Body

- Focal bronchiectasis due to obstruction distal to the lesion (e.g., obstructing tumor, foreign body, or broncholith)
- Air trapping with lucent lung in the affected lung segment or lobe

Clinical Issues

Patients with CF have a progressively worsening clinical course, with recurrent pneumonias and chronic airway colonization. Even with lung transplantation and modern antibiotic therapies, average life expectancy of CF patients remains limited to young adulthood.

Non-CF-related bronchiectasis can cause chronic cough and recurrent lung infection. Pulmonary function testing often reveals evidence of obstruction.

Treatment of patients with mild to moderate bronchiectasis involves supportive care with bronchodilators, antibiotics, and other medical therapy. Surgical resection is uncommon and usually reserved for cases of significant bronchiectasis limited to a single region of the lungs (e.g., a particular lobe or segment).

Key Points

- Bronchiectasis is irreversible localized or diffuse bronchial dilatation, a result of repeated bronchial injury and inflammation, coupled with obstruction and further injury and inflammation.
- Clues to the etiology of bronchiectasis can be derived from the distribution of findings, the pattern of ancillary findings (e.g., nodules), and the patient's clinical history.

Suggested Reading

Cantin L, Bankier AA, Eisenberg RL. Bronchiectasis. *AJR Am J Roentgenol.* 2009;193(3):W158–W171.

Hansell DM. Bronchiectasis. *Radiol Clin North Am.* 1998;36:107–128.

Javidan-Nejad C, Bhalla S. Bronchiectasis. *Radiol Clin North Am.* 2009;47:289–306.

Lynch DA, Travis WD, Muller NL, et al. Idiopathic interstitial pneumonias: CT features. *Radiology.* 2005;236:10–21.

McGuinness G, Naidich DP. CT of airways disease and bronchiectasis. *Radiol Clin North Am.* 2002;40:1–19.

CHAPTER 56

Emphysema

Travis S. Henry and Brent P. Little

Definition

Emphysema is defined by the American Thoracic Society as the abnormal, *permanent* enlargement of airspaces distal to the terminal bronchioles, accompanied by destruction of alveolar walls, but without obvious fibrosis. Emphysema is a leading cause of pulmonary morbidity and patient mortality worldwide, and as of 2011, an estimated 4.7 million people in the United States had been diagnosed with the disease. Chronic obstructive pulmonary disease (COPD) is a spectrum of obstructive lung diseases that includes emphysema and chronic bronchitis—diseases that frequently coexist, especially in smokers.

Clinical Features

The hallmark of emphysema, and COPD in general, is slowly progressive airflow obstruction. The airflow obstruction in COPD is at least partially irreversible, in contradistinction to asthma, which may respond to bronchodilators. The clinical diagnosis of COPD is confirmed with pulmonary function tests (PFTs), and there are two commonly used criteria for the diagnosis of COPD—"NICE" and "GOLD." The specifics of each criterion are slightly different, but in general PFT findings in COPD include the following:

- Decreased FEV_1
- Decreased FEV_1/FVC ($\leq$70% of predicted)
- Decreased DLCO

where FEV_1 is the forced expiratory volume in 1 second, FVC is forced vital capacity, and DLCO is diffusion capacity for carbon monoxide.

Patients with mild emphysema may be asymptomatic or have chronic cough ("smoker's cough") and may experience worsening dyspnea (especially on exertion), cough, and sputum production as the disease progresses. Physical examination may reveal decreased breath sounds and wheezing. In severe cases, digital clubbing and polycythemia may be present, but cyanosis is usually absent. Cor pulmonale may be a late manifestation of the disease.

Anatomy and Physiology

Emphysema is a disease of the small airways and alveoli, with a complex and incompletely understood pathophysiology. The most commonly accepted theory is that lung inflammation caused by cigarettes and other inhaled toxins results in an imbalance of protease and antiprotease (e.g., α_1-antitrypsin) that results in destruction of structural proteins in the lungs (e.g., elastin and collagen), leading to a characteristic enlargement of the distal airspaces.

There are three types of emphysema based on the anatomic location of lung destruction, with respective CT imaging patterns that are usually distinguishable on CT except in very severe cases.

Centrilobular (syn. *centriacinar*) emphysema is the most common type of emphysema and is highly associated with cigarette smoking. Histologically, it is characterized by destruction of the proximal respiratory bronchioles with preservation of the distal alveolar ducts and sacs. Macroscopically, centrilobular emphysema most severely affects the upper lobes and superior segments of the lower lobes (Fig. 56.1).

Panlobular (*panacinar*) emphysema represents near-uniform destruction of the pulmonary acinus and is classically associated with α_1-antitrypsin deficiency, with predominant involvement of the lower lobes. It may also occur in smokers (Fig. 56.2).

Paraseptal (*distal acinar*) emphysema represents an enlarged airspace in the periphery of the acinus, usually in the posterior upper lobes. Paraseptal emphysema may occur in isolation, but it often coexists with centrilobular or panacinar emphysema. Paraseptal emphysema is considered a precursor of bullous emphysema (Fig. 56.3), and it is also a well-recognized cause of spontaneous pneumothorax in young adults.

How to Approach the Image

Chest Radiograph

- *Are the lungs hyperinflated?* If the diaphragm appears flattened, or the anterior seventh ribs are visible above the diaphragm, the lungs are considered hyperinflated.
- *Is there a paucity of vessels?* Look for increased lucency with decreased peripheral vessels. Findings may be symmetric or asymmetric and may be predominant in the upper or lower lung zones. Look for a pleural line, which would indicate a pneumothorax.

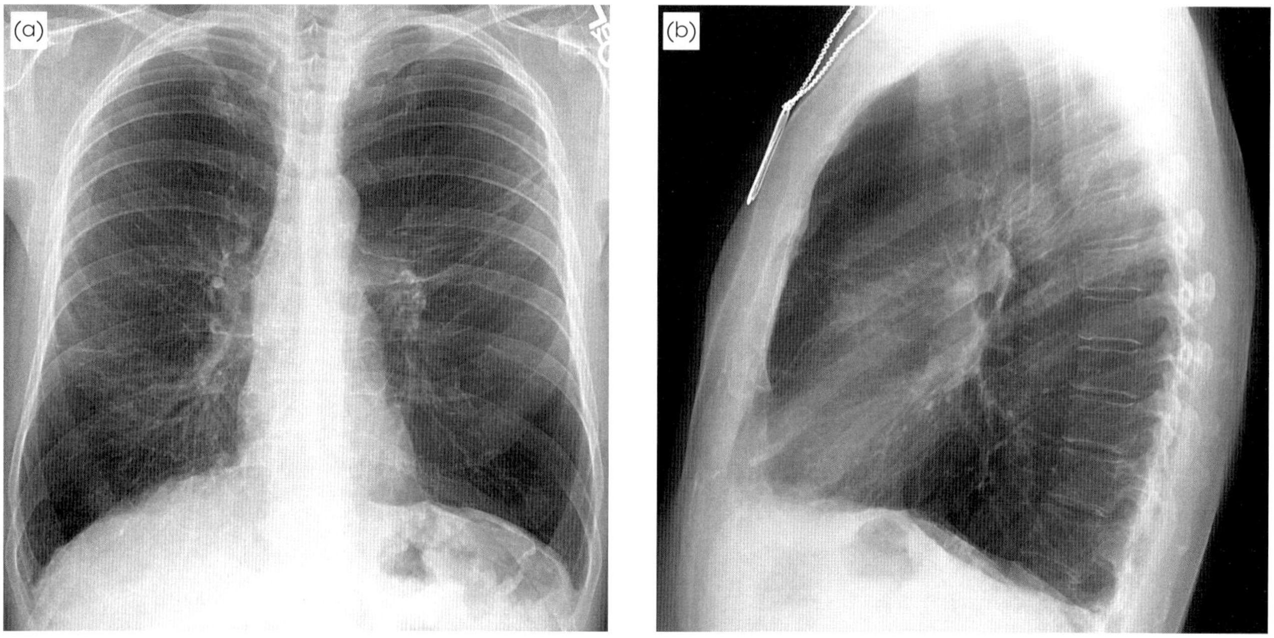

Figure 56.1. Severe emphysema on chest radiography. (a) Posteroanterior (PA) chest radiograph of a 50-year-old man with severe emphysema and a long history of cigarette smoking shows hyperinflated lungs with hyperlucency and a paucity of vessels in the upper lobes. (b) Lateral chest radiograph shows the hyperinflation, with increased anteroposterior diameter of the thorax, prominence of the retrosternal clear space, and flattened hemidiaphragms (diaphragmatic height <2.7 cm).

- *Is there a nodule?* Have a low threshold for recommending CT to evaluate a suspected nodular opacity because the incidence of lung cancer is increased in patients with emphysema.
- *Does the emphysema cause a common pathology* (pulmonary edema or pneumonia) *to look atypical?* Emphysema, particularly with bullous changes, may cause pulmonary consolidation to appear cavitary ("Swiss cheese lung"). Pulmonary edema may manifest with relative sparing of emphysematous lung and may lead to an asymmetric, patchy appearance on the chest radiograph.

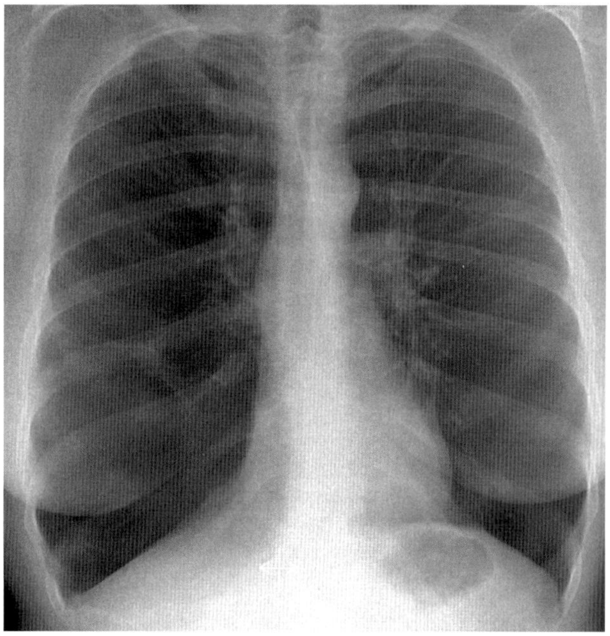

Figure 56.2. Panlobular emphysema (α_1-antitrypsin deficiency). PA radiograph of a 49-year-old woman with α_1-antitrypsin deficiency shows hyperinflated lungs with hyperlucency in the lower lung zones and near absence of normal vascular structures. The patient underwent successful lung transplantation.

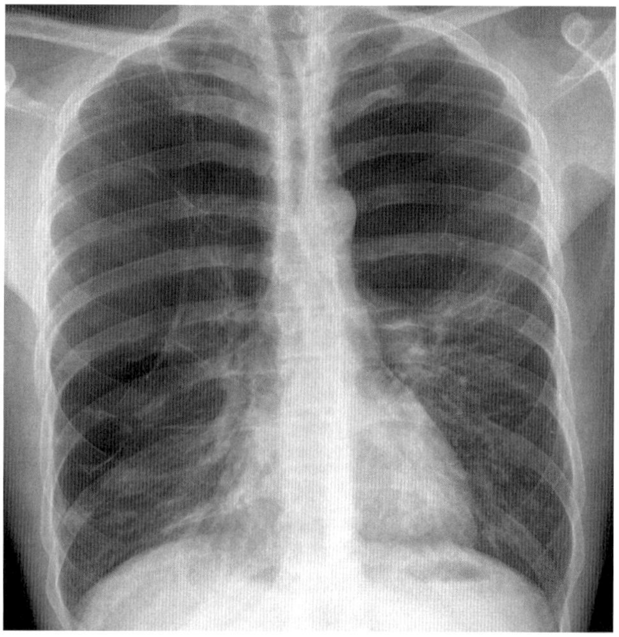

Figure 56.3. Giant bullous emphysema. PA radiograph of a 39-year-old man with giant bullous emphysema (vanishing lung syndrome). Bullae occupy more than one-third of the thorax and affect the right lung more than the left. Note crowding of vessels inferiorly in the relatively normal lower lobes. The patient was treated with bullectomy and experienced symptomatic relief.

Thin-section CT is the most sensitive test for detection, classification, and quantification of emphysema and its mimics.

- *Do the "holes" have walls?* Lung cysts have perceptible walls, whereas centrilobular emphysema does not.
- *What is the microscopic distribution* (centrilobular, paraseptal, panlobular)?
- *What is the macroscopic distribution* (upper vs. lower zone predominant)?
- *Are there complications?* Lung cancer, pulmonary hypertension, pneumonia, and spontaneous pneumothorax are all more common in patients with emphysema than in the general population.

What Not to Miss

- Hyperinflation of the lungs may indicate underlying emphysema that is not apparent on chest radiography.
- Thin-section CT is the best imaging modality for the detection and characterization of emphysema.
- The presence of centrilobular and/or paraseptal emphysema indicates a history of cigarette smoking, and imaging studies should be carefully inspected for signs of lung cancer.

Differential Diagnosis

Common Forms of Emphysema

- Centrilobular emphysema: Most common type of emphysema; it is usually seen in adult smokers but also related to other inhaled toxins.
- Panlobular emphysema: Can be seen in smokers or patients with α_1-antitrypsin deficiency, rarely as a result of intravenous Ritalin injection; patients with α_1-antitrypsin deficiency present earlier (fourth and fifth decades) and are also at risk for cirrhosis.
- Paraseptal emphysema: Usually seen in association with centrilobular emphysema; uncommonly seen in isolation; rupture may result in spontaneous pneumothorax.

Less Common Forms of Emphysema

- Combined pulmonary fibrosis and emphysema: An incompletely understood entity in which emphysema and pulmonary fibrosis (usual interstitial pneumonitis (UIP) pattern) coexist in the same patient; associated with a high prevalence of pulmonary hypertension and an especially poor prognosis; patients have pseudonormal PFTs (balance of restriction and obstruction) but severely decreased DLCO.
- Giant bullous emphysema: Also known as vanishing lung syndrome, a rare entity usually seen in middle-aged male smokers (fourth through sixth decades); upper lobe predominant bullae occupy more than one-third of the thoracic cavity and compress normal lung tissue (Fig. 56.3).

Emphysema Mimics

- Cystic lung disease: Lymphangioleiomyomatosis occurs exclusively in women in their reproductive years and may be associated with tuberous sclerosis complex; pulmonary Langerhans cell histiocytosis is almost always seen in smokers and may coexist with emphysema; prior pneumocystis pneumonia may result in pulmonary cysts that predominantly involve the upper lobes.
- Fibrotic lung disease: UIP also occurs in smokers, but it is a restrictive lung disease that is typically diffuse, peripheral, and basilar in distribution.
- Constrictive bronchiolitis (syn. obliterative bronchiolitis): Bronchiolar inflammation and fibrosis with stenosis/occlusion results in air trapping; may be focal or diffuse; it may be idiopathic, post-infectious (e.g., Swyer–James syndrome), result from toxic inhalation, or occur following transplantation.
- Aging lung: Normal lung changes occur with aging, with dilation of alveolar ducts and respiratory bronchioles; distinguished from emphysema by the lack of lung destruction; FEV_1 in never-smokers steadily declines at a rate much less than that of patients with emphysema, and it almost never produces symptoms.

Imaging Findings

Centrilobular Emphysema

- Focal lucent areas in lung parenchyma *without definable walls* most often with an upper lobe predominance (Fig. 56.4)
- Lucencies often surround the centrilobular artery that appears as a small central dot (Fig. 56.4)
- May become confluent and compress adjacent lung parenchyma, which can simulate a wall along part of the border
- In severe cases, may be indistinguishable from panlobular emphysema (Figs. 56.5 and Fig 56.7)

Paraseptal Emphysema

- Parenchymal lucencies in a subpleural location, most common along the lung apices (Fig. 56.6)
- Often demarcated by interlobular septa, which appear as thin walls
- Typically form a single row along the pleural surface, distinguishing it from honeycombing (typically multiple, stacked rows of thick-walled cysts)
- Measure up to 1 cm in diameter; if greater than 1 cm, then called a bulla
- Frequently coexists with centrilobular emphysema
- Ruptured paraseptal emphysema or bulla results in spontaneous pneumothorax

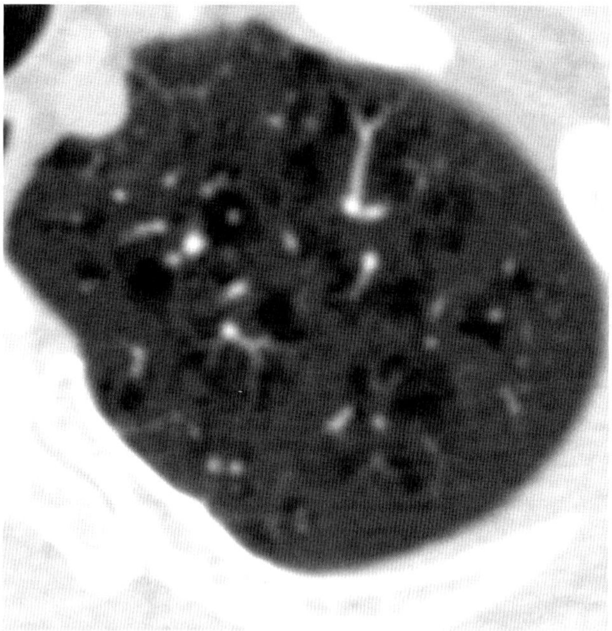

Figure 56.4. Centrilobular emphysema. Contrast-enhanced chest CT of left lung apex of a 67-year-old man with moderate centrilobular emphysema shows focal areas of low attenuation with imperceptible walls, with small centrilobular arteries passing through many of these areas. The imperceptible walls of centrilobular emphysema are a distinguishing feature from the thin-walled lung cysts that occur in other lung diseases (e.g., lymphangioleiomyomatosis and Langerhans cell histiocytosis).

Panlobular Emphysema

- Panlobular destruction results in a generalized decrease in lung attenuation in secondary pulmonary lobules and regions of affected lung (Fig. 56.7).

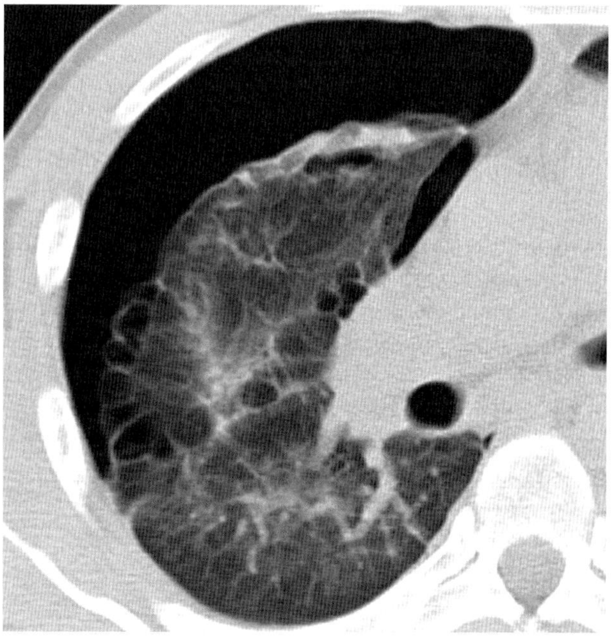

Figure 56.5. Paraseptal emphysema. Chest CT of a 30-year-old man shows paraseptal emphysema manifesting as a single tier of subpleural lucencies demarcated by thin walls representing interlobular septa and a pneumothorax. Ground-glass opacity and focal patchy consolidation in the lung parenchyma represent associated atelectasis.

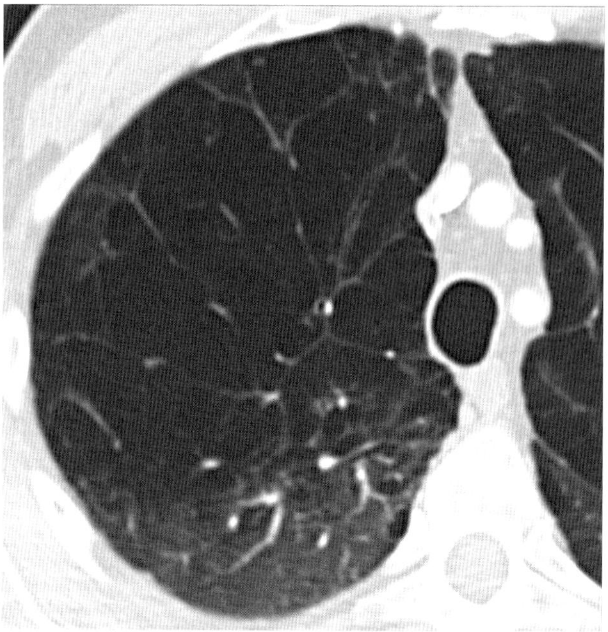

Figure 56.6. Severe centrilobular emphysema. Contrast-enhanced chest CT of a 50-year-old man with severe centrilobular emphysema shows large emphysematous spaces adjacent to areas of low attenuation with imperceptible walls. Some of the large spaces are partially lined by vessels or septae that may be confused for cysts.

- Lower lobe predominant (as opposed to centrilobular emphysema, although severe, diffuse cases may be indistinguishable).
- Lower lobe predominant bronchiectasis and scarring may also be present.

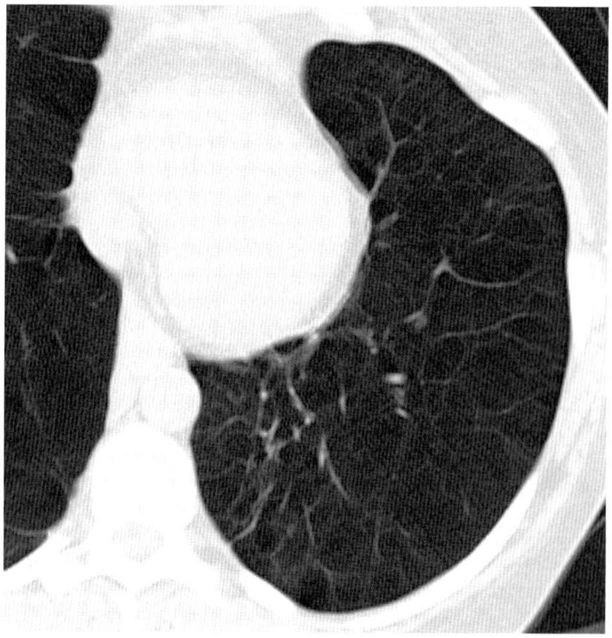

Figure 56.7. Panlobular emphysema (α_1-antitrypsin deficiency). Chest CT of a 49-year-old woman with α_1-antitrypsin deficiency shows panlobular emphysema with uniform destruction of the lung parenchyma and simplification of the lung architecture. These findings were bilateral and symmetric in distribution, predominantly affecting the lower lobes.

- In α_1-antitrypsin deficiency, a nodular liver contour is suggestive of associated fibrosis (cirrhosis).

Giant Bullous Emphysema

- Large bullae occupy a significant portion of the thoracic cavity (at least one-third by strict definition).
- Bullae form in the upper lobes, displacing lung tissue inferiorly (Fig. 56.3).
- May be symmetric or disproportionately affect one lung.

Clinical Issues

- Acute complications of emphysema include COPD exacerbation, pneumonia, and spontaneous pneumothorax. Acute exacerbation is usually secondary to worsening airway obstruction or infection, and only a minority of patients have an acute abnormality (e.g., pneumonia) on chest radiography.
- Chronic complications of emphysema include lung cancer and pulmonary hypertension, which may progress to cor pulmonale.
- CT is useful for surgical planning in advanced cases of emphysema. Lung volume reduction surgery can be effective in patients with bullous disease by resecting the overinflated, nonfunctioning lung tissue. The use of one-way endobronchial valves is a promising, minimally invasive technique that blocks the airway to overinflated lung and reduces its volume. In end-stage cases, lung transplantation may be considered.
- Multiple software vendors offer automated, quantitative analysis of distribution and severity of emphysema using a threshold value on CT scans (usually <950 HU). However, because emphysema is only part of the clinical spectrum of COPD, severity on imaging does not always correlate with clinical symptoms.

Key Points

- Emphysema is an extremely common disease, and in most cases the diagnosis is established with clinical data including PFTs. CT may be helpful for clarifying the diagnosis in mild cases or if another disease process (e.g., interstitial lung disease) is suspected.
- The three different types of emphysema (centrilobular, paraseptal, and panlobular) affect different parts of the secondary pulmonary lobule and are easily distinguished on CT.
- Emphysema distorts the normal lung anatomy and can cause superimposed processes (e.g., pneumonia or pulmonary edema) to look atypical on chest radiography and CT. Similarly, lung cancer may have an unusual morphology when it arises within emphysematous lung.
- Cystic lung disease and honeycombing in pulmonary fibrosis should not be confused with emphysema. Cysts and honeycombing have defined walls on CT, whereas centrilobular emphysema manifests as areas of low attenuation without perceptible walls.

Suggested Reading

Foster WL, Gimenez EI, Roubidoux MA, et al. The emphysemas: Radiologic–pathologic correlations. *RadioGraphics*. 1993;13(2):311–328.

Kemp SV, Polkey MI, Shah PL. The epidemiology, etiology, clinical features, and natural history of emphysema. *Thorac Surg Clin North Am*. 2009;19(2):149–158.

Sharma N, Justaniah AM, Kanne JP, Gurney JW, Mohammed TLH. Vanishing lung syndrome (giant bullous emphysema): CT findings in 7 patients and a literature review. *Journal Thorac Imaging*. 2009;24(3):227–230.

CHAPTER 57

Bronchiolitis

Brent P. Little and Travis S. Henry

Definition

In children, the term *bronchiolitis* refers to an acute respiratory illness caused by bronchiolar infection, typically by respiratory syncytial virus (RSV) or other viruses. In adults, the term refers to a primarily bronchiolar pattern of infection or inflammation caused by many pulmonary infections, systemic inflammatory conditions, inhaled irritants, certain systemic conditions, and accompanying several congenital diseases. Imaging may be helpful to assess the extent and severity of bronchiolitis and to establish a differential diagnosis based on the distribution of imaging findings, their respective morphologies, and any ancillary findings.

Clinical Features

Infections with viruses such as influenza, parainfluenza, adenovirus, and RSV can cause pneumonias with a significant bronchiolar component. Patients may present with "flu-like" symptoms, including cough, fever, myalagias, and malaise. Laboratory evaluation may include viral cultures and testing for specific nucleic acids or proteins using nasopharyngeal or bronchoalveolar lavage samples. However, in most cases of presumed viral bronchiolitis/pneumonia, a specific viral agent is not identified. Atypical bacterial pneumonias such as mycoplasma and chlamydia, mycobacterium tuberculosis, and atypical mycobacterial infections can also exhibit a bronchiolitis pattern on imaging.

Inhalational causes of bronchiolitis include respiratory bronchiolitis, a disease of smokers caused by chronic irritation of bronchioles, and hypersensitivity pneumonitis, caused by an immune-mediated inflammatory response to inhaled antigens such as fungi, certain bacteria, and avian proteins. Chronic hypersensitivity pneumonitis can lead to fibrosis. A subset of "inhalational" bronchiolitis is aspiration bronchiolitis, often seen in patients with an impaired swallowing mechanism, significant gastroesophageal reflux, or neurological compromise.

Congenital conditions with faulty bronchiolar function, such as cystic fibrosis and primary ciliary dyskinesia, can lead to a chronic bronchiolitis due to a combination of impaired clearance of secretions and chronic infection/colonization with characteristic organisms (e.g., *Pseudomonas* in cystic fibrosis). Patients have chronic respiratory symptoms punctuated by episodes of recurrent pneumonia.

Systemic and Idiopathic Causes

Bronchiolitis obliterans (BO) (obliterative bronchiolitis or constrictive bronchiolitis) is a disease of submucosal/peribronchiolar fibrosis. Patients typically present with gradually increasing shortness of breath; pulmonary function tests show an obstructive pattern. BO is the histology of chronic rejection in lung transplantation, and it is the major source of long-term morbidity/mortality in these patients. BO can also occur as a complication of any solid organ or bone marrow transplantation. Other causes include severe pneumonia (usually viral) and systemic diseases such as rheumatoid arthritis. BO can also be idiopathic.

Diffuse panbronchiolitis is an idiopathic chronic bronchiolitis occurring almost exclusively in Japanese men aged 30–50 years, with recurrent pneumonias, frequent *Pseudomonas* colonization, and progressive airflow obstruction with hypoxemia.

Follicular bronchiolitis involves lymphoid hyperplasia of the bronchus, and it arises most commonly in the setting of collagen vascular and immunodeficiency diseases. Patients with these conditions can present with progressive dyspnea, cough, and hypoxemia.

Anatomy and Physiology

Subsegmental bronchi branch multiple times into small noncartilagenous airways with diameters of 0.3–1.0 mm called bronchioles. With the exception of the final order (respiratory) bronchioles, bronchioles do not participate in gas exchange. Preterminal bronchioles divide over several generations into smaller, thinner-walled terminal bronchioles, which give rise to several respiratory bronchioles, opening to two or three alveolar ducts which in turn give rise to the alveolar sacs.

The normal centrilobular bronchiole is not visible on CT. In bronchiolitis, inflammation within and around the bronchiole manifests on CT as hazy nodules usually less than 10 mm in diameter, known as "centrilobular" nodules. Because these nodules arise at the center of the secondary pulmonary lobule, they are very even in their distribution and do not extend to the pleural/fissural surfaces. A special subset of the centrilobular pattern of nodules—the "tree-in-bud" pattern—can be seen when pus, liquid, or mucous distends the distal bronchioles and alveolar ducts. Clusters of branching linear structures correspond to impacted centrilobular bronchioles, and tiny nodules at the ends of the branches represent distended alveolar ducts.

How to Approach the Image

Are Radiographs Adequate or Should CT Be Performed?

In many cases of bronchiolitis, the chest radiograph is normal, or there are nonspecific findings such as a patchy or diffuse nodular or reticulonodular pattern (Fig. 57.1). CT can help clarify the pattern and extent of the abnormality when clinical findings are confusing.

What Is the Distribution?

Upper lobe predominant bronchiolitis is often caused by hypersensitivity pneumonitis, smoking-related lung disease, or infection such as tuberculosis, whereas lower lobe bronchiolitis should suggest the possibility of aspiration.

What Is the Chronicity?

Chronic bronchiolitis may suggest secondary to indolent infection (e.g., chronic atypical mycobacterial infections such as *Mycobacterium avium-intracellulare*) or chronic mucous plugging (cystic fibrosis and primary ciliary dyskinesia)

Is There Air Trapping?

Air trapping may be indicative of bronchiolitis obliterans (Fig. 57.2).

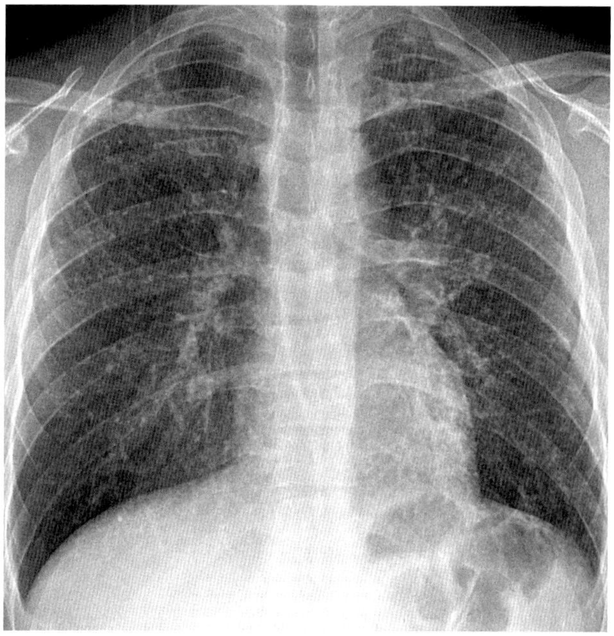

Figure 57.1. A 27-year-old man with frequent travel to Mexico: active tuberculosis with endobronchial spread. Chest radiograph shows a slight upper lobe predominance of extensive bilateral reticulonodular pattern in all lobes. Scattered large nodules are faintly seen, some of which could be cavitary.

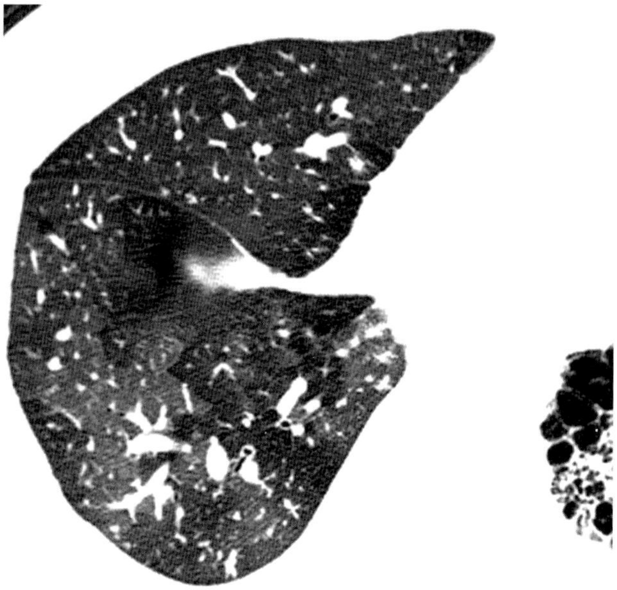

Figure 57.2. A 50-year-old man with bronchiolitis obliterans with slowing increasing obstruction on pulmonary function tests after unilateral right lung transplant. Axial CT at inspiration shows subtle mosaic attenuation. Expiratory image near the same level shows an increase in attenuation in areas of normal lung. The lucent regions remain lower attenuation, representing air trapping. Notice the smaller vessel caliber in areas of air trapping, reflecting hypoxemic vasoconstriction.

What Not to Miss

Although cavities are common in pulmonary tuberculosis, a bronchiolitis pattern can also occur as an isolated or associated finding. In the appropriate clinical setting, clustered nodularity with an upper lung predominance on chest radiography or a tree-in-bud pattern on chest CT should raise concern for endobronchial spread of tuberculosis.

A vascular tree-in-bud pattern can be misinterpreted as bronchiolitis on chest CT. Although uncommon, a variety of vascular disorders, including endovascular metastases, can manifest with this pattern. Irregularity or "beading" of adjacent pulmonary arteries may be a clue to the vascular nature of the imaging findings.

Hypersensitivity pneumonitis (HP) should be suspected on the basis of imaging findings of centrilobular ground-glass nodules, patchy ground-glass opacity, and air trapping on chest CT. It is important to suggest the possibility of this diagnosis to the patient's health care team because removal of the offending exposure may improve symptoms and prevent progression to chronic HP and fibrosis.

Differential Diagnosis

Because arterioles parallel the course of bronchioles in the center of the secondary pulmonary lobule, several diseases involving the small vessels can lead to a pattern indistinguishable from bronchiolitis.

Pulmonary Vasculitis

- Periarteriolar inflammation with centrilobular distribution
- Usually hazy, ground-glass nodules
- May exhibit a tree-in-bud appearance

Pulmonary Hypertension

- Ground-glass, centrilobular nodules
- Mosaic attenuation, geographic or lobular alternating areas of high and low attenuation within the lungs
- Enlarged pulmonary arteries

Endovascular Tumor Metastases

- Vascular tree-in-bud pattern can occur from endovascular tumor metastases or due to a vascular reaction to the emboli called thrombotic microangiopathy.
- Most commonly from hematogenous spread of renal cell carcinoma and certain adenocarcinomas

Talc/Cellulose Embolism

- Large particles from compositional binders in injected crushed tablets can lodge in the distal arterioles.
- Granulomatous periartiolar reaction with a vascular tree-in-bud pattern (excipient lung)

Pulmonary Capillary Hemangiomatosis

- Rare cause of pulmonary hypertension with proliferation of abnormal capillaries in the peribronchovascular interstitium
- Hazy centrilobular ground-glass nodules indistinguishable from subacute hypersensitivity pneumonitis

Imaging Findings

Infectious Bronchiolitis

Viral Bronchiolitis

- A common cause of infectious bronchiolitis
- Tree-in-bud and ground-glass centrilobular nodules on CT, often accompanied by diffuse or patchy ground-glass opacities
- Air trapping sometimes seen on CT due to distal airway obstruction (Fig. 57.3)

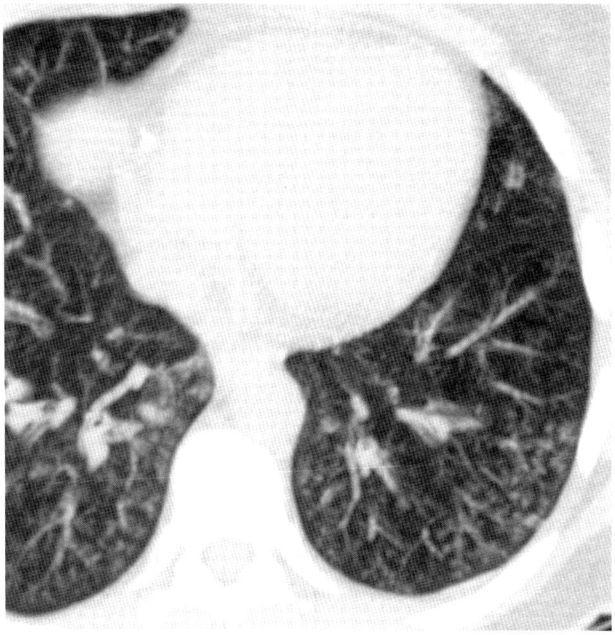

Figure 57.3. Viral Bronchiolitis. A 43-year old man with shortness of breath and viral bronchiolitis. Axial CT shows centrilobular nodules and tree-in-bud opacities.

Bacterial Bronchiolitis

- Bronchiolitis may accompany any bacterial pneumonia, either typical (streptococcal and others) or atypical (mycoplasma and chlamydia).
- Centrilobular/tree-in-bud nodules are seen on CT.
- A bronchopneumonia pattern of airways-centered patchy consolidation or more extensive consolidation can be seen on chest radiography and CT.

Tuberculosis

- Tree-in-bud nodules on CT, representing endobronchial spread of infection
- Bronchiectasis and bronchial wall thickening
- Upper lobes and superior segments of lower lobes usually involved
- Nodular consolidation can be seen
- Cavities and fistulous connections between airways and cavities common (Fig. 57.4)

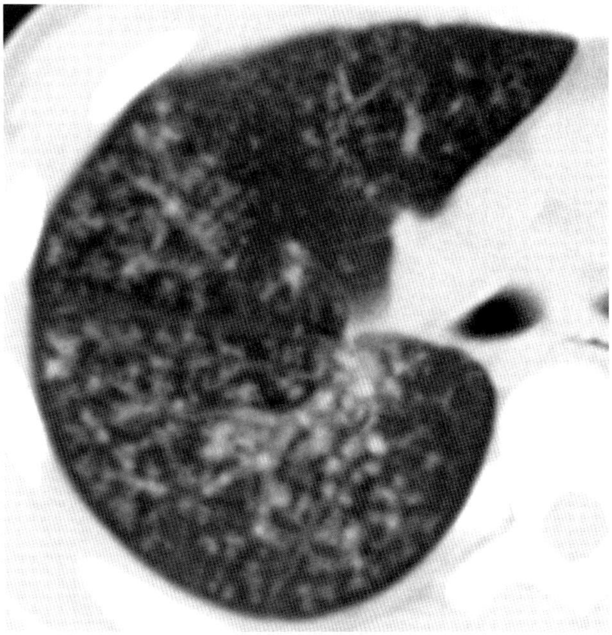

Figure 57.4. A 27-year-old man with frequent travel to Mexico: active tuberculosis with endobronchial spread. Axial CT image shows extensive nodules in a tree-in-bud pattern throughout the lungs. Several thick-walled cavities were present (not shown) in the left lung.

Atypical Mycobacterial Infection

- Classic type: Upper lung zone predominant, associated with cavities and tree-in-bud nodules, volume loss and architectural distortion, mimics postprimary tuberculosis
- Nonclassic type: Tree-in-bud nodules with right middle lobe and lingular predominance; chronic linear scarring/atelectasis and bronchiectasis in the same distribution common; usually elderly women

Fungal Infection

- Tree-in-bud nodules at CT, with or without cavities
- Consolidation often present
- Ground-glass opacities surrounding nodules (halo sign) suggestive of invasive fungal infection (often aspergillus) in an immunocompromised patient

Aspiration-Related Bronchiolitis

- Clustered centrilobular ground-glass or solid nodules at CT
- Dependent/lower lobe distribution common
- Diffuse pattern can involve even nondependent lungs
- Dependent bronchiectasis can be seen in chronic aspiration
- Common finding after trauma or surgery for certain head and neck cancers (Fig. 57.5)

Bronchiolitis Due to Inhaled Substances

Respiratory Bronchiolitis

- Respiratory bronchiolitis (RB) is a frequent finding in smokers.
- Chest radiographs may be normal or show evidence of only chronic obstructive pulmonary disease.
- CT shows hazy, ground-glass centrilobular nodules, upper lobe predominant; it is often best seen with narrow windows.
- "Pure" centrilobular nodules are common; tree-in-bud pattern is often absent.
- RB-associated interstitial lung disease (RB-ILD) is a term applied to RB with respiratory symptoms.
- It is often seen in conjunction with other smoking-related diseases (desquamative interstitial pneumonia and emphysema) (Fig. 57.6).

Hypersensitivity Pneumonitis

- Subacute HP often has a bronchiolitis pattern; radiographs can be normal or exhibit a subtle micronodular appearance.
- CT can show upper and mid zone predominant "pure" centrilobular ground-glass nodules.

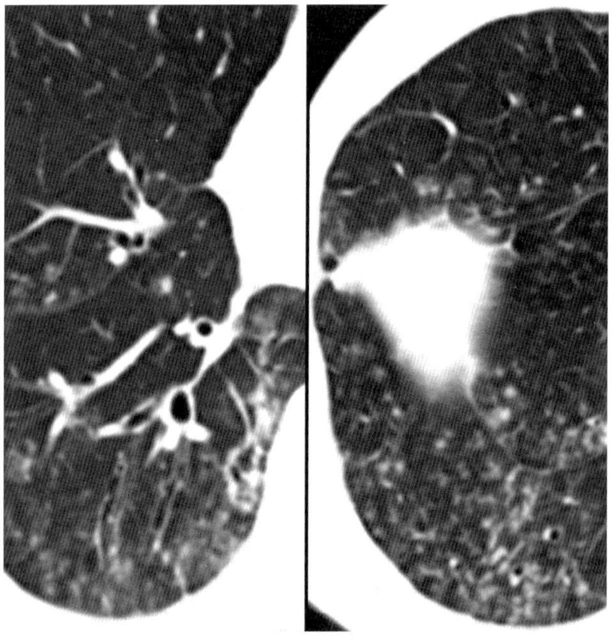

Figure 57.5. A 69-year-old man with recurrent aspiration. (Left) Axial CT image shows ground-glass nodules and patchy ground-glass opacity in a dependent distribution in the superior segment of the right upper lobe. Note the accompanying mild traction bronchiectasis, a finding commonly seen in chronic aspiration. (Right) Image from the same CT shows numerous clusters of dependent nodules in a tree-in-bud pattern in the right middle lobe and right lower lobe. Image through the right lung base shows a continuation of the extensive tree-in-bud bronchiolitis pattern.

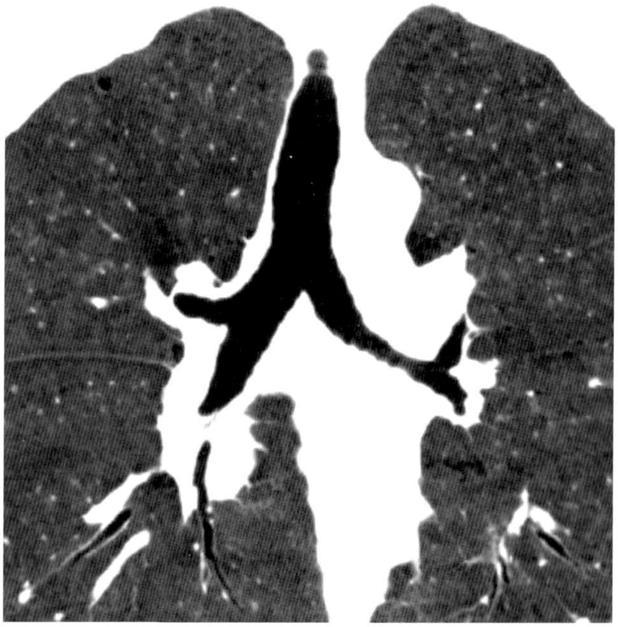

Figure 57.6. A 52-year-old one-pack-a-day smoker with respiratory bronchiolitis. Coronal reformatted minimum intensity projection (MinIP) CT image shows widely distributed ground-glass nodules in all lobes, with a slight upper lobe predominance. The nodules spare the pleural/fissural surfaces and have a "pure centrilobular" appearance, usually seen in airways inflammation such as respiratory bronchiolitis or hypersensitivity pneumonitis. The tree-in-bud pattern is more common in infection and refers to well-defined branching opacities with usually sharply defined terminal nodules, which usually represent bronchioles and alveolar ducts distended with fluid/pus. There is much overlap in etiologies of these two patterns, and the patterns can coexist.

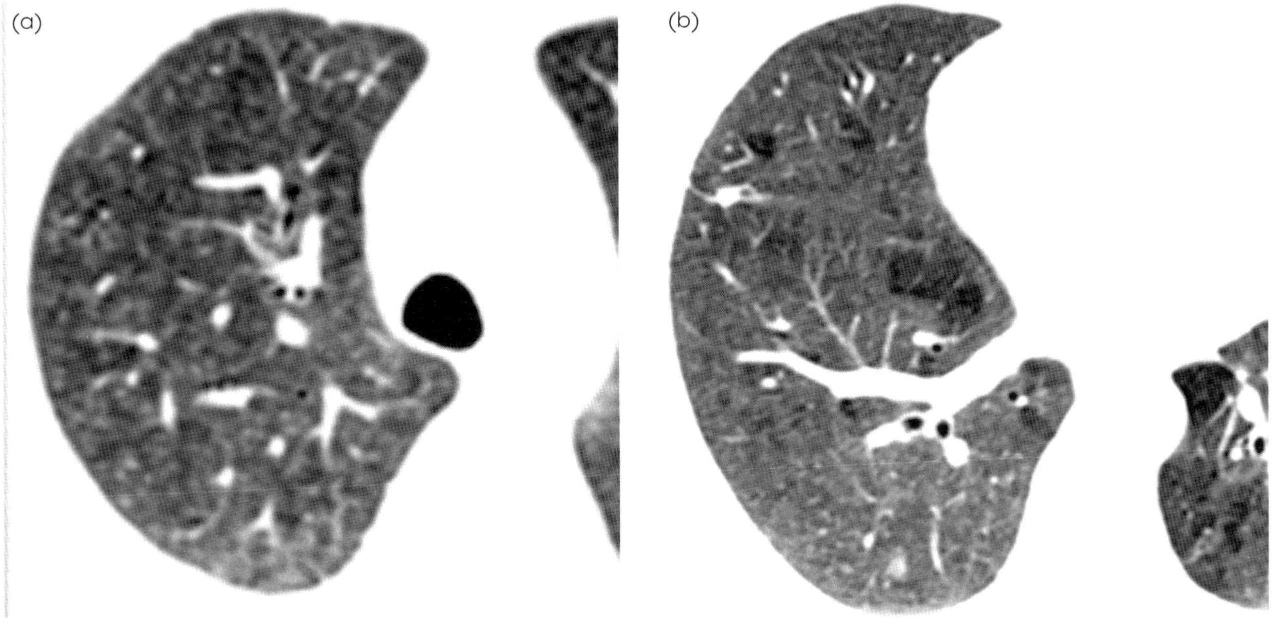

Figure 57.7. A 42-year-old woman with persistent dry cough and dyspnea: biopsy-proven hypersensitivity pneumonitis. The patient had a pet bird at home. (a) Axial CT at inspiration shows ill-defined diffuse centrilobular pattern of ground-glass nodules throughout the upper lobes. (b) Axial CT image from the same CT through the lower lobes shows a mosaic pattern of attenuation, with a "headcheese" appearance: Well-defined lucent areas represent air trapping, intermediate attenuation represents relatively normal lung, and the higher attenuation areas (ground-glass) represent inflammation.

- A "mosaic attenuation" pattern at CT (areas of alternating high and low attenuation in the lungs) representing air trapping is common, especially at expiratory imaging (Fig. 57.7b).
- Ground-glass opacities are often present (Fig. 57.7a). The combination of ground-glass and air trapping is known as the "headcheese" pattern.

Congenital Causes of Bronchiolitis

Primary Ciliary Dyskinesia/Kartagener's Syndrome

- Bronchiectasis and tree-in-bud nodules at the lung bases, predominantly the middle lobe and lingula
- Dextrocardia or complete situs inversus

Cystic Fibrosis

- Upper lobe predominant bronchiectasis
- Mucoid bronchial impaction and bronchial wall thickening
- Patchy tree-in-bud bronchiolitis pattern with air trapping throughout the lungs

Bronchiolitis Related to Systemic or Idiopathic Causes

Bronchiolitis Obliterans

- Air trapping at expiratory CT is the most sensitive finding. Lucent lung that does not increase in attenuation on expiratory imaging causes a "mosaic attenuation" pattern.
- Bronchiectasis and centrilobular/tree-in-bud nodules can be seen.

Follicular Bronchiolitis

- Associated with rheumatoid arthritis
- Tree-in-bud nodules at CT, often peripheral, represent a lymphoid interstitial infiltrate; can progress to fibrosis

Panbronchiolitis

- Idiopathic chronic obstructive disease affecting mainly Asians
- Diffuse tree-in-bud pattern of centrilobular nodules at CT

Allergic Bronchopulmonary Aspergillosus

- Fungal colonization and immune response leads to airway damage, with mid to upper lung, central bronchiectasis, and tree-in-bud nodules at CT.

Clinical Issues

- Infectious bronchiolitis can present with acute symptoms such as shortness of breath, fever, and cough. Whereas viral bronchiolitis is often self-limiting in the immunocompetent patient, treatment of other infections that cause bronchiolitis varies according to etiology.
- Patients with bronchiolitis often have pulmonary function tests indicative of obstruction, especially in chronic conditions such as bronchiolitis obliterans or for any of the congenital causes of bronchiolitis.
- Bronchiolitis obliterans is the most common long-term cause of death after lung transplantation.

Key Points

- The presence of cavities or architectural distortion with a bronchiolitis pattern, especially in the upper lungs, should prompt consideration of tuberculosis.
- Aspiration bronchiolitis is a common finding in patients with severe reflux or with impaired swallowing mechanisms.
- Early diagnosis of hypersensitivity pneumonitis can lead to prompt identification of the offending antigen.
- In cases with pure centrilobular nodules, smoking history is paramount: Smokers get RB, whereas nonsmokers have a higher likelihood of hypersensitivity pneumonitis.

Suggested Reading

Gosset N, Bankier AA, Eisenberg RL. Tree-in-bud pattern. *AJR Am J Roentgenol.* 2009;193(6):W472–W477.

Gotway MB, Reddy GP, Webb WR, Elicker BM, Leung, JW. High-resolution CT of the lung: Patterns of disease and differential diagnoses. *Radiol Clin North Am.* 2005;43(3):513–542.

Matar LD, McAdams HP, Sporn TA. Hypersensitivity pneumonitis. *AJR Am J Roentgenol.* 2000;174(4):1061–1066.

Rossi SE, Franquet T, Volpacchio M, Gimenez A, Aguilar G. Tree-in-bud pattern at thin-section CT of the lungs: Radiologic–pathologic overview. *RadioGraphics.* 2005;25(3):789–801.

Section XI

Connective Tissue Disorders and Autoimmune Conditions

CHAPTER 58

Introduction to Connective Tissue Disorders and Autoimmune Conditions

Santiago Martínez-Jiménez

Introduction

A variety of pathologic processes affect the connective tissues. The chapters in this section address some of these conditions, with an emphasis on autoimmune disorders (e.g., rheumatoid arthritis, scleroderma, systemic lupus erythematosus, dermatomyositis/polymyositis, Sjögren syndrome, mixed connective tissue disease, and vasculitis), amyloidosis, and eosinophilic lung disease.

Autoimmune Diseases

An autoimmune response is an immune response that targets an antigen within the host and attacks healthy body tissues (Fig. 58.1). This often involves T and B lymphocytes in a response that is very similar to an allergic reaction. Although the presence of an autoantibody is often an essential component of the autoimmune response, its mere presence does not define the disease. In addition to the presence of autoantibodies, the presence of soft tissue damage is required; thus, autoantibodies may be present in the absence of an inflammatory process. There is much debate about what can trigger an autoimmune response and whether the culprit can be endogenous or exogenous. In some cases, the answer has been fully elucidated, but in many cases it remains elusive and only hypotheses can be found.

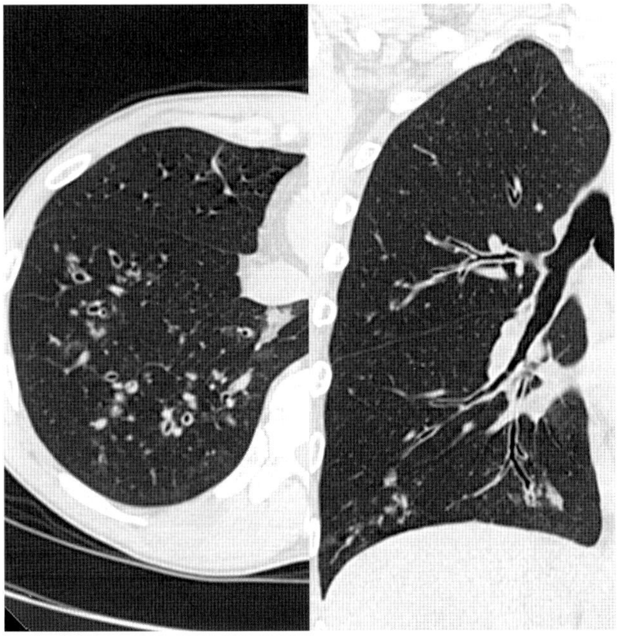

Figure 58.1. Bronchiectasis in ulcerative colitis. Composite image of a patient with ulcerative colitis with axial (left) and coronal (right) unenhanced chest CT shows bronchiectasis, bronchial wall thickening, mucoid plugging, and centrilobular nodules.

A unique model of autoimmunity is celiac disease, in which a genetic predisposition, an environmental factor, and autoantibodies have been fully identified. This autoimmune condition is known to be triggered by peptides (generically called prolamins) that occur naturally in the seeds of several grasses, including wheat, rye, and barley. In celiac disease, these exogenous peptides may elicit an autoimmune response in genetically predisposed individuals (e.g., HLA DQ2 and DQ8) that often targets the small intestine, leading to classic symptoms of diarrhea and failure to thrive. Interestingly, symptoms may occur exclusively outside the gastrointestinal tract (e.g., dermatitis herpetiformis), making the diagnosis challenging. The pathophysiologic events that lead to an autoimmune response in celiac disease are beyond the scope of this work but have been firmly established. In fact, it is postulated that this inflammatory response toward prolamins might be involved in the development of other autoimmune conditions (e.g., type 1 diabetes mellitus, autoimmune thyroid disease, autoimmune liver disease, rheumatoid arthritis, systemic lupus erythematosus, Addison disease, ankylosing spondylitis, and Sjögren syndrome), malignancies, and neurologic and psychiatric diseases.

In some cases, the development of autoimmunity is not well recognized, and extensive reports have linked it with viruses, bacteria, and medications. Although autoimmune diseases have a tendency to involve a certain organ(s), it seems clear that they are also part of an inflammatory response often with multisystemic compromise. Extensive research has been directed to a better understanding of autoimmune diseases with the hope of increasing the likelihood of successful treatment. For example, removal of exposure to prolamins often results in complete resolution of symptoms for patients with celiac disease.

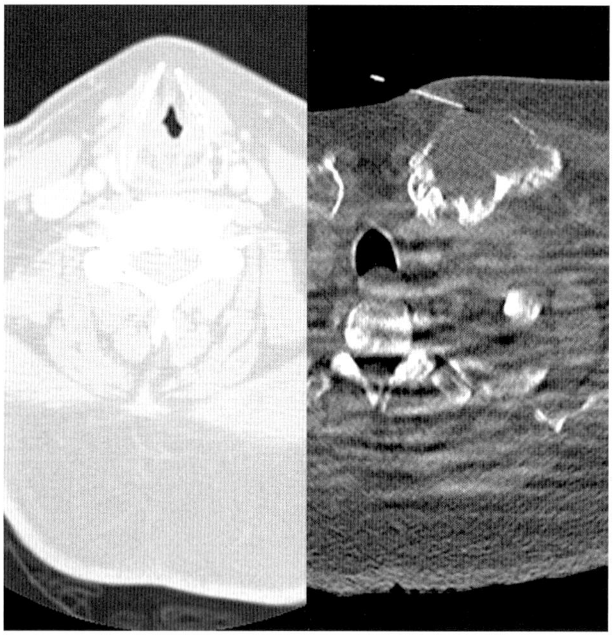

Figure 58.2. Primary amyloidosis associated with plasmacytoma. Composite image with contrast-enhanced chest CT shows subglottic stenosis (left) and an expansile lytic lesion in the medial left clavicle (right).

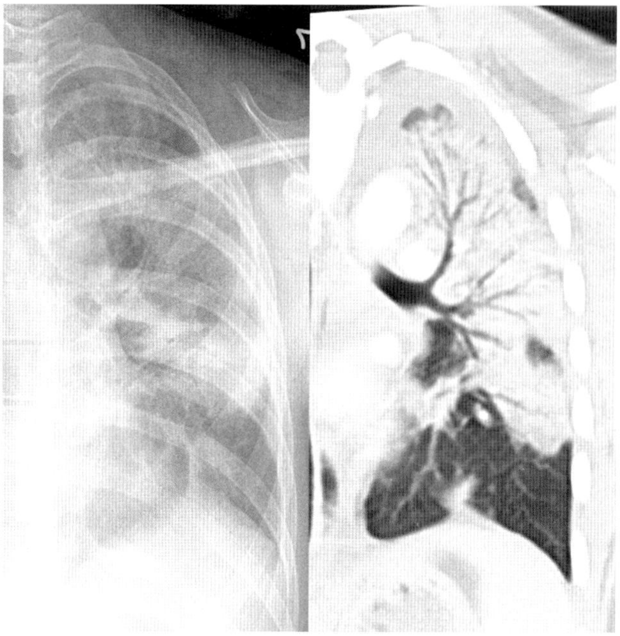

Figure 58.3. Chronic eosinophilic pneumonia. Composite image with posteroanterior chest radiograph (left) and contrast-enhanced chest CT (right) shows extensive multifocal airspace disease.

Amyloidosis

Amyloidosis is a pathologic entity with protean manifestations, often thought of as a single disease rather a group of diseases that share a similar pathophysiologic event: the deposition of proteins within the soft tissues. Amyloidosis can be hereditary or can be associated with plasma cell dyscrasia (e.g., multiple myeloma, Waldestrom macroglobulinemia, and non-Hodgkin lymphoma) or with chronic systemic inflammation (e.g., rheumatoid arthritis and inflammatory bowel disease) (Fig. 58.2).

Protein deposition is often associated with organ dysfunction. This may be a multisystemic event or may affect an isolated organ. Clinical manifestations frequently depend on the nature of the deposited protein as well as the affected tissue and the degree of deposition. Given the protean nature of amyloidosis, radiologists must be familiar with its most common imaging manifestations.

Eosinophilic Lung Disease

The term *eosinophilic lung disease* encompasses a wide variety of pathologic conditions that range from idiopathic diseases to systemic vasculitides (e.g., eosinophilic granulomatosis with polyangiitis) and in some cases a response to parasitic infestation (e.g., ascariasis, strongyloidiasis, and paragonimiasis) (Figs. 58.3 and 58.4). These entities are discussed together because they manifest with blood and/or soft tissue eosinophilia. The presence of eosinophilia is critical for the prospective diagnosis of these diseases, and many of these conditions would not be suspected in the absence of this feature. Thus, it is imperative for the radiologist to seek detailed clinical and laboratory information in order to suggest the diagnosis.

Chapter 63 summarizes important information about common eosinophilic lung diseases, with emphasis on allergic bronchopulmonary aspergillosis (ABPA), acute and

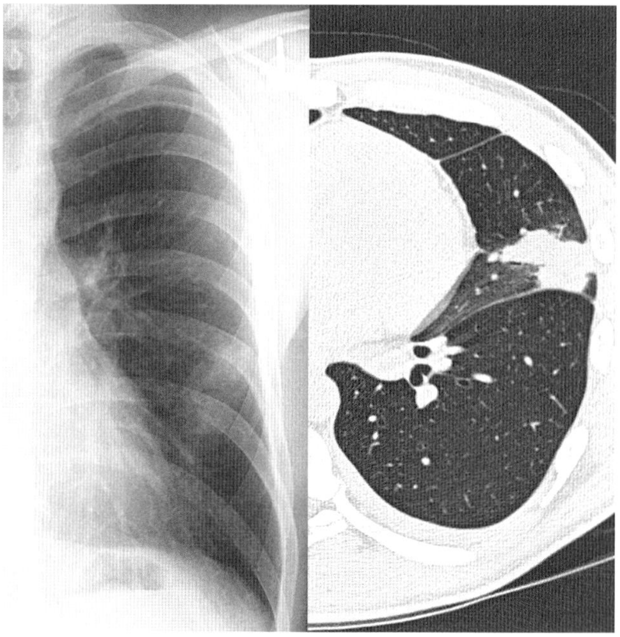

Figure 58.4. Paragonimiasis. Composite image with posteroanterior chest radiograph (left) and unenhanced chest CT (right) shows an ill-defined opacity in the left mid lung zone corresponding to a polylobular lingular nodule and an associated small left pleural effusion.

chronic eosinophilic pneumonia, and parasitic infection. Eosinophilic granulomatosis with polyangiitis (also known as Churg–Strauss syndrome) is discussed in Chapter 61.

Suggested Reading

Aylwin AC, Gishen P, Copley SJ. Imaging appearance of thoracic amyloidosis. *J Thorac Imaging.* 2005 Feb;20(1):41–46.

Li H, Groshong SD, Lynch S, Brown KK, Frankel SK. Eosinophilic lung disease. *Clin Pulm Med.* 2010;17:66–74.

Seaman DM, Meyer CA, Gilman MD, McCormack FX. Diffuse cystic lung disease at high-resolution CT. *AJR Am J Roentgenol.* 2011;196(6):1305–1311.

CHAPTER 59

Rheumatoid Arthritis

Felipe Martínez

Definition

Rheumatoid arthritis (RA) is a progressive chronic systemic autoimmune disorder characterized by symmetric deforming erosive synovitis. The disease affects 1% of the population. Pulmonary involvement occurs in 18% of all patients, is one of the most common extra-articular manifestations of the disease, and is a major cause of morbidity and mortality.

The most common pleuropulmonary manifestations of RA include rheumatoid-associated interstitial lung disease (RA-ILD), drug-related lung disease, infection secondary to immunosuppression, necrobiotic nodules, organizing pneumonia, upper and lower airway disease, pulmonary vascular disease (vasculitis and pulmonary hypertension), and serositis (i.e., pleural and/or pericardial effusions).

Clinical Features

Progressive exertional dyspnea is the main symptom associated with intrathoracic involvement by RA. Although it is difficult to accurately estimate the prevalence of pleuropulmonary involvement, respiratory abnormalities are thought to develop in up to half of patients with RA. Pleuritic chest pain secondary to pleurisy or pleural effusion can also be present.

RA has a well-known predilection to affect women. Clinically significant RA-ILD is slightly more common in women, and it is more common in patients with severe disease. RA-ILD may lead to pulmonary fibrosis in up to 35% of patients. Usual interstitial pneumonia (UIP) pattern is more common than nonspecific interstitial pneumonia (NSIP). Fibrosis and pulmonary hypertension may progress to cor pulmonale, a major cause of mortality in affected patients.

Anatomy and Physiology

RA results from a combination of inherited and random events. Among genetic events, certain human leukocyte antigens (HLAs) are clearly linked to the disease. Among random events, tobacco use appears to be a common preventable association.

When the autoimmune response has developed, the synovium reacts as an invasive tissue that can compromise the cartilage and bone. Increased vascularity leads to joint effusions and chemotaxis of inflammatory cells. Autoantibodies may trigger or enhance joint inflammation. Complement activation and immune complexes also appear to have an important role. The pathogenesis of RA-ILD is poorly understood and appears to be multifactorial. Tobacco abuse increases the risk of RA as well as RA-ILD.

How to Approach the Image

- A normal chest radiograph does not exclude RA-ILD. As disease progresses, radiographic abnormalities may become more apparent.
- Thin-section or high-resolution computed tomography (HRCT) is the study of choice to assess RA-ILD.
- Imaging findings of RA-ILD are no different than those of other idiopathic interstitial pneumonias, hence the importance of correlation with clinical history and laboratory findings. Likewise, all patients with ILD should undergo evaluation for autoimmune disorders, including RA.

What Not to Miss

- Early or mild lung involvement may be present in patients with normal chest radiographs.
- Early signs of ILD and pulmonary fibrosis, such as subtle subpleural reticular and/or ground-glass opacities on HRCT, may be difficult to differentiate from dependent atelectasis. Prone CT imaging as part of HRCT is important because abnormalities of RA-ILD persist in the prone position.
- There is an increased incidence of lung cancer in patients with ILD. Radiologists must carefully scrutinize images for discrete nodules and masses.

Differential Diagnosis

- Idiopathic ILD (e.g., UIP and NSIP), other autoimmune diseases associated with ILD, and asbestosis are included in the differential diagnosis. These entities are indistinguishable from each other on imaging. Esophageal dilatation should raise concern for scleroderma. Asbestosis may be associated with

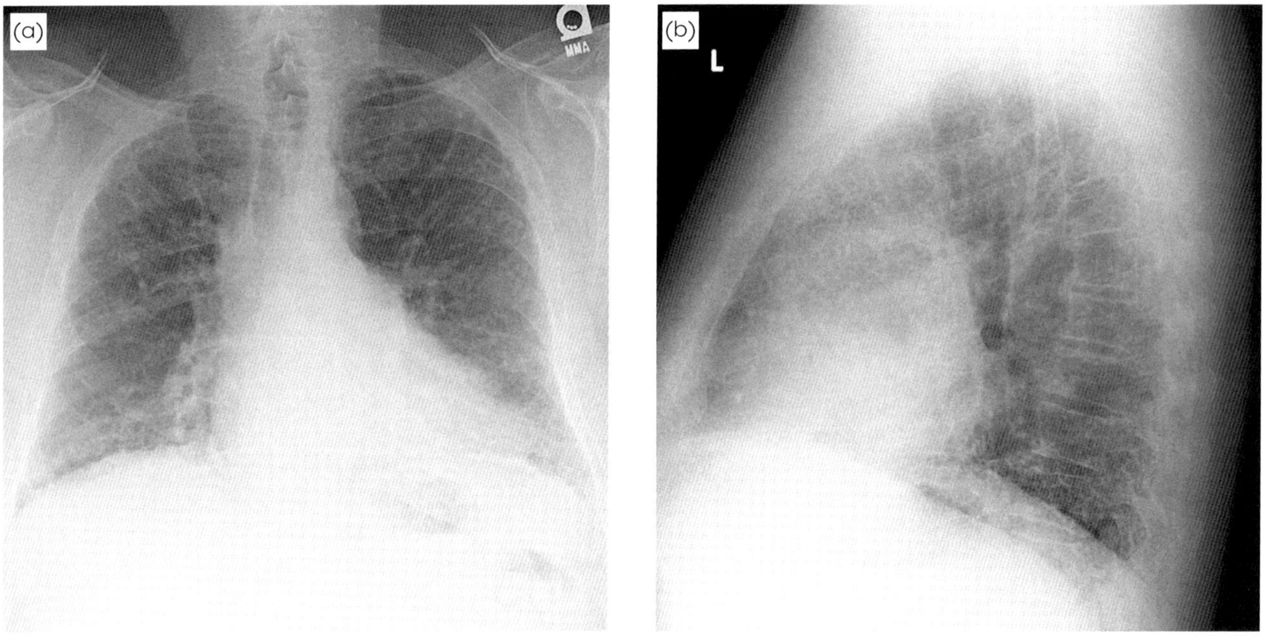

Figure 59.1. RA-ILD. (a) posteroanterior and (b) lateral chest radiographs of a patient with long-standing RA and progressive dyspnea shows bilateral lower lobe predominant volume loss, coarse reticular opacities, and peripheral bronchiectasis and honeycombing.

discontinuous calcified pleural plaques (asbestos-related pleural disease).

- Peribronchovascular upper lobe predominant fibrosis and honeycombing should suggest end-stage sarcoidosis or hypersensitivity pneumonitis.
- Constrictive bronchiolitis may occur as a manifestation of the post-infectious process, inhalational injury, and rejection after transplantation (e.g., bone marrow and lung transplant).
- Multifocal airspace disease and/or ground-glass opacities such as those seen in organizing pneumonia may be manifestations of chronic eosinophilic pneumonia, lymphoma, and multifocal lung adenocarcinoma.
- Macrobiotic RA nodules may cavitate, resolve, or grow. Cavitation should also suggest vasculitis (e.g., granulomatosis with polyangiitis or Wegener), septic embolism, and metastatic disease.

Imaging Findings

RA-ILD (UIP and NSIP)

- Chest radiography: Fine reticular opacities with lower lobe predominance and volume loss (Fig. 59.1). Ancillary findings include pulmonary hypertension such as dilated pulmonary trunk and pulmonary artery pruning.
- Thin-section CT: Lower lobe predominant subpleural reticulation and ground-glass opacities (GGO). With more advanced disease, there is traction bronchiectasis, architectural distortion, honeycombing, and volume loss (Figs. 59.2 and 59.3).

Small Airways Disease in RA

- Bronchiectasis (Fig. 59.4), constrictive bronchiolitis, and follicular bronchiolitis
- Normal chest radiograph or subtly abnormal nonspecific radiographic abnormalities (i.e., reticulonodular opacities)

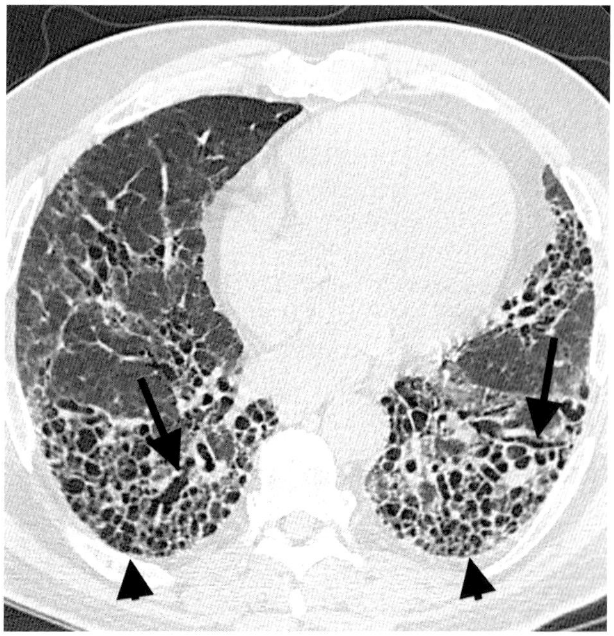

Figure 59.2. RA-ILD, UIP pattern. Chest CT of a patient with RA who presented with progressive dyspnea shows coarse reticular opacities, bronchiectasis (arrows), honeycombing (arrowheads), and lower lobe predominant volume loss.

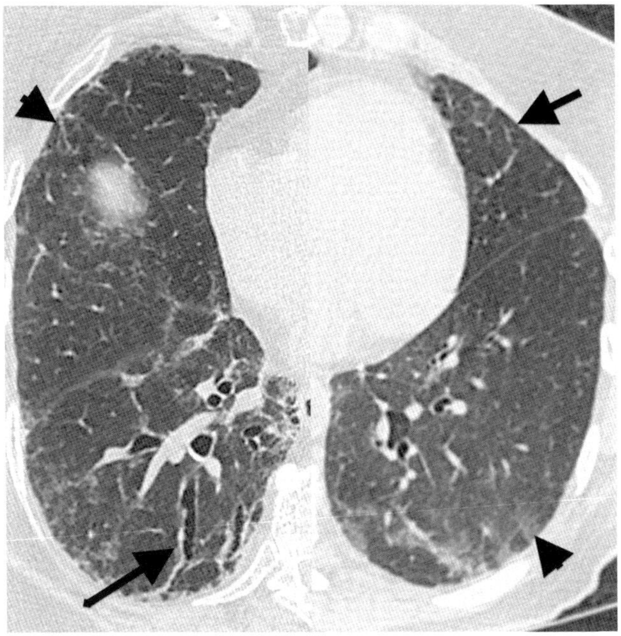

Figure 59.3. RA-ILD, NSIP pattern. Composite image with chest CT of two patients with long-standing lung involvement by RA manifesting as fibrosing NSIP (left) with traction bronchiectasis (arrow), coarse peripheral reticulation (arrowhead), and GGO and as cellular NSIP (right) characterized by fine peripheral reticulation (arrow) and GGO (arrowhead).

- Constrictive bronchiolitis: Subtle mosaic attenuation on inspiratory CT and air trapping on expiratory imaging (Fig. 59.5); associated bronchial wall thickening and bronchiectasis

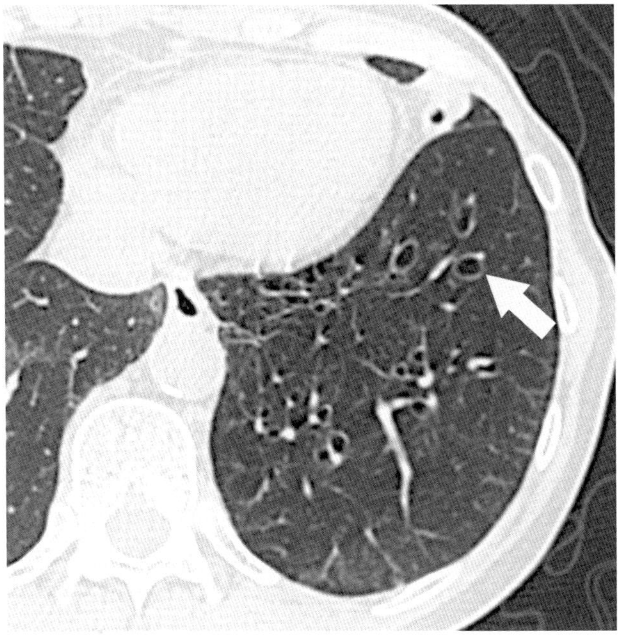

Figure 59.4. Bronchiectasis in RA. Chest CT scan of a patient with advanced RA and worsening chronic cough shows left lower lobe cylindrical bronchiectasis manifesting with the classic "signet-ring" sign (arrow) produced by the bronchiectatic airway and the adjacent pulmonary artery.

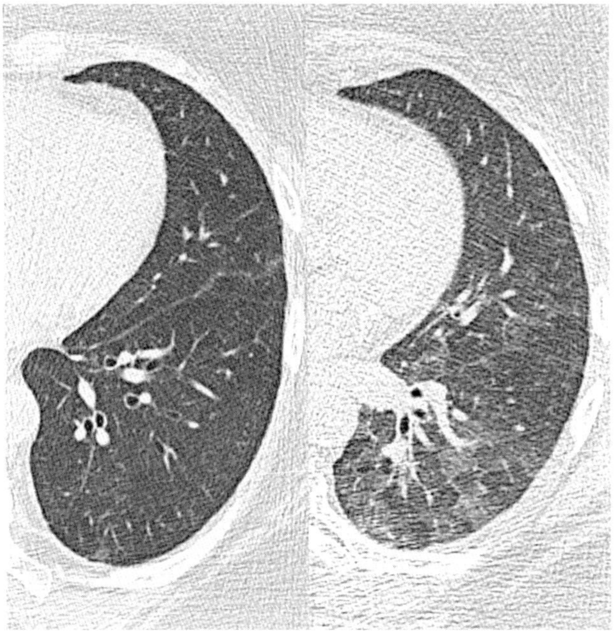

Figure 59.5. Constrictive bronchiolitis in RA. Composite image with inspiratory (left) and expiratory (right) thin-section chest CT of a 45-year-old woman with chronic dyspnea shows subtle mosaic attenuation (left) and findings of expiratory air trapping (right).

- Follicular bronchiolitis: Centrilobular nodules, peribronchovascular nodules, bronchial wall thickening, and occasionally bronchiectasis and cysts (Fig. 59.6)
- Bronchiectasis: May occur as an isolated finding in patients with RA

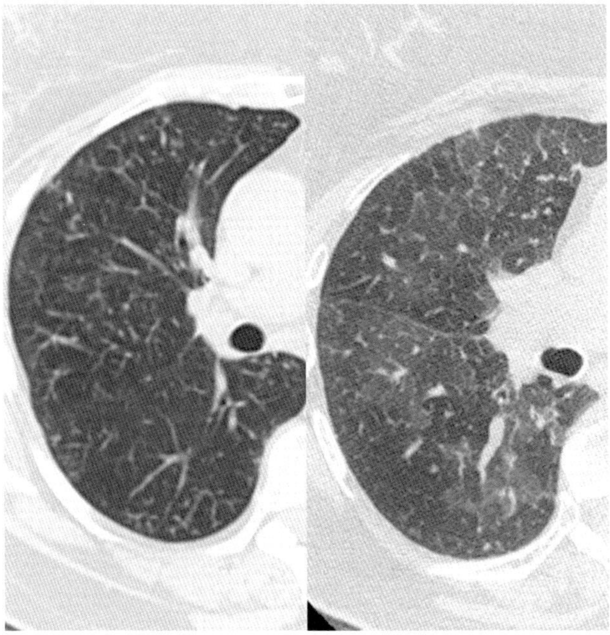

Figure 59.6. Follicular bronchiolitis in RA. Composite image with inspiratory (left) and expiratory (right) chest CT of a 53-year-old woman with chronic dyspnea and cough shows centrilobular micronodules and tree-in-bud opacities (left) and expiratory air trapping (right) consistent with small airways disease.

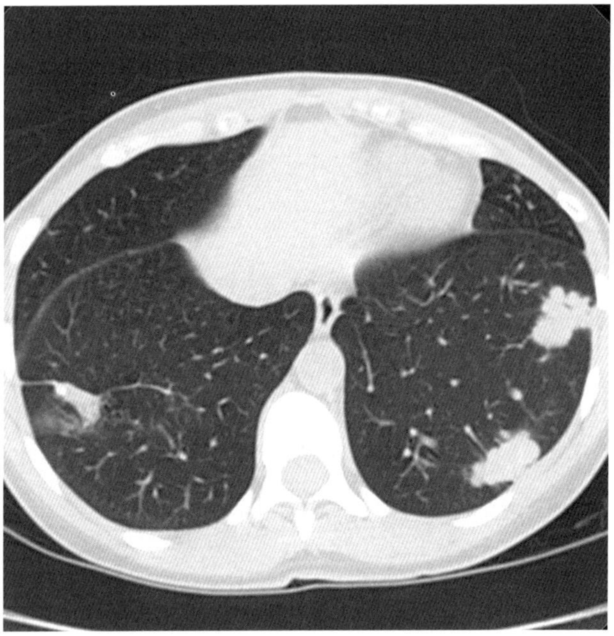

Figure 59.7. Necrobiotic nodules in RA. Chest CT of a male patient with RA shows bilateral lobulated, solid, noncalcified peripheral subpleural pulmonary nodules that demonstrated cavitation on follow-up imaging (not shown).

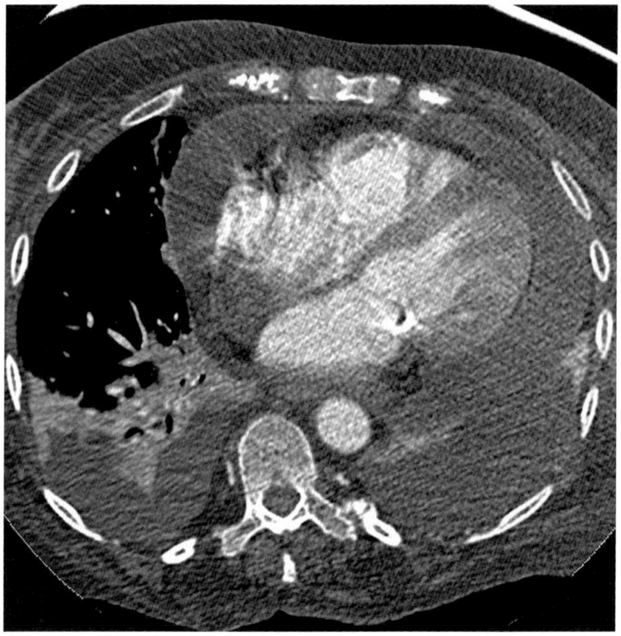

Figure 59.8. Pleural and pericardial disease in RA. Contrast-enhanced chest CT of a patient with RA flare-up shows bilateral nonspecific pleural effusions and a moderate pericardial effusion.

- Drug-induced lung disease: A variety of drugs can cause lung toxicity in the setting of RA, including gold salts, penicillamine, and methotrexate. Common patterns of involvement include organizing pneumonia, constrictive bronchiolitis, and diffuse alveolar damage.

Nodules

- Necrobiotic nodules: Single or multiple nodules, ranging from a few millimeters to 7 cm, often subpleural or associated with interlobular septa (Fig. 59.7). May increase or decrease in size according to disease activity. Cavitation may lead to infection, pneumothorax, or bronchopleural fistula. Calcification may occur and is common in Caplan syndrome (i.e., RA in the setting of coal worker's pneumoconiosis).
- Pleural and pericardial disease: Pleural thickening and effusions are the most common thoracic manifestations of RA with a prevalence of up to 70%, but imaging findings are nonspecific (Fig. 59.8).
- Osseous changes: Symmetric erosions in the distal clavicles and humeral heads may provide a helpful clue to the diagnosis of pulmonary involvement by RA (Fig. 59.9).
- Large airway involvement: There are cricoarytenoid abnormalities in up to 75% of patients with RA due to the presence of a true synovial surface in this joint. Erosions, subluxation, prominence or abnormal position of the vocal cord, vocal cord nodules, or submucosal masses also occur.

Clinical Issues

- RA-ILD is a common complication of patients with RA. Imaging features of UIP and NSIP related to RA are identical to those of their idiopathic counterparts.

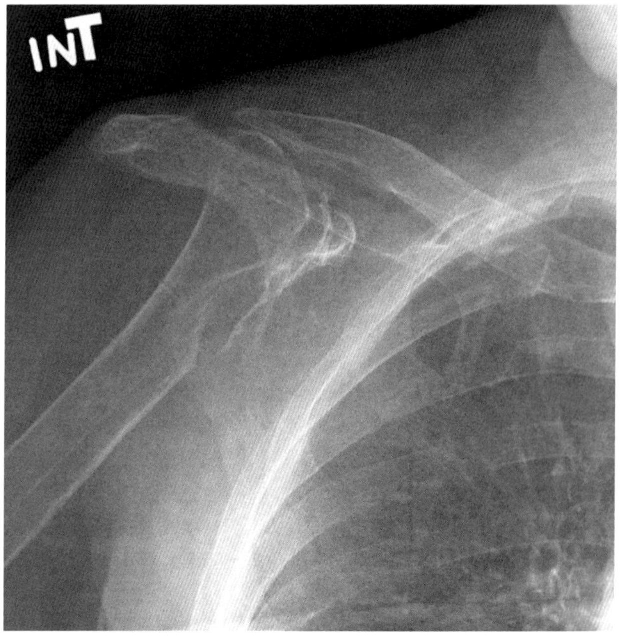

Figure 59.9. Osseous changes seen on chest radiograph in RA. Posteroanterior chest radiograph of a patient with RA coned down to the right upper lobe shows marked right glenohumeral joint deformity with partial humeral head resorption and marked joint space narrowing.

- It is not uncommon for patients' autoimmune disease to present with ILD even months to years before RA-related clinical symptoms occur.
- Discrete nodules in RA should undergo follow-up imaging to determine malignant potential.
- Typically, necrobiotic nodules are more common in men who are smokers, have subcutaneous nodules, and have a positive rheumatoid factor.

Key Points

- Pleuropulmonary involvement in patients with RA is common even in the absence of symptoms.
- Pulmonary involvement by RA can manifest as RA-ILD, pulmonary nodules, and small airways disease (e.g., bronchiectasis, constrictive bronchiolitis, and follicular bronchiolitis). Thin-section or HRCT is the study of choice for evaluation of these findings.
- Worsening symptoms could represent disease progression, superimposed infection, or drug toxicity.

Suggested Reading

Capobianco J, Grimberg A, Thompson BM, Antunes VB, Jasinowodolinski D, Meirelles GS. Thoracic manifestations of collagen vascular diseases. *RadioGraphics*. 2012;32(1):33–50.

Demir R, Bodur H, Tokoglu F, et al. High resolution computed tomography of the lung in patients with rheumatoid arthritis. *Rheumatol Int.* 1999;19:19–22.

Kim EJ, Elicker BM, Maldonado F, Webb WR, Ryu JH, Van Uden JH, et al. Usual interstitial pneumonia in rheumatoid arthritis-associated interstitial lung disease. *Eur* Respir J. 2010;35(6):1322–1328.

Tanaka N, Kim JS, Newell JD, et al. Rheumatoid arthritis-related lung disease: CT findings. *Radiology.* 2004;232:81–91.

Tanoue LT. Pulmonary manifestations of rheumatoid arthritis. *Clin Chest Med.* 1998;19:667–682.

CHAPTER 60

Systemic Sclerosis

Felipe Martínez

Definition

Systemic sclerosis (SSc), or scleroderma, is a chronic autoimmune disorder of small vessels and connective tissue characterized by organ fibrosis, small vessel vasculopathy, and disease-specific antibodies. It results in multisystem organ fibrosis and affects predominantly the skin and frequently the lungs, heart, and the gastrointestinal and renal systems.

Clinical Features

Up to 80% of patients with SSc have limited cutaneous disease that typically involves the face and extremities. The other 20% may have diffuse disease with more severe multisystem manifestations. Women in the third to fifth decades of life are affected more commonly than men.

Although clinically evident pulmonary disease is seen in 25% of patients, autopsy reports demonstrate some degree of pulmonary involvement in all patients with systemic disease. Pulmonary disease is second only to esophageal fibrosis and has surpassed renal disease as the leading cause of death. The most frequent symptoms of pulmonary involvement include progressive cough, dyspnea, and hemoptysis. Systemic sclerosis-associated interstitial lung disease (SSc-ILD) and pulmonary hypertension are the two major lung manifestations of SSc, and the latter is the leading cause of death.

Esophageal dilatation is highly prevalent among patients with SSc, and it is frequently associated with aspiration pneumonia and bronchiolitis. Patients with SSc have an increased incidence of malignancy, including lung and breast cancer.

Anatomy and Physiology

The pathophysiology of SSc is complex and incompletely understood. Factors that may play a role include immune activation, vascular damage, and increased synthesis and deposition of collagen.

How to Approach the Image

Chest radiography may be insensitive to the presence of early or mild pulmonary disease. Radiographs are often normal during early disease stages. As disease progresses, volume loss, reticular opacities, and traction bronchiectasis develop.

Due to accurate characterization of interstitial lung disease, thin-section or high-resolution computed tomography (HRCT) is the imaging modality of choice for the evaluation and follow-up of patients with SSc. Ancillary findings such as esophageal dilatation and lymphadenopathy are helpful in suggesting the diagnosis. Esophageal dilatation may also be associated with acute or recurrent aspiration pneumonia and bronchiolitis.

What Not to Miss

- A normal chest radiograph does not exclude SSc-ILD.
- It is important to identify imaging abnormalities of early SSc-ILD, such as ground-glass opacity (GGO) and reticulation, due to proven favorable response to treatment with cyclophosphamide and/or corticosteroids. In the setting of SSc, GGO is indicative of microscopic fibrosis rather than active alveolitis. Untreated GGO may lead to overt fibrosis (i.e., honeycombing). Evaluation of the extent of pulmonary fibrosis is also important. Patients with extensive disease on HRCT, defined as involvement of more than 20% of the lungs, have a significantly higher mortality than those with lesser or no involvement.
- Aspiration in the form of either aspiration pneumonia or bronchiolitis is common in patients with SSc.
- Lung cancer is a common complication and should always be excluded on imaging studies.

Differential Diagnosis

- Idiopathic interstitial lung diseases: Usual interstitial pneumonia (UIP) and nonspecific interstitial pneumonia (NSIP) may exhibit findings identical to those of ILD related to SSc. Other autoimmune diseases may also manifest with ILD, including rheumatoid arthritis, polymyositis/dermatomyositis, systemic lupus erythematosus, and Sjögren syndrome. Moderate to marked esophageal dilatation should suggest SSc.
- Honeycombing may occur in end-stage sarcoidosis and chronic hypersensitivity pneumonitis. Fibrosis in

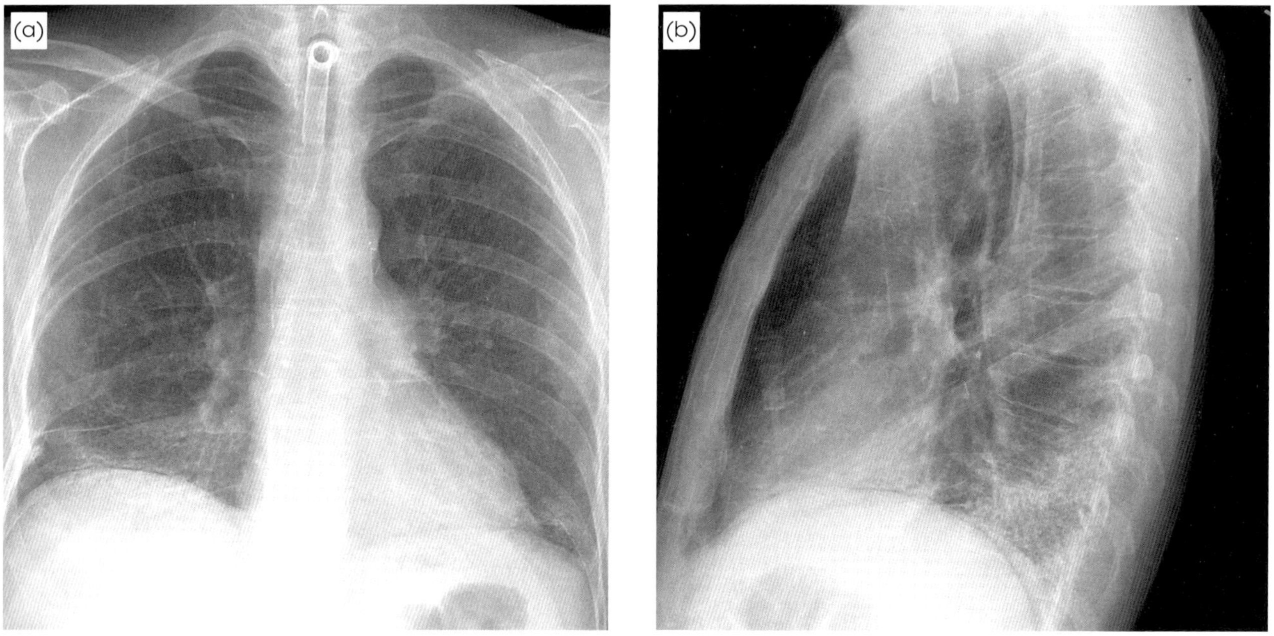

Figure 60.1. SSc-ILD. (a) Posteroanterior and (b) lateral chest radiographs of a 51-year-old woman with known SSc and progressive dyspnea show signs of SSc-ILD manifesting as bilateral symmetric volume loss and bilateral lower lobe predominant reticular opacities and bronchiectasis.

these cases exhibits a peribronchovascular rather than subpleural distribution. Asbestosis with honeycombing may be identical to UIP, but it is often associated with discontinuous calcified pleural plaques.

- Esophageal dilatation may occur in achalasia and esophageal malignancy. These diseases are not associated with ILD but are often associated with aspiration bronchiolitis, which may simulate ILD. Aspiration bronchiolitis typically manifests with centrilobular nodules (or tree-in-bud opacities), bronchiectasis, bronchial wall thickening, mucoid plugging, and mosaic attenuation or frank air trapping.

Imaging Findings

Nonspecific Interstitial Pneumonia

- Chest radiography: Low lung volume; bibasilar hazy, reticular, or reticulonodular opacities (Fig. 60.1); esophageal dilatation.
- Thin-section or HRCT: Subpleural, basilar predominant, posterior GGO and/or reticulation (Fig. 60.2). Bronchovascular distribution of abnormalities with subpleural sparing is a specific pattern of NSIP. GGO may be subtle, and differentiation from dependent atelectasis may be challenging; persistence of GGO on prone imaging confirms pulmonary involvement (Fig. 60.3).

Usual Interstitial Pneumonia

- Chest radiography: Similar to NSIP; usually coarser opacities, but sensitivity of radiography in differentiating NSIP from UIP is poor.
- Thin-section or HRCT: Subpleural, basilar predominant, posterior reticulation and honeycombing (Fig. 60.4). Cystic bronchiectasis may simulate honeycombing (Fig. 60.5); multiplanar reformations and minimal-intensity projection (MinIP) reformations are helpful to demonstrate tubular appearance of bronchiectasis.

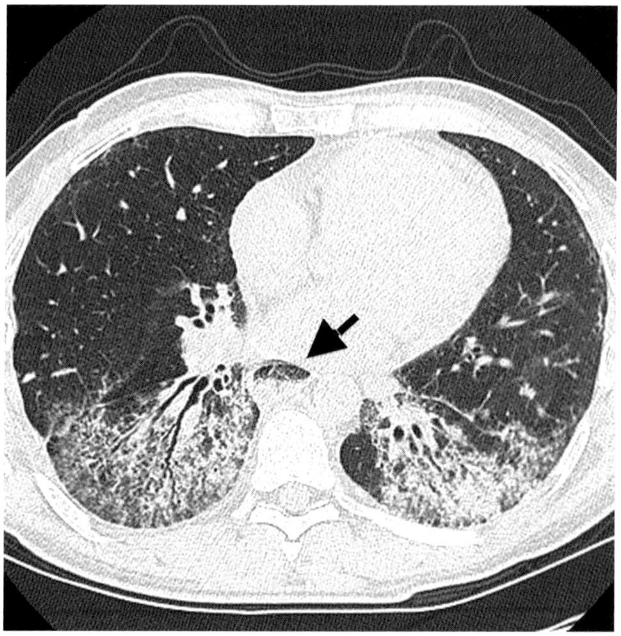

Figure 60.2. SSc-ILD, NSIP pattern. Unenhanced chest CT of a patient with SSc shows features of NSIP characterized by bilateral lower lobe predominant peripheral reticulation and ground-glass opacities with traction bronchiectasis and peribronchial opacities. Note a dilated esophagus with internal debris (arrow).

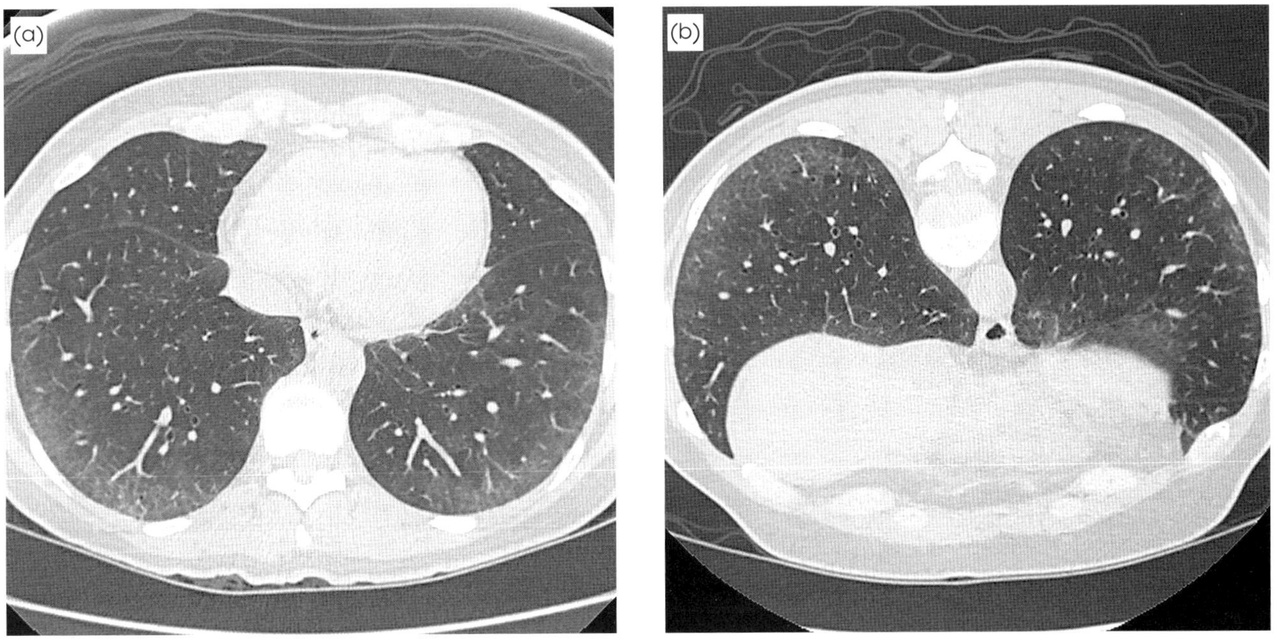

Figure 60.3 SSc-ILD, NSIP Pattern. A 45-year-old patient with recently diagnosed SSc shows an NSIP pattern of lung involvement. (a) Supine thin-section chest CT shows peripheral-dependent lower lobe ground-glass opacities. (b) Prone thin-section chest CT shows persistence of abnormalities consistent with early ILD.

Pulmonary Vascular Disease

- Pulmonary hypertension is the most common manifestation of pulmonary vascular disease.
- Chest radiograph: Enlarged pulmonary trunk, dilated interlobar pulmonary arteries, and pulmonary arterial pruning.
- Thin-section or HRCT: Dilated pulmonary trunk (>3.0 cm) (Fig. 60.6); cardiomegaly and pericardial effusion are common ancillary findings.
- Esophageal dilatation is present in the vast majority of patients.

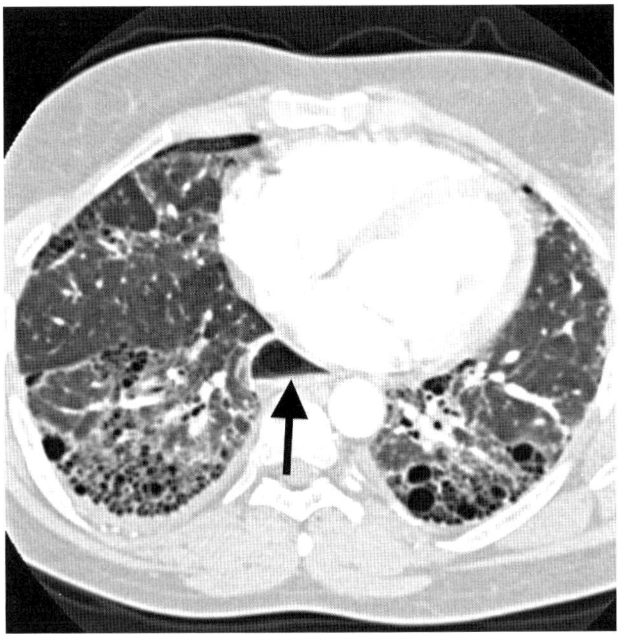

Figure 60.4. SSc-ILD, UIP pattern. Thin-section chest CT of a 52-year-old patient with long-standing SSc and worsening dyspnea shows lower lobe predominant bronchiectasis, bronchiolectasis, and honeycombing with associated bilateral coarse reticulation and ground-glass opacities. Note dilated esophagus with internal debris and an air–fluid level (arrow).

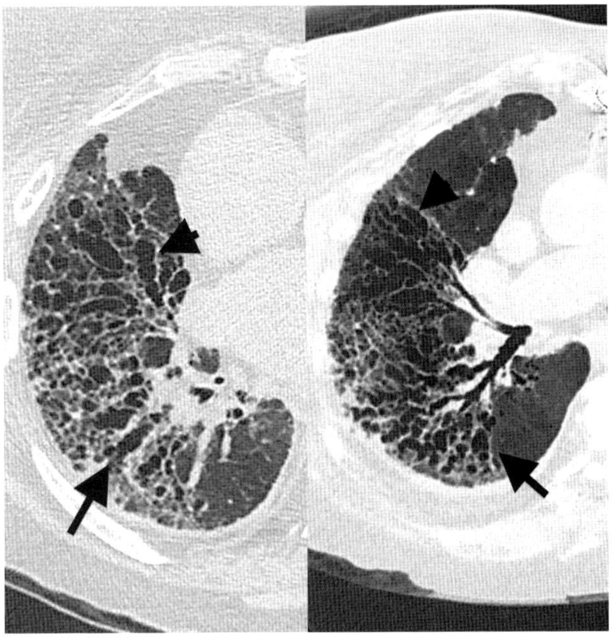

Figure 60.5. Systemic sclerosis with SSc-ILDC. Composite image with thin-section CT (left) and MinIP reformation (right) of a patient with SSc shows extensive cylindrical (arrow) and varicose (arrowhead) bronchiectasis and bronchiolectasis, better appreciated on the MinIP reformation.

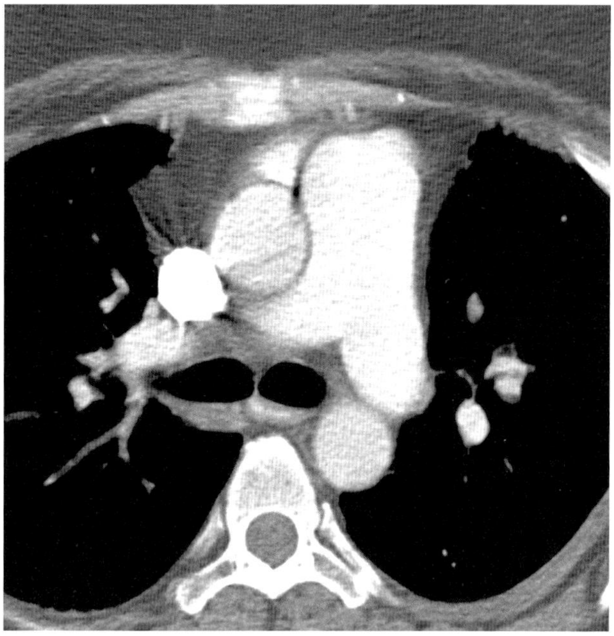

Figure 60.6. Pulmonary hypertension. Contrast-enhanced chest CT of a 60-year-old patient with SSc shows an enlarged pulmonary trunk consistent with pulmonary hypertension.

- Infection: Pneumonia is common due to immunosuppression often related to therapy; imaging findings are not different from those of pneumonias of other etiologies.
- Pleural disease: Pleural effusion and thickening.
- Lymphadenopathy: Common, often reactive.

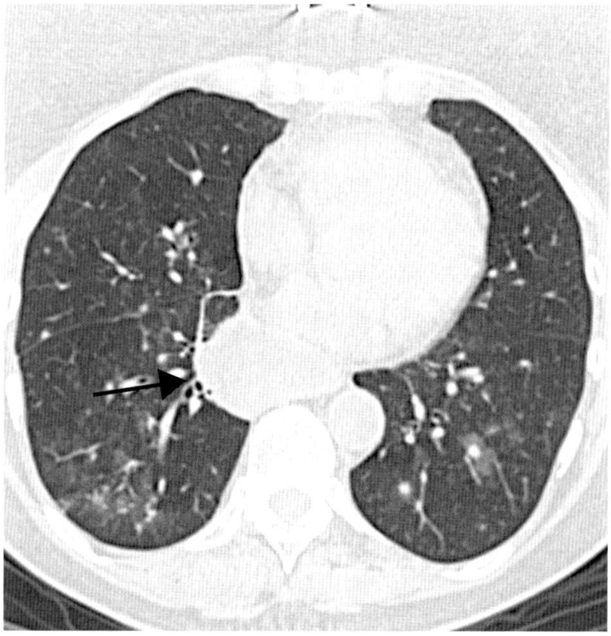

Figure 60.7. Aspiration bronchiolitis. Unenhanced chest CT of a patient with SSc shows bilateral ground-glass nodules, dilated esophagus (arrow) and opacities predominant centrilobular distribution associated with mild bronchial wall thickening from biopsy-proven aspiration bronchiolitis.

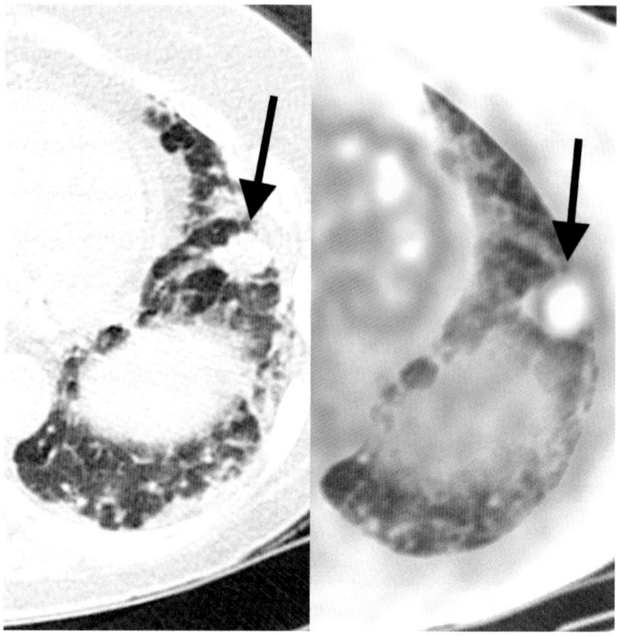

Figure 60.8. Lung adenocarcinoma in SSc. Composite image with chest CT (left) and PET/CT (right) of a patient with SSc and an enlarging left lower lobe nodule shows a small left lower lobe nodule (left; arrow) that is FDG avid on PET/CT (right; arrow).

Aspiration

- Aspiration pneumonia: Indistinguishable from infectious pneumonia with focal or multifocal airspace disease.
- Aspiration bronchiolitis: Chest radiography may be normal or may show reticulonodular opacities. Thin-section CT or HRCT shows centrilobular nodules with or without tree-in-bud opacities, bronchiectasis and bronchiolectasis, bronchial wall thickening, mosaic attenuation, and expiratory air trapping (Fig. 60.7).

Malignancy

- Imaging: Nodules or masses with or without lymphadenopathy and/or metastases.
- Coalescent fibrosis may be very difficult to differentiate from malignancy, particularly because most patients with SSc have hilar and mediastinal lymphadenopathy. Follow-up CT or further evaluation with PET/CT may be helpful (Fig. 60.8).

Clinical Issues

- Patients with SSc should undergo further evaluation with thin-section CT or HRCT regardless of the radiographic findings.
- Clinical and radiologic manifestations of aspiration are common but frequently overlooked in patients with SSc. They must always be suspected and actively excluded.
- Lung cancer is a common complication of SSc.
- NSIP pattern is more prevalent than UIP and entails a better prognosis.

Key Points

- HRCT should be part of the initial evaluation of patients with SSc even when pulmonary symptoms are not present.
- The radiologist should be able to recognize signs of early fibrosis and pulmonary hypertension on radiography and HRCT due to the proven benefit of adequate therapy in the overall outcome and mortality.
- GGO are not indicative of active alveolitis but may represent microscopic fibrosis. If left untreated, GGO may progress to overt fibrosis (i.e., honeycombing).
- HRCT and histopathological features of SSc-ILD represent overlapping features of NSIP and UIP, but NSIP is the most common pattern.
- The radiologist must always consider and actively search for other complications of SSc, such as aspiration and malignancy.

Suggested Reading

Capobianco J, Grimberg A, Thompson BM, Antunes VB, Jasinowodolinski D, Meirelles GS. Thoracic manifestations of collagen vascular diseases. *RadioGraphics*. 2012;32(1):33–50.

Hant FN, Herpel LB, Silver RM. Pulmonary manifestations of scleroderma and mixed connective tissue disease. *Clin Chest Med*. 2010;31:433–449.

Strollo D, Goldin H. Imaging lung disease in systemic sclerosis. *Curr Rheumatol Rep*. 2010;12:156–160.

CHAPTER 61

Pulmonary Vasculitis

Felipe Martínez

Definition

Vasculitis refers to inflammation of blood vessel walls that results in vascular wall destruction and ischemic injury to the affected organ. Common vasculitides include Takayasu arteritis (TAK), giant cell arteritis (GCA), anti-neutrophil cytoplasmic antibody (ANCA)-associated vasculitides such as granulomatosis with polyangiitis (GPA) and eosinophilic granulomatosis with polyangiitis (EGPA), and anti-glomerular basement membrane (anti-GBM) disease or Goodpasture syndrome.

Diffuse alveolar hemorrhage (DAH), a common manifestation of vasculitis, is considered a syndrome rather than a specific entity, but it is discussed in this chapter. However, note that DAH may also result from nonvasculitic etiologies.

Clinical Features

TAK is a progressive vasculitis of unknown etiology that affects individuals younger than age 50 years. It characteristically involves the aorta and its major branches. The pre-pulseless phase of the disease manifests with nonspecific systemic symptoms such as fever, malaise, fatigue, and weight loss. The vascular inflammatory phase of the disease is characterized by diminished or absent pulses.

GCA typically affects individuals older than age 50 years and classically involves the aorta and its branches with a predilection for the carotid and vertebral arteries. Systemic and musculoskeletal symptoms such as malaise, low-grade fever, weight loss, polymyalgia rheumatica, and tenosynovitis are more frequently present than in other vasculitides.

GPA (Wegener granulomatosis) is an uncommon multisystem necrotizing vasculitis that usually manifests as a clinical triad of upper and lower respiratory involvement and glomerulonephritis. The respiratory tract (lung parenchyma and airways) is involved in most patients. Aortic and cardiac involvement may be present. Without treatment, mortality is high.

EGPA (Churg–Strauss syndrome) is a vasculitis characterized by eosinophilic and necrotizing granulomatous inflammation and primarily affects the lungs. In most cases, EGPA exhibits three clinical phases. The first phase is characterized by relatively late-onset (adult) asthma that is usually preceded by allergic rhinitis. The second phase is characterized by marked peripheral eosinophilia and eosinophilic tissue infiltration. The third (late) phase is that of overt systemic vasculitis, which may be life-threatening and may also affect the skin and heart.

Anti-GMB disease (Goodpasture syndrome) is a small-vessel vasculitis resulting from deposition of anti-GMB autoantibodies that leads to pulmonary DAH and glomerulonephritis.

DAH is a syndrome resulting from vasculitic and non-vasculitic etiologies that is classically defined as diffuse pulmonary opacities, hypoxemic respiratory failure, and decreased hematocrit. Although common, hemoptysis may be absent. Vasculitides that manifest with DAH include ANCA-associated vasculitides, Goodpasture syndrome, and systemic lupus erythematosus. Nonvasculitic etiologies include idiopathic pulmonary hemosiderosis, coagulopathies, mitral stenosis, inhalational injury, bone marrow transplantation, and drug toxicity.

Anatomy and Physiology

Vasculitides are further subcategorized depending on the size of the predominantly affected vessel as large-, medium-, and small-vessel vasculitis. The size of the involved vessels strongly influences the clinical and radiological features of the disease. Intrathoracic involvement is more common in small- and large-vessel vasculitides.

TAK and GCA are progressive systemic large-vessel vasculitis. GCA has historically been referred to in the medical literature as temporal arteritis. However, this term should be avoided because GCA temporal arteritis may be absent and also because other vasculitides may manifest with temporal artery involvement.

GPA and EGPA are examples of small-vessel vasculitides. GPA and EGPA are commonly associated with positive ANCA titters, a feature that plays an important role in the diagnosis. The Chapel Hill Consensus recommends avoiding the terms Wegener granulomatosis and Churg–Strauss syndrome.

The term anti-GMB disease is inaccurate because antibodies are reactive not only against the glomerular basement membrane but also toward the pulmonary alveolar capillary membrane. Despite this, the term remains in use and is accepted by the Chapel Hill Consensus.

How to Approach the Image

Although some vasculitides are often considered in the differential diagnosis of pulmonary infection and malignancy, a high index of clinical suspicion is required to consider the diagnosis. Although imaging findings may support the diagnosis of EGPA, this etiology is rarely considered in the absence of a history of asthma. Elderly patients commonly exhibit mild aortic thickening secondary to atherosclerosis, but GCA is rarely considered if an appropriate clinical scenario is not present (e.g., polymyalgia rheumatica or systemic symptoms).

What Not to Miss

- The aortic wall thickness and the caliber of the head and neck vessel origins must always be evaluated on contrast-enhanced chest CT in order to consider the diagnosis of TAK and GCA, which frequently affect these vessels.
- Multifocal cavitary consolidations, nodules, or masses are frequent in GPA, especially if the patient is not very sick or septic (i.e., necrotizing multifocal infection or septic embolism).
- A patient with asthma and pulmonary opacities almost always has a pulmonary infection. However, EGPA should be considered in the absence of signs and symptoms of infection.
- A patient with acute respiratory symptoms and diffuse pulmonary opacities may have diffuse pulmonary infection. However, DAH should be considered in the setting of a decreasing hematocrit, even if hemoptysis is absent.

Differential Diagnosis

- Aortic intramural hematoma (IMH) and severe atherosclerosis are the main differential considerations in TAK and GCA. Classically, TAK and GCA do not exhibit the classic hyperdense wall thickening on unenhanced CT seen in IMH.
- Cavitary opacities are common in necrotizing infection, septic embolism, and multifocal malignancy. Patients with necrotizing infection are usually septic. Septic embolism should be considered in a septic patient when an infected source is known (e.g., cardiac valve vegetation). Multifocal cavitary malignancy may exhibit an indolent course.
- Atypical infection (e.g., *Pneumocystis jirovecii* pneumonia) and pulmonary edema may mimic DAH on imaging. However, hemoptysis and decreasing hematocrit should help suggest the diagnosis.
- Large airway stenosis may occur in GPA. Focal airway lesions are more common in GPA than in amyloidosis. Relapsing polychondritis and tracheobronchopathia osteochondroplastica may manifest with tracheobronchial narrowing but typically spare the posterior tracheal membrane.

Imaging Findings

TAK

- Early stage: Contrast-enhanced CT shows wall thickening and stranding of surrounding fat. Contrast-enhanced MRI is superior in demonstrating wall enhancement.
- With progressive vascular inflammation, luminal narrowing/occlusion and mural calcifications develop and may result in vessel stenosis or aneurysm formation.
- Late-stage disease may affect the pulmonary arteries, with stenoses and occlusions more frequently involving the segmental and subsegmental branches and, to a lesser extent, the lobar or main pulmonary arteries (Figs. 61.1 and 61.2).

GCA

- Contrast-enhanced CT and MRI are the imaging studies of choice.
- Wall thickening in the acute phase may lead to stenoses, wall calcification, and occlusions in the late phase.
- MRA is superior for demonstrating vessel wall enhancement (Figs. 61.3 and 61.4).

GPA

- Pulmonary nodules, masses, or consolidations that may exhibit intrinsic cavitation (Figs. 61.5 and 61.6).

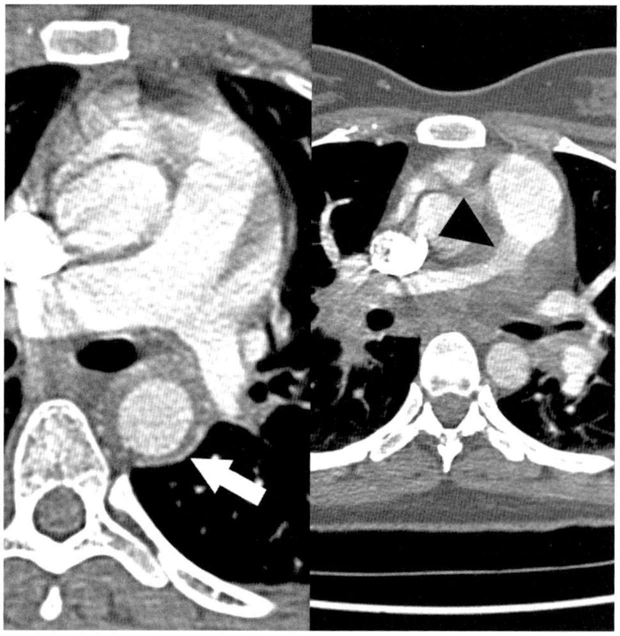

Figure 61.1. Takayasu arteritis. Composite image with contrast-enhanced chest CT of two patients with TAK shows early disease manifesting with diffuse concentric mural thickening and abnormal enhancement of the descending aorta (arrow) and infiltration of the mediastinal fat (left). Marked luminal narrowing of the pulmonary trunk (arrowhead) and bilateral pulmonary arteries with significant soft tissue attenuation in the mediastinum in a patient with late-stage disease (right).

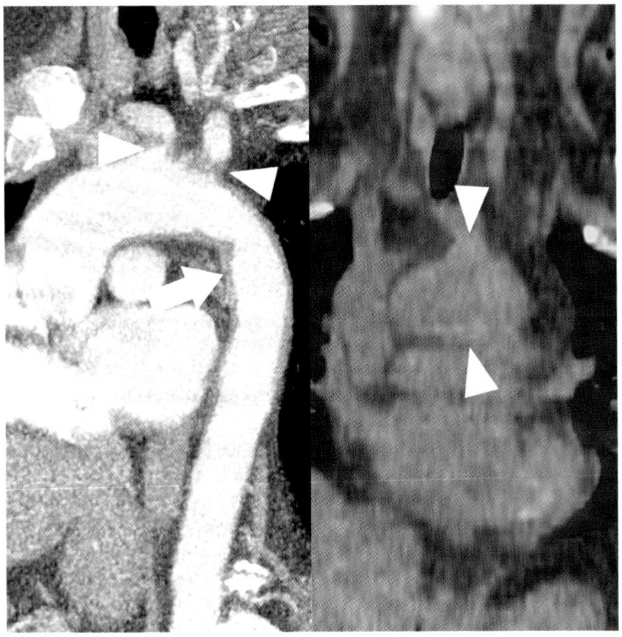

Figure 61.2. Takayasu arteritis. Composite image with oblique sagittal chest CT (left) and coronal FDG PET/CT (right) of a young woman with TAK and progressive constitutional symptoms shows concentric mural thickening and mild aortic lumen narrowing (arrow) of the distal arch and proximal descending aorta and severe stenosis of the right brachiocephalic and left subclavian arteries (left; arrowheads). Note abnormal moderately increased mural FDG uptake in the aortic arch (right; arrowheads) consistent with active inflammation.

Waxing and waning behavior of these abnormalities is common regardless of treatment. Lesions may heal with focal scarring often manifesting as band-like opacities.

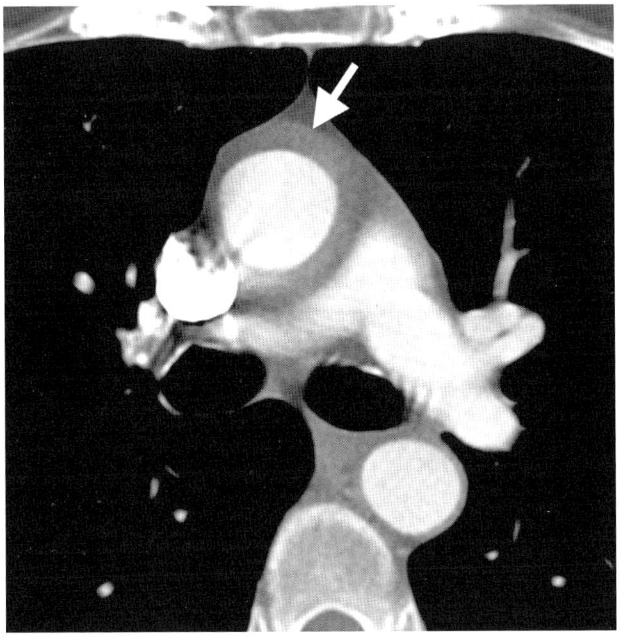

Figure 61.3. Giant cell arteritis. Contrast-enhanced chest CT of a 65-year-old man with polymyalgia rheumatica and chest pain shows concentric wall thickening of the ascending aorta (arrow) and mild stranding of the periaortic fat consistent with acute inflammation.

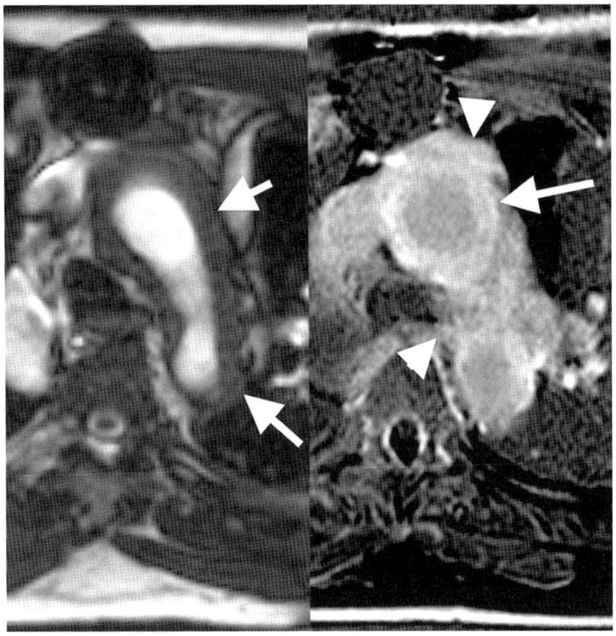

Figure 61.4. Giant cell arteritis. Composite image with steady-state free precession (SSFP) MRI (left) and delayed contrast-enhanced MRI (right) of a patient with exacerbation of GCA. SSFP MRI shows concentric mural thickening of the ascending aorta and aortic arch (arrows). Delayed contrast-enhanced MRI shows aortic wall thickening and abnormal enhancement (arrow) with periaortic mediastinal inflammatory changes (arrowheads).

- DAH may manifest as diffuse peribronchial ground-glass opacities (GGO) and consolidations that may mimic atypical infection, which is also common in patients with GPA.

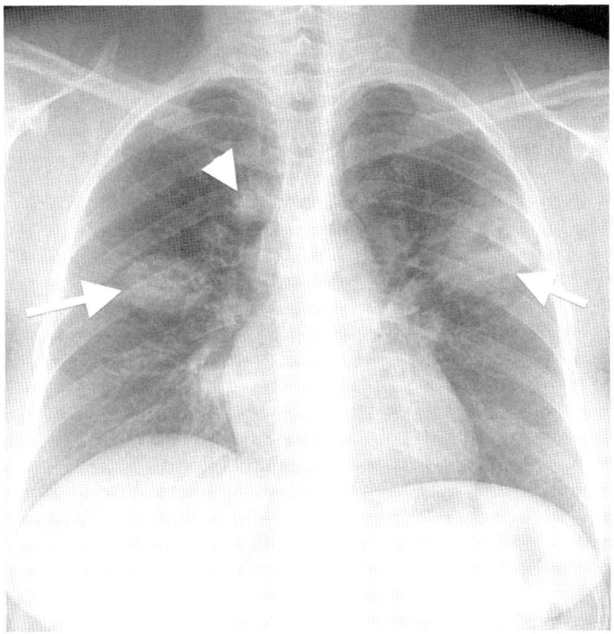

Figure 61.5. Granulomatosis with polyangiitis. Posteroanterior (PA) chest radiograph of a patient presenting with sinusitis and cough shows bilateral cavitary (arrows) and noncavitary nodular opacities (arrowhead).

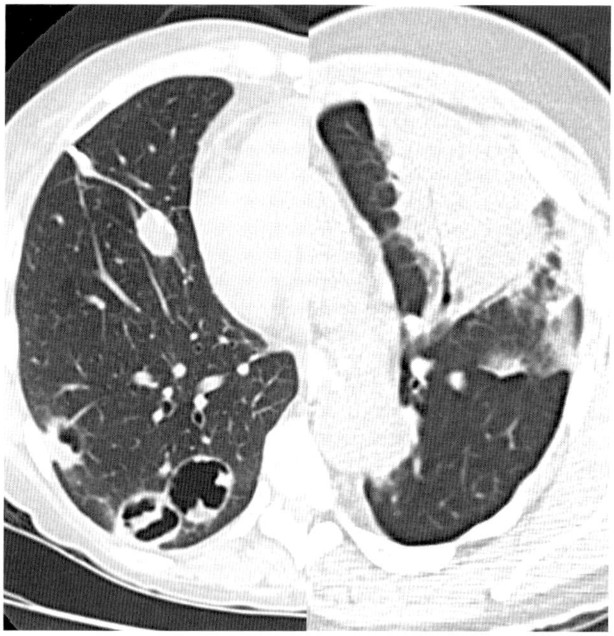

Figure 61.6. Granulomatosis with polyangiitis. Composite image with chest CT of two different patients with GPA shows cavitary and noncavitary lung nodules (left) and left lung upper lobe consolidation (right).

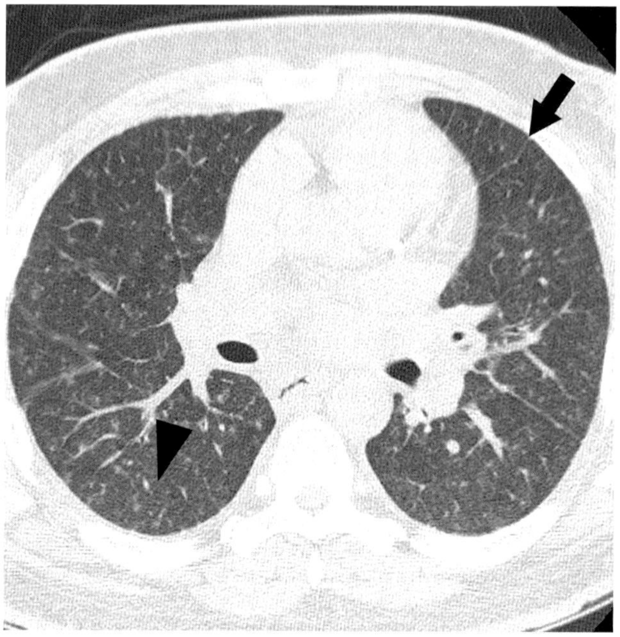

Figure 61.7. Eosinophilic granulomatosis with polyangiitis. Thin-section chest CT of a young man with EGPA and worsening pulmonary symptoms shows interlobular septal thickening (arrows), centrilobular nodules (arrowheads), and bronchiolar wall thickening—common findings in EPGA.

- Tracheobronchial involvement is characterized by concentric smooth or nodular mural thickening of the tracheobronchial tree often involving the membranous posterior segment.

EGPA

- Transient scattered bilateral parenchymal consolidations without lobar predominance are the most common imaging finding. This is better defined on CT with peripheral predominant GGO and consolidation, often with a waxing and waning behavior.
- Interlobular septal thickening, also common, may be related to edema or septal eosinophilic infiltration (Fig. 61.7).
- Airway abnormalities including tree-in-bud nodules and bronchiolar wall thickening as manifestations of asthma are almost always present in patients with EGPA.

Anti-GBM Disease and DAH

- Chest radiography: Diffuse bilateral opacities, although hemorrhage may also be focal.
- Chest CT: In the acute phase, there are centrilobular nodules and GGO that may progress to airspace consolidations. In the subacute phase, after resorption of alveolar hemorrhage and accumulation of interstitial hemosiderin-laden macrophages, interlobular septal thickening develops and may manifest with the "crazy paving" pattern (Figs. 61.8–61.10).
- DAH often resolves within 2 weeks after the acute episode. Chronic or repeated episodes of DAH may result in pulmonary hemosiderosis that may range from interlobular septal thinking and reticulation to lung fibrosis with traction bronchiectasis and peripheral honeycombing.

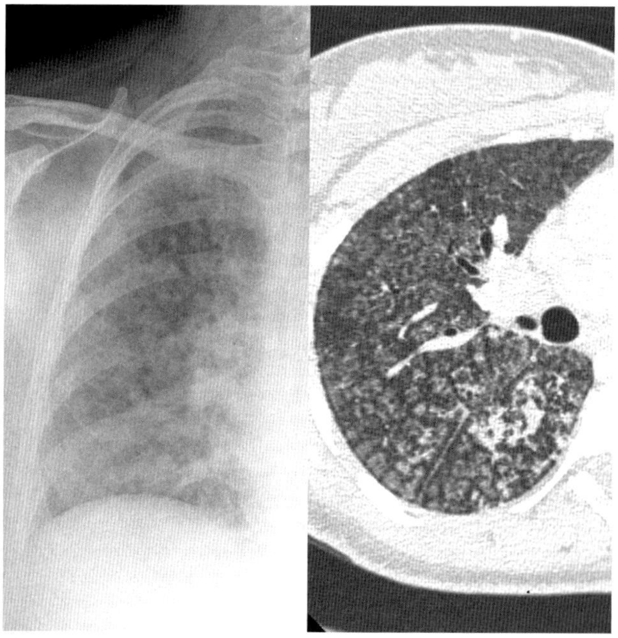

Figure 61.8. Anti-GBM disease and diffuse alveolar hemorrhage. Composite image with PA chest radiograph (left) and thin-section chest CT (right) of a patient with hemoptysis shows diffuse multifocal nodular opacities that manifest as diffuse ground-glass centrilobular nodules on chest CT.

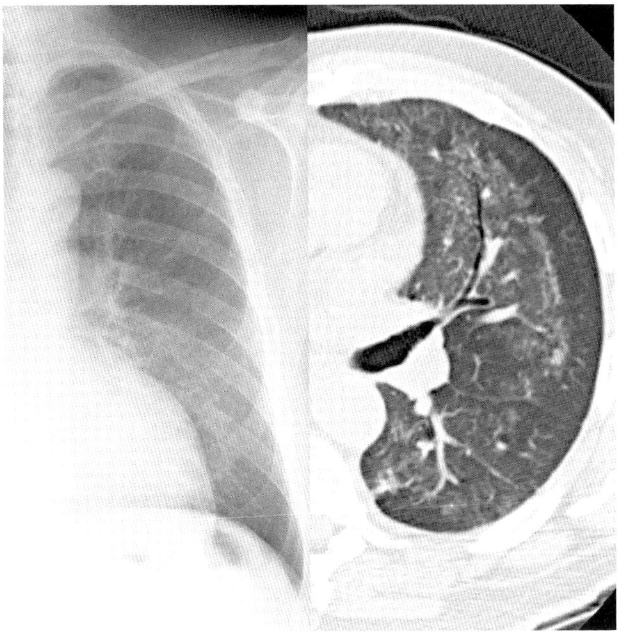

Figure 61.9. Diffuse alveolar hemorrhage due to GPA. Composite image with PA chest radiograph (left) and chest CT (right) of a patient with GPA and hemoptysis shows faint radiographic opacities with a central distribution corresponding to peribronchovascular GGO on CT.

Clinical Issues

- Given imaging and clinical heterogeneity of the vasculitides and the relative low frequency of these diseases, the diagnosis may not be considered without knowledge of the clinical findings.

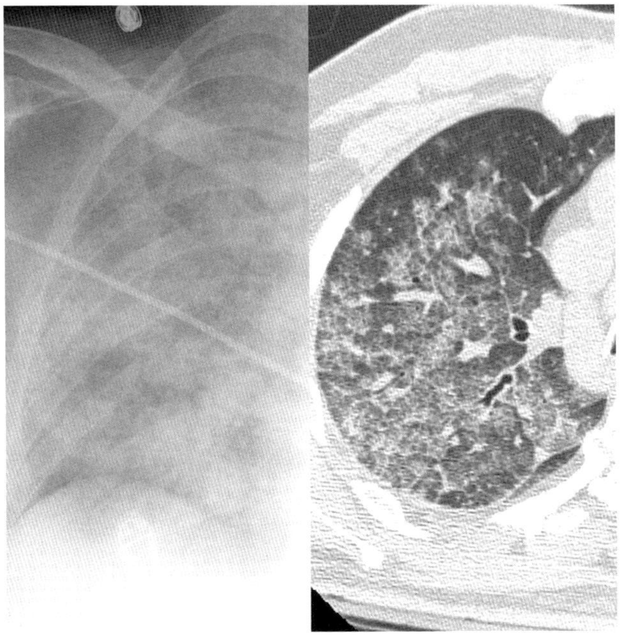

Figure 61.10. Diffuse alveolar hemorrhage, drug-induced. Composite image with AP chest radiograph (left) and chest CT (right) of a young patient with methotrexate-induced lung injury shows diffuse consolidations that manifest as GGO with interlobular septal thickening on CT, the so-called "crazy paving" pattern.

- Aortic involvement in GCA is usually asymptomatic during the early phase of disease and may result in significant late complications such as aneurysms and dissections.

Key Points

- The diagnosis and workup of patients with primary vasculitides is challenging and requires close collaboration between the clinician, the radiologist, and the pathologist.
- The diagnosis of vasculitis may be delayed because other common diseases may exhibit similar imaging findings. Early diagnosis is critical given the high morbidity and mortality of affected patients.
- Multifocal cavitary opacities are very common in GPA.
- CT and MR are the imaging modalities of choice in the assessment of vascular mural thickening and enhancement for the diagnosis of TAK and GCA.
- DAH should be considered in patients with diffuse pulmonary opacities and decreasing hematocrit with or without hemoptysis.

Suggested Reading

Capobianco J, Grimberg A, Thompson BM, Antunes VB, Jasinowodolinski D, Meirelles GS. Thoracic manifestations of collagen vascular diseases. *RadioGraphics*. 2012;32(1):33–50.

Demir R, Bodur H, Tokoglu F, et al. High resolution computed tomography of the lung in patients with rheumatoid arthritis. *Rheumatol Int*. 1999;19:19–22.

Kim EJ, Elicker BM, Maldonado F, et al. Usual interstitial pneumonia in rheumatoid arthritis-associated interstitial lung disease. *Eur Respir J*. 2010;35(6):1322–1328.

Tanaka N, Kim JS, Newell JD, et al. Rheumatoid arthritis-related lung disease: CT findings. *Radiology*. 2004;232:81–91.

Tanoue LT. Pulmonary manifestations of rheumatoid arthritis. *Clin Chest Med*. 1998;19:667–682.

CHAPTER 62

Other Autoimmune Diseases

Santiago Martínez-Jiménez

Definition

Autoimmune disease is defined as the development of autoantibodies against the host's own tissues. Several autoimmune diseases have been described. In addition to rheumatoid arthritis (RA), scleroderma or progressive systemic sclerosis (PSS), and vasculitis (discussed elsewhere), other autoimmune diseases may affect the chest. Examples include systemic lupus erythematosus (SLE), dermatomyositis/polymyositis (DM/PM), Sjögren syndrome (SS), and mixed connective tissue disease (MCTD).

Clinical Features

SLE is a common autoimmune disease that predominantly affects women of reproductive age. Symptoms vary according to the affected thoracic organ. Pleural involvement is common, often manifesting with pleural effusion or thickening and associated with pleuritic chest pain. Pneumonia is also common and can be related to common pathogens typical of community-acquired pneumonia, but atypical microorganisms are common, including various mycobacteria, *Pneumocystis jirovecii*, cytomegalovirus, *Aspergillus* spp., and *Nocardia* spp. Diffuse alveolar hemorrhage (DAH) and lupus pneumonitis (LP) are uncommon life-threatening complications of SLE, and affected patients often present with fever, dyspnea, and hypoxemia. Infection, DAH, and LP have similar manifestations both clinically and on imaging. Patients with SLE may also have cardiac disease/failure and renal disease/failure that can lead to hydrostatic pulmonary edema. Interstitial lung disease may also complicate SLE, including nonspecific interstitial pneumonia (NSIP) and usual interstitial pneumonia (UIP).

DM/PM affects the skeletal muscle and may frequently result in hypoventilation and respiratory failure (respiratory muscle involvement) and aspiration (laryngeal involvement). Interstitial lung disease is also frequent, and NSIP and organizing pneumonia are the most common patterns.

SS typically affects women in the fourth and fifth decades of life. Classic symptoms include xerophtalmia and xerostomia. Interstitial lung disease is among the most common thoracic manifestations, and although NSIP, UIP, organizing pneumonia, and amyloidosis can occur, lymphocytic interstitial pneumonia (LIP) is the classic form of interstitial lung disease in SS.

MCTD combines clinical features of RS, SLE, PSS, and PM/DM. Thoracic involvement is common often in the form of pulmonary arterial hypertension and interstitial lung disease (NSIP or, less frequently, UIP and LIP).

Anatomy and Physiology

All autoimmune diseases have particular target antigens and consequently have particular autoantibodies that are immunologically detectable in the laboratory and are helpful in diagnosis.

How to Approach the Image

- As with interstitial lung diseases not related to autoimmune disease, chest radiography is frequently normal, and abnormalities may be nonspecific. Therefore, radiologists must have a high index of suspicion when evaluating a patient with known autoimmune disease, thoracic symptoms, and abnormal pulmonary function tests, in the setting of a normal chest radiograph.
- Thin-section or high-resolution computed tomography (HRCT) is the imaging modality of choice for the evaluation and follow-up of patients with autoimmune disorders and those with interstitial lung disease.

What Not to Miss

- Patients with SS should be carefully evaluated for pulmonary cysts.
- Pulmonary infection, lupus pneumonitis, and DAD are clinically and radiologically identical in patients with SLE. Differentiation of these entities requires laboratory tests and often bronchoalveolar lavage.
- The radiologist must look for signs of pulmonary hypertension on imaging of patients with autoimmune diseases because it often denotes a worse prognosis.

Differential Diagnosis

- Idiopathic interstitial lung diseases (ILD) may manifest as UIP or NSIP, and imaging findings may be identical to those of ILD related to autoimmune disease.
- LIP is always considered in the differential diagnosis of cystic lung diseases, which also includes lymphangioleiomyomatosis and pulmonary Langerhans cell hystiocytosis.

- The differential diagnosis of pulmonary hypertension is extensive. Common causes of pulmonary hypertension should be excluded, including left heart failure and chronic obstructive pulmonary disease.

Imaging Findings

Interstitial Lung Disease

- Overall, NSIP is the most common ILD in patients with autoimmune disease. Chest radiographs may be normal or may exhibit lower lobe predominant subpleural reticular opacities. HRCT shows subpleural lower lobe predominant reticular and ground-glass opacities that may be associated with peripheral traction bronchiectasis and honeycomb cysts. A characteristic feature of NSIP is relative subpleural sparing, but it is not always seen (Figs. 62.1–62.3).
- UIP is also seen in autoimmune disease and is indistinguishable from idiopathic pulmonary fibrosis. Chest radiographs show low lung volume and fine basilar reticular opacities. HRCT shows characteristic basilar predominant honeycombing, defined as clustered cystic spaces that share their walls. Predominant honeycombing in a typical distribution on imaging indicates UIP.

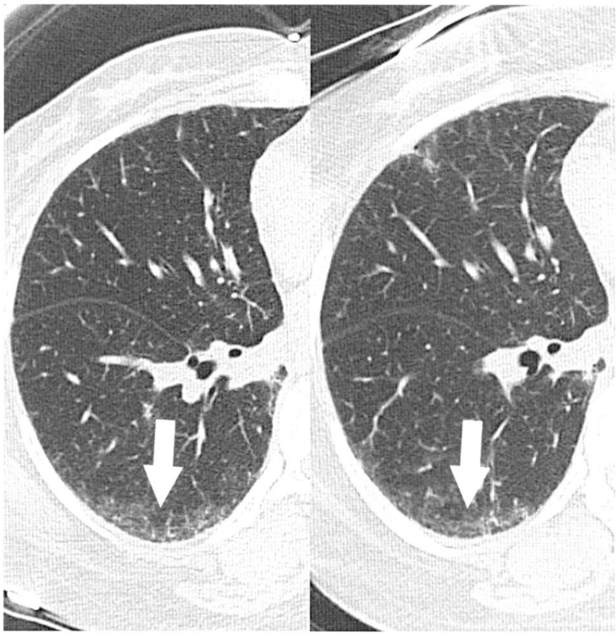

Figure 62.2. Polymyositis, cellular NSIP. Composite image with supine (left) and prone (right) chest CT of a 37-year-old woman with polymyositis, chronic cough, and dyspnea shows right lower lobe subpleural reticular and ground-glass opacities (arrows) that persist on prone imaging.

SLE

- DAH (Fig. 62.4) in patients with SLE manifests on chest radiography as nonspecific diffuse airspace disease. Chest CT findings are also nonspecific and are characterized by diffuse ground-glass or airspace opacities with or without interlobular septal thickening and occasionally diffuse centrilobular nodules. Diffuse opacities associated with decreasing hemoglobin may be the only clue to the correct diagnosis.

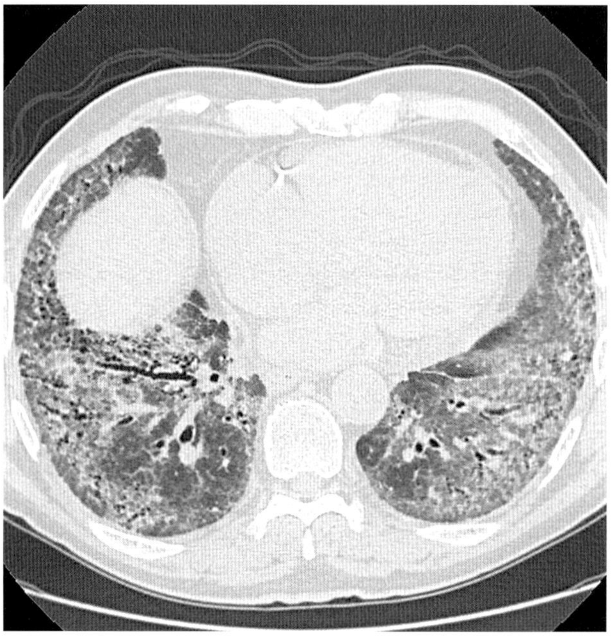

Figure 62.1. SLE, NSIP. HRCT of a 42-year-old man with chronic cough and increasing dyspnea shows extensive subpleural reticulation, ground-glass opacities, and traction bronchiectasis diagnosed on biopsy as fibrosing NSIP.

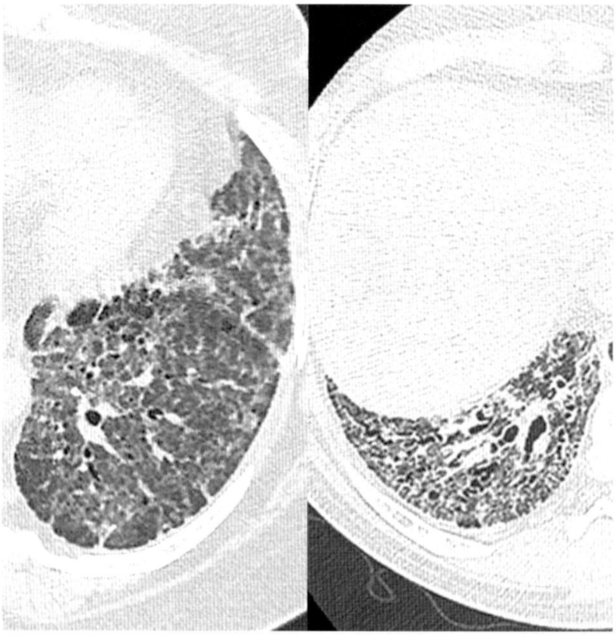

Figure 62.3. Mixed connective tissues disease and polymyositis, fibrosing NSIP. Composite image with chest CT of two different patients with NSIP in the setting of mixed connective tissue disease (left) and polymyositis (right). HRCT (left) shows diffuse reticular and ground-glass opacities and bronchiectasis without honeycombing. HRCT (right) shows lower lobe predominant subpleural reticular and ground-glass opacities with associated traction bronchiectasis.

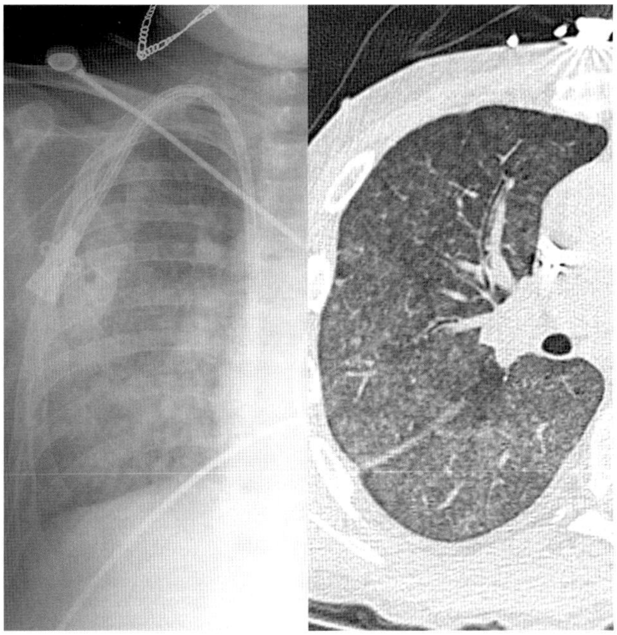

Figure 62.4. SLE, DAH. Composite image with anteroposterior (AP) chest radiograph (left) and unenhanced chest CT (right) of a 47-year-old man with hemoptysis and decreasing hemoglobin shows extensive heterogeneous opacities that manifest as diffuse ground-glass opacities and centrilobular micronodules on CT.

- Lupus pneumonitis (Fig. 62.5), pulmonary hemorrhage, and diffuse pulmonary infection have imaging findings similar to those of DAH. Differentiation based solely on imaging is not possible.

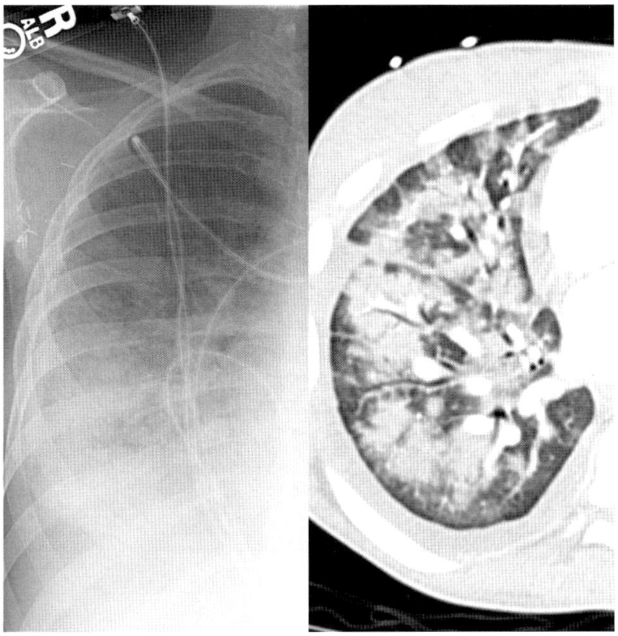

Figure 62.5. SLE, lupus pneumonitis. Composite image with AP chest radiograph (left) and chest CT (right) of a 35-year-old woman with acute dyspnea shows extensive heterogeneous opacities that manifest on CT as multifocal consolidations with air bronchograms. Note small right pleural effusion.

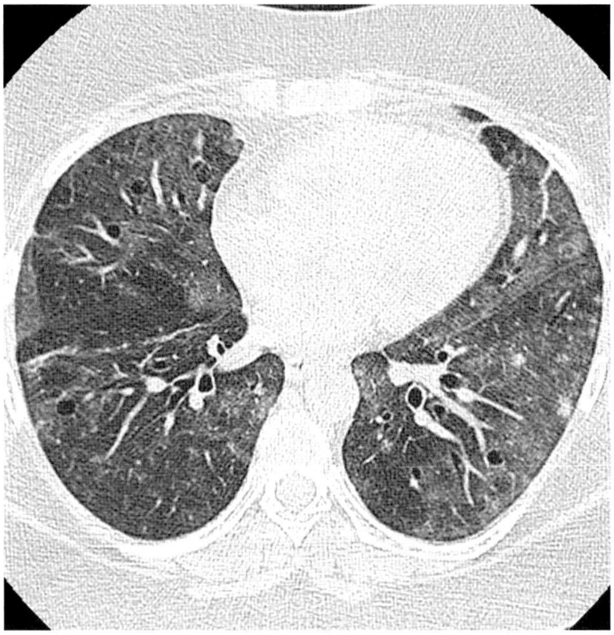

Figure 62.6. Sjögren syndrome, LIP. Thin-section chest CT of a 29-year-old man with Sjögren syndrome, cough, and dyspnea demonstrates diffuse bilateral ground-glass opacities, a few ill-defined pulmonary nodules, and scattered thin-walled cysts.

SS-LIP

- Chest radiography may show diffuse nonspecific reticular opacities in patients with pulmonary cysts. HRCT is helpful in demonstrating characteristic thin-walled cysts that may be associated with ground-glass opacities, small nodules, and interlobular septal thickening (Fig. 62.6).

Infection

Patients with autoimmune diseases are more prone to infection, given the disease itself and/or the immunosuppressant therapy. This can vary from community-acquired pneumonia to fungal infections such as *P. jirovecii* and *Aspergillus* spp. Imaging findings range from bronchopneumonia airspace disease to lobar consolidation, diffuse parenchymal opacities, and cavitary disease (nodules and/or consolidation) (Fig. 62.7). As previously mentioned, infection can be impossible to differentiate from alveolar hemorrhage or lupus pneumonitis.

The following are additional findings of autoimmune disease:

- Pulmonary hypertension (Fig. 62.8) may be isolated or associated with ILD. Enlarged pulmonary trunk and central pulmonary arteries with abrupt peripheral tapering may be seen on chest radiography. On CT, a pulmonary trunk diameter greater than 30 mm correlates well with pulmonary hypertension. Common ancillary findings include pericardial effusion and enlarged right heart chambers.

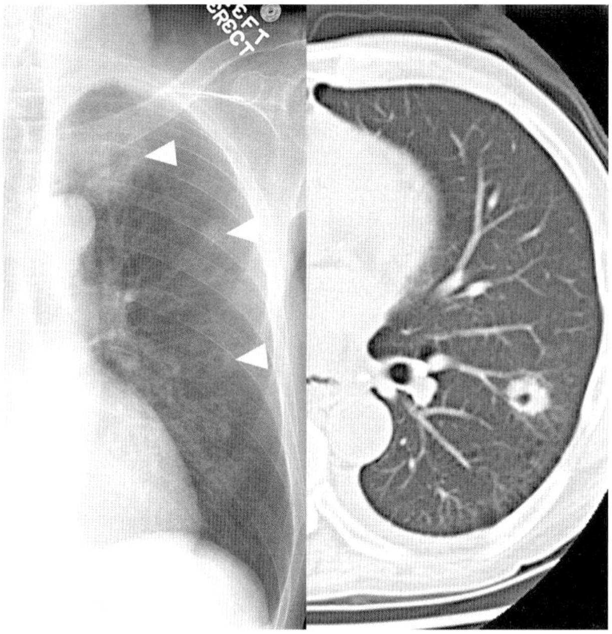

Figure 62.7. SLE, angioinvasive aspergillosis. Composite image with AP chest radiograph (left) and unenhanced chest CT (right) of a 37-year-old man with SLE, fever, and chronic steroid therapy shows multifocal cavitary lung nodules (arrowheads). Chest CT (right) shows a left lower lobe nodule with cavitation and a small left pleural effusion.

- Lymphadenopathy (Fig. 62.8) is a common nonspecific finding seen in autoimmune disease. Enlarged intrathoracic lymph nodes typically measure greater than 1.0 cm in their short axis.

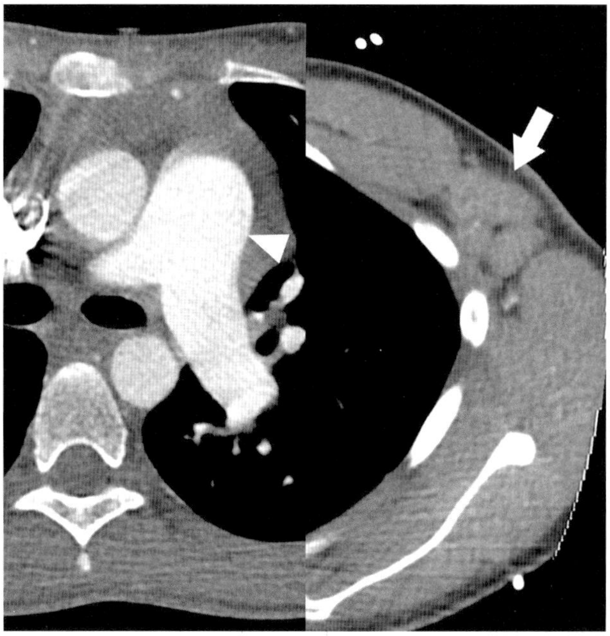

Figure 62.8. SLE, pulmonary hypertension and axillary lymphadenopathy. Composite image with contrast-enhanced chest CT of a 31-year-old man with SLE shows a dilated pulmonary artery (arrowhead) consistent with pulmonary hypertension and left axillary lymphadenopathy (arrow).

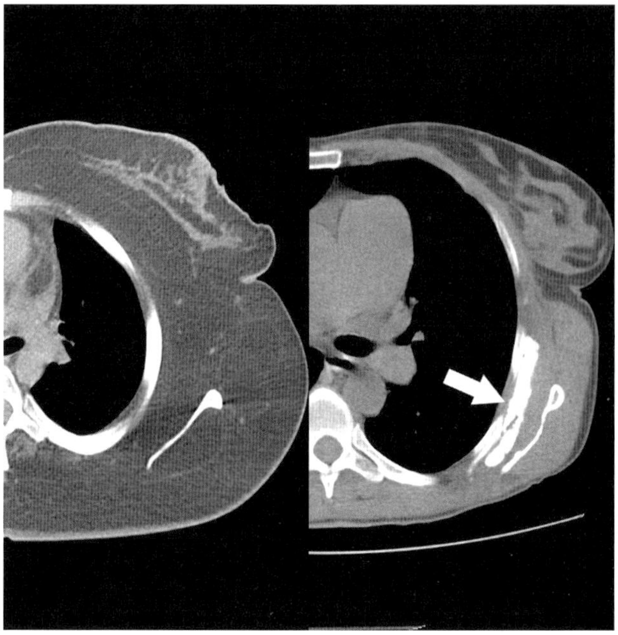

Figure 62.9. Polymyositis with muscle atrophy and fat replacement and dermatomyositis with soft tissue calcifications. Composite image with chest CT of two different patients shows common soft tissue findings in polymyositis (left) and dermatomyositis (right). Note the absence of chest wall muscles due to fat replacement (left) and left chest wall soft tissue calcifications (arrow).

- Muscle atrophy and soft tissue calcification are common polymyositis and dermatomyositis respectively (Fig. 62.9)
- Pleural and pericardial effusions (Fig. 62.10) are nonspecific findings frequently seen in autoimmune diseases.

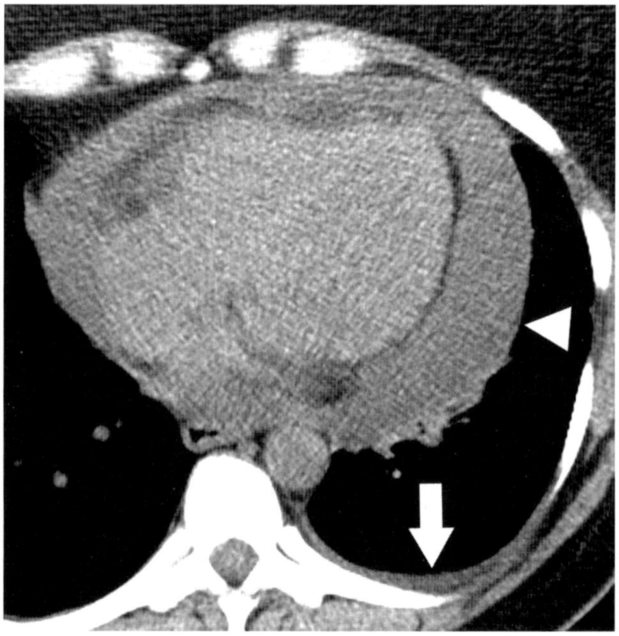

Figure 62.10. SLE, serositis. Contrast-enhanced axial chest of a 42-year-old woman with SLE and chest pain shows a moderate pericardial effusion (arrowhead) and trace left pleural effusion (arrow).

Clinical Issues

- Infection, ILD, and pulmonary hypertension cause the greatest morbidity and mortality in patients with autoimmune disease.

Key Points

- Pulmonary edema, lupus pneumonitis, diffuse alveolar hemorrhage, and infection—common in patients with SLE—have similar findings on imaging.
- Interstitial lung disease in patients with autoimmune disease is typically NSIP and, less frequently, UIP. HRCT is the imaging modality of choice for evaluating interstitial lung disease.
- LIP, classically associated with Sjögren syndrome, typically manifests with thin-walled cysts at thin-section chest CT.
- Pulmonary hypertension may occur as an isolated finding or in association with ILD in patients with autoimmune disease and entails a worse prognosis.

Suggested Reading

Capobianco J, Grimberg A, Thompson BM, Antunes VB, Jasinowodolinski D, Meirelles GS. Thoracic manifestations of collagen vascular diseases. *RadioGraphics*. 2012;32(1):33–50.

Lynch DA. Lung disease related to collagen vascular disease. *J Thorac Imaging*. 2009 Nov;24(4):299–309.

Mayberry JP, Primack SL, Müller NL. Thoracic manifestations of systemic autoimmune diseases: Radiographic and high resolution CT findings. *RadioGraphics*. 2000 Nov–Dec;20(6):1623–35.

Eosinophilic Lung Diseases

Santiago Martínez-Jiménez

Definition

Eosinophilic lung diseases (ELD) are a group of diseases that affect the lungs and manifest with blood and/or tissue eosinophilia. ELD may be secondary to a variety of conditions, such as infection by parasites (e.g., ascariasis, strongyloidoiasis, and paragonimiasis), drug reaction, allergic bronchopulmonary aspergillosis (ABPA), and malignancy. ELD may also be primarily either limited to the lung (e.g., acute and chronic eosinophilic diseases) or part of a systemic disorder (e.g., allergic granulomatosis with polyangiitis or hypereosinophilic syndromes).

Clinical Features

ELD should be considered in patients with peripheral blood eosinophilia. Symptoms are usually nonspecific and rarely lead to a clinical diagnosis. Important clues include recent travel to areas where parasites are endemic, history of asthma, and treatment with certain drugs. The diagnosis of ELD is rarely considered in patients without eosinophilia.

ABPA often occurs in the setting of asthma and cystic fibrosis, and it results from a hypersensitivity reaction to *Aspergillus* spp. antigens. Affected patients present with cough, wheezing, low-grade fever, malaise, and sputum production.

A very large list of drugs (e.g., antibiotics) are associated with ELD. Drug-related ELD is often suspected when a patient presents with shortness of breath, cough, and fever after starting on drug therapy.

Many parasites are associated with ELD. Strongyloidiasis (*Strongyloides stercoralis*), in contrast with other helminth infections, may reinfect the human host from the gastrointestinal tract. This may lead to the so-called hyperinfection syndrome, a life-threatening complication often seen in immunocompromised patients (e.g., patients with AIDS and patients on chronic corticosteroids). These patients often present with the systemic inflammatory response syndrome. Diagnosis is made by identifying larvae in the bronchoalveolar lavage fluid.

Acute eosinophilic pneumonia (AEP) is frequent in young individuals and often related to initiation of smoking. Affected patients present acutely with pneumonia-like symptoms. Eosinophilia is often initially absent but develops at later stages of the disease.

Chronic eosinophilic pneumonia (CEP) is an idiopathic interstitial pneumonia that develops over weeks to months. Affected patients often present with cough, dyspnea, and constitutional symptoms. Peripheral blood eosinophilia is common.

Allergic granulomatosis with polyangiitis or Churg–Strauss syndrome is further discussed in Chapter 61.

Hypereosinophilic syndrome (HES) is defined as eosinophilia for more than 6 months in the absence of any known cause and with or without symptoms of end-organ damage. Entities considered within the spectrum of HES are complex and are beyond the scope of this work.

Anatomy and Physiology

Eosinophils are an important part of type 1 hypersensitivity reactions (i.e., allergic reactions). Whereas mast cells are involved with early phase allergic reaction (minutes to hours), eosinophils are more related to late-phase allergic reaction (days to months), being a more readily available marker of allergy.

How to Approach the Image

Imaging diagnosis of ELD relies on correlation with the clinical scenario—that is, an appropriate history, the presence of eosinophilia, or other abnormal laboratory results (e.g., anti-neutrophil cytoplasmic antibodies in allergic granulomatosis with polyangiitis). The diagnosis should be considered in patients with multifocal pulmonary opacities in whom pulmonary infection is not suspected. If ELD is suspected, the radiologist should review the medical record for associated abnormalities, drug therapy, and documentation of peripheral eosinophilia.

What Not to Miss

- The so-called "photographic negative of pulmonary edema" pattern is specific but not sensitive for the diagnosis of CEP.
- ELD should be considered in patients with peripheral, migratory, or waxing and waning consolidations or ground-glass opacities.

Differential Diagnosis

- Mucus plugging within central bronchiectasis may mimic ABPA but may also be seen in bronchial atresia, cystic fibrosis, and endoluminal lung cancer or other neoplasm. Although the presence of asthma always suggests ABPA, lung cancer should be excluded.
- ELD associated with parasitic infection may mimic organizing pneumonia. Pulmonary opacities in ELD associated with parasites tend to be self-limited and often resolve without treatment.
- The main differential consideration of AEP is acute interstitial pneumonia (i.e., idiopathic acute respiratory distress syndrome (ARDS)). Both have very similar clinical and radiologic findings.
- The main differential diagnosis of CEP is organizing pneumonia. The latter does not commonly exhibit eosinophilia.
- Because ELDs cause parenchymal opacities, bacterial pneumonia is within the differential diagnosis. Typically, the clinical presentation of infection is more characteristic with acute symptoms including fever, cough, and purulent sputum.

Imaging Findings

ABPA

- Chest radiography: Tubular branching opacities that may exhibit the "finger-in-glove" sign (i.e., inspissated mucus within dilated central bronchi); migratory parenchymal opacities (Figs. 63.1–63.3).

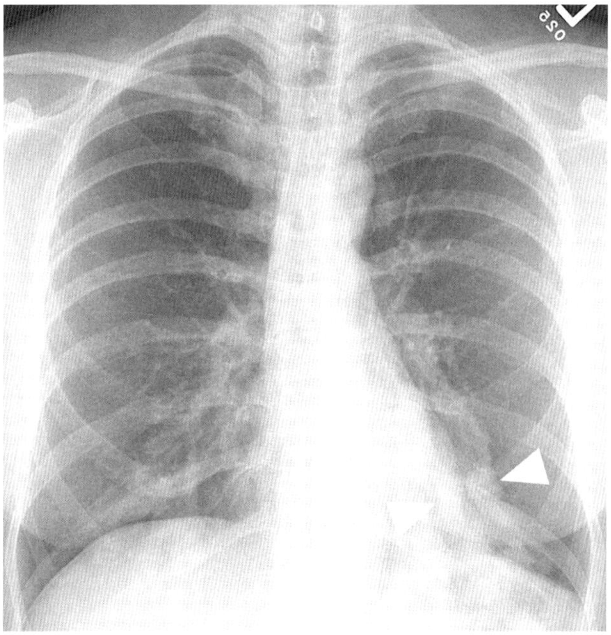

Figure 63.1. ABPA. Posteroanterior (PA) chest radiograph of a 57-year-old woman with a history of asthma shows tubular branching opacities in the bilateral lower lobes (arrowheads), demonstrating the so-called finger-in-glove sign, from inspissated mucus within bronchiectasis.

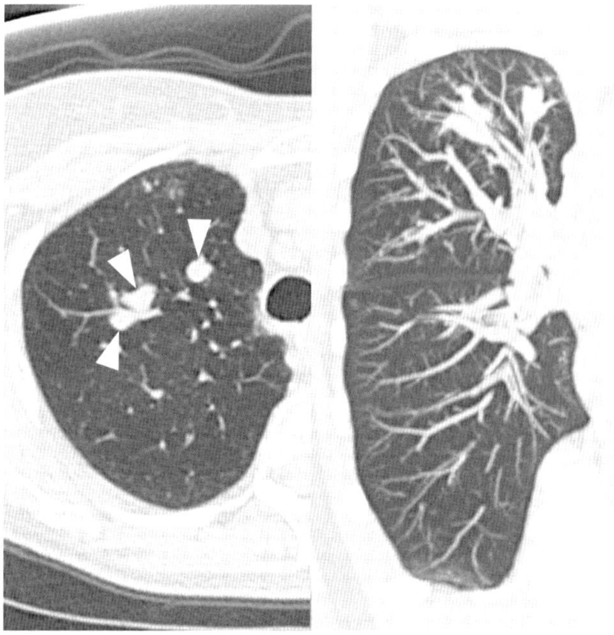

Figure 63.2. ABPA. Composite image with unenhanced chest CT of a 53-year-old woman with asthma shows mucus-fluid right upper lobe bronchiectasis manifesting as nodules (arrowheads) adjacent to pulmonary arteries (left). Coronal maximum intensity projection reformation shows branching opacities consistent with inspissated mucus within bronchiectasis.

- Chest CT: Endoluminal inspissated mucus within bronchiectatic airways is often hypodense but may be hyperdense due to the deposition of calcium salts. Other nonspecific findings, such as

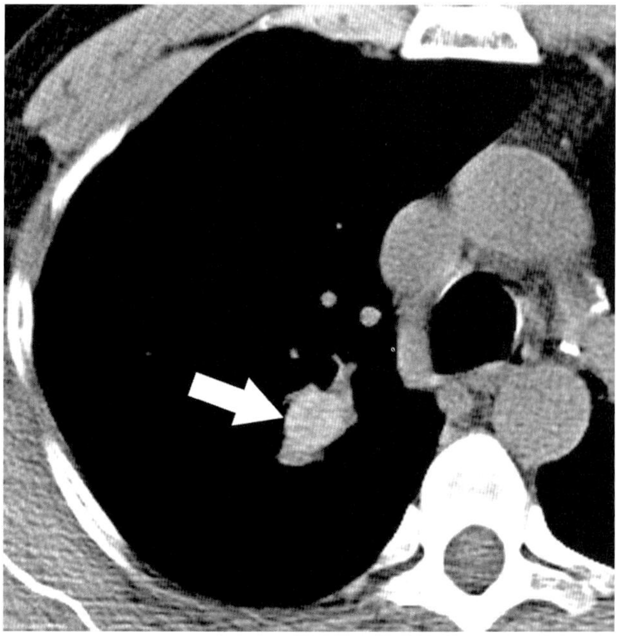

Figure 63.3. ABPA. Unenhanced chest CT of a 47-year-old man with asthma shows hyperdense mucus (arrow) within a right upper lobe bronchiectatic airway related to calcium salt deposition in the mucus.

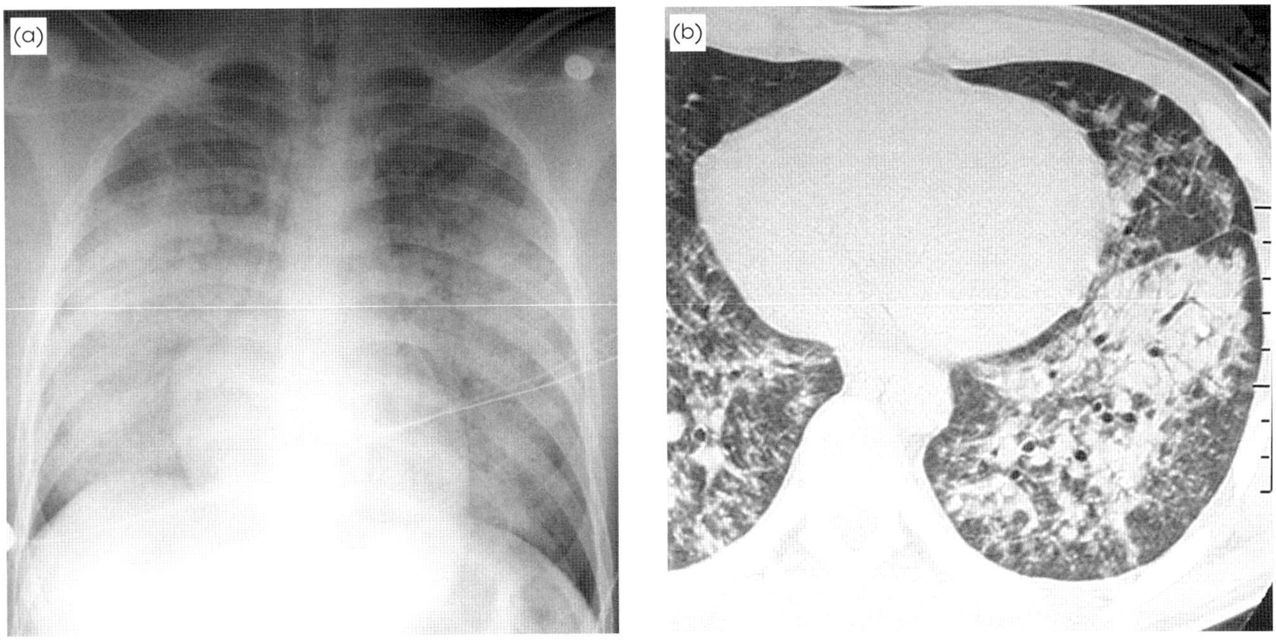

Figure 63.4. Strongyloidiasis. (a) Anteroposterior (AP) chest radiograph of a 27-year-old man with end-stage renal failure on chronic corticosteroid therapy and acute respiratory failure shows diffuse bilateral heterogeneous opacities. (b) Unenhanced chest CT of the same patient confirms diffuse bilateral heterogeneous opacities that correlated with coexistent alveolar hemorrhage and ARDS.

migratory parenchymal opacities, may be seen on imaging.

Strongyloidiasis

- Chest radiography: Multifocal pulmonary opacities affecting all pulmonary lobes (Fig. 63.4).
- Chest CT: Ground-glass opacities, consolidations, or both. A dominant focal segmental opacity should raise suspicion of bacterial superinfection.

AEP

- Chest radiography: Mimics cardiogenic pulmonary edema (Fig. 63.5)
- Chest CT: Ground-glass opacities, interlobular septal thickening, and pleural effusion

CEP

- Chest radiography: Classic features are bilateral, peripheral, upper lobe opacities, often referred as

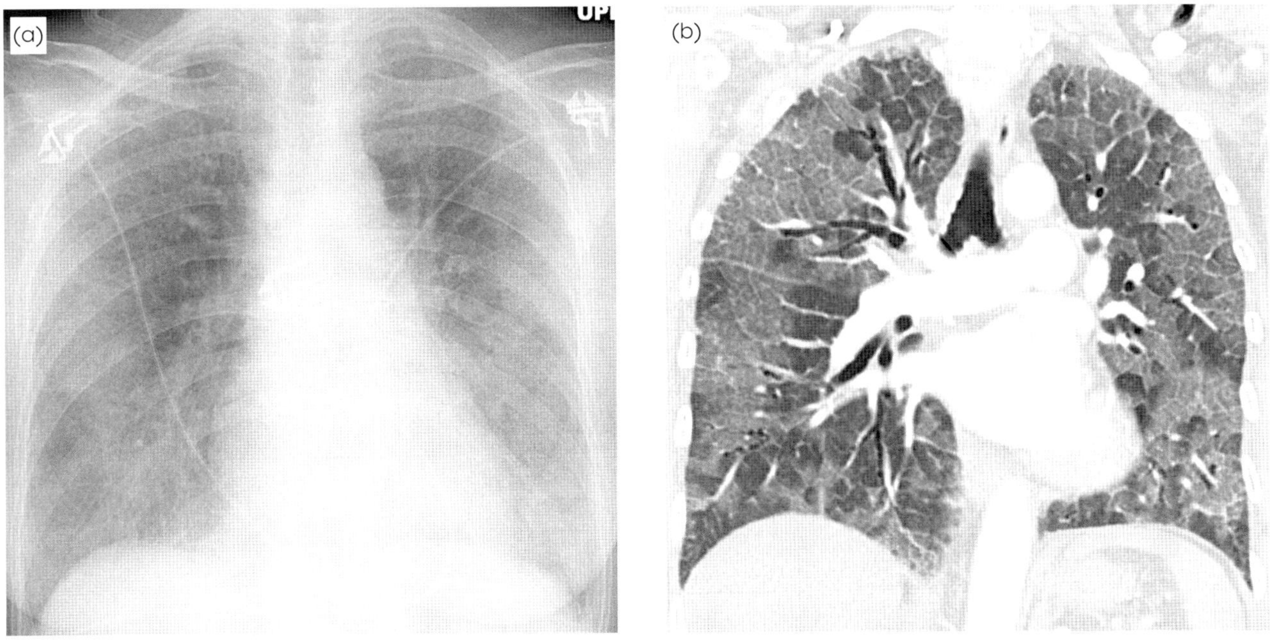

Figure 63.5. AEP. (a) AP chest radiograph of a 62-year-old patient with acute respiratory failure shows diffuse hazy opacities affecting all lobes. (b) Coronal contrast-enhanced chest CT shows extensive ground-glass opacities and interlobular septal thickening.

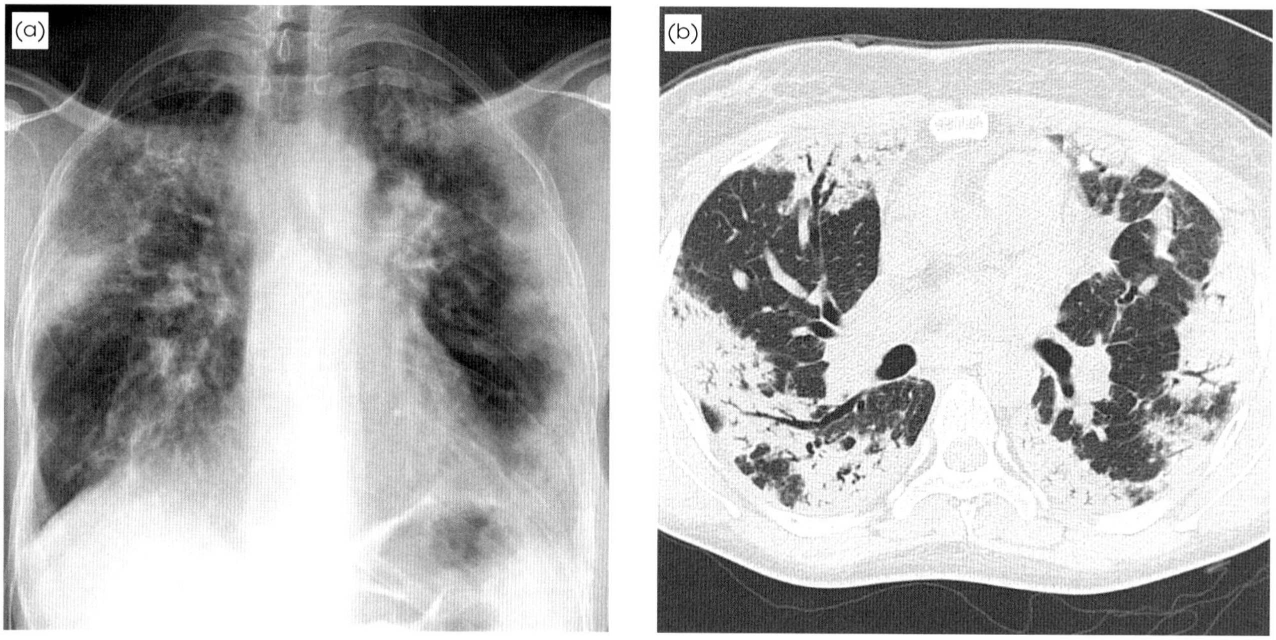

Figure 63.6. Chronic eosinophilic pneumonia. (a) AP chest radiograph of a 54-year-old woman with insidious dyspnea and constitutional symptoms shows bilateral upper lobe peripheral consolidations manifesting with the classic "photographic negative of pulmonary edema." (b) HRCT shows multifocal peripheral consolidations with intrinsic air bronchograms.

the "photographic negative of pulmonary edema." Nonspecific scattered opacities and nodules are more frequent findings (Fig. 63.6).

- Chest CT: Coexistent consolidations and ground-glass opacities. Migratory opacities may be seen on follow-up imaging (Fig.63.7).

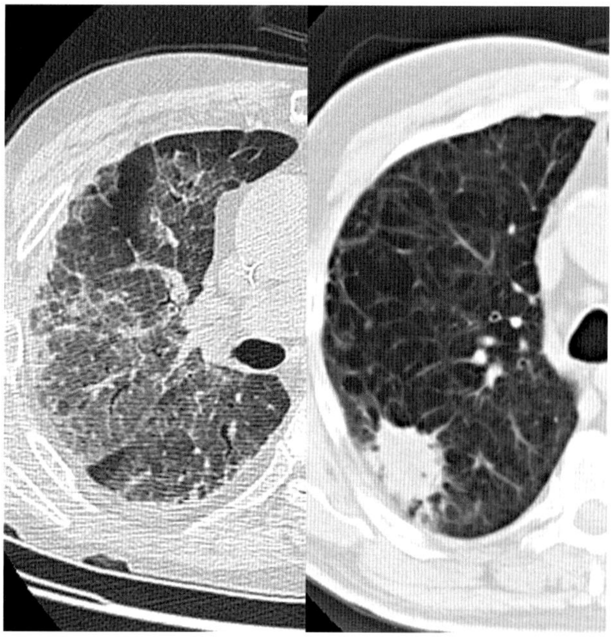

Figure 63.7. Chronic eosinophilic pneumonia. Composite image with chest CT of two different patients with CEP shows diffuse ground-glass opacities (left) and a spiculated right upper lobe nodule mimicking lung cancer on a background of emphysema, the latter a rather uncommon presentation (right).

Clinical Issues

- Eosinophilia may be absent in blood and may require time to be reported in tissue. Thus, ELD may not be considered before the performance of imaging studies. A high index of suspicion on the part of the radiologist is required to direct management and further testing.

Key Points

- Consider ELD in the setting of peripheral and/or tissue eosinophilia.
- ABPA typically manifests with branching opacities that produce the finger-in-glove sign on chest radiography.
- Strongyloidiasis is a diagnosis of exclusion often made by the identification of larvae in the bronchoalveolar lavage fluid.
- Consider AEP in a patient with diffuse pulmonary opacities after recent initiation of cigarette smoking.
- The "photographic negative of pulmonary edema" is a classic pattern in CEP, but it is not commonly seen.

Suggested Reading

Jeong YJ, Kim KI, Seo IJ, Lee CH, Lee KN, Kim KN, et al. Eosinophilic lung diseases: A clinical, radiologic, and pathologic overview. *RadioGraphics.* 2007;27(3):617–637.

Li H, Groshong SD, Lynch S, Brown KK, Frankel SK. Eosinophilic lung disease. *Clin Pulm Med.* 2010;17:66–74.

Martínez S, Restrepo CS, Carrillo JA, Betancourt SL, Franquet T, Varón C, et al. Thoracic manifestations of tropical parasitic infections: A pictorial review. *RadioGraphics.* 2005 Jan–Feb;25(1):135–155.

CHAPTER 64

Amyloidosis

Felipe Martínez

Definition

Amyloidosis is a group of disorders characterized by overexpression and extracellular deposition of amyloid with resultant organ dysfunction. Amyloid is an insoluble protein aggregate that is apple-green birefringent when stained with Congo red and viewed under polarized light. At least 15 different amyloid proteins derive from different precursors. Some of these proteins are morphologically similar to immunoglobulins.

Clinical Features

The heart is the most commonly involved organ in the chest. Progressive systolic dysfunction in a patient with left ventricular hypertrophy is a common manifestation. Up to one-third of patients with primary amyloidosis develop heart failure secondary to myocardial amyloid deposition, which has a high mortality with a life expectancy of 12 months or less.

Pulmonary involvement is relatively rare and is more common in the localized form of the disease. Patients usually present with recurrent pneumonia secondary to bronchial or bronchiolar obstruction due to deposition along the bronchial walls or, less commonly, due to an amyloidoma. Pulmonary involvement is not a major cause of mortality.

Anatomy and Physiology

Amyloidosis produces significant morbidity and mortality, and its prevalence is increasing. The disease is clinically significant when organ function is impaired due to either loss of normal cell structure or mass effect from accumulating amyloid. A total of 85% of amyloid is composed of fibrillar protein, which defines the type of amyloidosis and varies depending on the underlying disease. The remaining 15% of amyloid is composed of other proteins and glycoproteins common to all types of amyloidosis.

The current classification of amyloidosis is based on the different types of fibrillar proteins that define organ involvement and disease manifestations. There are systemic and localized forms of the disease, with the systemic forms being more common. The four major categories of systemic amyloidosis are (1) primary or immunoglobulin light chain disease, (2) secondary or amyloid protein A disease, (3) hereditary or mutant transthyretin disease, and (4) dialysis-associated or β_2 microglobulin disease. Localized amyloidosis accounts for 15% of cases and includes amyloid deposits associated with Alzheimer disease, isolated atrial amyloidosis, diabetes type 2, and medullary islet cell tumors.

How to Approach the Image

- Chest radiography is often the first imaging study performed in affected patients who are often evaluated for dyspnea. Unfortunately, chest radiography findings are nonspecific in cases of thoracic amyloidosis.
- High-resolution CT is the modality of choice in the evaluation of patients with suspected tracheopulmonary amyloidosis.
- Cardiac MRI is the imaging modality of choice in the evaluation of patients with suspected amyloid cardiomyopathy.

What Not to Miss

It is very important to differentiate calcified and noncalcified amyloidomas from benign or malignant primary or secondary lung neoplasms such as bronchogenic carcinoma, chondroma, and metastatic disease from mucinous adenocarinoma or osteosarcoma.

Differential Diagnosis

Airway Involvement

- Granulomatosis with polyangiitis (Wegener) may produce circumferential large airway wall thickening.
- Relapsing polychondritis may produce airway wall thickening but typically spares the posterior tracheal wall.
- Tracheobronchopathia osteochondroplastica manifests with calcified or ossified tracheal wall nodules and spares the posterior tracheal membrane.

Lung Parenchymal Involvement

- Nodular parenchymal amyloidosis may mimic lung cancer, metastatic disease, pulmonary ossification, granulomatous disease, rheumatoid arthritis, and granulomatosis with polyangiitis.

- Fine linear or reticulonodular opacities in amyloidosis may mimic other common interstitial lung diseases, including usual interstitial pneumonia, autoimmune disorders (e.g., scleroderma and rheumatoid arthritis), and drug toxicity.
- Amyloidosis with diffuse or multifocal calcification may mimic granulomatous disease, metastatic calcification, silicosis, and alveolar microlithiasis.
- Lymphadenopathy, common in amyloidosis, may also occur in sarcoidosis, tuberculosis, fungal infection, and metastatic malignancy.

Imaging Findings

Chest radiography may be normal in the majority of patients with thoracic amyloidosis. When abnormal, findings are nonspecific and include reticular or reticulonodular opacities, atelectasis, and consolidation.

Pulmonary Amyloidosis

- Tracheobronchial pattern: Most common pattern of respiratory involvement. CT may show focal or segmental involvement characterized by submucosal amyloid deposition in the trachea or segmental airways resulting in nodules, plaques, or concentric discontinuous thickening with intrinsic calcification (Figs. 64.1 and 64.2). This may result in atelectasis, hyperinflation, and post-obstructive pneumonia.
- Nodular parenchymal pattern: Usually seen in the localized form of the disease. Single or multiple pulmonary nodules (amyloidomas) typically with subpleural or peripheral distribution. Amyloidomas exhibit multiple shapes and sizes (up to several centimeters), may be calcified or ossified in up to 50% of cases, and are characterized by slow growth with no regression. Cavitation is very rare (Figs. 64.3–64.5).

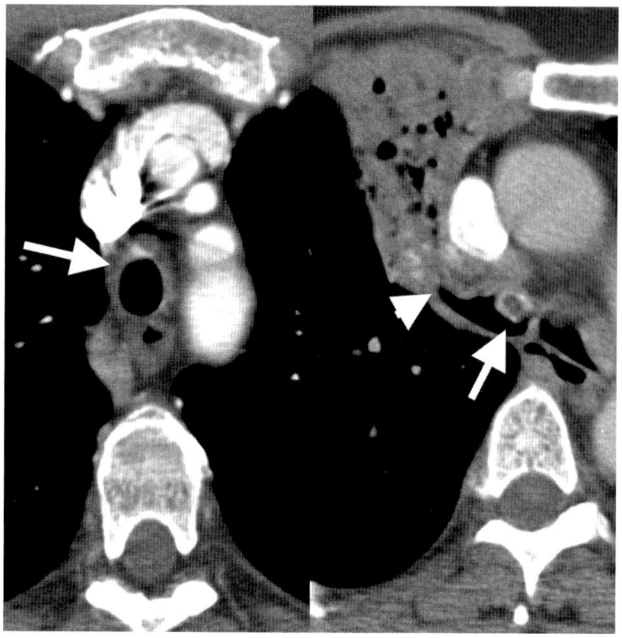

Figure 64.2. Amyloidosis, tracheal and bronchial involvement. Composite image with contrast-enhanced chest CT of a patient with amyloidosis shows nodular concentric mural thickening of the distal trachea (arrow) with intrinsic calcification (left) and a peripherally calcified endobronchial lesion in the right mainstem bronchus (arrow), concentric mural thickening, and occlusion of the right upper lobe bronchus (arrowhead) resulting in lobar collapse (right).

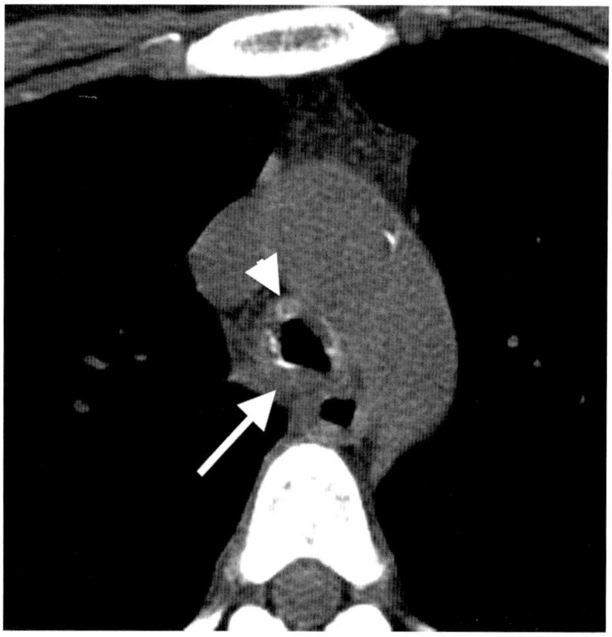

Figure 64.1. Amyloidosis, tracheal involvement. Unenhanced chest CT of a patient with progressive dyspnea shows nodular concentric mural thickening of the distal trachea (arrow) with areas of mural calcification (arrowhead) and luminal narrowing.

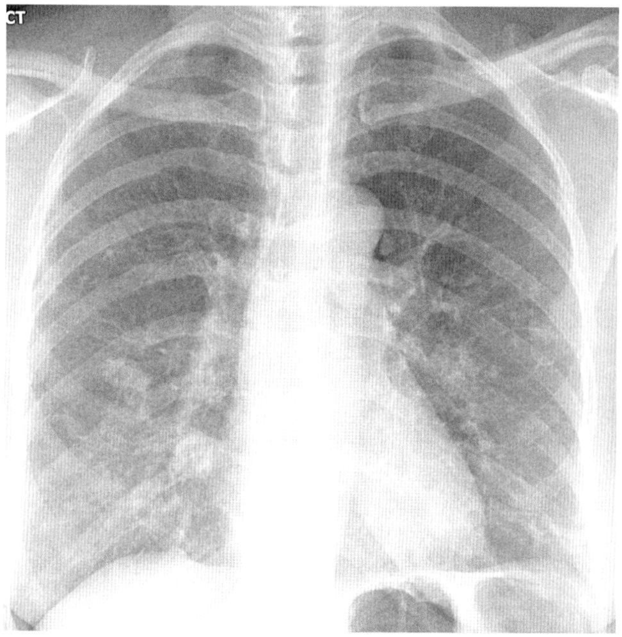

Figure 64.3. Amyloidosis, nodular parenchymal pattern. Posteroanterior (PA) chest radiograph of a patient with pulmonary amyloidosis shows bilateral calcified and noncalcified lung nodules.

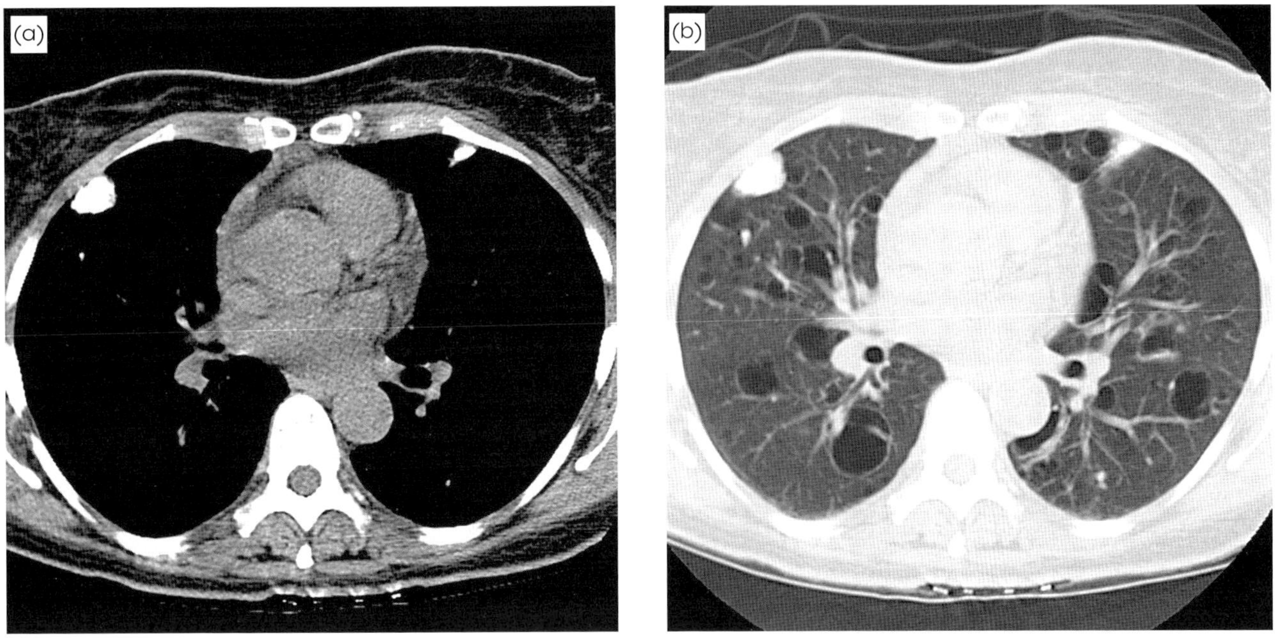

Figure 64.4. Amyloidosis, nodular parenchymal pattern. Unenhanced chest CT of a patient with nodular amyloidosis and Sjögren syndrome shows (a) bilateral calcified pulmonary nodules (amyloidomas) and (b) thin-walled cysts that are thought to result from associated lymphoid interstitial pneumonia.

- Diffuse alveolar septal pattern: Least common pattern frequently related to systemic disease and is often subclinical. CT shows reticulation and interlobular septal thickening often associated with micronodules secondary to amyloid deposition (Figs. 64.6 and 64.7). Less common findings include ground-glass opacities, traction bronchiectasis, and honeycombing. When present, it is a marker for cardiac amyloid deposition.
- Although nonspecific, mediastinal and hilar lymphadenopathy may be an important finding in amyloidosis, which together with interlobular interstitial thickening help suggest systemic disease.

Cardiac Amyloidosis

- Echocardiography and cardiac MRI are the modalities of choice for evaluation of suspected cardiac

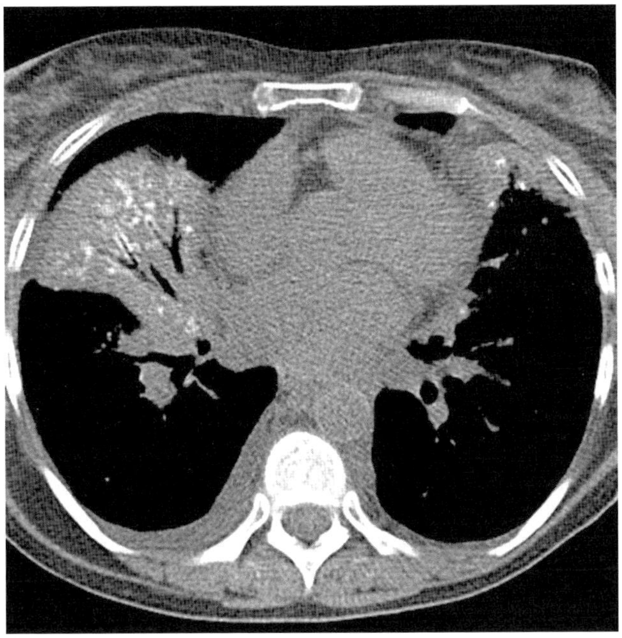

Figure 64.5. Amyloidosis, nodular parenchymal pattern. Unenhanced chest CT of a patient with pulmonary amyloidosis shows a large mass-like consolidation in the middle lobe with extension to the hilum and intrinsic punctate calcifications.

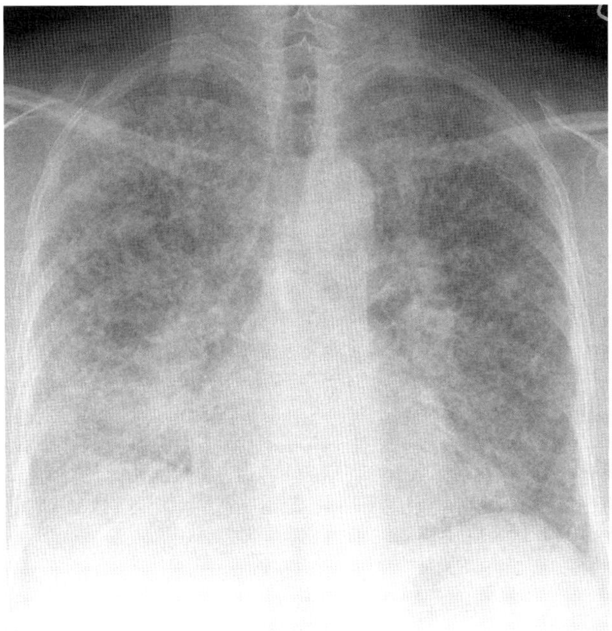

Figure 64.6. Amyloidosis, diffuse alveolar septal pattern. PA chest radiograph of a patient with pulmonary amyloidosis and progressive dyspnea shows decreased lung volumes and diffuse bilateral reticulation and nodular and perihilar opacities.

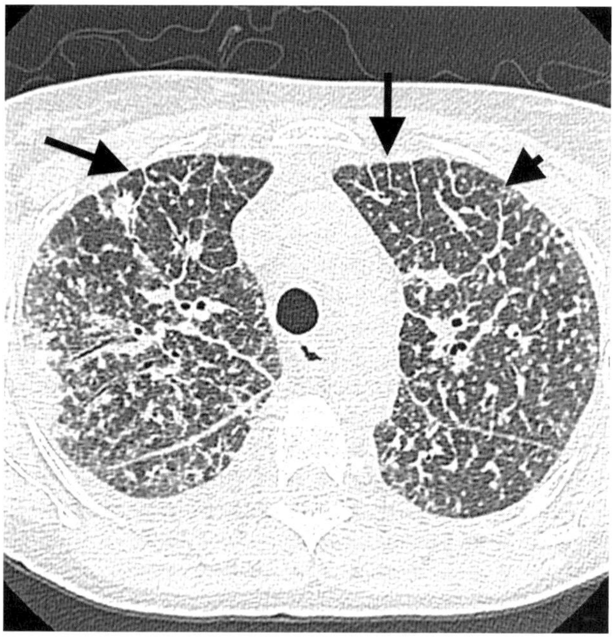

Figure 64.7. Amyloidosis, diffuse alveolar septal pattern. Unenhanced chest CT of a patient with pulmonary amyloidosis and progressive dyspnea shows bilateral reticulation with interlobular septal thickening (arrows) and scattered micronodules (arrowhead) and nodular opacities.

amyloidosis, and they show concentric left ventricular wall thickening and diastolic and subsequently systolic dysfunction.

- On echocardiography, a speckled or granular appearance of the myocardium, although not specific, is very characteristic and should raise concern for myocardial amyloid deposition.

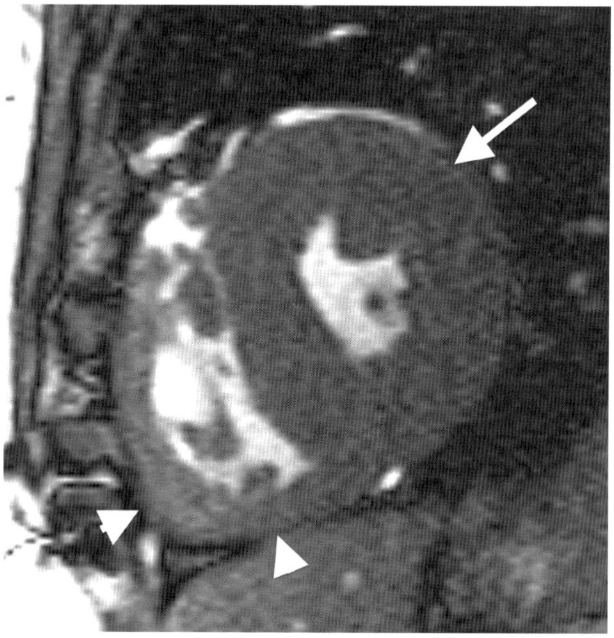

Figure 64.8. Cardiac amyloidosis, concentric biventricular hypertrophy. Static steady-state free precession cardiac MRI, short-axis view, of a patient with diastolic heart failure shows marked concentric left ventricular wall thickening (arrow) and, to a lesser extent, right ventricular wall thickening (arrowheads) secondary to myocardial amyloid deposition.

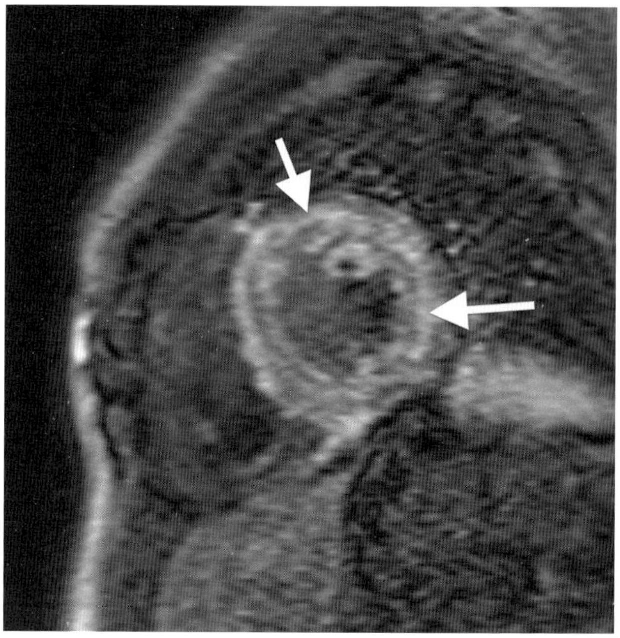

Figure 64.9. Cardiac amyloidosis, subendocardial late gadolinium enhancement. Double inversion recovery cardiac MRI after intravenous gadolinium, short-axis view, of a patient with suspected amyloid cardiomyopathy shows poor myocardial nulling with characteristic concentric ring-like subendocardial late gadolinium enhancement (arrows).

- Cardiac MR with intravenous contrast and delayed imaging provides functional and morphological information as well as tissue characterization. Cine MR may exhibit marked myocardial hypertrophy (Fig. 64.8). Poor myocardial nulling on inversion recovery images is a classic finding. Late enhanced images may exhibit diffuse myocardial enhancement, with subendocardial predominance and patchy enhancement (Fig. 64.9).

Clinical Issues

- Amyloidosis is an uncommon disease that requires a high index of clinical suspicion in order to be considered in the differential diagnosis.
- Thoracic amyloidosis has protean clinical and imaging manifestations and may mimic other more common entities.
- Cardiac amyloid deposition may be subclinical.

Key Points

- Pulmonary involvement in patients with amyloidosis is common, but the clinical outcome is highly variable. The nodular parenchymal form of the disease exhibits a slow progression and rarely requires intervention.

- Amyloidosis should always be considered in patients with tracheal narrowing; large calcified parenchymal nodules; and coexistent interlobular thickening (i.e., septal lines) and pulmonary nodules, especially when pulmonary edema is clinically unlikely.
- Cardiac amyloidosis, although not common, carries high morbidity and mortality. MRI is the test of choice to assess for myocardial compromise.

Suggested Reading

Aylwin AC, Gishen P, Copley SJ. Imaging appearance of thoracic amyloidosis. *J Thorac Imaging*. 2005 Feb;20(1):41–46.

Berk JL, O'Regan A, Skinner M. Pulmonary and tracheobronchial amyloidosis. *Semin Respir Crit Care Med.* 2002;23:155–165.

Georgiades CS, Neyman EG, Barish MA, et al. Amyloidosis: Review and CT manifestations. *RadioGraphics.* 2004;24:405–416.

Gillmore JD, Hawkins PH. Amyloidosis and the respiratory tract. *Thorax.* 1999;54:444–451.

Maceira AM, Joshi J, Prasad SK, Moon JC, Perugini E, Harding I, et al. Cardiovascular magnetic resonance in cardiac amyloidosis. *Circulation.* 2005 Jan 18;111(2):186–193.

Urban BA, Fishman EK, Goldman SM, et al. CT evaluation of amyloidosis: Spectrum of disease. *RadioGraphics.* 1993;13:1295–1308.

Section XII

Pneumoconiosis

CHAPTER 65

Pneumoconiosis

Sanjeev Bhalla

Introduction

Lung disease related to dust inhalation is referred to as *pneumoconiosis.* Inhaled particles tend to produce a pulmonary reaction that may result in fibrosis, as with asbestosis or silicosis, or in a macrophage-mediated reaction with little fibrosis, as with stannosis (tin) or baritosis (barium). Because these dusts are associated with the workplace, the term *occupational lung disease* may sometimes be used to include pneumoconiosis. This term is broader than pneumoconiosis and includes work-related asthma, sick building syndrome, and hypersensitivity pneumonitis from inhaled organic dusts.

Clinical Features

Symptoms depend on the degree of pulmonary involvement by fibrosis and on whether there is a superimposed infection or neoplasm. Certain pneumoconioses are more commonly associated with fibrosis, including asbestosis, silicosis, coal worker's pneumoconiosis, berylliosis, and talcosis. Hard metal inhalation (tungsten or cobalt) is associated with obliterative bronchiolitis and fibrosis from giant cell interstitial pneumonia. Other pneumoconioses, such as stannosis, baritosis, and siderosis (iron oxide), are not associated with fibrosis. Both silicosis and coal worker's pneumoconiosis are associated with an increased risk of tuberculosis. Coal worker's pneumoconiosis has a high association with obstructive lung disease that may contribute to dyspnea. Asbestosis and silicosis have a higher association with lung cancer. Asbestos exposure also has an association with malignant pleural mesothelioma.

Approach to Pneumoconioses

Three key features must be addressed in a potential case of pneumoconiosis: history of exposure, location of imaging abnormalities, and pattern of distribution of abnormalities. Mining, quarrying, and tunneling are associated with silicosis. Ceramic workers may be exposed to beryllium and arc welders to iron. Talcosis may be seen in the manufacturing of textiles, rubber, and paper.

As with any diffuse lung disease, the key to making the diagnosis of pneumoconiosis will rely on localization of the imaging abnormality to the lung and its appearance and distribution in relation to the secondary pulmonary lobule. Both silicosis and coal worker's pneumoconiosis exhibit a posterior and upper lobe predilection and manifest with tiny nodules (2–5 mm) typically in a perilymphatic distribution (Fig. 65.1). The nodules may coalesce into larger opacities known as progressive massive fibrosis.

Asbestosis exhibits a predilection for the lower lobes (Fig. 65.2). In its early stages, asbestosis may manifest with fine reticulation with interlobular septal thickening, intralobular lines, and cystic spaces. In advanced cases, honeycombing similar to that seen in usual interstitial pneumonia (UIP) may occur. Berylliosis is characterized by noncaseating granuloma formation and may mimic sarcoidosis (Fig. 65.3) with its upper lung predominance. Inhaled talcosis tends to spare the apices and the lung bases near the costophrenic sulci. Siderosis tends to affect peribronchovascular lymphatics and may manifest with vague centrilobular nodules (Fig. 65.4).

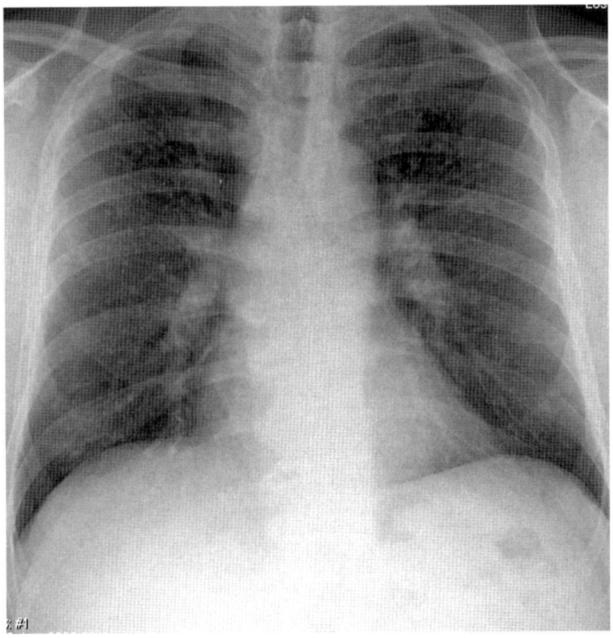

Figure 65.1. Silicosis. Posteroanterior (PA) chest radiograph of a 65-year-old man with a long history of working in a foundry with exposure to silica shows multiple tiny pulmonary nodules with an upper lung distribution.

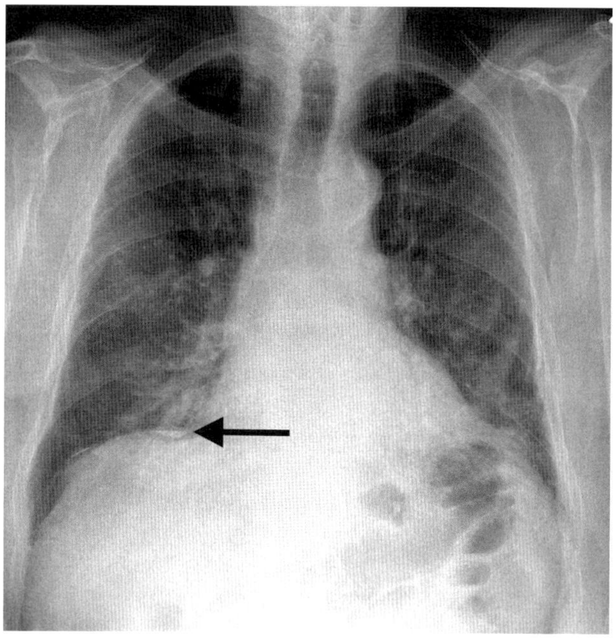

Figure 65.2. Asbestosis. PA chest radiograph of a 73-year-old man with occupational exposure to asbestos shows multiple pleural plaques, including one over the right hemidiaphragm (arrow), and mild basilar reticulation.

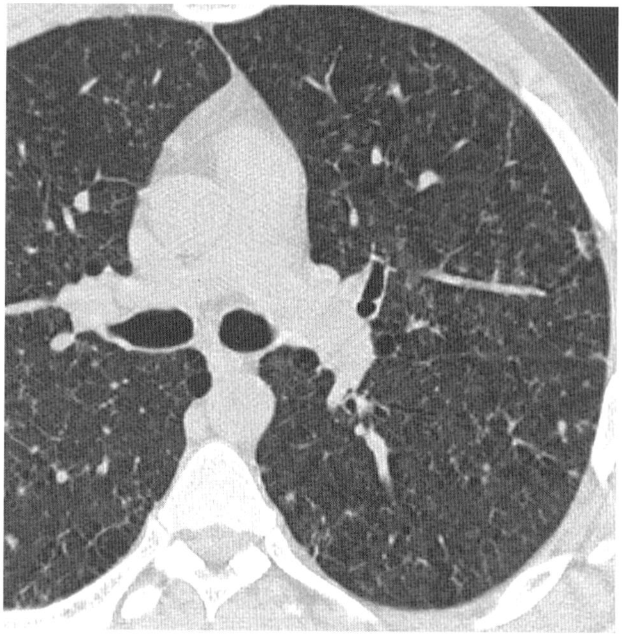

Figure 65.4. Siderosis. Unenhanced chest CT of a 43-year-old man with biopsy-proven siderosis as a result of working as a welder shows vague centrilobular nodules with areas mimicking tree-in-bud. The occupational history is key in determining the etiology.

Differential Diagnoses

Silicosis and Coal Worker's Pneumoconiosis

The main differential diagnosis is sarcoidosis. All three conditions may exhibit perilymphatic nodules, upper lobe predominance, and progressive massive fibrosis.

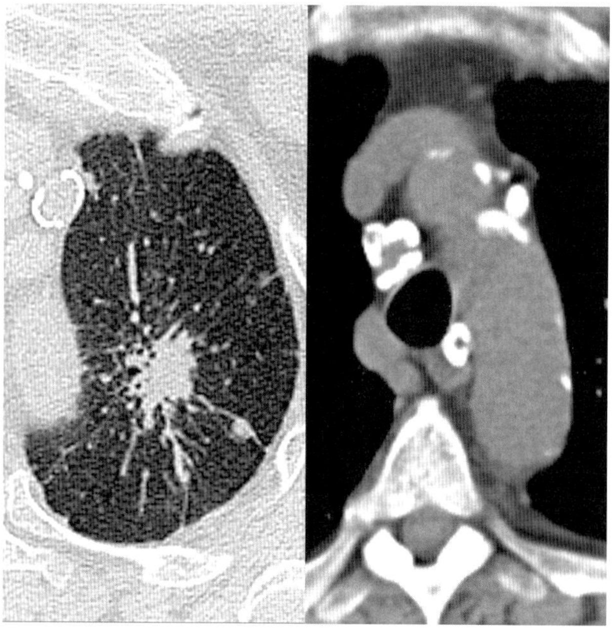

Figure 65.3. Berylliosis. Unenhanced chest CT of a 68-year-old man with berylliosis as a result of working in a nuclear power plant. The CT features mimic sarcoidosis with upper lobe progressive massive fibrosis and eggshell calcified lymph nodes. The key to the diagnosis is the occupational exposure history.

Lymph nodes exhibiting eggshell calcification are more common with sarcoidosis and silicosis, and they are unusual with coal worker's pneumoconiosis.

Asbestosis

Early asbestosis can mimic nonspecific interstitial pneumonia. Later stages of the disease may take on an appearance more typical of UIP. The presence of pleural plaques favors asbestosis.

Berylliosis

The main differential diagnosis is sarcoidosis. Small nodules in a perilymphatic distribution may be associated with lymphadenopathy, occasionally with progressive massive fibrosis, and rarely with honeycombing.

Hard Metal Pneumoconiosis

Early disease manifests with obliterative bronchiolitis and can mimic obliterative bronchiolitis from other conditions, such as prior infection, collagen vascular diseases, and other exposures. Advanced disease manifests with interstitial fibrosis that can mimic nonspecific interstitial pneumonia and UIP.

Inhaled Talcosis

Exposure to talc contaminated with silica or asbestos results in pneumoconiosis typical of the latter because talc is less pathogenic. Exposure to isolated talc manifests with early disease characterized by ground-glass centrilobular nodules that mimic respiratory bronchiolitis and hypersensitivity pneumonitis. Advanced disease may manifest with a pattern that resembles berylliosis with sparing of the lung bases near the costophrenic angles. High attenuating consolidation may occur and may mimic the findings of amiodarone exposure and amyloidosis.

Patients with pneumoconioses may present with very subtle imaging abnormalities. Care must be taken to assess the lungs for nodules and interstitial fibrosis. Often, high-resolution CT will be performed to further characterize radiographic abnormalities. Conversely, patients without pneumoconiosis may present with overlapping features. The diagnosis rests on matching the clinical history, exposure history, and radiologic findings. When areas of cavitation are seen, tuberculosis must be considered in patients with silicosis and coal worker's pneumoconiosis. Any noncalcified nodule must be carefully assessed to exclude lung cancer.

Suggested Reading

Chong S, Lee KS, Chung MJ, Han J, Kwon OJ, Kim TS. Pneumoconiosis: Comparison of imaging and pathologic findings. *RadioGraphics*. 2006 Jan–Feb;26(1):59–77.

Flors L, Domingo ML, Leiva-Salinas C, Mazón M, Roselló-Sastre E, Vilar J. Uncommon occupational lung diseases: High-resolution CT findings. *AJR Am J Roentgenol*. 2010 Jan;194(1): W20–W26.

CHAPTER 66

Asbestosis

Joseph T. Azok

Definition

Asbestosis (asbestos-induced pulmonary fibrosis) is a fibrotic pneumoconiosis associated with exposure to asbestos. For nearly 100 years, inhalation of asbestos fibers has been known to cause pleural and lung disease. Due to its physical properties, asbestos has been widely used in insulation, brake pads, flooring, and electrical wiring. Exposure is either primary (mining and acquisition of asbestos) or secondary (manufacturing, construction, and shipbuilding). Although asbestos has been banned in many countries, the prevalence of asbestos-related disease has increased during the past several decades, likely due to the long latency period between initial exposure and the development of biological effects that may occur 30–40 years following exposure.

Clinical Features

Patients exposed to asbestos typically remain asymptomatic for more than 10–20 years. The earliest manifestation of asbestos exposure is a pleural effusion, which occurs in a minority of patients and may develop as early as 1 year after exposure. Most are small, and affected patients are typically asymptomatic. Pleural plaques are the most common imaging manifestation of asbestos exposure and occur 20–30 years after initial exposure. Pleural plaques are not premalignant and do not produce symptoms. Diffuse pleural thickening associated with restrictive lung disease is related to the magnitude of asbestos exposure.

Prolonged high-level exposure may result in pulmonary fibrosis (asbestosis) characterized by insidious dyspnea that progresses in the absence of continued exposure. Clinical deterioration is associated with a progressive decline in vital and diffusion capacities.

Asbestos exposure is associated with an increased risk of lung cancer, which is exacerbated by cigarette smoking due to the synergistic effects of both carcinogens. The average latency period is thought to be more than 40 years. The association between asbestos exposure and mesothelioma is strong, also with a prolonged latency period of more than 40 years.

Anatomy and Physiology

The association between asbestos and its biological effects is complex and poorly understood. Inhaled asbestos fibers are deposited in the distal airways and alveoli. With increased exposure, asbestos fibers accumulate in a subpleural location. An inflammatory response is incited, leading to fibrosis. Asbestos-related disease affects the pleura (Figs. 66.1 and 66.2) and the lung. Pleural plaques and other nonfibrotic sequelae, such as rounded atelectasis (Fig. 66.3), are merely reflective of asbestos exposure. The term *asbestosis* should be reserved for pulmonary fibrosis secondary to asbestos inhalation (Fig. 66.4).

How to Approach the Image

Any imaging study performed to evaluate a patient with asbestos exposure must focus on a detailed analysis of the pleural surfaces. Pleural thickening can easily be overlooked and, when calcified, can be confused for a rib. On radiography, the pleural plaques will often be vague on one projection and better defined on the other. The lung parenchyma should be evaluated for any reticulation or honeycombing. These can be more common in the dependent regions. Although the International Labor Organization developed a classification system to describe and quantitate parenchymal and pleural radiographic abnormalities provoked by inhaled particulates, several studies have shown that high-resolution CT is more sensitive and specific for the diagnosis of asbestosis. Finally, all mass lesions should be carefully interrogated for any indication of volume loss, swirling of vessels, or mass effect.

What Not to Miss

Asbestos exposure is well associated with two thoracic malignancies: mesothelioma and lung cancer. The former can be insidious and may present as a recurrent pleural effusion. However, most often, a nodular pleural surface is seen. When soft tissue extension into the subpleural fat is encountered, mesothelioma is strongly favored over a bland plaque. Lung cancer must be differentiated from rounded atelectasis. When the lesion has mass effect and no appreciable volume loss or swirled vessels, cancer becomes a concern. Sometimes PET/CT or biopsy is needed to distinguish between the two.

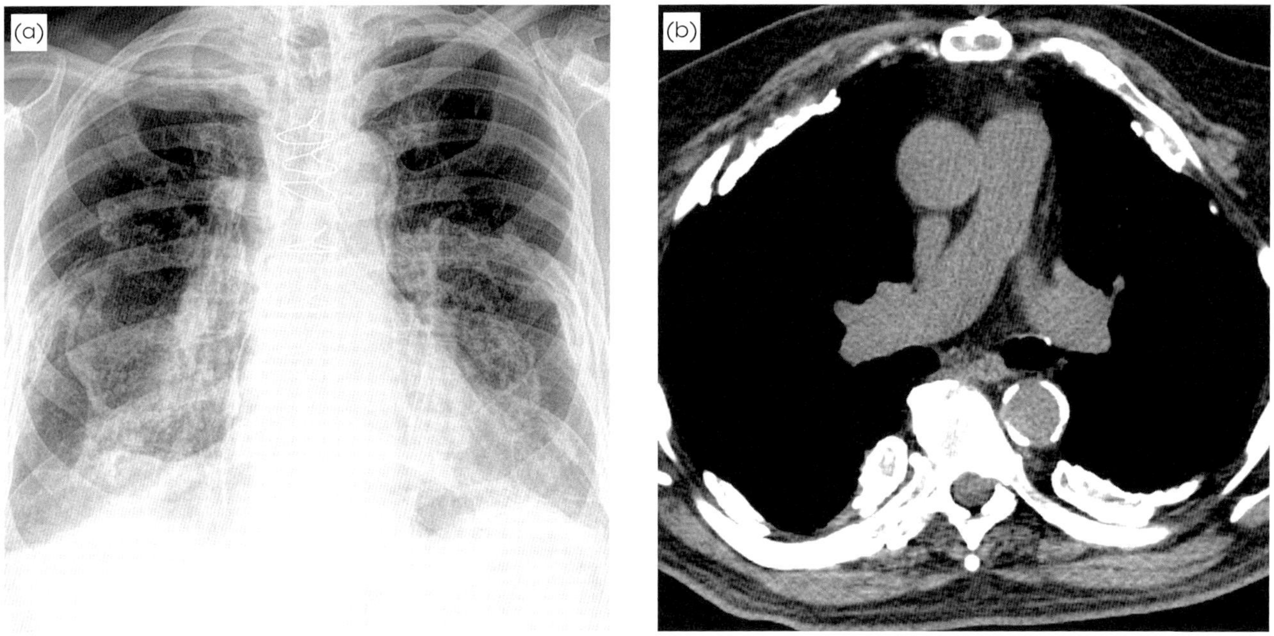

Figure 66.1. Asbestos-related pleural plaques. (a) Posteroanterior chest radiograph of an 83-year-old man with an occupational exposure to asbestos shows bilateral amorphous calcifications with a vertical linear orientation when seen in tangent and an irregular nodular or mass-like appearance en face. (b) Unenhanced chest CT confirms well-circumscribed symmetric multifocal discontinuous areas of pleural thickening with calcification.

Differential Diagnosis

Pleura

- Prior hemothorax and prior empyema may result in pleural plaques that often calcify. These are usually unilateral, unlike the asbestos-related plaques, which tend to be bilateral.
- Mediastinal pleural involvement, circumferential distribution, and nodular pleural thickening all favor malignancy. Differential diagnosis includes metastatic disease (typically adenocarcinoma), lymphoma, or invasive thymoma.

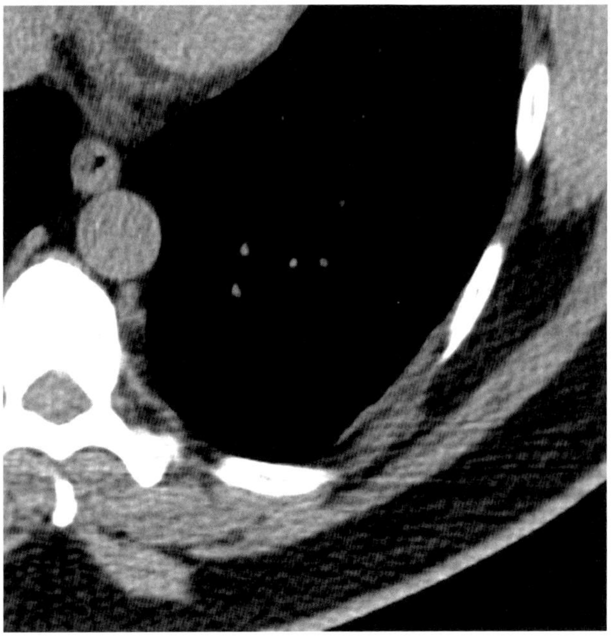

Figure 66.2. Asbestos-related pleural plaques. Unenhanced chest CT of a 54-year-old man with asbestos exposure shows a well-circumscribed area of pleural thickening along the posterolateral left hemithorax separated from the underlying rib and soft tissue by a thin layer of fat consistent with a noncalcified pleural plaque.

Parenchyma

- Atelectasis can simulate early fibrosis but should disappear with prone imaging.
- Advanced asbestosis can simulate usual interstitial pneumonia or nonspecific interstitial pneumonia. The patterns may be idiopathic or seen with drug toxicities or collagen vascular disease. The presence of plaques and an exposure history favor asbestosis.
- Lung cancer or any pulmonary nodule may mimic rounded atelectasis. Care must be taken to look for the characteristic swirling of vessels and a component of volume loss. If those are not seen, biopsy or PET/CT may be required.

Imaging Findings

Pleural Abnormalities

Pleural Plaques

- Well-circumscribed foci of pleural thickening, a minority of which are calcified
- Typically bilateral, most common along the posterolateral chest wall and central diaphragm, and spare the apical and costophrenic sulcus pleura

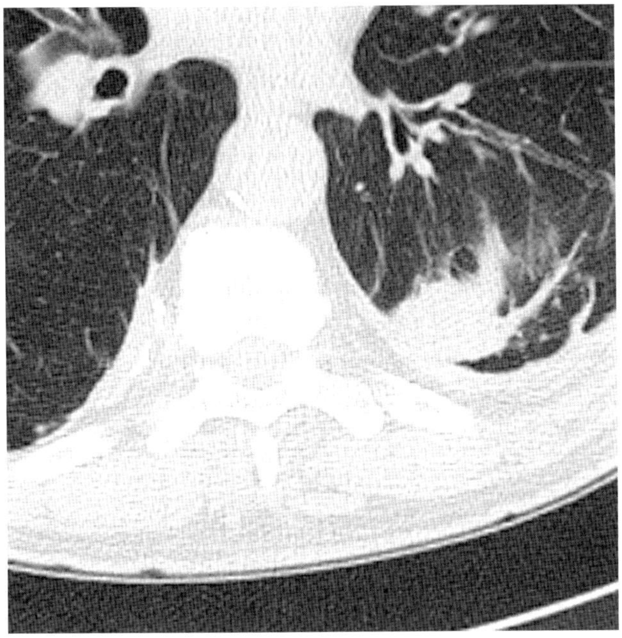

Figure 66.3. Rounded atelectasis. Unenhanced chest CT of an asymptomatic 71-year-old heavy smoker shows a peripheral left lower lobe subpleural opacity adjacent to pleural thickening. Note the curvilinear orientation of the bronchovascular markings toward the lesion, virtually diagnostic of rounded atelectasis. The right-sided calcified pleural plaque confirms asbestos exposure.

- On radiography, the plaques tend to be angled and elongated with a portion of the border being obscured (due to their pleural origin). This appearance has been termed the "holly leaf" sign.

Pleural Effusions

- Typically small, unilateral or bilateral

Diffuse Pleural Thickening

- Smooth pleural thickening extending for 5 cm axially and 8 cm longitudinally
- Involves the pleura of the costophrenic angles

Mesothelioma

- Ipsilateral volume loss
- Unilateral pleural effusion
- Circumferential, nodular pleural thickening involving the fissures and mediastinal pleura (Fig. 66.5)
- Often associated with other features of asbestos exposure
- May produce local invasion into the chest wall and mediastinum

Parenchymal Abnormalities

Asbestosis

- Radiography: Fine reticular opacities that may be subtle or not radiographically visible in early disease

CT

- Predominantly posterior lower lobe reticulation.
- With increasing fibrosis, honeycombing, traction bronchiectasis, and architectural distortion can develop.
- The presence of pleural plaques (often better seen on CT) is an important finding that may help differentiate asbestosis from other idiopathic pneumonias.

Rounded Atelectasis

- Peripheral atelectasis adjacent to pleural thickening
- "Comet tail" sign—vessels and bronchi curve into rounded opacity
- Associated volume loss

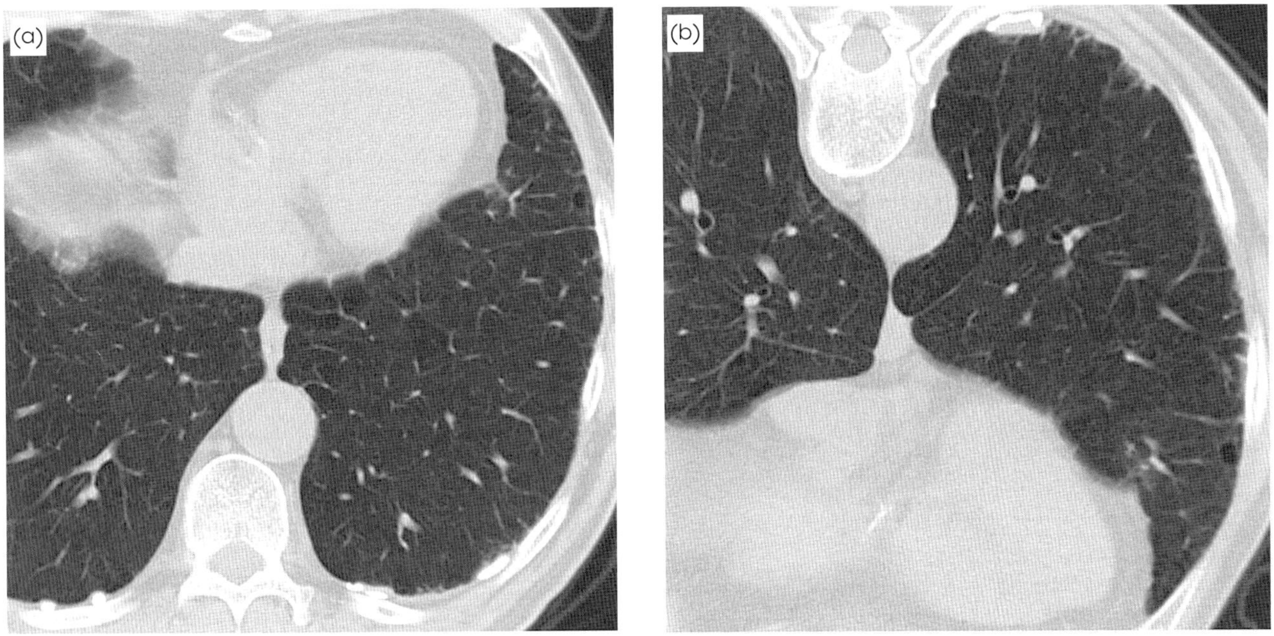

Figure 66.4. Asbestosis. (a) CT in an 85-year-old man with occupational asbestos exposure shows subtle basilar reticular opacities and pleural plaques. (b) Prone image confirms the presence of the reticulation, in keeping with asbestosis.

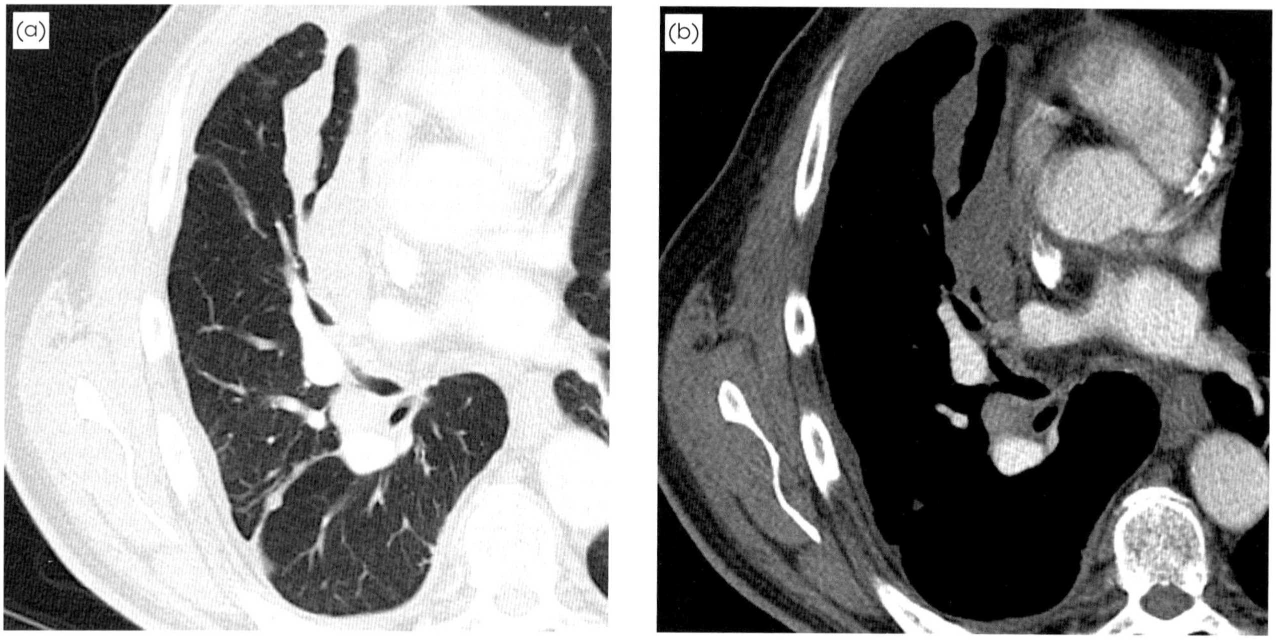

Figures 66.5. Mesothelioma. Unenhanced chest CT of a 72-year-old man with asbestos exposure and recently diagnosed mesothelioma shows (a) right hemithorax volume loss and (b) circumferential nodular pleural thickening involving the mediastinal and fissural pleura.

Primary Lung Cancer

- Similar to non-asbestos-related lung cancer
- Most commonly occurs in the peripheral lower lobes
- Early detection challenging due to the wide range of concurrent pleural and parenchymal asbestos-related abnormalities

Clinical Issues

- Pleural effusions from asbestos exposure are typically exudative, but they may be hemorrhagic.
- A recurrent effusion should raise concern for mesothelioma in a patient with asbestos exposure.
- Rounded atelectasis may result from any pleural effusion with adjacent pleural thickening.
- Absence of typical features of rounded atelectasis should prompt further evaluation with biopsy or PET/CT to exclude malignancy.

Key Points

- Pleural plaques are the most common manifestation of asbestos exposure and are not premalignant.
- Pleural plaques typically occur along the posterolateral chest wall or central diaphragm and are often visible on radiography, but CT is more sensitive and can concurrently provide assessment for other asbestos-related pleural or parenchymal diseases.
- Asbestosis refers to pulmonary fibrosis secondary to inhaled asbestos particles and manifests initially as subpleural reticulation that mimics nonspecific interstitial pneumonia but may progress to honeycombing mimicking usual interstitial pneumonia.
- When there is clinical concern for asbestosis, prone imaging may help identify early fibrosis that can be obscured by dependent atelectasis on supine imaging.
- A peripheral lower lobe mass-like opacity adjacent to pleural thickening associated with the comet tail sign should suggest rounded atelectasis. However, if characteristic imaging features are absent, biopsy or PET/CT may be warranted to exclude a primary lung cancer.
- Circumferential nodular pleural thickening involving the fissures and mediastinal pleura should suggest pleural malignancy and specifically mesothelioma in asbestos-exposed individuals. Asbestos-related diffuse pleural thickening may mimic mesothelioma.

Suggested Reading

Chong S, Lee KS, Chung MJ, Han J, Kwon OJ, Kim TS. Pneumoconiosis: Comparison of imaging and pathologic findings. *RadioGraphics*. 2006;26:59–77.

International Labour Organization (ILO). *Guidelines for the Use of the ILO International Classification of Radiographs of Pneumoconioses*, rev. ed. Geneva: ILO; 2011.

Kim KI, Kim CW, Lee MK, Lee KS, Park CK, Choi SJ, et al. Imaging of occupational lung disease. *RadioGraphics*. 2011; 21:1371–1391.

CHAPTER 67

Silicosis and Coal Worker's Pneumoconiosis

Joseph T. Azok

Definition

Silicosis and coal worker's pneumoconiosis (CWP) are occupational lung diseases associated with exposure to free silica and coal dust, respectively. Occupations associated with silicosis include mining, tunneling, and sandblasting. CWP is seen almost exclusively in coal workers.

Clinical Features

The clinical presentation of silicosis is variable depending on the duration and magnitude of exposure. Patients most commonly present with classic silicosis and develop symptoms 10–20 years following initial exposure generally to low concentrations of silica over a long time period. Cough and dyspnea are the most common symptoms. Concomitant emphysema is hypothesized to be a major cause of disability in these patients. With pulmonary fibrosis, pulmonary hypertension develops, leading to cor pulmonale. Other processes associated with silicosis include mycobacterial infection, lung cancer, and connective tissue disease.

Acute silicosis (silicoproteinosis) and accelerated silicosis are less common presenting manifestations of silica exposure. Acute silicosis results from high silica exposure over a short time period, and affected patients present with acute dyspnea and cough complicated by cyanosis. Despite aggressive treatment, this condition is typically fatal. Accelerated silicosis and classic silicosis are radiographically and pathologically indistinguishable. However, patients with accelerated silicosis become symptomatic within 5–10 years of exposure and rapidly progress to death within 5 years after the development of symptoms.

Exposure to coal dust can result in CWP, emphysema, Caplan syndrome, and silicosis (due to the silica content within coal). However, the most common presentation is either simple or complicated CWP. Most patients with simple CWP are asymptomatic, but symptomatic subjects typically present with chronic cough. With increased and prolonged exposure to coal dust, progressive massive fibrosis may develop (complicated CWP). Dyspnea increases, and cough becomes productive of black sputum. Pulmonary hypertension can develop, resulting in respiratory failure. Similar to silicosis, patients with CWP are at increased risk of developing tuberculosis and nontuberculous mycobacterial infections. An association between CWP and rheumatoid arthritis is well known. The presence of peripheral rheumatoid-like lung nodules without an apical–basilar gradient is known as Caplan syndrome.

Anatomy and Physiology

Free silica is inhaled and deposited within respiratory bronchioles. Silica particles are cleared rapidly from the lower lobes by lymphatics. Hence, similar to many other pneumoconioses, deposition occurs primarily within the upper lobes. Macrophages take up silica not cleared by lymphatics, inciting an inflammatory response, leading to pulmonary fibrosis. In classic silicosis, small, round, 2- to 5-mm nodules are deposited in the peribronchiole and perivascular interstitium (Figs. 67.1 and 67.2). With longer and

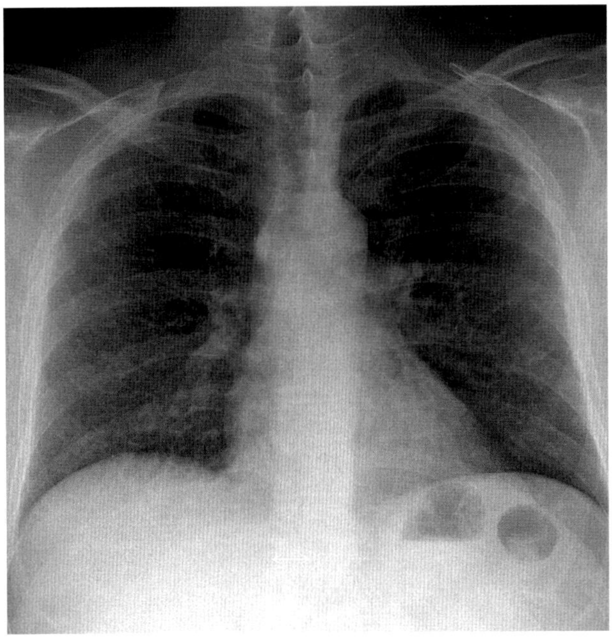

Figure 67.1. Simple silicosis. Posteroanterior (PA) chest radiograph of a 50-year-old quarry worker demonstrates small subcentimeter bilateral upper lobe predominant reticulonodular opacities.

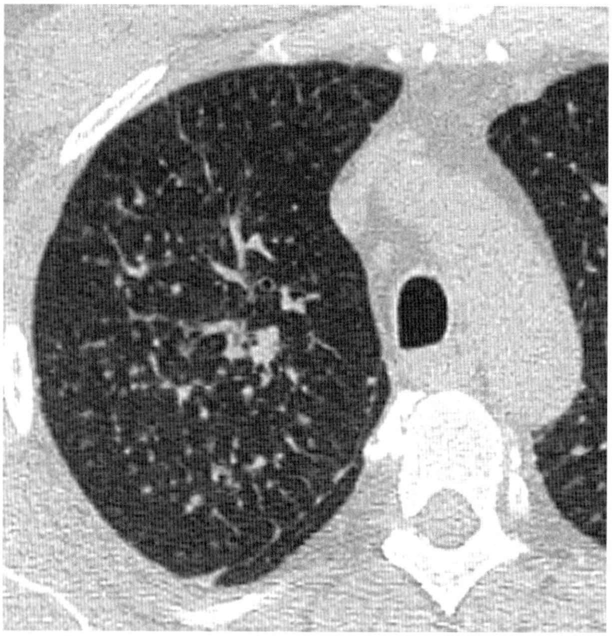

Figure 67.2. Simple silicosis. Unenhanced chest CT of a 48-year-old foundry worker shows innumerable small (<1 cm) upper lobe predominant pulmonary nodules in a perilymphatic distribution.

increased rates of exposure, nodules can coalesce, resulting in larger conglomerate nodules (>1 cm), referred to as progressive massive fibrosis (PMF).

CWP, although different from silicosis, results in similar imaging findings. Inhaled coal particles are deposited predominantly in respiratory bronchioles and subsequently taken up by macrophages. The macrophage is surrounded by fibrotic material, termed a coal macule, the hallmark of simple CWP. Macules enlarge with continued coal dust exposure, coalescing to result in pulmonary fibrosis. When nodules become larger than 1 cm, they result in complicated CWP or CWP with PMF (Fig. 67.3).

How to Approach the Image

Although histologically distinct, the imaging features of silicosis and CWP are similar and not reliably distinguished on radiography.

- Chest radiographs are relatively insensitive and nonspecific in early diagnosis.
- If radiographs are normal but a pneumoconiosis is suspected, chest CT should be performed.

What Not to Miss

In reading cases of silicosis or CWP, the key is to look for mass lesions or areas of cavitation. These may be indicative of a more active process such as tuberculosis or a lung cancer. Both have a higher association with these pneumoconioses, especially when there is a history of smoking. Cavitation in the conglomerate masses of PMF should raise the suspicion for tuberculosis. Although ischemia may result in cavitation, this diagnosis should be one of exclusion. PET/CT or biopsy may be needed to exclude malignancy.

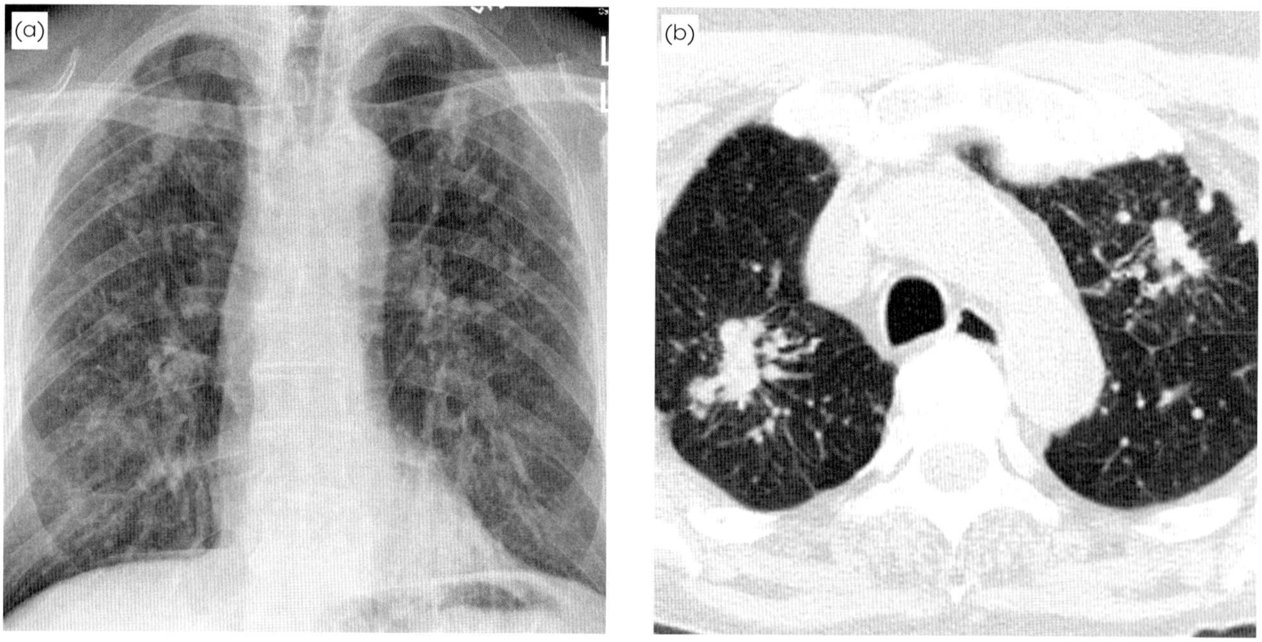

Figure 67.3. Complicated CWP. (a) PA chest radiograph of a 69-year-old male retired coal miner shows mid and upper lobe predominant bilateral nodular opacities, several of which are greater than 1 cm in diameter. (b) Unenhanced chest CT of the same patient demonstrates conglomerate upper lobe opacities and surrounding smaller subcentimeter nodules in a perilymphatic distribution consistent with complicated CWP with PMF.

Differential Diagnosis

- For micronodules in a perilymphatic distribution, the main differential diagnosis consists of sarcoidosis and lymphangitic carcinomatosis. The absence of septal thickening, pleural effusion, and malignancy makes lymphangitic carcinomatosis less likely.
- For masses in the upper lobes, the main consideration is PMF from another process such as sarcoidosis or a lung cancer. PMF may be calcified and often takes a rhomboid or rectangular shape.
- For the calcified lymphadenopathy, the differential includes sarcoidosis and treated lymphoma (usually Hodgkin). When the nodes are totally calcified, one should consider prior histoplasmosis infection.

Imaging Findings

Simple Silicosis or Simple CWP

- Small (2–5 mm) pulmonary nodules in upper and posterior lung zones. Silicosis nodules tend to be better defined and more homogeneous than CWP nodules.
- Mild cases may spare lower lobes.
- Perilymphatic distribution is typical.
- Calcification occurs in 20% of nodules.
- Pleural effusions are rare.

Complicated Silicosis or Complicated CWP

- Nodular opacities greater than 1 cm are known as PMF and typically have irregular borders and commonly calcify. Some have described their rhomboid shape as akin to angel wings.
- Most commonly affect posterior and apical segments of the upper and lower lobes, usually within the outer third of the lung.
- Lesions slowly migrate toward the hilum, resulting in upper lobe volume loss and adjacent architectural distortion.
- Cavitation is typically from secondary concomitant infection such as tuberculosis (Fig. 67.4) but rarely from ischemic necrosis.
- Emphysema that develops between PMF and the pleura is referred to as paracicatricial emphysema (adjacent to pulmonary scarring or fibrosis) (Fig. 67.5).

Lymph Nodes

- Lymph node involvement is common in silicosis and CWP.
- Mediastinal and hilar lymph nodes in approximately 50% of cases exhibit uniform calcification (Fig. 67.6).
- Calcification may manifest as a thin peripheral calcified rim, known as eggshell calcification, which occurs in less than 10% of patients and is more typical of silicosis than CWP (Fig. 67.7).

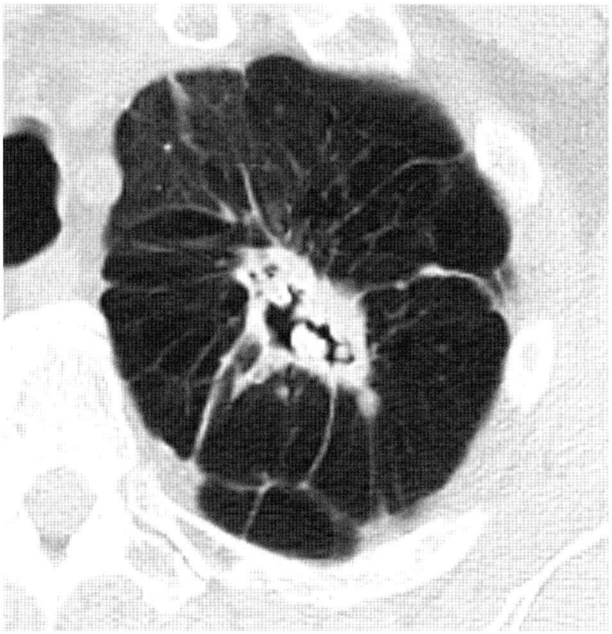

Figure 67.4. Mycobacterial infection. Unenhanced chest CT of a 56-year-old retired foundry worker shows a left upper lobe cavitary mass, consistent with complicated silicosis/silicosis with progressive massive fibrosis. *Mycobacterium kansasii* was recovered on bronchoscopy.

Acute Silicosis (Silicoproteinosis)

- Resembles pulmonary alveolar proteinosis and pulmonary edema on radiography.
- Rapid (weeks to months) development of diffuse bilateral ground-glass opacities.

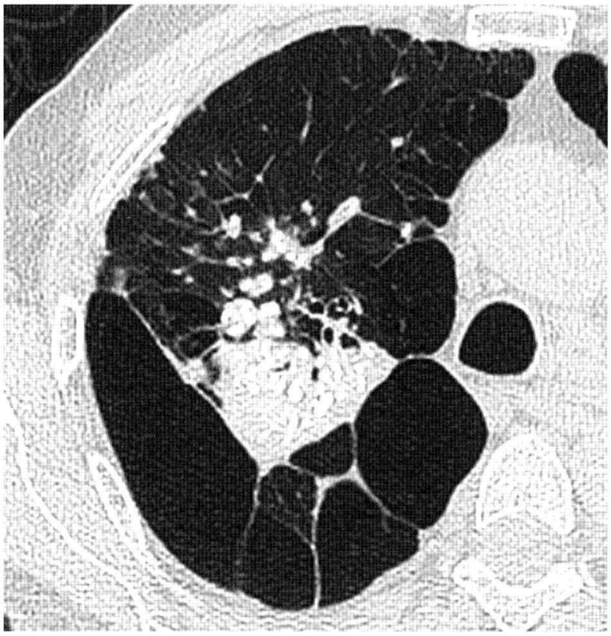

Figure 67.5. Paracicatricial emphysema. Unenhanced chest CT of a 63-year-old iron foundry worker with a long (>30 year) smoking history shows a right upper lobe mass consistent with PMF and large airspaces between the mass and pleura representing paracicatricial emphysema secondary to surrounding fibrosis.

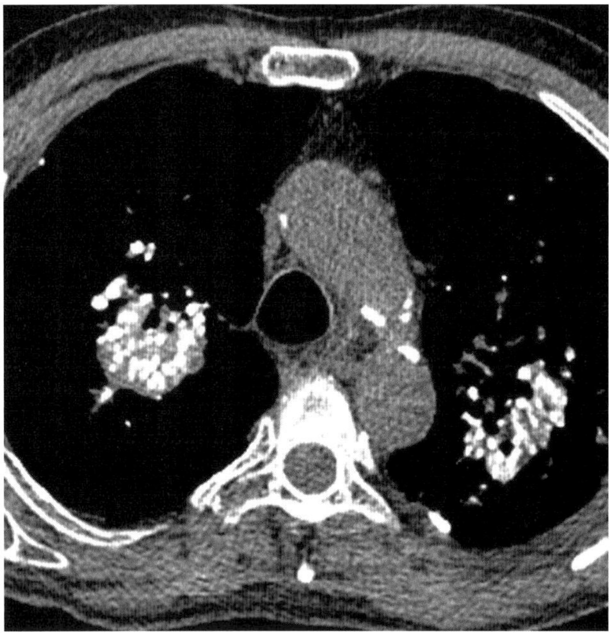

Figure 67.6. PMF. Unenhanced chest CT of a 63-year-old retired foundry worker shows conglomerate bilateral upper lobe masses with intrinsic nodular calcifications consistent with progressive massive fibrosis.

- *Accelerated silicosis* is indistinguishable from classic silicosis except for the time frame, with imaging findings developing more than 5 years earlier than for classic silicosis.

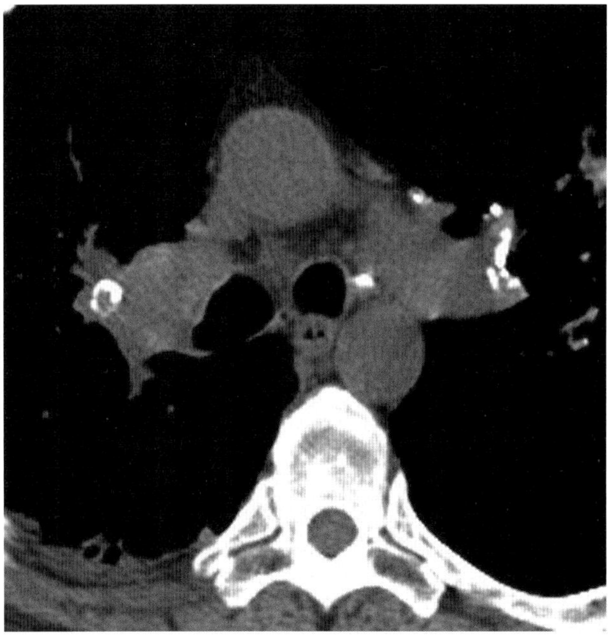

Figure 67.7. Eggshell calcification. Unenhanced chest CT of a 56-year-old man with complicated silicosis shows eggshell calcification in a right hilar lymph node and diffuse calcification of left hilar lymph nodes.

Clinical Issues

- Acute silicosis or silicoproteinosis is typically fatal within 2 years.
- Because silicosis and CWP often cannot be reliably distinguished on imaging, eliciting a history of occupational exposure is important in determining the diagnosis.

Key Points

- Silicosis and CWP are occupational lung diseases secondary to chronic exposure to inhaled silica and coal dust.
- Radiography is relatively insensitive and nonspecific in early diagnosis of simple silicosis and simple CWP, and chest CT should be obtained if there is high clinical suspicion for a pneumoconiosis.
- Simple silicosis and CWP manifest with small, upper lobe predominant, occasionally calcified nodules in a perilymphatic distribution.
- PMF (complicated silicosis and complicated CWP) is characterized by conglomerate upper lobe nodules or masses greater than 1 cm with associated upper lobe volume loss, upward retraction of the hila, and paracicatricial emphysema.
- Mediastinal and hilar lymphadenopathy is common (~50%) in patients with silicosis and CWP. Eggshell calcifications are classic in silicosis but occur in less than 10% of affected patients.
- Cavitation can occur in conglomerate masses in the setting of progressive massive fibrosis secondary to ischemic necrosis. However, tuberculosis can coexist and needs to be excluded.
- Lung cancer rarely is confused with silicosis or CWP. However, lung cancer can coexist. Occasionally, PET/CT or biopsy is needed to distinguish PMF from a mass.

Suggested Reading

Chong S, Lee KS, Chung MJ, Han J, Kwon OJ, Kim TS. Pneumoconiosis: Comparison of imaging and pathologic findings. *RadioGraphics*. 2006;26:59–77.

Kim KI, Kim CW, Lee MK, Lee KS, Park CK, Choi SJ, et al. Imaging of occupational lung disease. *RadioGraphics*. 2011;21:1371–1391.

Shah SH, Nagymanyoki Z, Ramaiya NH, Howard S. AIRP best cases in radiologic–pathologic correlation. *RadioGraphics*. 2012;32:2047–2052.

Section XIII

Iatrogenic Conditions

CHAPTER 68

Introduction to Iatrogenic Conditions

Sanjeev Bhalla

Introduction

Post-therapy imaging interpretation can be challenging. In most practices, the main thoracic interventions include drug therapy, surgery, and radiation therapy. In certain practices, especially in the absence of stereotactic radiation, radiofrequency ablation (RFA) and cryoablation may be seen and may produce perplexing pulmonary abnormalities.

Conditions Associated with Treatment

Post-therapeutic changes in the lung may be classified into two main categories: local and diffuse. Local changes are usually seen with radiation and percutaneous therapies, usually represent localized injury, and may exhibit a variety of imaging abnormalities based on the type of therapy. Traditional radiotherapy may manifest with linear consolidation that follows the radiation port instead of anatomic structures. When more focused radiation is used as with stereotactic therapy, the result may be focal consolidation and fibrosis. Percutaneous treatments may result in a variety of appearances, including a variation of the halo (nodule with surrounding ground-glass opacity) or reverse halo (ground-glass opacity within the nodule) signs.

Abnormalities found in the immediate postoperative period include focal edema or atelectasis, pleural effusion, and pneumothorax. Complications include bronchopleural fistula, empyema, pneumonia, hemothorax, chylothorax, retained foreign body, and, rarely, lobar torsion. Occasionally, local vascular complications occur, including venous thrombosis and arterial injury, and may be associated with unusual patterns of edema or infarction.

Postsurgical diffuse alveolar damage has been well reported. For unknown reasons, patients post lobectomy or pneumonectomy may present with a noncardiogenic edema pattern that results in profound hypoxia. Rarely, post-pneumonectomy patients will present with contralateral stenosis of the main bronchus from the torqueing effect of the mediastinal shift (post-pneumonectomy syndrome).

Distant changes may also follow radiation and drug therapy and usually manifest with organizing pneumonia (OP). OP may be seen in the radiation port but also in other parts of the lung. Studies suggest that radiation may sensitize the recipient to OP anywhere in the lung. Drug therapy may produce diffuse abnormalities that typically manifest as OP, diffuse alveolar hemorrhage or damage, or nonspecific interstitial pneumonia (NSIP) (Fig. 68.1).

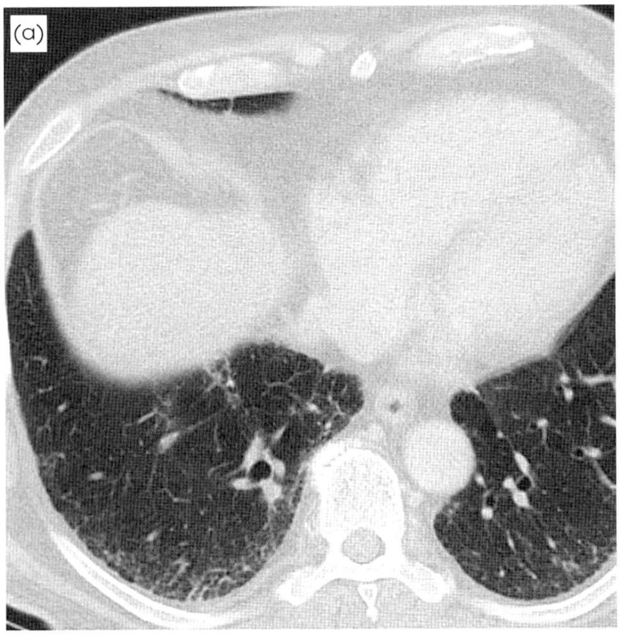

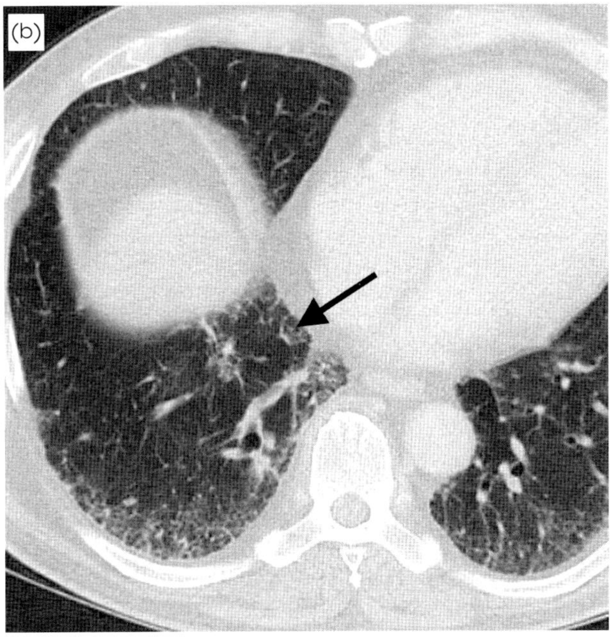

Figure 68.1. NSIP. Unenhanced chest CT of a 43-year-old man with esophageal carcinoma on chemotherapy and worsening dyspnea shows basilar subpleural ground-glass opacity and reticulation (a) that progresses in the medial basal segment of the right lower lobe (b; arrow), suggestive of NSIP.

Of course, recurrence of malignancy remains one of the major concerns.

Approach to the Post-therapy Patient

Two key questions must be answered when dealing with the treated patient: What was the prior therapy? and When was the treatment? Both questions help determine the significance of the imaging abnormalities. For example, consolidation in a radiation port a few months after completion of therapy is almost certainly radiation pneumonitis, but distant consolidation or new consolidation a few years after the therapy is more likely to represent infectious pneumonia.

In many practices, radiography and CT are the standard for assessing the postsurgical patient (Fig. 68.2). In the immediate post-therapy period, the radiologist must understand the nature of the surgery and expected appearance because small effusions, volume loss, and pneumothoraces are fairly common. Knowing that a lobectomy

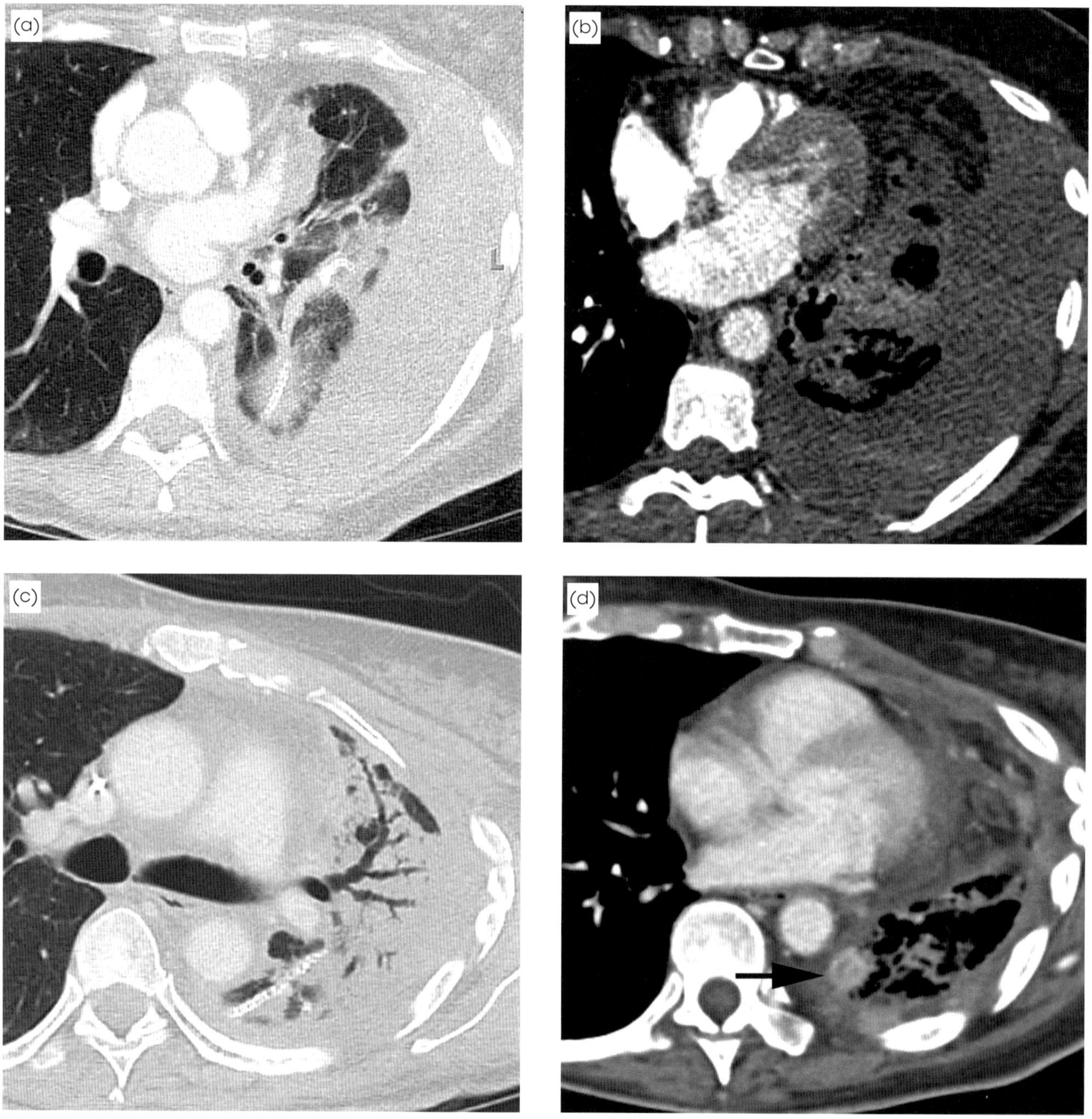

Figure 68.2. Evolution of post-treatment abnormalities. (a, b) Contrast-enhanced chest CT of a 72-year-old woman 2 weeks post left lower lobe wedge resection for lung cancer shows the surgical staple line (black arrow) and high-attenuation pleural effusion (b) consistent with hemothorax. (c, d) Contrast-enhanced chest CT of the same patient obtained 1 year later shows a left upper lobe consolidation consistent with radiation fibrosis (c) and an enhancing nodule (d; arrow) outside of the radiation field. Biopsy confirmed recurrent carcinoma.

was performed, for example, might explain greater volume loss than would be seen with a wedge resection. Further out from therapy, comparison to prior imaging is of paramount importance. If possible, comparison to more than just the most recent study should be undertaken because subtle changes, such as a slowly growing recurrence, may be difficult to appreciate over a short interval. Currently, there is no national guideline for the imaging follow-up of post-cancer resection patients, so time between follow-up examinations will vary based on practice.

Patients on targeted therapies (stereotactic radiation, percutaneous RFA, or cryoablation) and chemotherapy are typically followed with cross-sectional imaging (CT). Imaging aims to identify tumor recurrence (local or distant), and diagnosis rests on comparison with prior imaging to assess for change. Occasionally, patients present for imaging because of symptoms. In these cases, the findings may not be subtle. Accurate diagnosis relies on knowledge of prior therapies. For example, peripheral ground-glass opacities might be indicative of OP in a patient treated with chemotherapy, but OP would be unusual post RFA.

Differential Diagnosis

The differential diagnosis is based on understanding whether the imaging abnormalities are expected post-treatment changes or not. In the case of unexpected abnormalities, one must decide whether or not the finding is related to therapy.

In the hospital setting, the surgical patient is exposed to all of the risks of being an inpatient, including pneumonia (sometimes aspiration-related) and pulmonary infarcts from pulmonary emboli. When unexpected imaging findings are encountered, these must be considered in addition to treatment complications.

In the outpatient setting, pneumonia and pulmonary emboli remain important diagnostic considerations. In fact, in an outpatient cancer setting, pulmonary thromboemboli may be seen in up to 5% of patients being imaged for restaging. Finally, in the outpatient setting, recurrent or metachronous neoplasm should be considered when a new abnormality is seen.

Suggested Reading

Choi YW, Munden RF, Erasmus JJ, et al. Effects of radiation therapy on the lung: Radiologic appearances and differential diagnosis. *RadioGraphics*. 2004;24:985–997.

Krishnam M, Suh R, Tomasian A, et al. Postoperative complications of lung transplantation: Radiologic findings along a time continuum. *RadioGraphics*. 2007;27:957–974.

Rossi SE, Erasmus JJ, McAdams HP, Sporn TA, Goodman PC. Pulmonary drug toxicity: Radiologic and pathologic manifestations. *RadioGraphics*. 2000 Sep;20(5):1245–1259.

CHAPTER 69

Radiation Pneumonitis and Fibrosis

Travis S. Henry and Brent P. Little

Definition

Radiation pneumonitis and radiation fibrosis encompass a spectrum of side effects of therapeutic radiation on normal lung tissue. Radiation pneumonitis is an acute/subacute response to injury that is generally reversible and occurs within the first 6 months after completion of therapy. Radiation fibrosis represents chronic remodeling of lung tissue that may evolve 6–24 months after radiation. Doses of at least 20 Gy and usually greater than 40 Gy are required to cause these side effects. Lung cancer is the most common indication for thoracic therapeutic radiation and is the main focus of this chapter. However, radiation therapy for other malignancies including Hodgkin lymphoma and also breast, esophageal, and head/neck cancers may also injure the lungs and have characteristic injury patterns.

Clinical Features

Who Receives Radiation Therapy for Lung Cancer?

Radiation therapy is a viable treatment option in many different patient populations. Radiation is potentially curative in medically inoperable (e.g., severe lung or cardiac disease precluding surgery) stage I and stage II lung cancers. In locally advanced cases, radiation may be potentially curative or used as an adjunct therapy if there is nodal involvement or unresectable locally invasive tumor (stage IIIA). In patients with metastatic disease, radiation may be used as palliation to relieve pain and improve quality of life.

Radiation Pneumonitis

Acute radiation pneumonitis occurs 1–6 months after completion of radiation therapy. Affected patients may present with dyspnea, cough, low-grade fever, and/or chest discomfort. Approximately 13–37% of patients who undergo three-dimensional conformal radiation therapy (3D-CRT) for lung cancer develop symptoms (only 4% with stereotactic body radiation therapy (SBRT)). Symptoms usually resolve spontaneously, but corticosteroid treatment results in prompt symptomatic relief in approximately half of patients.

Radiation Fibrosis

Radiation fibrosis begins 6–12 months after completion of radiation, and imaging findings may evolve for up to 24 months after therapy. Radiation fibrosis produces symptoms less frequently than pneumonitis and may occur with or without antecedent pneumonitis. The most common symptoms include dyspnea and persistent dry cough.

Risk Factors

Risk factors for development of radiation pneumonitis and fibrosis include lung performance status, the presence of preexisting lung disease, and administration of concomitant chemotherapy (especially actinomycin D, adriamycin, bleomycin, or busulfan). Treatment-related factors include total radiation dose, dose fractionation (smaller doses with a protracted schedule reduce biologic effects), total irradiated volume, and beam arrangement. Tumor location near the mediastinum or major nerves may also increase morbidity/mortality.

Anatomy and Physiology

Radiation causes diffuse alveolar damage and, similar to other etiologies, the lung injury evolves through three phases: the acute exudative phase, the organizing/proliferative phase, and the chronic fibrotic phase. The first two phases correlate with the time frame of radiation pneumonitis and manifest as cellular infiltration in the lung (predominantly macrophages). The third stage represents radiation fibrosis and, histologically, demonstrates collagen deposition and fibrotic changes.

Radiation Techniques

Conventional radiation therapy for lung cancer uses parallel beams with opposite orientation (i.e., anteroposterior and posteroanterior without or with obliquity) and delivers daily doses of 2 Gy over several weeks, with a total treatment dose of approximately 60 Gy. The large amount of normal tissue exposed to the radiation field limits the total dose that can be delivered to the tumor and is a major limitation of this technique. Oblique beams are used to boost the dose and reduce dose to critical structures such as the spinal cord.

3D-CRT has largely replaced conventional therapy for delivering more radiation to the tumor volume with less effect on surrounding tissues. 3D-CRT uses the images from a CT scan to create a 3D tumor volume, and a computer generates multiple oblique radiation fields that pass through the tumor from different angles. Each field dose can be less than 2 Gy per day (limiting the effects on normal tissue), but the cumulative dose to the tumor is much higher (≥70 Gy),resulting in a greater therapeutic dose to the tumor but less toxicity to normal tissue.

SBRT is a conformal technique used to accurately treat small (T1 or T2) tumors. A stereotactic body frame is used to localize a tumor and concentrate high doses of radiation into a small tumor volume.

Any radiation therapy technique may result in radiation pneumonitis or fibrosis, although the distribution of lung involvement will vary based on the number and orientation of radiation ports. Reference times for development of radiation pneumonitis and radiation fibrosis are calculated beginning at the completion of radiation therapy.

How to Approach the Image

Is There a History of Radiation?

Knowledge of the type of radiation and treatment timeline is essential. Radiation pneumonitis occurs within the first 6 months. Radiation fibrosis can evolve for up to 2 years after completion of radiation therapy.

What Is the Distribution of Parenchymal Abnormalities?

- Anteroposterior or oblique, spanning from one pleural surface to another and crossing fissures: Conventional radiation therapy for lung cancer (3D-CRT may exhibit a similar but less extensive distribution) (Fig. 69.1)
- Focal, not spanning the entire lung parenchyma: 3D-CRT or SBRT for lung cancer treatment
- Bilateral paramediastinal: Mantle radiation for lymphoma (Fig. 69.2)
- Unilateral paramediastinal: Radiation for lung cancer lymph node metastases or esophageal cancer
- Biapical: Head and neck cancer radiation
- Unilateral apical: Axillary radiation for lymph node metastases (most commonly breast)
- Unilateral anterolateral tangential: Breast cancer radiation

If you see an unusual/confusing pattern on a radiograph or CT, ask, “Could this be from radiation?” A history of radiation may not be available, but it should always be considered when a pattern of abnormality does not conform to anatomic boundaries.

What Not to Miss

Clearly, a follow-up study in a patient with lung cancer should not overlook a recurrent tumor or second neoplasm. A careful approach can avoid this potential trap.

Is There Recurrence?

Recurrence generally will occur along the margin of a radiation field. Findings that suggest recurrence include the following:

- New mass growing along/within radiation field
- New convex margin of radiation field

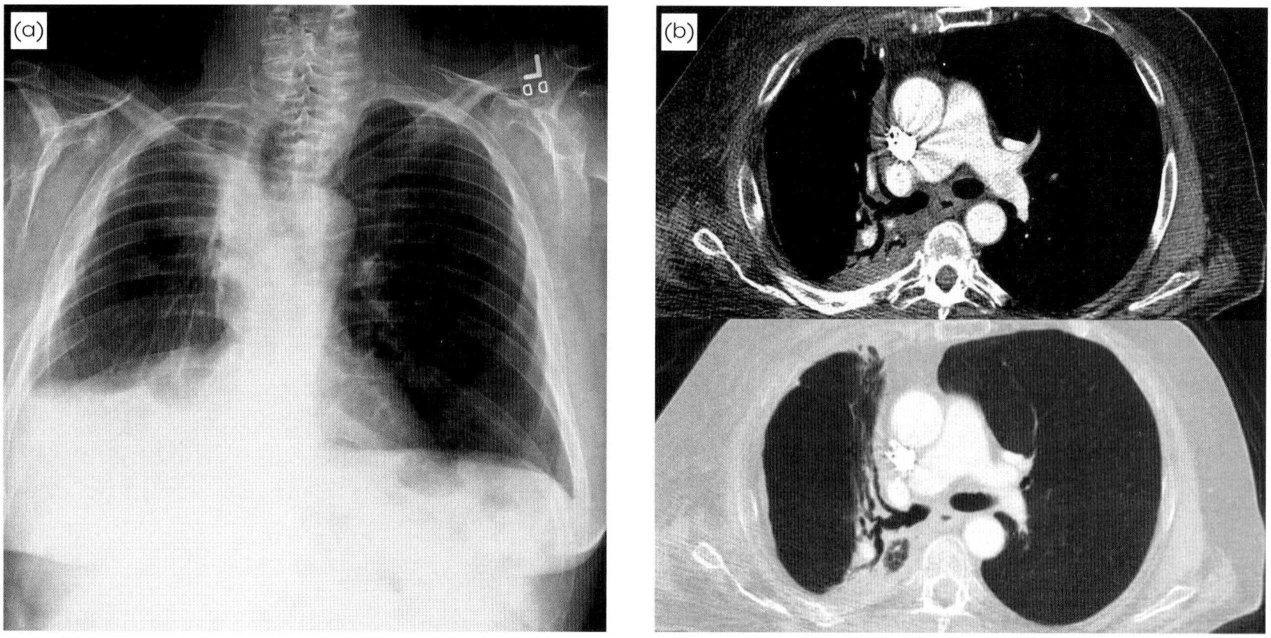

Figure 69.1. Radiation fibrosis. (a) Posteroanterior chest radiograph of a 69-year-old man 3.5 years status post completion of conventional radiation therapy for right upper lobe lung cancer and hilar lymph node metastasis with anteroposterior/posteroanterior and oblique radiation and a total dose of 63 Gy shows severe right upper lobe volume loss, rightward mediastinal shift, and right hemidiaphragm elevation. (b) Composite image with contrast-enhanced chest CT with soft tissue (top) and minimum intensity projection lung window (bottom) geographic right paramediastinal cicatricial atelectasis with traction bronchiectasis that does not exert mass effect on the pulmonary vasculature.

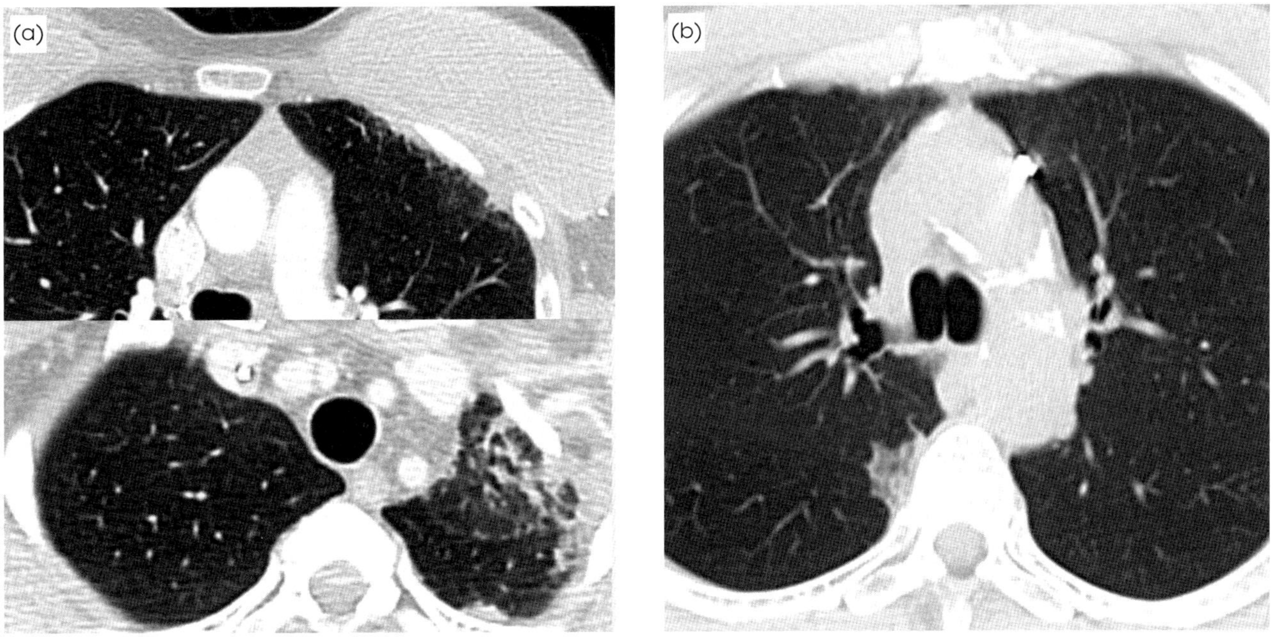

Figure 69.2. Various patterns of radiation fibrosis. (a) Composite image of CT images in two different patients. The top image of a 36-year-old woman shows tangential radiation fibrosis along the anterolateral left lung. Note ancillary findings of breast cancer treatment including mastectomy/implant. The bottom image demonstrates left apical radiation fibrosis and volume loss in a 42-year-old woman treated for metastatic left axillary lymph nodes in breast cancer. (b) CT showing subtle bilateral paramediastinal fibrosis with volume loss and traction bronchiectasis in a 53-year-old man who underwent mantle radiation for Hodgkin lymphoma approximately 20 years prior. The most notable finding is the advanced atherosclerotic disease that was localized to the radiation port (including the coronary arteries and thoracic aorta).

- New mass effect on/filling in of traction bronchiectasis
- New pleural effusion (after long-term stability without effusion)

Are There Complications/Sequelae of Radiation?

The entire radiation field (everything in the path including soft tissues and bones) should be inspected for complications:

- Bones: Radiation osteonecrosis
- Pleura/pericardium: Effusion, pleuritis, pericarditis
- Vessels: Accelerated atherosclerotic disease may develop within radiation field. Radiation at a young age may be complicated by earlier than expected complications, including myocardial infarction. Valvular dysfunction if valve is included in the field (e.g., aortic valve).
- Lymph nodes: Calcified lymph nodes may represent treated disease (especially lymphoma).
- Esophagus: Esophageal strictures

Is There a Second Primary Malignancy Within the Radiation Field?

A new mass occurring several years after radiation may represent a second primary malignancy rather than recurrence—typically new lung cancer, sarcomas (e.g., osteosarcoma, chondrosarcoma, and undifferentiated soft tissue sarcomas), breast cancer, and lymphoma.

Differential Diagnosis

Infection

Infection may mimic radiation pneumonitis both clinically and on imaging. Findings that favor infection include the following:

- Ground-glass opacity (GGO) or consolidation that develops before completion of radiation therapy
- Tree-in-bud opacities (as with tuberculosis) or cavitation
- Bilateral/diffuse abnormalities distant from the radiation field
- Rapid development of new abnormality (steroid withdrawal may precipitate rapid development of radiation pneumonitis)

Recurrent Tumor

Recurrent tumor usually occurs within 2 years of completing radiation therapy (Fig. 69.3). Modern 3D-CRT and SBRT therapies have lower recurrence rates because of higher radiation doses delivered to the tumor. Findings suggesting recurrence include the following:

- New soft tissue nodule/mass within radiation field
- Filling in of air bronchograms with soft tissue
- Alteration in contour of the fibrosis (e.g., a new convex border and new mass effect on structures)

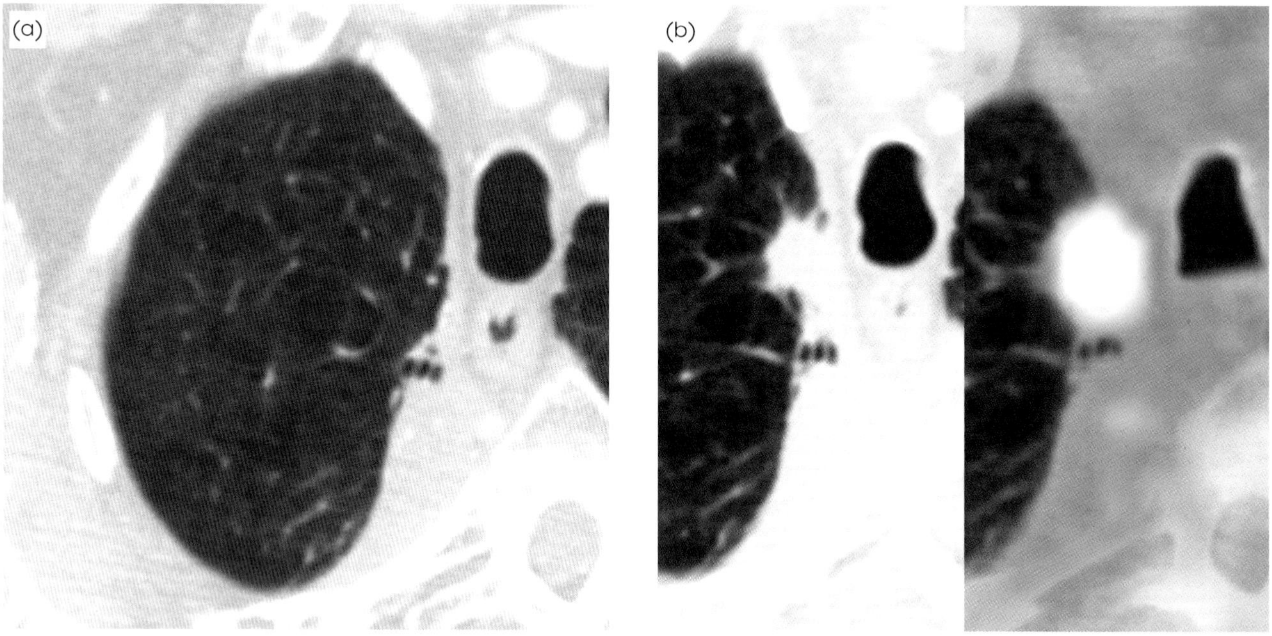

Figure 69.3. Recurrent tumor. (a) CT in a 64-year-old man undergoing routine surveillance CT shows typical findings of radiation fibrosis, including geographic consolidation with sharp margins, volume loss, and traction bronchiectasis. (b) Composite image from a surveillance CT 12 months later demonstrates a new spiculated nodule along the superolateral margin of the radiation field (left). PET/CT (right) demonstrates increased metabolic activity, and subsequent biopsy confirmed recurrent squamous cell carcinoma.

- New nodules along radiation field margin or outside radiation field
- New lymphadenopathy
- New pleural effusion long after completion of therapy

Lymphangitic Carcinomatosis

Lymphangitic carcinomatosis (LC) usually occurs with severe and rapidly progressing dyspnea rather than radiation fibrosis. Imaging findings supporting LC include the following:

- Septal thickening (smooth or nodular)
- Peribronchovascular thickening
- New lymphadenopathy
- New pleural effusion

Radiation-Induced Tumor

Radiation may induce a second malignancy with a median time of approximately 10 years later.

Imaging Findings

Radiation pneumonitis and fibrosis are typically confined to the radiation field. Whereas conventional radiation therapy causes changes spanning from one pleural surface to another (e.g., anterior to posterior), 3D-CRT and SBRT may cause unusual patterns of pneumonitis/fibrosis based on the number and orientation of radiation ports.

- Radiation pneumonitis: Transient; 1–6 months after completion of therapy; may progress to radiation fibrosis
  - GGO and/or consolidation
  - Non-anatomic abnormalities (i.e., cross fissures and span segments/lobes)
  - GGO and consolidation outside of radiation field in 20% of cases
  - Pleural/pericardial effusion from pleuritis/pericarditis
- Radiation fibrosis—Permanent; 6 months after completion of therapy; may continue to evolve for up to 2 years
  - Geographic consolidation with traction bronchiectasis
  - Architectural distortion (e.g., displacement of fissures and loss of normal anatomic landmarks)
  - Volume loss

Distribution of Fibrosis in 3D-CRT and SBRT

- Modified conventional: Linear distribution of fibrosis similar to conventional therapy, but fibrosis may not extend throughout the entire lung
- Mass-like: Fibrosis confined to a 2-cm margin around the tumor
- Scar-like: Linear fibrosis 1 cm or less in thickness (seen most often with SBRT) (Fig. 69.4)

Clinical Issues

What if There Is Uncertainty About Recurrence?

- Follow-up CT can be helpful in detecting recurrent tumor.

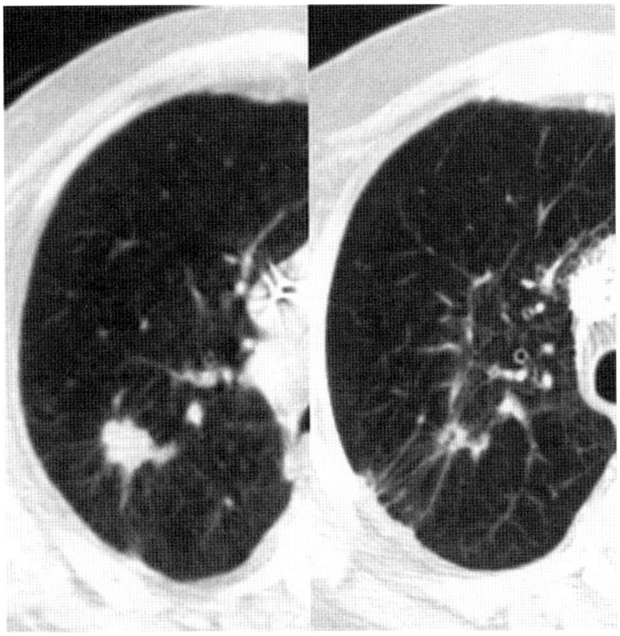

Figure 69.4. SBRT. Composite image with contrast-enhanced chest CT at diagnosis (left) and 1 year after completion of SBRT (right) in a 71-year-old man with right upper lobe lung cancer shows a spiculated right upper lobe nodule (left) that resolves after completion of therapy, with residual linear fibrosis affecting a small region of the right upper lobe.

- PET/CT should not be performed within the first 3 months after completion of radiation therapy because of the potential for false positives from uptake in early radiation pneumonitis.
- Although radiation pneumonitis/fibrosis may be metabolically active, the maximum standardized uptake value of tumor is generally higher.

Key Points

- Radiation changes (especially fibrosis) are common on imaging and usually clinically asymptomatic.
- Different diseases are treated with varying radiation fields. Recognizing the distributions of fibrosis can suggest underlying diagnosis (mantle radiation for Hodgkin lymphoma, anterolateral tangential for breast cancer, etc.).
- Knowing how to distinguish recurrence from the normal evolution of radiation pneumonitis/fibrosis on follow-up scans is one of the radiologist's most important roles. Prior imaging and radiation therapy completion date are the two most useful tools a radiologist can employ to make a confident diagnosis.

Suggested Reading

Choi YW, Munden RF, Erasmus JJ, et al. Effects of radiation therapy on the lung: Radiologic appearances and differential diagnosis. *RadioGraphics*. 2004;24:985–997.

Larici AR, del Ciello A, Maggi F, et al. Lung abnormalities at multimodality imaging after radiation therapy for non-small cell lung cancer. *RadioGraphics*. 2011;31:771–789.

Park HJ, Kim KJ, Park SH, Kay CS, Oh JS. Early CT findings of tomotherapy-induced radiation pneumonitis after treatment of lung malignancy. *AJR Am J Roentgenol*. 2009;193: W209–W213.

CHAPTER 70

Drug-Induced Lung Disease

Travis S. Henry and Brent P. Little

Definition

Hundreds of drugs (therapeutic and illicit) may produce lung disease with significant respiratory-associated morbidity and mortality. Although clinical and radiographic presentation is often nonspecific, certain patterns of injury are most commonly encountered, and some drugs may cause more than one pattern of lung disease. Definitive diagnosis of drug-induced lung disease (DILD) depends on the following:

- Temporal relationship between drug exposure and onset of respiratory symptoms
- Radiologic findings compatible with DILD
- Histologic evidence (if biopsy is performed) of lung injury
- Exclusion of other causes of lung damage, such as infection, radiation pneumonitis/fibrosis, or progression of primary disease

Clinical Features

The clinical presentation of patients with DILD is variable and nonspecific. Presenting symptoms include cough, fever, dyspnea, hypoxemia, and/or pleuritic chest pain. Pulmonary function tests usually show decreased diffusion capacity of carbon monoxide and a restrictive pattern. These features overlap with a myriad of more common entities, including infection, heart failure, collagen vascular disease, malignancy, and pulmonary embolism. DILD typically begins after institution of a new drug, and cessation of the offending agent is the first step of treatment. In early cases, the symptoms may be reversible. In severe cases, treatment with corticosteroids may be necessary. Amiodarone or nitrofurantoin may cause insidious lung disease that worsens over years.

Biopsy is not routinely performed, and the diagnosis relies on clinical presentation and imaging findings. Prompt recognition of DILD is crucial because cessation of the offending agent may result in complete resolution of injury, or at least arrest of progression.

Anatomy and Physiology

DILD can cause one of many pathologic reactions in the lung. Histopathologic findings from drug reactions are indistinguishable from other causes of these entities. The most common patterns include the following:

- Diffuse alveolar damage and acute respiratory distress syndrome (ARDS)
- Organizing pneumonia OP
- Eosinophilic pneumonia
- Hypersensitivity reaction
- Interstitial pneumonitis/fibrosis
- Alveolar hemorrhage
- Pulmonary vasculitis/pulmonary hypertension
- Bronchiolitis obliterans (sometimes referred to as constrictive bronchiolitis)
- Sarcoid-like reaction

How to Approach the Image

DILD should be considered when any of the previously mentioned patterns of lung injury is encountered. Thin-section and high-resolution CT are more sensitive than radiography for the detection of DILD and can more fully characterize the abnormalities to narrow the differential diagnosis. Two key questions must be answered in cases of suspected DILD:

- Are the findings acute, subacute, or chronic? In the acute/subacute setting, knowledge of recently started drugs will be most important. If findings are subacute/chronic, the patient may have started treatment long before presentation due to slow deterioration.
- Can the radiologic pattern be classified? Because drug reactions produce nonspecific patterns of lung injury, often with overlapping appearance, one must try to characterize the findings to the extent possible.

In cases of suspected DILD, the radiologist must promptly communicate with the referring clinician to determine any recent changes to the patient's medication list. Because drugs may cause more than one pattern of injury, and because new therapeutics (especially monoclonal antibodies) are continually being approved, one cannot expect to recall all DILDs. The website http://www.pneumotox.com is an extremely helpful resource because it includes a continually updated DILD database.

What Not to Miss

As with any parenchymal process, the key is not to become so focused on the medication that one forgets to consider common entities such as infectious pneumonia, cardiogenic pulmonary edema, and lung cancer. Symptoms and clinical history can be very helpful. Acute onset or fever in a patient with no recent change in medications is unlikely to be medication related.

Differential Diagnosis

- In the acute setting, the differential diagnosis includes infection, pulmonary edema or hemorrhage from another cause, and progression of underlying systemic disease (e.g., malignancy and collagen vascular disease).
- Chronic DILD usually manifests as a fibrosing lung disease, and the differential diagnosis includes idiopathic interstitial pneumonia, collagen vascular disease, other exposures (chronic hypersensitivity pneumonitis), and radiation pneumonitis/fibrosis.

Imaging Findings

Diffuse Alveolar Damage/ARDS

Diffuse alveolar damage (DAD)/ARDS is one of the most common patterns of DILD (Fig. 70.1). CT findings are indistinguishable from other causes of DAD and include the following:

- Exudative stage (first week after injury): Bilateral consolidation, typically in the mid and lower lung zones; septal thickening is generally absent.
- Organizing stage (occurs 1 or 2 weeks after injury): Findings of exudative stage may stabilize, improve, or progress; fibrosis begins with architectural distortion and traction bronchiectasis; may progress to end-stage fibrosis with reticulation and honeycombing.

Organizing Pneumonia

OP is a common pattern of DILD (Fig. 70.2). With the exception of amiodarone (discussed later), CT findings are indistinguishable from other causes of OP:

- Patchy or nodular consolidation or ground-glass opacity in a bronchiolocentric or subpleural distribution
- Usually mid and lower lung zone predominant
- Reverse halo or atoll sign may be present

Nonspecific Interstitial Pneumonia

Imaging findings may overlap/coexist with OP or DAD (Fig. 70.3) and include the following:

- Ground-glass opacities with varying amounts of reticulation and traction bronchiectasis/bronchiolectasis
- Honeycombing should be absent
- May have a subpleural or bronchocentric distribution
- Usually mid and lower lung zone predominant

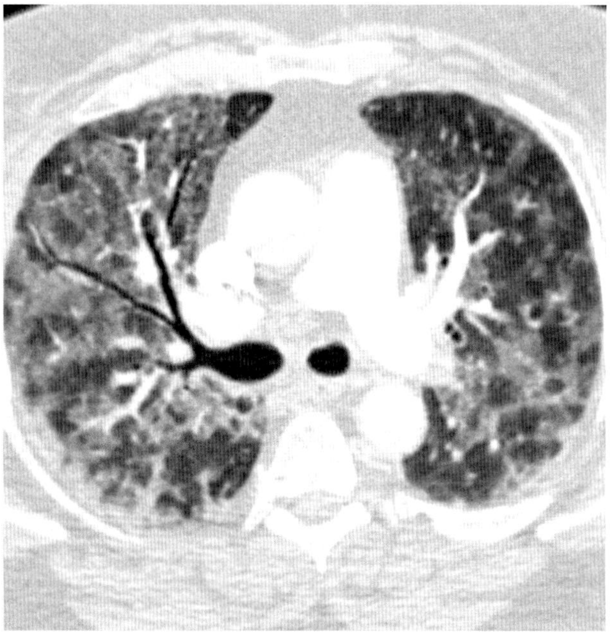

Figure 70.1. DAD. Contrast-enhanced chest CT of a 71-year-old man undergoing treatment for Hodgkin lymphoma with bleomycin toxicity and diffuse alveolar damage shows patchy ground-glass opacities and consolidations in the absence of pleural effusion. Bronchial dilatation suggests the organizing stage of DAD.

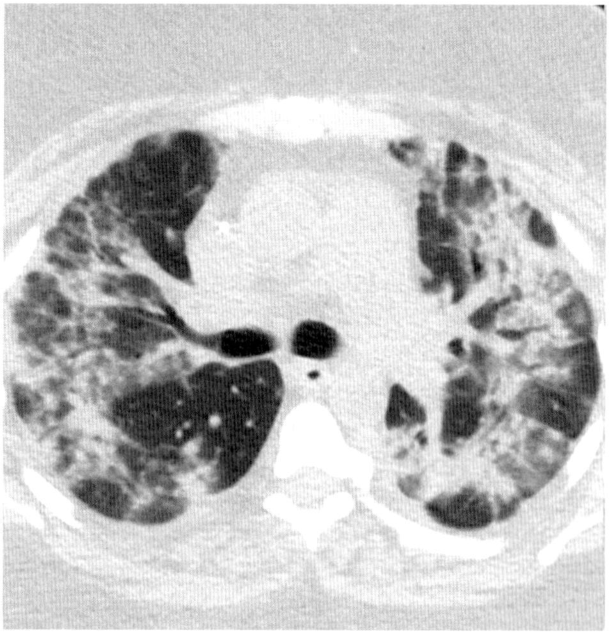

Figure 70.2. Organizing pneumonia. Unenhanced chest CT of a 56-year-old woman on a monoclonal antibody clinical trial shows symmetric consolidation that is mostly bronchiolocentric and peripheral. These opacities improved with drug cessation and steroids.

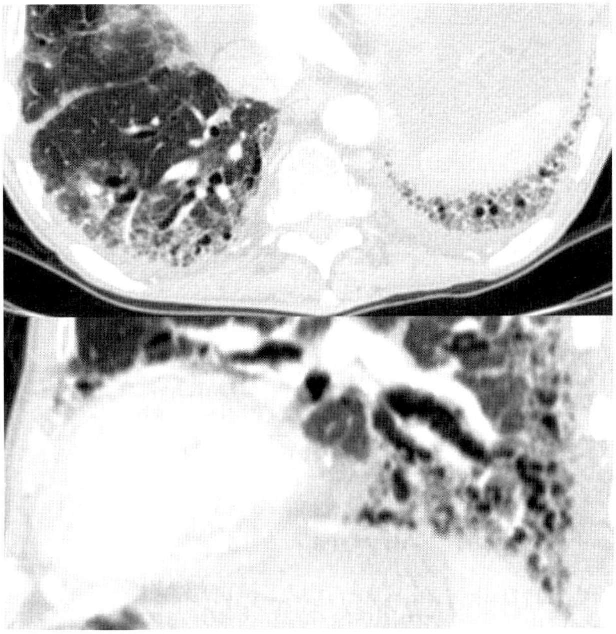

Figure 70.3. Nonspecific interstitial pneumonia. Composite of an unenhanced chest CT in a 64-year-old man undergoing treatment for pancreatic cancer that shows basilar predominant traction bronchiectasis/bronchiolectasis on axial images (top) and ground-glass opacities, which developed during a 6-month period. The vertical distribution may be better appreciated on the sagittal image (bottom).

Usual Interstitial Pneumonia

The usual interstitial pneumonia (UIP) pattern is a rare manifestation of DILD (Fig. 70.4). CT findings are similar to other causes of UIP and include the following:

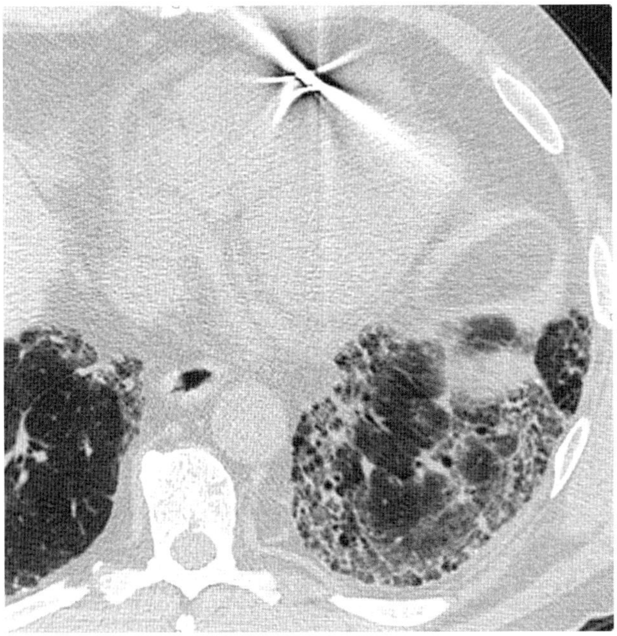

Figure 70.4. UIP. Unenhanced chest CT of a 73-year-old man with a 15-year history of amiodarone treatment shows basilar subpleural reticulation and mild honeycombing, in keeping with a UIP pattern.

- Basilar and peripheral predominant honeycombing, reticulation, and traction bronchiectasis/bronchiolectasis
- Ground-glass opacity should be minimal

Hypersensitivity Pneumonitis/Eosinophilic Pneumonia

DILD is a common cause of an eosinophilic pneumonia pattern but a relatively uncommon cause of hypersensitivity pneumonitis. Imaging findings overlap those of other causes for each respective entity (Fig. 70.5) and include ground glass or consolidation with a peripheral predilection.

Alveolar Hemorrhage

Alveolar hemorrhage may be acute or chronic (Fig. 70.6). The appearance is nonspecific and overlaps with other causes of pulmonary hemorrhage on CT. Pleural effusions are generally absent.

Sarcoid-like Reaction

Recognition of this pattern is especially important in the setting of malignancy because this may be mistaken for metastatic disease. Imaging findings are typical of sarcoid and include perilymphatic micronodules, usually with an upper lung predominance (Fig. 70.7), and mediastinal lymphadenopathy that resolves after cessation of the offending agent or steroid therapy.

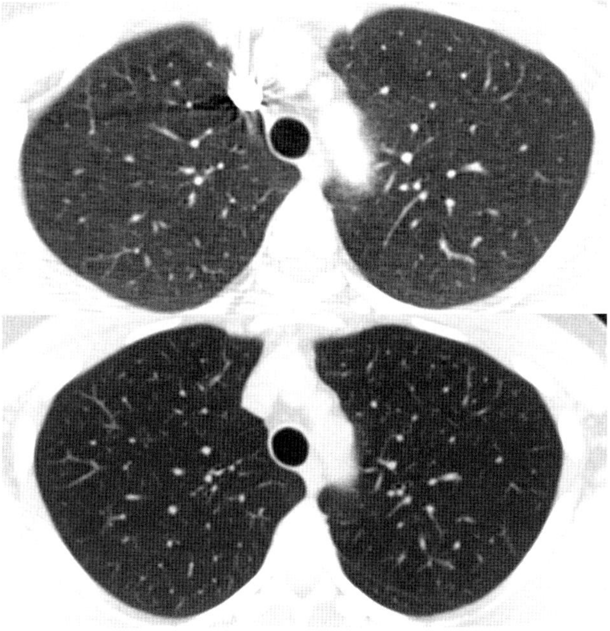

Figure 70.5. Hypersensitivity pneumonitis. Composite image with unenhanced chest CT of a 42-year-old woman on 6-mercaptopurine therapy shows diffuse ill-defined centrilobular ground-glass opacities that developed 8 weeks after initiation of therapy (top) and that resolved 3 months after cessation of treatment (bottom).

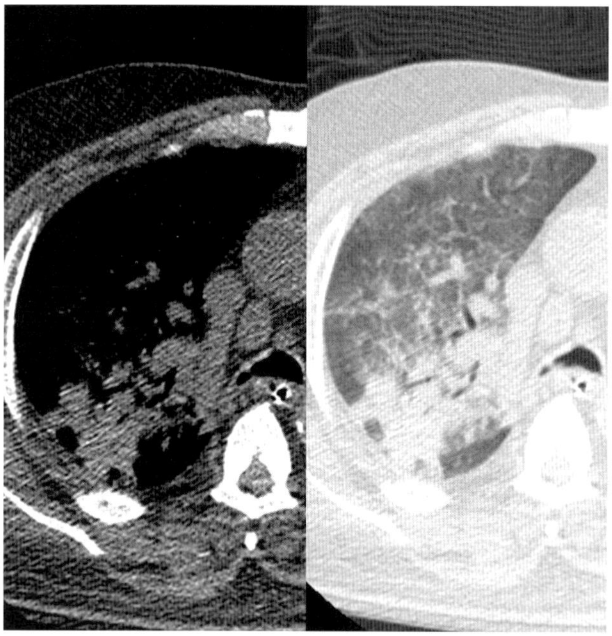

Figure 70.6. Pulmonary hemorrhage. Unenhanced chest CT of a 64-year-old man on nitrofurantoin therapy shows multifocal consolidation and ground-glass opacities in the absence of pleural effusions. Pulmonary hemorrhage was confirmed on biopsy.

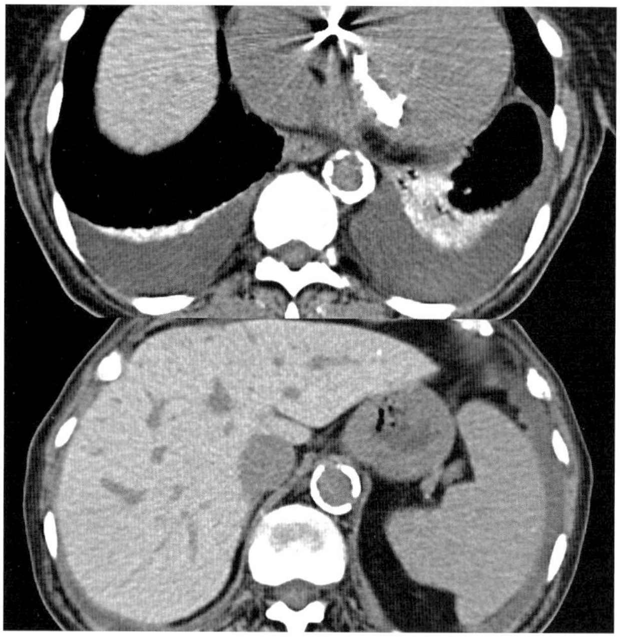

Figure 70.8. Amiodarone toxicity. Composite image with unenhanced chest CT of a 73-year-old woman on chronic amiodarone therapy shows high-attenuation consolidation (top) and high attenuation of the liver (bottom), which are typical of amiodarone. The defibrillator is another clue to the diagnosis.

Amiodarone

Amiodarone has unique CT findings because it contains iodine, which results in high-attenuation consolidation and higher than expected attenuation of the liver or spleen (Fig. 70.8). Ancillary clues include cardiomegaly or the presence of a pacemaker/defibrillator (signs of cardiac dysfunction that would necessitate amiodarone administration).

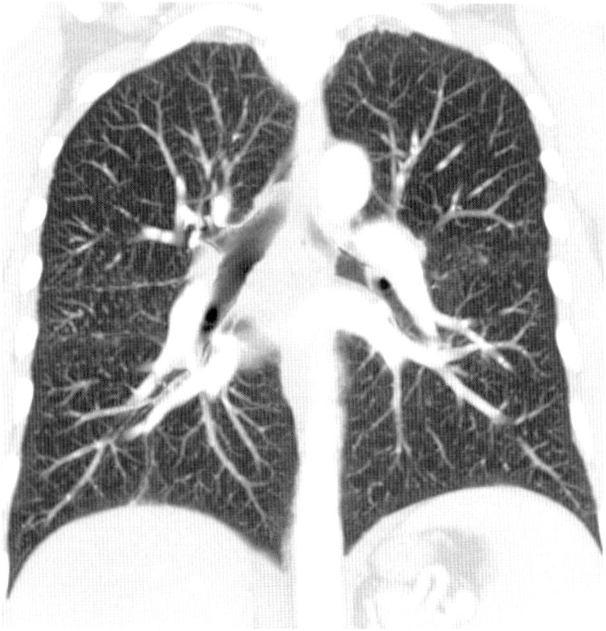

Figure 70.7. Sarcoid-like reaction. Coronal maximum intensity projection contrast-enhanced chest CT of a 42-year-old man treated with interferon for melanoma shows numerous perilymphatic micronodules that prompted open lung biopsy due to suspicion of metastases.

Clinical Issues

- Early recognition of a DILD with prompt cessation of the offending agent is important because the radiologic/pathologic abnormalities may completely resolve, or at least stabilize.
- Because imaging features of DILD are nonspecific, it is largely a diagnosis of exclusion. A temporal relationship between initiation of therapy and onset of symptoms is crucial, but the diagnosis is usually not confirmed until after the drug is stopped and the symptoms improve.
- Drugs that commonly cause a DAD pattern include cytotoxic agents (busulfan, cyclophosphamide, carmustine, and bleomycin), methotrexate, aspirin, narcotics, and amiodarone.
- The most common causes of medication-induced OP include amiodarone, bleomycin, interferon, cyclophosphamide, methotrexate, and nitrofurantoin.
- A nonspecific interstitial pneumonia pattern is commonly caused by cytotoxic agents, amiodarone, methotrexate, nitrofurantoin, and hydrochlorothiazide.
- A UIP pattern is commonly associated with long-term nitrofurantoin use.
- Peripheral eosinophilia or increased eosinophils on bronchial lavage are typical findings of drug-induced eosinophilic pneumonia/hypersensitivity.

- Alveolar hemorrhage is usually from anticoagulants, amphotericin B, cyclophosphamide, cytosine arabinoside, penicillamine, and crack cocaine. Hemoptysis is usually absent.
- Sarcoid-like reaction is an unusual drug reaction that has been described in two distinct clinical scenarios:
  - Interferon therapy—used for treatment of malignant and nonmalignant disease, including melanoma and hepatitis C
  - Tumor necrosis factor-α antagonists—used for treatment of inflammatory arthropathies

Key Points

- Drug reactions can manifest with either acute or subacute/chronic symptoms, and the radiologic and pathologic findings are usually indistinguishable from other causes of the specific pattern of DILD.
- Almost all drugs can cause some pulmonary toxicity, and new drugs, especially novel chemotherapeutic agents, are constantly being introduced. The website http://www.pneumotox.com is a helpful reference that is constantly updated with new drugs and patterns of injury they cause.
- Drug reaction should always be considered in the differential diagnosis of unexplained pulmonary abnormalities.

Suggested Reading

Isabela C, Silva S, Müller NL. Drug-induced lung diseases: Most common reaction patterns and corresponding high-resolution CT manifestations. *Semin Ultrasound CT MRI.* 2006 Apr;27(2): 111–116.

Matsuno O. Drug-induced interstitial lung disease: Mechanisms and best diagnostic approaches. *Respir Res.* 2012 May 31;13(1):1–1.

Ravenel JG, McAdams HP, Plankeel JF, Butnor KJ, Sporn TA. Sarcoidosis induced by interferon therapy. *AJR Am J Roentgenol.* 2001 Jul;177(1):199–201.

Rossi SE, Erasmus JJ, McAdams HP, Sporn TA, Goodman PC. Pulmonary drug toxicity: Radiologic and pathologic manifestations. *RadioGraphics.* 2000 Sep;20(5):1245–59.

CHAPTER 71

Postoperative Complications

Brent P. Little and Travis S. Henry

Definition

Patients may be imaged after a procedure to establish a new baseline or because of a suspected complication, usually based on symptoms. Most post-procedural complications are classified as acute (during hospitalization), intermediate, and long term (there is not a strict distinction between the latter two).

Clinical Features

Lung Resection

The most common complications of lung resection are pneumonia (in up to 20% of patients), empyema, and hemorrhage.

Lung Transplantation

Double lung transplantation has a higher long-term survival rate than single lung transplantation. The 1-year survival rate after transplantation is approximately 80%, and the 5-year survival rate approaches 50%. The most common cause of death within 6 months of transplant is infection leading to sepsis, and the most common cause of mortality at 5 years is chronic rejection (bronchiolitis obliterans).

Common Adult Cardiac and Open Vascular Surgeries

Intrathoracic complications of invasive vascular surgeries include infections such as sternitis, mediastinitis, graft infection, or empyema. Pseudoaneurysms or hemorrhage from dehiscence at an anastomotic site can also occur.

Anatomy and Physiology

Lung Resection

Pneumonectomy and lobectomy are usually performed with an incision in the fifth intercostal space. An intrapleural pneumonectomy involves removal of the lung and visceral pleura, with ligation of the bronchus, pulmonary artery, and veins at the hilum. Extrapleural pneumonectomy consists of removal of visceral and parietal pleurae, pericardium, and diaphragm, and it is usually performed to treat early stage mesothelioma.

Surgery can often be performed via video-assisted thorascopic surgery with a scope and instruments inserted through small incisions in the chest wall. Wedge resection is typically reserved for lesions in the outer one-third of the lung. Segmentectomy can be used for some nodules/masses deeper within the lung. In a sleeve lobectomy, a lobe is resected with an airway segment and an anastomosis is created between the distal and proximal bronchi by telescoping the narrower portion of the bronchus into the wider one.

Lung Transplantation

Double lung transplantation is most frequently performed. Single lung transplantation is performed through a posterolateral thoracotomy, whereas double lung transplantation is usually performed with a transverse or clamshell thoracosternotomy. Donor and recipient hilar structures are dissected, and bronchial, pulmonary arterial, and pulmonary venous anastomoses are created.

Common Adult Cardiac and Open Vascular Surgeries

Common invasive adult cardiovascular surgeries include coronary artery bypass graft surgery (CABG), thoracic aneurysm repair, and cardiac valve repair or replacement. Traditionally, CABG, valve replacement, and ascending aorta/arch repair are performed through a vertical median sternotomy, whereas descending aortic surgeries are performed through a left thoracotomy. However, an increasing number of minimally invasive surgeries are performed through smaller (3 or 4 cm) sternal and/or intercostal incisions.

Open thoracic aortic repair is performed with a synthetic graft made of Dacron or other related material. The target portion of the native aorta is excised, and the graft is interposed. Sutures at proximal and distal anastomotic sites are reinforced by felt. Complex ascending/hemi-arch repairs employ multiple anastomoses to the arch vessels.

Many invasive thoracic cardiovascular surgeries are performed under cardiopulmonary bypass, with arterial cannulation sites in the ascending aorta and venous cannulation sites in the vena cavae or right atrium; felt pledgets are typically sewn to these sites to reinforce closure upon removal of the cannulae.

How to Approach the Image

Imaging should be approached with the following considerations:

- What was the type of surgery and surgical technique?
  - Know the types of surgeries performed at your institution.
  - Review the surgeon's preoperative assessment and operative notes.
  - Assess all surgical anastomoses.
- When did the surgery occur?
  - Some complications occur in the immediate postoperative period, others within the first week, and others weeks to months later. This is especially important in imaging assessment of lung transplantation.
- Is this an expected postsurgical appearance or a complication?
  - Gain familiarity with the expected postsurgical appearance of chest surgeries to distinguish normal postoperative findings from complications.

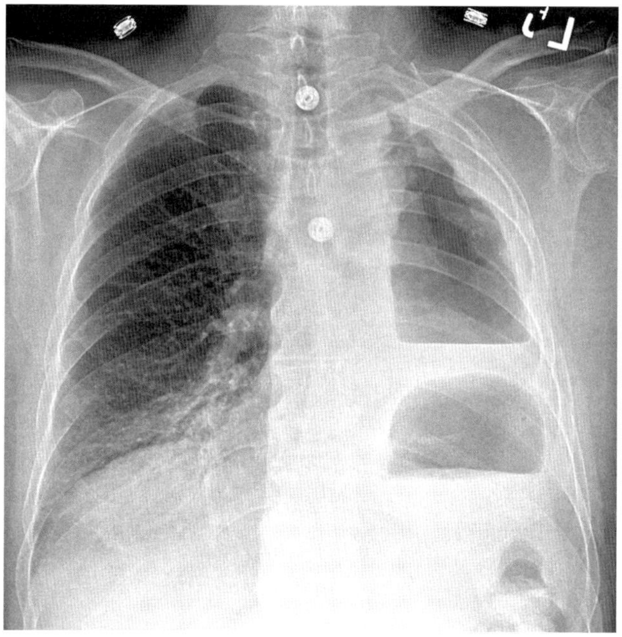

Figure 71.1. Empyema and bronchopleural fistula. Posteroanterior (PA) chest radiograph of a 60-year-old man status post left pneumonectomy for non-small cell lung cancer shows a large amount of air in the pneumonectomy space months after surgery consistent with bronchopleural fistula from a dehiscent left mainstem bronchus stump. Cultures grew *Klebsiella* and *Aspergillus fumigatus*.

What Not to Miss

Although the imaging study should focus on detecting any complications of the specific surgery, common general postoperative complications should not be overlooked. These include the following:

- Pneumothorax, hemothorax, and mediastinal hemorrhage in the immediate postoperative period
- Central line and tube malposition
- Pneumonia, empyema, sternal wound infection, and mediastinitis
- Pulmonary emboli due to immobility
- Retained needles, surgical sponges, line fragments, and other materials that may result in an inflammatory reaction with formation of a mass-like phlegmonous reaction (gossypiboma)

Differential Diagnosis

Lung Resection

- Hemothorax or chylothorax
- Noncardiogenic pulmonary edema (usually 2 or 3 days after surgery)
- Bronchopleural fistula
  - Rare immediately post surgery; most occur weeks to months after surgery due to infection, anastomosis dehiscence, or, less commonly, tumor recurrence (Fig. 71.1).
- Postoperative infection
  - Empyema (Fig. 71.2)
  - Pneumonia in up to 20% of post-thoracotomy patients, usually due to aspiration
- Post-pneumonectomy syndrome
  - Mediastinal shift to side of pneumonectomy with resultant bronchial stretching and compression between mediastinal structures; more common after right pneumonectomy (Fig. 71.3)

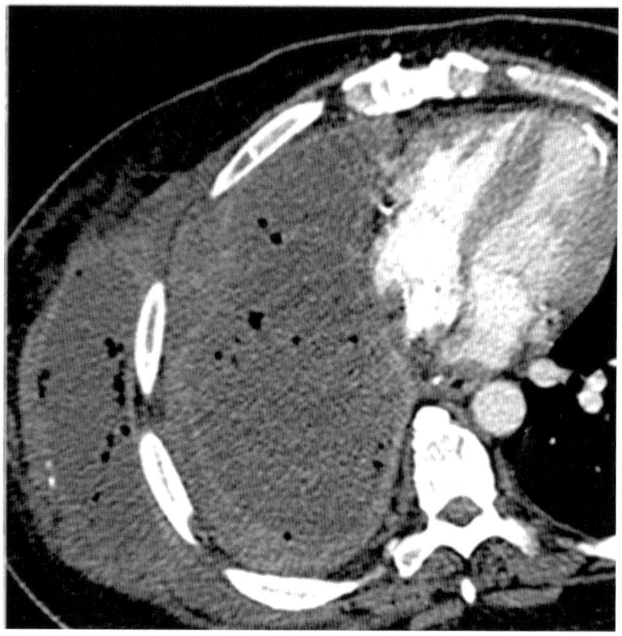

Figure 71.2. Empyema and empyema necessitatis. Contrast-enhanced CT in a 55-year-old man status post right pneumonectomy shows enhancement of parietal pleura and gas bubbles in the pneumonectomy space, with extension of fluid and gas into the adjacent chest wall consistent with empyema.

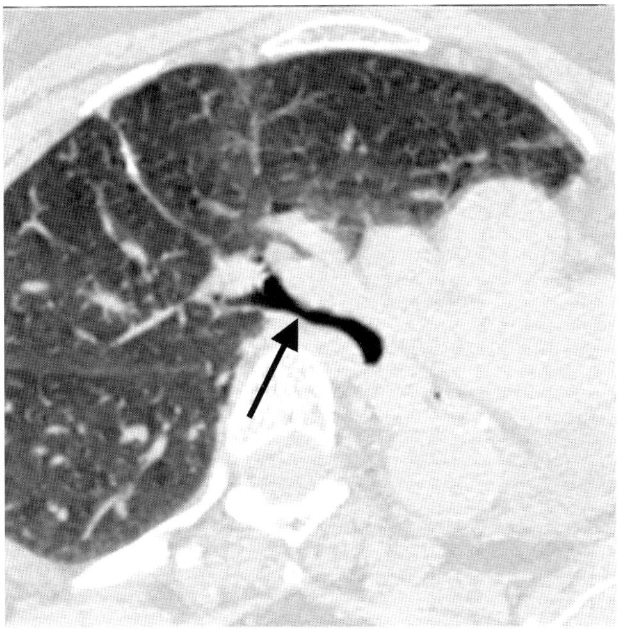

Figure 71.3. Post-pneumonectomy syndrome. Unenhanced chest CT of a 56-year-old woman with 3 months of increasing dyspnea and chest pain 12 years after left pneumonectomy for severe tuberculosis shows complete mediastinal shift into the left pneumonectomy space with stretching and compression of the right tracheobronchial tree (arrow).

- Lung torsion
  - Rare
  - Affected lobe twists on its vascular pedicle, resulting in ischemia, congestion, and ultimately necrosis.

Lung Transplantation

- Early complications (within first week)
  - Hyperacute rejection
  - Reimplantation edema
  - Empyema
- Intermediate complications (after first week to 2 months)
  - Infections (Fig. 71.4): Bacterial infections are most common (up to 75% of patients), usually in the first month. Fungal, tuberculous, pneumocystis, and other infections are less common.
  - Acute rejection: Affects 30–60% of patients but is usually self-limited (Fig. 71.5).
  - Bronchial dehiscence: Caused by ischemia or infection at/near anastomosis, usually within 1 month of transplantation (1–32%).
- Late complications (≥2 months)
  - Infections: Cytomegalovirus common (peak 1–4 months after lung transplantation). Other viruses, such as influenza, respiratory syncytial virus, and adenovirus, are more common more than 9 months after surgery.
  - Bronchial stenosis
  - Bronchomalacia

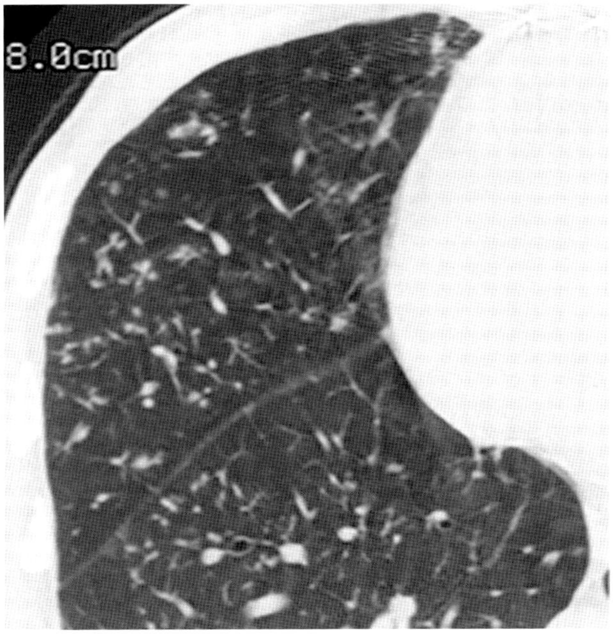

Figure 71.4. Post-transplantation infection. Unenhanced chest CT of a patient with respiratory syncytial virus pneumonia following lung transplantation shows right middle and lower lobe centrilobular micronodules and tree-in-bud opacities.

  - Chronic rejection (bronchiolitis obliterans): Most common long-term complication (>50% of patients at 5 years) (Fig. 71.6)
  - Post-transplant lymphoproliferative disorder (PTLD)

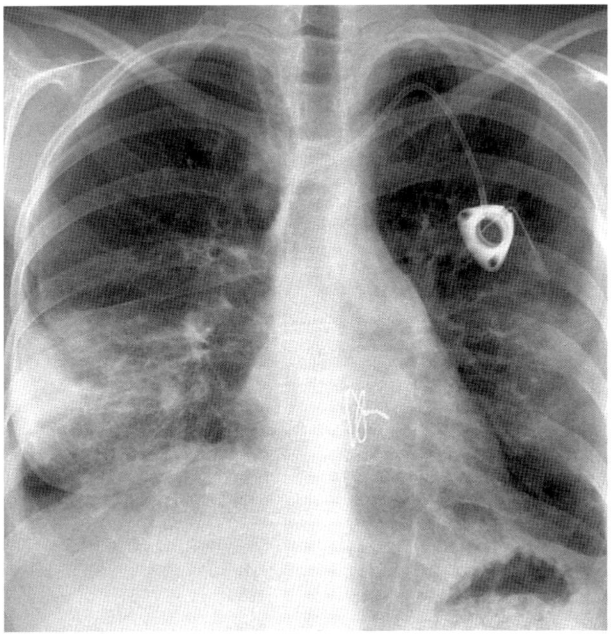

Figure 71.5. Acute rejection. Portable radiograph in a 33-year-old woman 1 month after bilateral lung transplant has an appearance similar to asymmetric pulmonary edema with a small effusion and increased interstitial markings. Biopsy confirmed acute rejection.

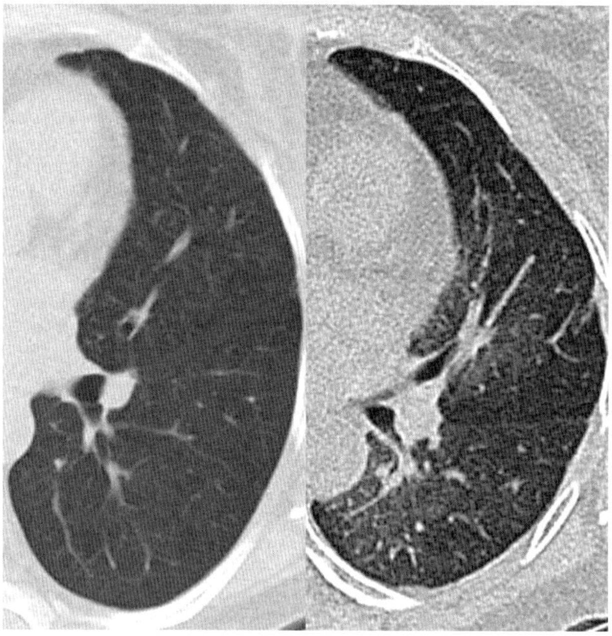

Figure 71.6. Chronic rejection. Composite CT in a 56-year-old woman 4 years after bilateral lung transplant. Inspiration (left) image is nearly normal with very subtle mosaic attenuation. Exhalation (right) shows areas of air trapping. Pulmonary function testing confirmed worsening obstruction.

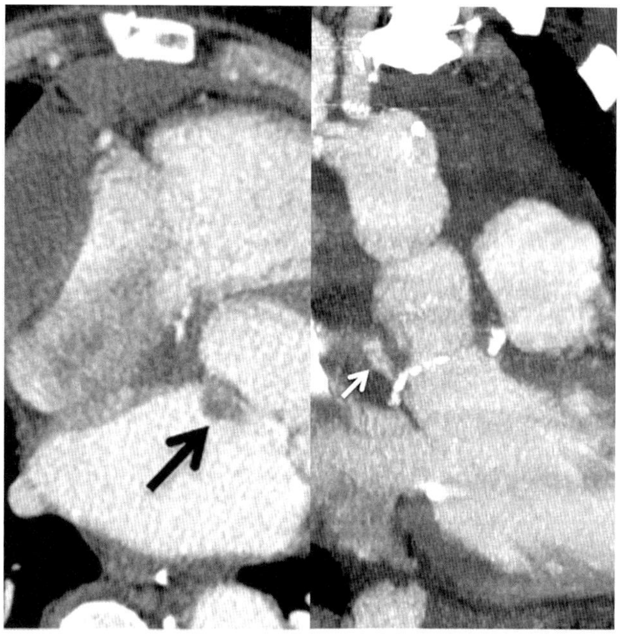

Figure 71.7. Aortic root dehiscence from endocarditis. Contrast-enhanced chest CT of a 49-year-old woman after aortic valve replacement and aortic root, ascending aortic, and arch repair shows hemopericardium and vegetation along anterior mitral leaflet (black arrow) and contrast extravasation (white arrow) from the aortic root at the site of high-attenuation suture line and felt.

Cardiac and Vascular Surgery

- Injury to other organs: Stroke, renal damage, and spinal infarcts leading to paralysis from embolization of vessel thrombi or atherosclerotic plaque
- Arterial injury
- Suture line dehiscence/pseudoaneurysms: Hemorrhage and pseudoaneurysms are uncommon but typically arise from a suture/anastomotic site (Fig. 71.7).
- Cardiopulmonary bypass cannulation complications: Pseudoaneurysms and infections can occur at the ascending aortic arterial cannulation sites used for cardiopulmonary bypass (Fig. 71.8).
- Graft infection: Can occur in the perioperative period or months after open aortic surgical graft repair
- Sternitis/mediastinitis: Usually in the intermediate postoperative period, days to weeks after surgery
- Coronary artery graft occlusion

Imaging Findings

Mediastinum

- Normal postsurgical appearance
  - Enlarged cardiomediastinal silhouette on radiography from supine imaging, postoperative edema, small volume hemopericardium, or mediastinal hematoma
  - Mild stranding, pneumomediastinum, and fluid normal in the early postoperative period
- Mediastinal hematoma
  - Pronounced mediastinal widening on the first postoperative radiograph
  - Rapid increase in mediastinal width on successive postoperative radiographs

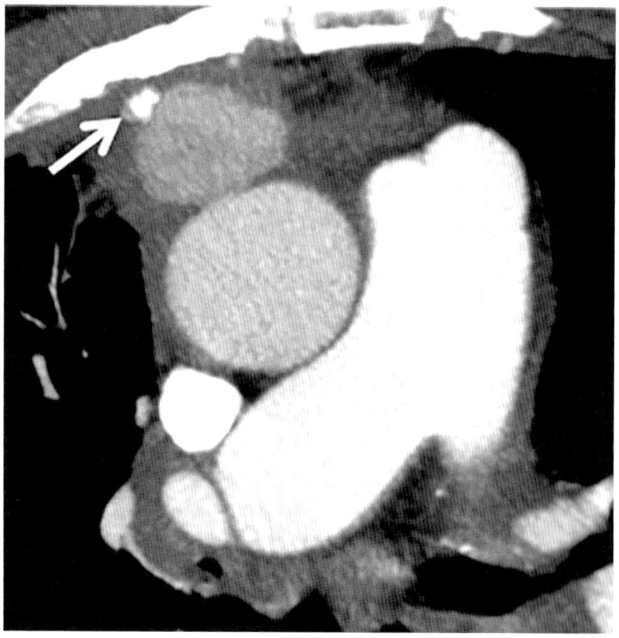

Figure 71.8. Pseudoaneurysm. Contrast-enhanced chest CT of a 63-year-old man after bilateral lung transplantation shows a pseudoaneurysm manifesting as a round contrast collection at the ascending aortic arterial cannulation site posterior to the felt pledget used to reinforce the arteriotomy site.

- CT: high-attenuation fluid in the mediastinum. Search for focus of active extravasation with attention to anastomotic or cannulation sites; increased sensitivity on delayed imaging.
- Mediastinitis
  - Mediastinal widening on radiography
  - CT: Mediastinal fluid, rim enhancing fluid collections, fat stranding, and/or gas. Look for mediastinal extension of sternal wound infection.

Pleura

- Normal postsurgical appearance
  - Small pleural effusions or pneumothoraces can be expected following many thoracic surgeries.
- Pleural air collections
  - Pneumothorax from line placement or chest tube malposition
  - Persistent pneumothorax resistant to chest tube drainage suggests a bronchopleural fistula from infection or bronchial suture line dehiscence. A connection between pleura and bronchus is not always visible.
- Pleural fluid collections
  - Rapidly increasing pleural fluid on radiography suggests hemothorax or chylothorax.
  - CT: High-attenuation layering or loculated pleural fluid or organized clot in hemothorax. Chylothorax may manifest as a water attenuation collection.
  - Pleural enhancement and thickening surrounding pleural fluid suggests empyema in the setting of infection (the "split pleura" sign). Loculation can be seen.
- Filling of pneumonectomy space
  - Fluid should gradually fill the pneumonectomy space, occupying approximately half the space in 4 or 5 days, and should continue to increase over several weeks; thereafter, the volume of the affected hemithorax should decrease, and the mediastinum should shift toward the pneumonectomy space. The entire space usually fills 2 or 3 months after surgery.
  - Increasing air within the pneumonectomy space or new air in previously fluid-filled pneumonectomy space suggest a bronchopleural fistula.

Lungs

- Normal postsurgical appearance
  - Immediately post surgery, basilar atelectasis and small pleural effusions are common.
  - After cardiac surgery, interstitial edema is often due to aggressive hydration.
- Focal increased pulmonary opacity
  - Overlapping appearances of pneumonia, aspiration, atelectasis, and asymmetric or focal edema.
  - Volume loss with mediastinal and fissural shift with uniform increase in opacity suggest atelectasis, often from mucous plugging.
  - Patchy or confluent opacities without volume loss suggest pneumonia.
  - Aspiration may be focal or diffuse and suggested by lower zone distribution.
  - Asymmetric edema may cause rapidly changing airspace opacities (usually with a parahilar predominance) and interstitial thickening.
  - Focal edema due to venous congestion and/or venous infarct can be seen in cases of pulmonary vein stenosis or lobar torsion.
  - PTLD may manifest as multiple nodules, enlarged lymph nodes, septal thickening, and/or airspace opacities.
- Diffuse increased pulmonary opacity
  - Diffuse pneumonia, pulmonary edema, and alveolar damage can present as diffuse airspace opacities and/or interstitial thickening.
  - Post-transplant reperfusion edema: Bilateral opacities within the first day after surgery and improving during the next 5–7 days.
  - Hyperacute rejection can mimic noncardiogenic pulmonary edema.
    - Reimplantation edema (ischemic reperfusion injury, primary graft dysfunction): Pulmonary edema pattern develops 24 hours after transplant and resolves spontaneously in 5–7 days.
    - Acute rejection may mimic edema, but it more frequently occurs after the first postsurgical week.
- Other
  - The most sensitive finding for chronic rejection on CT is mosaic attenuation with air trapping on expiratory series. Tree-in-bud nodules can also be seen.

Airways

- Normal postsurgical appearance
  - Traditional lobectomies and pneumonectomies result in a bronchial stump, recognized at CT as a short segment of bronchus just proximal to the resected lung; sutures or clips mark the site.
  - Sleeve lobectomies and some lung transplantations employ end-to-end anastomoses, with a smooth contour of the resulting airway.
  - A telescoping anastomosis results in a small shelf of tissue manifesting with overlap of the bronchial edges; a small amount of air within this overlap is normal and does not signify dehiscence.
  - Small pneumomediastinum or pneumopericardium may be normal.
- Airway irregularity and peribronchial air collections
  - Increasing pneumomediastinum on radiography or small focal air collections adjacent to bronchial anastomoses on CT should suggest primary bronchial injury or anastomotic dehiscence. Knowledge of normal postsurgical bronchial appearance is important in order to avoid diagnostic confusion.

- Bronchomalacia post-transplant may be detected on expiratory exam, which can show significant (>50–70%) airway collapse.

Vessels

- Normal postsurgical appearance: Vascular anastamotic sites are usually visible due to radiopaque sutures or ligation clips or to felt reinforcement. Noncontrast exams may be useful to differentiate felt pledgets from anastamotic leaks.
- Perigraft fluid collections: A small volume of perigraft fluid is normal in the immediate postoperative period. Outside of the perioperative period, a new or enlarging fluid collection adjacent to a graft is concerning for infection. Peripheral enhancement of the collection or foci of gas can be seen.
- Contrast/blood collections: Extravasation of contrast is always abnormal, and it can be seen as either a linear jet of high attenuation extending from a surgical site or as a focal collection adjacent to a surgical site. Extravasated contrast and/or blood can collect in the mediastinum, pleura, or along vessels.
- Vessel occlusions or dissections: Coronary grafts should enhance in the aortic phase of contrast administration; the absence of contrast in these vessels indicates occlusion. Dissections and focal intimal injuries are uncommon; when they occur, the lead point is usually either a cannulation site or a suture line.

Bones and Soft Tissues

- Normal postsurgical appearance
  - A sharply marginated rib defect can be seen after thoracotomy.
  - Median sternotomy wires should align vertically on radiography, regardless of patient rotation.
  - At CT, corresponding sternal fragments should closely approximate each other, although complete sternal healing can take several months to occur. A transverse (clamshell) thoracosternotomy has a single set of adjacent wires within the lower sternum.
  - A small amount of stranding or fluid within the peristernal fat is a normal finding up to several weeks after surgery.
- Sternal wire displacement or sternal fluid collections
  - Deviation of one or more sternal wires compared to the other wires of a median sternotomy suggests sternal dehiscence.
  - CT confirmation of sternal fragment separation, focal fluid collections, and mediastinal fluid or stranding (seen in mediastinitis).
  - Dehiscence of a clamshell sternotomy is often best appreciated on lateral radiography and manifests with displacement of the inferior and superior fragments in relation to one another.

Clinical Issues

- Chylothorax may result from a thoracic duct injury and is usually confirmed on thoracentesis with pleural fluid triglyceride levels greater than 110 mg/dl.
- Noncardiogenic edema is rare after lung resection but is potentially lethal.
- Acute rejection is common post transplant but is rarely lethal.
- Post-transplant bronchial dehiscence is usually partial rather than total.
- Hyperacute rejection is very rare from preformed antibodies against allograft antigens and is often detected in the operating suite.
- Chronic rejection presents with progressive dyspnea and can lead to complete graft failure and death. Diagnosis is first suggested by obstructive pattern in pulmonary function tests. Transbronchial biopsy can be used for confirmation, but false-negative results are common.
- The ascending aortic cardiopulmonary bypass arteriotomy site or, less commonly, a suture line can serve as a lead point for arterial injury post cardiac surgery.
- The 10-year occlusion rate of venous bypass grafts is up to 50%; it is lower (~20%) for internal mammary grafts.
- Often unsuspected clinically in the perioperative period, sternal dehiscence is almost always due to infection and can be confirmed with CT.

Key Points

- Knowledge of specific complications of specialized chest surgeries is essential for prompt diagnosis. Familiarity with the normal expected postsurgical appearances of each surgery is important for avoiding misdiagnosis.
- Review of the surgical note is of paramount importance prior to image interpretation.
- Leaks can occur at any anastomosis (vascular or airway). A new fluid and/or gas collection outside the immediate postoperative period should prompt thorough interrogation of all surgical sites.
- Recognition of the time course of the abnormality as well as the steps and anatomic considerations of the surgical technique are essential for diagnosis of a complication.
- Aortotomy sites should not be confused with the normal appearance of felt pledgets used to reinforce the sites.
- Sternal dehiscence may be seen on imaging before it is suspected clinically. A thorough search pattern must include confirmation that sternotomy wires are aligned centrally.

Suggested Reading

Boasquevisque CHR, Yildirim E, Waddel TK, Keshavjee S. Surgical techniques: Lung transplant and lung volume reduction. *Proc Am Thorac Soc.* 2009;6:66–78.

Caruso S, Crino F, Milazzo M, et al. Thoracic complications following lung transplantation: 64-MDCT findings. *Clin Transplant.* 2011;25:673–684.

Krishnam M, Suh R, Tomasian A, et al. Postoperative complications of lung transplantation: Radiologic findings along a time continuum. *RadioGraphics.* 2007;27:957–974.

Li Ng Y, Paul N, Patsios D, Walsham A, Chung TB, Keshavjee S, et al. Imaging of lung transplantation: Review. *AJM Am J Roentgenol.* 2009;192:S1–S13.

Shepard JA. Imaging of lung transplantation. *Clin Chest Med.* 1999;20:827–844.

Soyer P, Devine N, Frachon I, Vinatier I, Stern M, Normand SL, et al. Computed tomography of complications of lung transplantation. *Eur Radiol.* 1997;7:847–853.

Section XIV

Diffuse Infiltrative Lung Disease

CHAPTER 72

Diffuse Infiltrative Lung Disease

Santiago Martínez-Jiménez

Introduction

Assessment of diffuse lung opacities (DLO) is one of the most common challenging tasks encountered by radiologists. The differential diagnosis of DLO is extensive, and as a result, radiologists must develop strategies to narrow the differential diagnosis. This section reviews some of the most important causes of DLO, with emphasis on a practical approach to the formulation of a concise and meaningful differential diagnosis.

Acute Versus Chronic

The most important discriminator when dealing with DLO is the acuity of abnormalities. The acuity of symptoms and availability of comparison studies are very helpful. For example, acute ground-glass opacities are often related to pulmonary edema, infection, or alveolar hemorrhage. On the other hand, chronic ground-glass opacities may be related to interstitial lung disease such as nonspecific interstitial pneumonia (NSIP) or desquamative interstitial pneumonia (Fig. 72.1). Unfortunately, in many cases, radiologists and clinicians are unable to determine whether an abnormality is acute or chronic. In those cases, a broader and less helpful differential diagnosis is typically provided. For example, alveolar proteinosis tends to follow an indolent and chronic course, but affected patients often have subclinical symptoms that they may fail to disclose. Thus, radiologists must make every possible effort to determine whether the abnormalities are acute or chronic. If this can be determined with certainty, the differential diagnosis should be formulated accordingly.

Airspace Versus Interstitial

An additional common challenge is to determine whether diffuse ground-glass opacities are a manifestation of airspace disease or interstitial thickening. This is difficult because the precise anatomic localization of the abnormalities may be below the resolution of CT. In these cases, determining the location and distribution of the abnormalities is helpful. For example, in NSIP, the ground-glass opacities are located mainly in the subpleural portions of the lower lobes. Identification of ancillary findings such as traction bronchiectasis and subpleural reticulation is very helpful because these are not typically seen in pulmonary edema, alveolar hemorrhage, or infection.

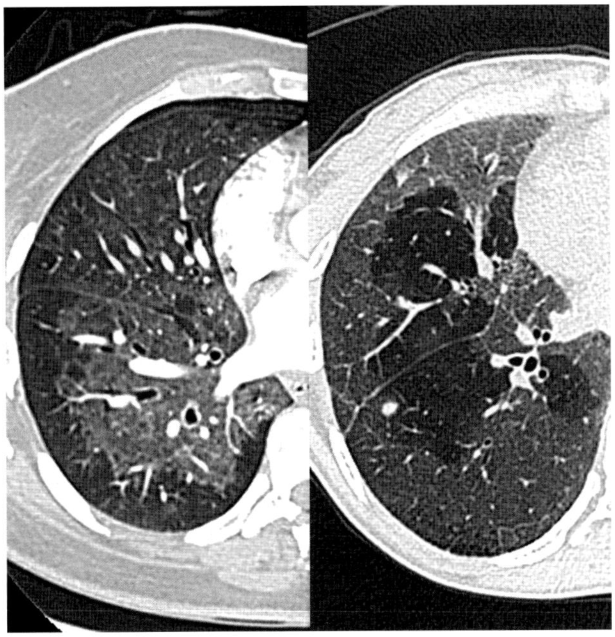

Figure 72.1. Ground-glass opacities—acute versus chronic. Composite image with chest CT of two different patients—one with AIDS and pneumocystis pneumonia (left), one with desquamative interstitial pneumonia (right), and both with diffuse ground-glass opacities—highlights the importance of determining acuity of imaging abnormalities in order to narrow the differential diagnosis.

Reticular Opacities

Reticular opacities may be identified on chest radiography and CT. The approach to reticular opacities is different on chest radiography versus chest CT. For example, patients with undiagnosed pulmonary emphysema and radiographic diffuse reticular opacities may show only emphysema on chest CT. In these cases, the reticular pattern on chest radiography is not truly an interstitial abnormality but, rather, artifactual and due to microatelectasis around the destroyed lung. Young women with undiagnosed lymphangioleiomyomatosis (LAM) often have a reticular pattern and hyperinflation on radiography, and it is nearly impossible to identify pulmonary cysts with

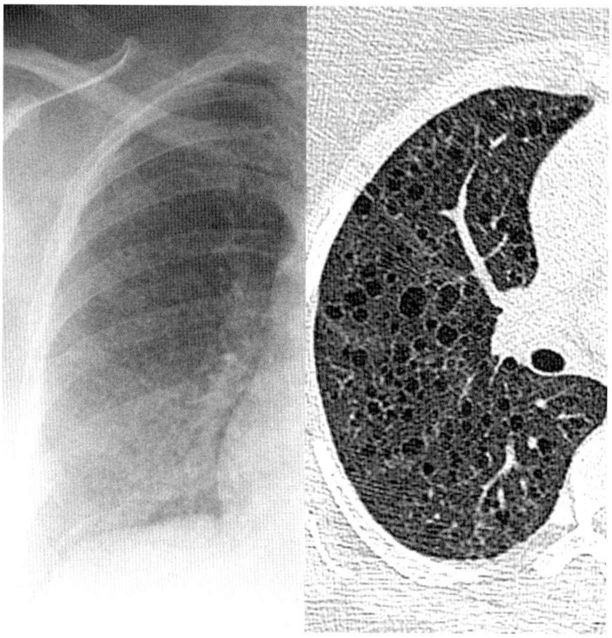

Figure 72.2. Reticular opacities on chest radiography. Composite image with posteroanterior chest radiograph (left) and thin-section chest CT (right) of a young woman with lymphangioleiomyomatosis shows a diffuse reticular pattern on radiography and innumerable thin-walled lung cysts on CT, emphasizing that cystic lung diseases may appear as reticular opacities on radiography.

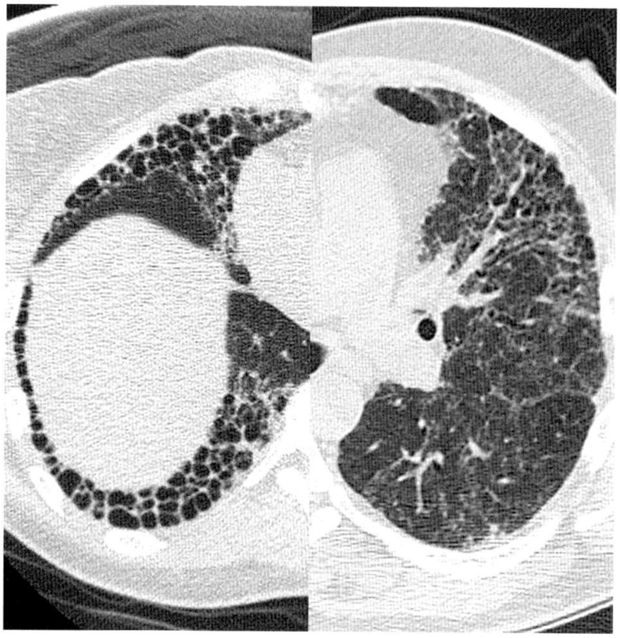

Figure 72.3. Distribution of reticulation on chest CT. Composite image with chest CT of two different patients, one with UIP (left) and one with cluster 2 hypersensitivity pneumonitis (HP) (right), shows subpleural honeycombing in UIP and upper lobe predominant peribronchovascular reticulation in HP.

certainty. Chest CT typically shows diffuse thin-walled cysts and not an interstitial process as suggested by the radiograph (Fig. 72.2. Finally, a patient with undiagnosed NSIP may have a normal chest radiograph and yet may exhibit extensive ground-glass and reticular opacities on CT. As a result, the question of when to further evaluate radiographic findings of reticular opacities remains open to discussion, but the following guidelines should be taken into consideration:

1. Reticular opacities on chest radiography may be artifactual (i.e., low lung volume) or may relate to emphysema.
2. It is extremely difficult to know when radiographic reticular opacities require further evaluation with CT, and a history of chronic symptoms may be helpful in making this decision.
3. Many patients with interstitial lung disease or diffuse infiltrative lung disease may have normal chest radiographs. Therefore, the radiologist must recognize the limitations of chest radiography in the assessment of reticular opacities.

Evaluation of reticular opacities on CT requires determination of the location and distribution of the abnormalities. Usual interstitial pneumonia (UIP) and NSIP exhibit a subpleural lower lobe predominance, whereas fibrosis from hypersensitivity pneumonitis or sarcoidosis exhibit a peribronchovascular upper lobe distribution (Fig. 72.3).

Cysts

The differential diagnosis of pulmonary cysts is straightforward once detected on CT. The challenge is to identify these findings on chest radiography, which is often not possible. Cysts may manifest as reticular opacities on chest radiography, which prompts evaluation with chest CT and definitive identification of pulmonary cysts. Note that a young female heavy smoker with thin-walled cysts on CT that simulate LAM may actually have centrilobular emphysema. Although there are several strategies for differentiating cysts from emphysema on CT, it may not always be easy to do so in practice. Visualization of a "central dot" sign within the "cyst" representing the centrilobular pulmonary artery is very helpful in making the diagnosis of emphysema. In addition, the so-called "cysts" of emphysema typically lack a perceptible wall on CT, but in some cases, emphysema may manifest with an appearance of perceptible walls due to microatelectasis at the periphery of the secondary pulmonary lobule surrounding the destroyed centrilobular lung parenchyma.

Micronodules

Chest CT is an extremely valuable diagnostic tool in the assessment of micronodules. Characterization of such nodules as having a centrilobular, perilymphatic, or random distribution allows differentiation of cellular bronchiolitis from sarcoidosis or metastases (Fig. 72.4). Although chest radiography may allow identification of the nodules, it is poor for establishing their distribution. It is generally

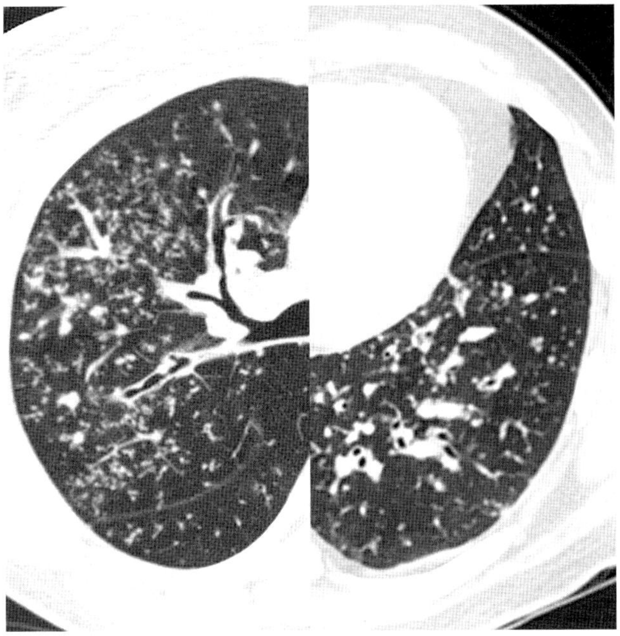

Figure 72.4. Distribution of micronodules on chest CT. Composite image with chest CT in two different patients, one with infectious bronchiolitis (left) and one with sarcoidosis (right), shows centrilobular and perilymphatic micronodules, respectively, highlighting the importance of micronodule distribution in the formulation of the differential diagnosis.

accepted that diffuse micronodules on chest radiography should be further evaluated with thin-section or high-resolution chest CT.

Suggested Reading

Al-Jahdali H, Rajiah P, Koteyar SS, Allen C, Khan AN. Atypical radiological manifestations of thoracic sarcoidosis: A review and pictorial essay. *Ann Thorac Med.* 2013 Oct;8(4):186–196.

Boitsios G, Bankier AA, Eisenberg RL. Diffuse pulmonary nodules. *AJR Am J Roentgenol.* 2010;194(5):W354–W366.

Seaman DM, Meyer CA, Gilman MD, McCormack FX. Diffuse cystic lung disease at high-resolution CT. *AJR Am J Roentgenol.* 2011;196(6):1305–1311.

CHAPTER 73

Ground-Glass Opacities

Juliana Bueno

Definition

Ground-glass opacity (GGO) is defined on thin-section CT as abnormally increased lung density in which vascular and bronchial margins remain visible. This contrasts with consolidation, in which the margins are typically obscured.

In the setting of diffuse lung disease, GGO may be related to airspace filling (e.g., fluid and cells), interstitial thickening (e.g., interstitial lung disease), or both (e.g., pulmonary edema and pulmonary proteinosis).

A few corollaries of diffuse GGO are helpful to recognize because they may be associated with a more specific diagnosis. The so-called "crazy paving" pattern is defined as the coexistence of GGO and reticular opacities, often in the form of interlobular and intralobular interstitial thickening. The "headcheese" pattern pertains to the coexistence of GGO and air trapping. The mosaic attenuation pattern is defined as the coexistence of geographic areas of increased and decreased lung density related to air trapping and/or focal oligemia.

Clinical Features

- Pathologic processes manifesting as diffuse GGO have widely varied symptoms according to the etiology. Nonspecific symptoms include cough, dyspnea, and shortness of breath. Clinical history has a critical role, and events such as inhalation exposure, smoking, long-term use of medications, and systemic diseases can be hints to diagnosis. Pulmonary function tests may be insensitive as well, with some diseases showing an obstructive pattern and others a restrictive pattern.
- Infection (e.g., *Pneumocystis jirovecii* pneumonia): Infection is often suspected in HIV patients with low CD4 count or patients with other immunocompromised states (e.g., chronic steroid therapy).
- Hemorrhage: Patients with diffuse alveolar hemorrhage may manifest with hemoptysis and/or decreasing hemoglobin and hematocrit.
- Pulmonary edema: Pulmonary edema often has a distinct clinical presentation in patients with risk factors.
- Hypersensitivity pneumonitis: Cluster 1 forms associated with systemic acute symptoms such as fever, cough and myalgias. Cluster 2 forms are more indolent symptoms associated with clubbing and inspiratory crackles.
- Organizing pneumonia (OP): Indolent course with often mild respiratory and systemic symptoms. It remains a diagnosis of exclusion because it can mimic various other conditions on imaging. Inflammatory serum markers such as erythrocyte sedimentation rate and C-reactive protein are usually elevated.
- Chronic eosinophilic pneumonia
  - Subacute respiratory symptoms
  - Peripheral eosinophilia
  - Eosinophilic bronchoalveolar lavage or pulmonary biopsy
- Pulmonary alveolar proteinosis: Rare diagnosis of exclusion. Often workup when crazy paving pattern is identified at high-resolution CT (HRCT). Milky bronchoalveolar lavage is fairly characteristic.
- Desquamative interstitial pneumonia (DIP): Any opacities in a symptomatic smoker often point toward a smoking-related disease. Diagnosis is often made on pathology.

Anatomy and Physiology

Alveolar filling and interstitial thickening seen on diffuse GGO occur at an anatomic level that is beyond the resolution of chest radiography and thin-section or HRCT. Whereas on chest radiography consolidations are typically denser and exhibit air brochogram, diffuse GGO may manifest with more subtle nonspecific hazy opacities or even normal chest radiographs. A similar phenomenon occurs on HRCT, which is a powerful tool to detect diffuse GGO but not to determine whether it is related to alveolar filling or interstitial thickening.

Awareness of the normal anteroposterior density gradient throughout the lungs in the supine position is helpful to avoid confusing dependent atelectasis for true GGO. Differentiation often requires complementary prone imaging in which atelectasis should resolve.

How to Approach the Image

If a patient with suspected diffuse lung disease has a normal chest radiograph or one with subtle abnormalities, an HRCT may be required for further evaluation.

Subtle radiographic abnormalities may be challenging to differentiate from some common technical artifacts, such as bronchovascular crowding from low lung volume (i.e., expiratory imaging) or increased attenuation in patients with large body habitus.

The assessment of diffuse GGO is primarily achieved with HRCT. Helpful features when establishing a differential diagnosis include chronicity, distribution of opacities, and ancillary findings.

What Not to Miss

- Diffuse GGO in a patient with thickened septal lines, pleural effusion, and cardiomegaly is often seen in pulmonary edema.
- Diffuse GGO in a patient with HIV is often related to *P. jirovecii* pneumonia.

Differential Diagnosis

- Acute diffuse GGO
  - Infection (e.g., *P. jirovecii* pneumonia): Commonly related to immunodeficiency such as AIDS, chronic corticosteroid therapy, and other states of immunosuppression.
  - Alveolar hemorrhage: Various etiologies; may be idiopathic or associated with capillaritis such as in autoimmunity (e.g., granulomatosis with polyangiitis, lupus).
  - Pulmonary edema: Both cardiogenic and noncardiogenic.
- Chronic diffuse GGO
  - Extensive differential diagnosis: Important considerations include the following:
    - HP: Allergic alveolitis related to inhalation of various antigens. In up to 50% of cases, the triggering agent cannot be determined.
    - OP: Polypoid plugs of granulation tissue within the airspace. It may be cryptogenic or represent a pattern of lung reaction toward various infectious/inflammatory noxa.
    - Chronic eosinophilic pneumonia: Eosinophilic accumulation within the lungs; often cryptogenic.
    - Pulmonary alveolar proteinosis (PAP): Alveolar accumulation of proteinaceous and lipid-rich surfactant-like material. It may be congenital, autoimmune, or secondary (e.g., silica exposure, hematologic malignancy, or immunodeficiency).
    - DIP: Within the spectrum of smoking-related lung diseases. It may improve or progress to pulmonary fibrosis.

Imaging Findings

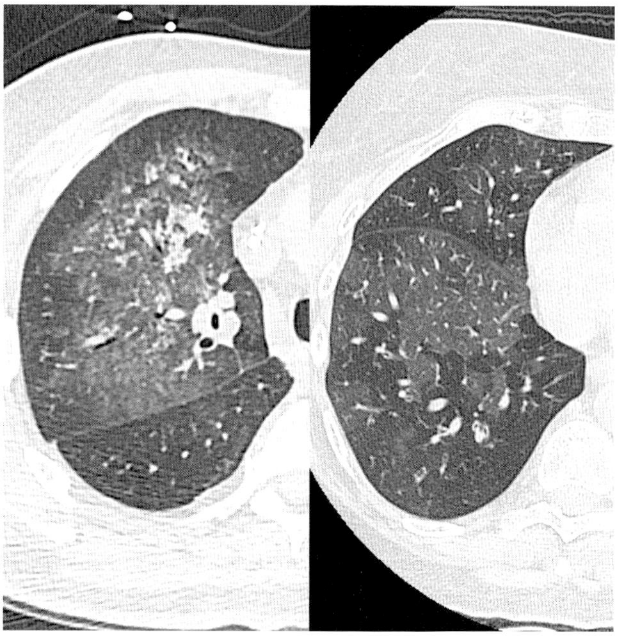

Figure 73.1. Differences between diffuse GGO and mosaic attenuation at thin-section chest CT. Composite image showing an alveolar hemorrhage and constrictive bronchiolitis. (Left) Thin-section chest CT shows diffuse GGO in this patient with alveolar hemorrhage. (Right) Expiratory thin-section chest CT shows mosaic attenuation in this patient with constrictive bronchiolitis. At first glance, the patterns may appear very similar. However, note conspicuous areas of decreased vascular caliber in constrictive bronchiolitis that make it possible to differentiate mosaic attenuation from GGO.

- Cases of diffuse GGO with geographic distribution may be difficult to differentiate from mosaic attenuation secondary to either air trapping or chronic occlusive pulmonary disease (e.g., chronic thromboembolic disease). The former scenario typically has pulmonary arteries with similar caliber in areas of GGO and spared lung. The latter scenario typically has vessels with decreased caliber within the areas of hypoattenuation (Fig. 73.1).
- Infection (e.g., *P. jirovecii* pneumonia) (Fig. 73.2)
  - Chest radiograph: Normal chest radiograph, diffuse hazy opacities
  - HRCT: Diffuse GGO; typically without pleural effusion or mediastinal/hilar lymphadenopathy
- Alveolar hemorrhage (Fig. 73.3)
  - Chest radiograph: Normal chest radiograph, diffuse hazy opacities
  - HRCT: Diffuse airspace or GGO; crazy paving pattern more frequent in subacute stages
- Pulmonary edema (Fig. 73.4)
  - Chest radiograph: Diffuse hazy and/or heterogeneous opacities, thickened septal lines, pleural effusions, cardiomegaly
  - HRCT: Diffuse GGO, thickened interlobar interstitium (septal lines), acinar nodules, pleural effusions
- Hypersensitivity pneumonitis (Fig. 73.5)
  - Chest radiograph: patients with cluster 1 HP may have a normal radiograph or present with subtle non-specific opacities whereas cluster 2 HP often demonstrate diffuse reticulation and fibrosis
  - HRCT: a typical appearance of cluster 1 HP is the presence of upper and middle lobepredominant

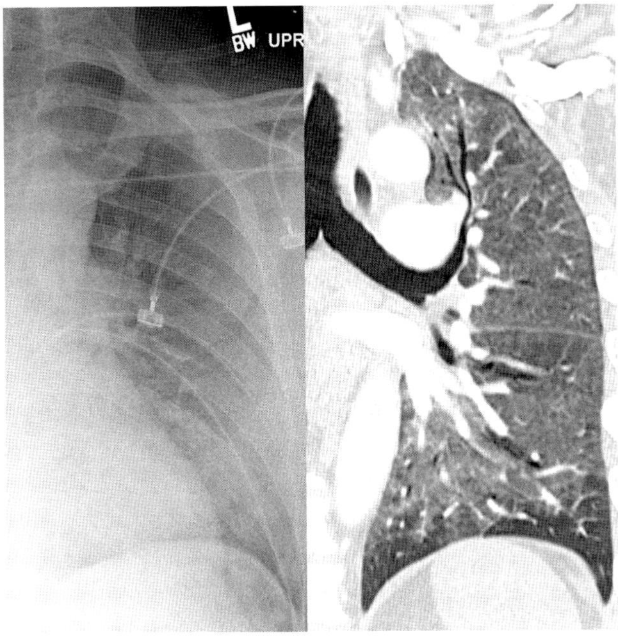

Figure 73.2. *Pneumocystis jirovecii* pneumonia. Composite image in a 34-year-old male with HIV and acute dyspnea and fever. (Left) Chest radiograph shows diffuse hazy opacities throughout the lungs. (Right) Thin-section chest CT (coronal reformation) demonstrates diffuse GGO.

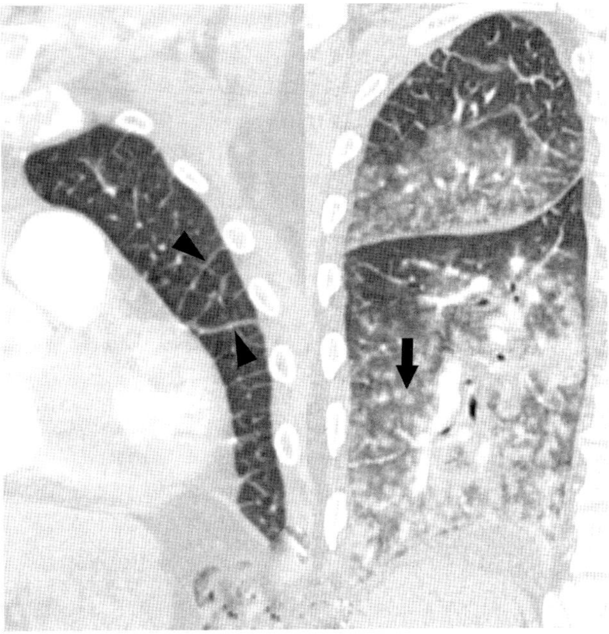

Figure 73.4. Cardiogenic pulmonary edema. Composite image in a 63-year-old male with acute shortness of breath. Thin-section chest CT coronal reformations at two different levels show scattered smooth thickened septal lines (arrowheads) with diffuse GGO and acinar nodules (arrows).

GGO and/or GG centrilobular nodules with associated lobular airtrapping on expiratory imaging (i.e. head-cheese pattern). These findings may be similar to respiratory bronchiolitis. Cluster 2 HP presents with reticulation or honeycombing (fibrosis) that could have upper lobe peribronchovascular distribution (similar to chronic burnout parenchymal sarcoidosis) or could be subpleural with lower lobe predominance, very similar to usual interstitial pneumonia.

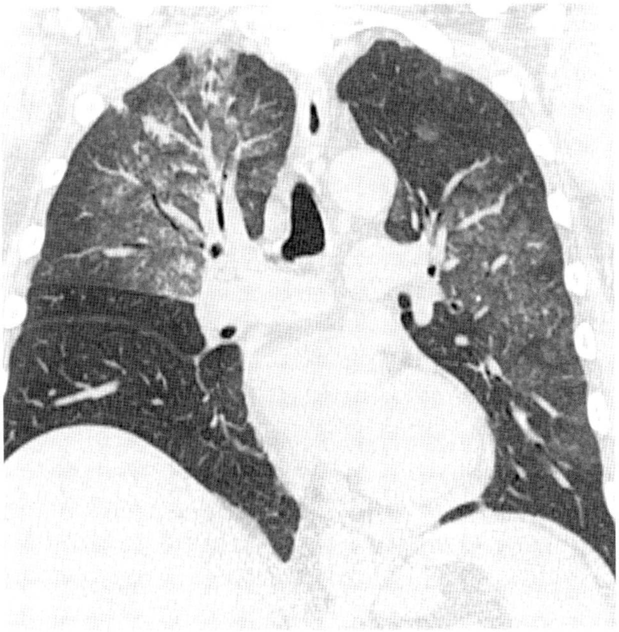

Figure 73.3. Diffuse alveolar hemorrhage with capillaritis. Image in a 37-year-old female with granulomatosis with polyangiitis (Wegener syndrome) and decreasing hematocrit. Thin-section coronal reformation from chest CT demonstrates scattered GGO throughout the lungs.

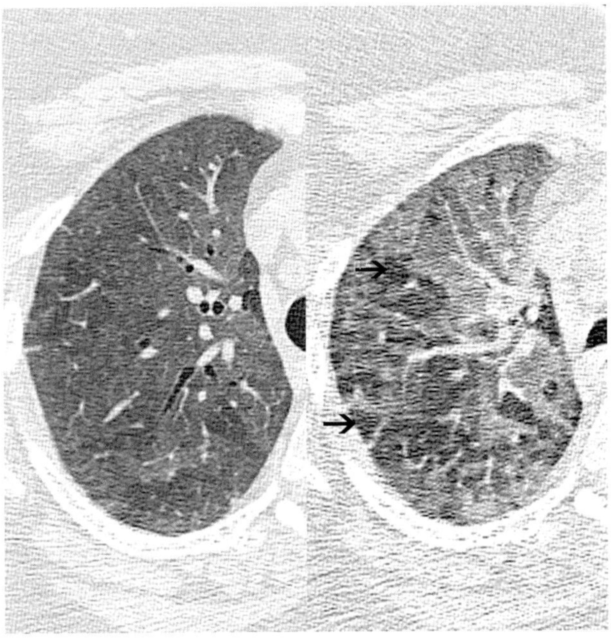

Figure 73.5. HP (Cluster 1) related to birds.

Composite image in a 33-year-old woman presenting with malaise, weight loss and dyspnea.

(left) Inspiratory thin-section chest CT demonstrates a mosaic attenuation pattern. (right)

Expiratory thin-section CT demonstrates lobular air-trapping (arrows), the so-called "headcheese" pattern.

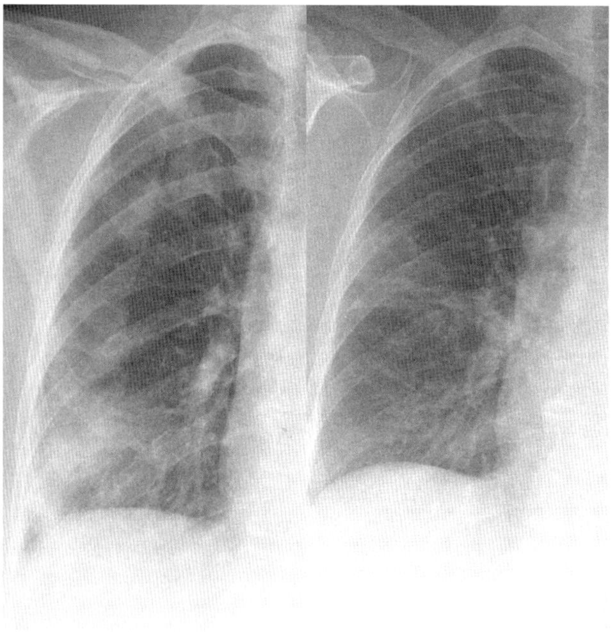

Figure 73.6. Cryptogenic organizing pneumonia (COP). Composite image in a 37-year-old with chronic cough and dyspnea. (Left) Initial chest radiograph shows multifocal airspace disease (solid arrows). (Right) Chest radiograph after several months shows resolution of previous areas of airspace disease with new areas (open).

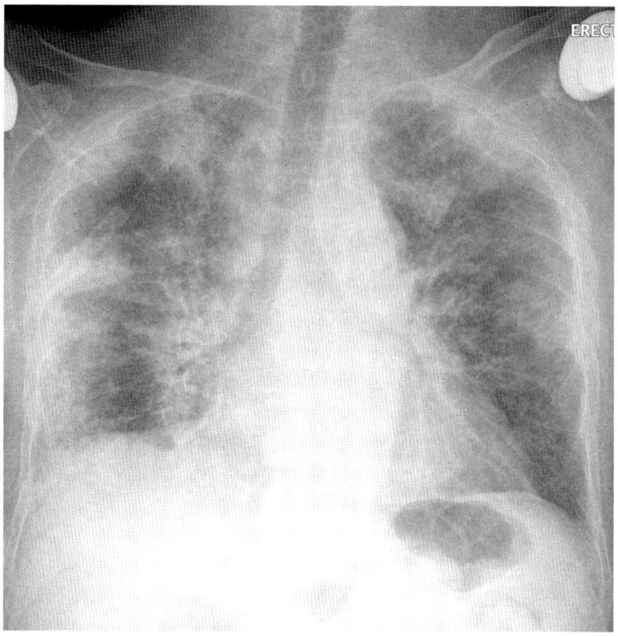

Figure 73.8. Chronic eosinophilic pneumonia. Image in a 41-year-old male with subacute dyspnea and eosinophilia. Chest radiograph demonstrates predominantly peripheral airspace disease with relatively more central sparing. the so-called "photographic negative of pulmonary edema."

- Organizing pneumonia (Figs. 73.6 and 73.7)
  - Chest radiograph: Migratory pulmonary opacities at serial radiographs
  - HRCT: Peripheral and asymmetric alveolar or GGO; waxing and waning nature on serial CTs; central areas of consolidation surrounded by GGO, the so-called CT "halo" sign; consolidation surrounding the GGO, the so-called "atoll" or "reversed halo" sign
- Chronic eosinophilic pneumonia (Figs. 73.8 and 73.9)
  - Chest radiograph: "Photographic negative of pulmonary edema" pattern with more peripherally

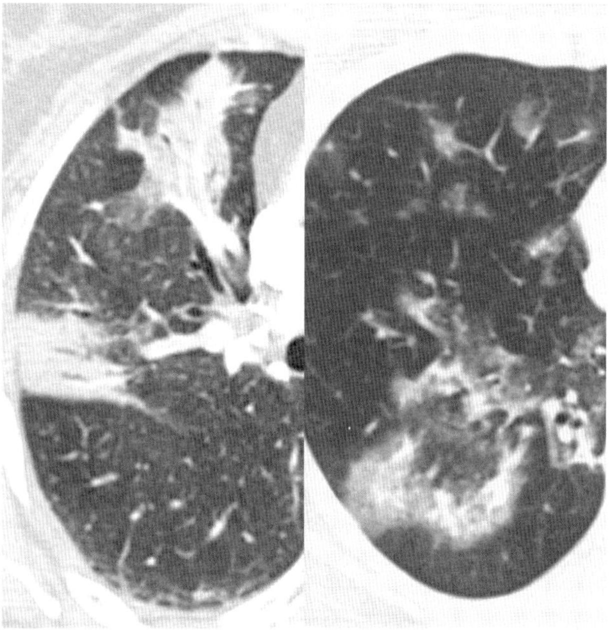

Figure 73.7. COP. Composite image in two different patients with COP. (Left) Thin-section chest CT shows multifocal subsegmental areas of consolidation. (Right) Thin-section chest CT shows airspace disease surrounding areas of GGO, the so-called "atoll" or "reverse halo" sign.

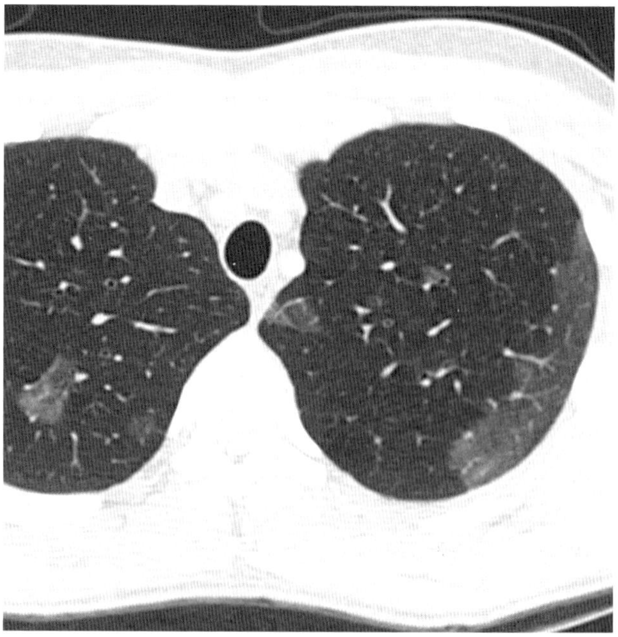

Figure 73.9. Chronic eosinophilic pneumonia. Image in a 35-year-old female with eosinophilia and normal chest radiograph. Thin-section chest CT shows bilateral, multifocal, somewhat peripheral, and sharply demarcated areas of GGO.

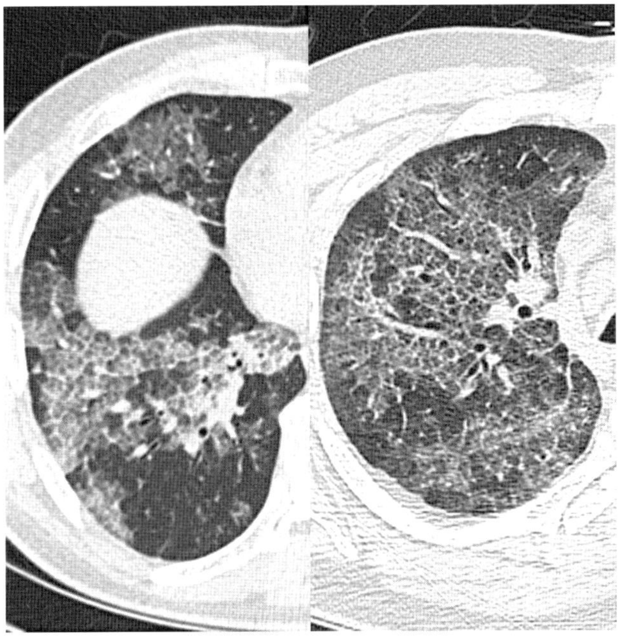

Figure 73.10. PAP and DIP. Composite image of two different patients with PAP and DIP. (Left) Thin-section chest CT demonstrates the "crazy paving" pattern. (Right) Thin-section chest CT demonstrates the "crazy paving" pattern.

distributed opacities; may mimic bacterial pneumonia or lung cancer
  - HRCT: Peripherally distributed GGO or airspace disease; may mimic organizing pneumonia, bacterial pneumonia, or lung cancer
- Pulmonary alveolar proteinosis (Fig. 73.10)
  - Chest radiograph: Nonspecific perihilar mid lung and basal predominant GG or heterogeneous opacities
  - HRCT: Diffuse geographic areas of GG opacities with diffuse intra- and interlobular thickening, the so-called crazy paving pattern; associated areas of consolidation should raise concern for superimposed infection
- Desquamative interstitial pneumonia (Fig. 73.10)
  - Chest radiograph: Ill-defined airspace opacities
  - HRCT: Basilar and peripheral GGO, scattered cysts; may coexist with areas of emphysema; can progress to severe architectural distortion, honeycombing, and pulmonary fibrosis

Clinical Issues

GGO is a nonspecific HRCT pattern that should always be interpreted in light of acuity of symptoms, specific clinical presentation, and laboratory results. Even when all the information is taken into consideration, differential diagnosis may remain elusive.

Key Points

- In contrast to consolidation, GGO do not obscure the pulmonary vasculature.
- GGO may be related to partial filling of the alveoli and/or interstitial thickening.
- When approaching a differential diagnosis, always consider diffuse GGO in the acute and the chronic setting.
- Clinical information may be the only clue to a more definitive diagnosis.
- Diffuse GGO coexisting with normal lung and mosaic attenuation occasionally may be difficult to differentiate; if a decrease in the caliber of pulmonary vessels is evident in areas of hypoattenuation, it is more likely mosaic attenuation due to focal hypoperfusion.

Suggested Reading

Attili A, Kazerooni EA, Gross BH, et al. Smoking-related interstitial lung disease: Radiologic–clinical–pathologic correlation. *RadioGraphics.* 2008;28:1383–1398.

Collins J, Stern EJ. Ground-glass opacity at CT: The ABCs. *AJR Am J Roentgenol.* 1997 Aug;169(2):355–367.

Jeong Y, Kim KI, Seo IJ, et al. Eosinophilic lung diseases: A clinical, radiologic and pathologic overview. *RadioGraphics.* 2007;27:617–639.

Screaton NJ, Hiorns MP, Müller NL. Differential diagnosis in chronic diffuse infiltrative lung disease on high-resolution computed tomography. *Semin Roentgenol.* 2002;37(1):17–24.

Silva CIS, Churg A, Muller NL. Hypersensitivity pneumonitis: Spectrum of high-resolution CT and pathologic findings. *AJR Am J Roentgenol.* 2007;188:334–344.

CHAPTER 74

Cystic Lung Disease

Juliana Bueno

Definition

The Fleischner Society defines a cyst as a round parenchymal lucency or low-attenuating area with a well-defined interface with normal lung and surrounded by an epithelial or fibrous wall that is often less than 2 mm in thickness. Cysts are often filled with air, but fluid and solid contents may also occur.

Several other conditions may mimic pulmonary cysts, including cavitation, pneumatocele, abscess, emphysema, and bronchiectasis. Differentiation of these conditions from cystic lung disease is usually feasible, but overlapping imaging findings may occur. For example, although emphysema classically lacks defined surrounding walls, surrounding microatelectasis may simulate a wall. Cavity walls are typically thick, but thin walls may also occur. A pneumatocele is a thin-walled gas-filled space thought to result from a combination of parenchymal necrosis and check-valve airway obstruction, and it may mimic a cyst.

Clinical Features

A heterogeneous group of diseases may manifest with cystic lung lesions. Symptoms include dyspnea, cough, and/or progressive dyspnea. Some of these diseases may be associated with recurrent pneumothorax, chylothorax, or hemoptysis. Affected patients are often asymptomatic until advanced disease ensues or abnormal pulmonary function tests are documented.

Anatomy and Physiology

Imaging analysis of cystic lung disease requires knowledge and recognition of normal anatomic structures and their geographic relationship to the cysts. Centrilobular emphysema may mimic cystic lung disease, particularly when occurring on a background of ground-glass opacity (e.g., associated pulmonary edema or pneumonia) or when there is surrounding atelectasis. In these circumstances, emphysema may exhibit discrete walls. Identification of the central lobular artery within the cyst-like structure (central dot sign) allows differentiation of centrilobular emphysema from true cysts (Fig. 74.1).

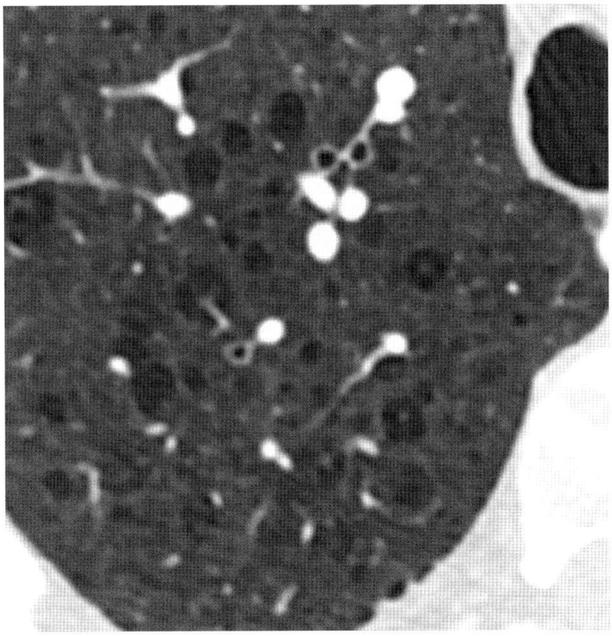

Figure 74.1. Emphysema. Coned-down thin-section chest CT of a 57-year-old smoker shows innumerable cystic lucencies, many of which demonstrate a central density—the so-called "central dot" sign diagnostic of centrilobular emphysema.

How to Approach the Image

Identification of cysts that are small and/or few in number on chest radiography is challenging and often not possible. Occasionally, cysts are recognized with certainty on radiography. Extensive and diffuse cystic lung disease in cases of lymphangioleiomyomatosis (LAM) or pulmonary Langerhans cell histiocytosis (PLCH) may manifest with normal radiographs, diffuse reticular opacities, or hyperinflation. Thin-section chest CT (and high-resolution CT) remains the imaging study of choice for identification and characterization of pulmonary cysts and allows differentiation from other cyst-like conditions. Detailed analysis of cyst morphology, distribution, and wall thickness is important in the formulation of a differential diagnosis.

- Distribution and localization: Cysts may be subpleural, perivascular, along fissures, or without geographic predominance.

- Morphology: Cysts may be round or may exhibit bizarre shapes (e.g., PLCH cysts typically exhibit bizarre or irregular shapes).
- Associated findings: Identification of coexisting emphysema, nodules, ground-glass opacities, pneumothorax, pleural effusion, renal angiomyolipomas, or other renal neoplasms may provide clues to the diagnosis.

What Not to Miss

- Chest radiography may be normal or may show subtle abnormalities.
- Reticular opacities and/or hyperinflation in young patients should raise suspicion of possible cystic disease.
- Symptoms and imaging findings may become more evident and characteristic as disease advances.

Differential Diagnosis

The differential diagnosis of true pulmonary cysts is narrow and includes LAM, PLCH, lymphoid interstitial pneumonia (LIP), and Birt–Hogg–Dubé (BHD) syndrome. Conditions that may mimic cystic lung disease include postinfectious pneumatoceles, tracheobronchial papillomatosis, cavitary disease (e.g., tuberculosis and fungal infection), bronchiectasis, and emphysema.

- LAM: Rare disorder characterized by abnormal smooth muscle proliferation in the lungs, mediastinum, and retroperitoneum. It affects women of childbearing age and may be associated with tuberous sclerosis. LAM is frequently associated with recurrent pneumothorax, chylous pleural effusions, and hemoptysis.
- PLCH: Idiopathic smoking-related disease of young and middle-aged individuals characterized by proliferation of Langerhans cells in the lung. Pneumothorax is not infrequent at presentation. Pulmonary function and chest radiographs may be initially normal, and findings may become more conspicuous and severe over time.
- LIP: Lymphocytic infiltration of the interstitium that may extend into the alveolar spaces and is classified as both an interstitial pneumonia and a lymphoproliferative disorder. It has a strong association with autoimmune disorders (e.g., Sjögren syndrome and rheumatoid arthritis), multicentric Castleman disease, and some immunodeficiencies (e.g., HIV and common variable immunodeficiency).
- BHD: Autosomal dominant genetic disorder involving the BHD gene, which encodes for folliculin. It has multiple nonpulmonary manifestations, such as follicular hamartomas, renal oncocytomas, and clear cell renal carcinomas.

Imaging Findings

LAM

Chest Radiography

- Early radiographic abnormalities may be subtle
- Increased lung volumes and/or fine reticular, reticular, or nodular opacities (Fig. 74.2)
- Characteristic diffuse and symmetric lung involvement
- Ancillary findings: Pneumothorax, pleural effusion (chylothorax)

CT

- Innumerable thin-walled rounded cysts with normal intervening lung parenchyma (Fig. 74.3)
- Diffuse involvement including the basilar lung near the costophrenic angles, which helps differentiation from PLCH
- Ancillary findings: Chylothorax, recurrent pneumothorax, lymphadenopathy, fat-containing renal lesions (angiomyolipomas)

PLCH (Figures 74.4 & 74.5)

Chest Radiography

- Lung volumes usually preserved but may be increased
- Early disease may manifest with small nodules, and cystic component may be less apparent

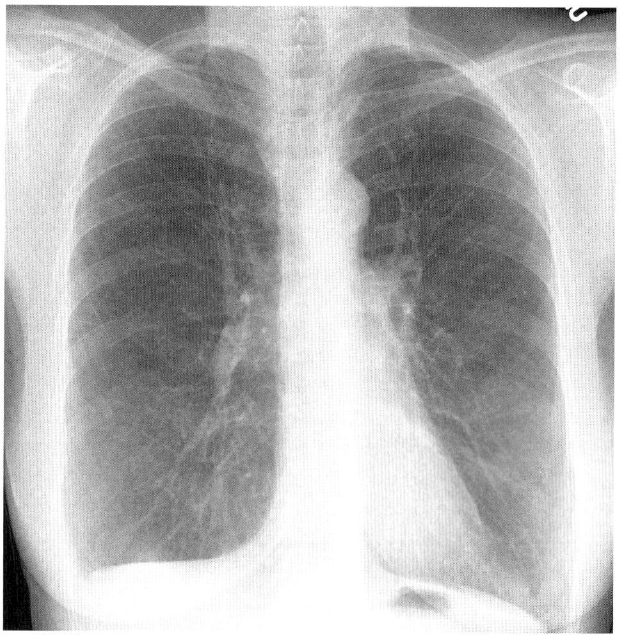

Figure 74.2. LAM. Posteroanterior chest radiograph of a 37-year-old woman with LAM shows hyperinflation, subtle bilateral reticular opacities, and a small right pleural effusion secondary to chylothorax.

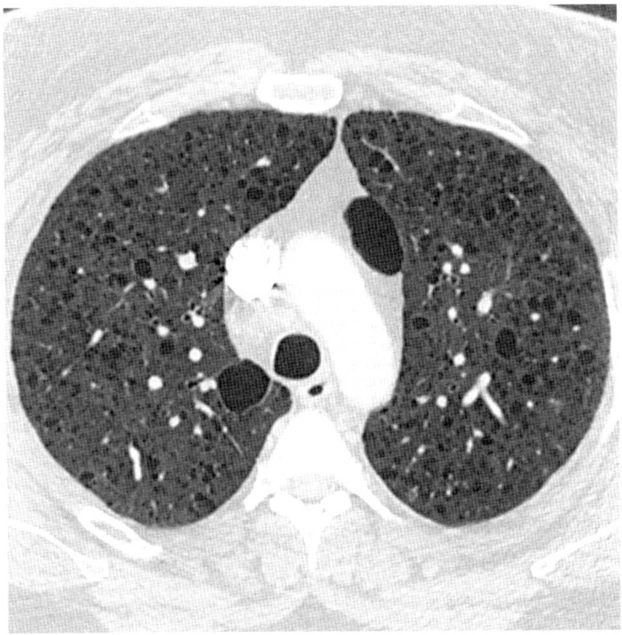

Figure 74.3. LAM. Contrast-enhanced chest CT of a 42-year-old woman with LAM shows innumerable bilateral, round thin-walled cysts of variable sizes.

- Characteristic mid and upper lung zone predominance with sparing of the basilar lung near the costophrenic angles (Fig. 74.4)

CT

- Upper lung zone predominant involvement
- Solid nodules measuring less than 10 mm with irregular shapes

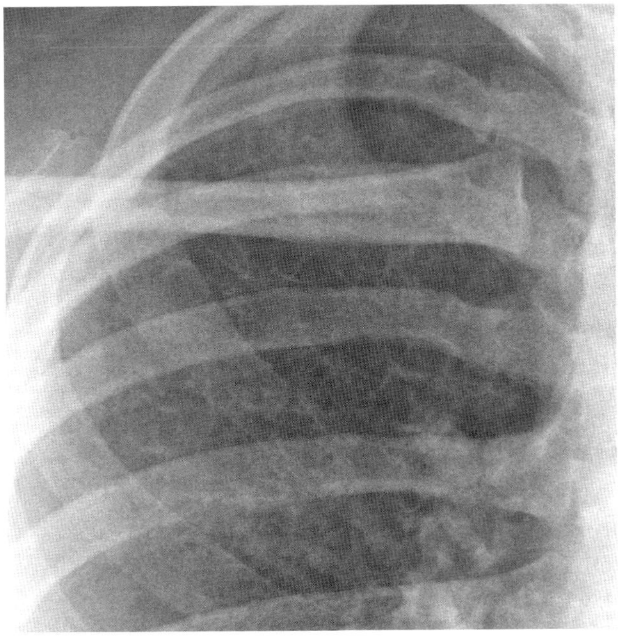

Figure 74.4. PLCH. Posteroanterior chest radiograph (coned down to the right upper lobe) of a 35-year-old woman smoker with dyspnea and cough shows thin reticular opacities that represented thin cyst walls.

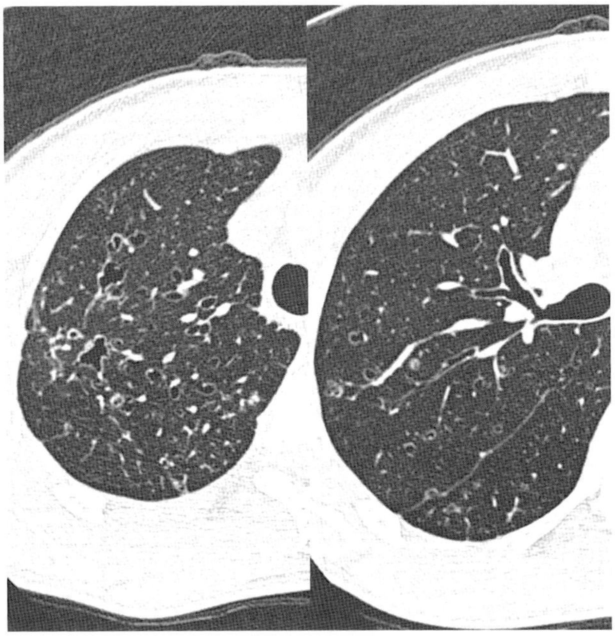

Figure 74.5. PLCH. Composite image with thin-section CT of a 27-year-old male smoker with weight loss shows multiple bizarre-shaped cysts and scattered small nodules with varying degrees of cavitation.

- Irregularly shaped cysts with variable wall thickness (Fig. 74.5)
- Coexistence of pulmonary cysts and small nodules
- Cysts become confluent, bizarre-shaped, and thin-walled in advanced disease
- Pulmonary hypertension (i.e., dilated pulmonary trunk) frequent in late disease

LIP

Chest Radiography

- Basilar predominant reticular or heterogeneous opacities

CT

- Ground-glass opacities or consolidation
- 2- to 4-mm poorly defined centrilobular and subpleural nodules
- Thin-walled cysts of variable size with peribronchovascular distribution (Fig. 74.6)
- Peribronchovascular and interlobular septal thickening
- Honeycombing in late disease

BHD

Chest Radiography

- Spontaneous and recurrent pneumothorax

CT

- Often an incidental diagnosis
- Bilateral lower lobe predominant, round, oval, or irregular, thin-walled cysts ranging from 3 mm to 8 cm Fig. 74.7)

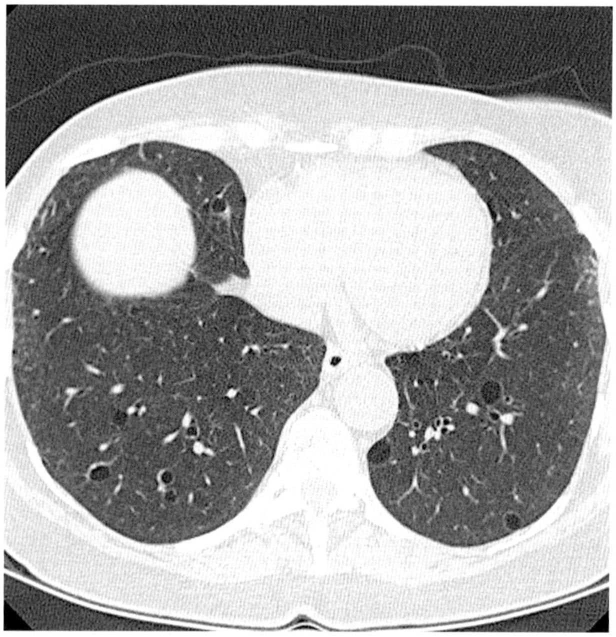

Figure 74.6. LIP. Thin-section chest CT of a 29-year-old man with Sjögren syndrome, cough, and dyspnea demonstrates subtle ground-glass opacities and a few scattered thin-walled cysts.

- Large cysts commonly multiseptated
- Cysts may abut or surround lower lobe pulmonary arteries or veins

Clinical Issues

- LAM and PLCH are rare, but they are the most frequently encountered cystic lung diseases. Patients with early disease may be asymptomatic and have normal pulmonary function.
- LAM is not classified as a neurocutaneous disorder, but pulmonary involvement in patients with tuberous

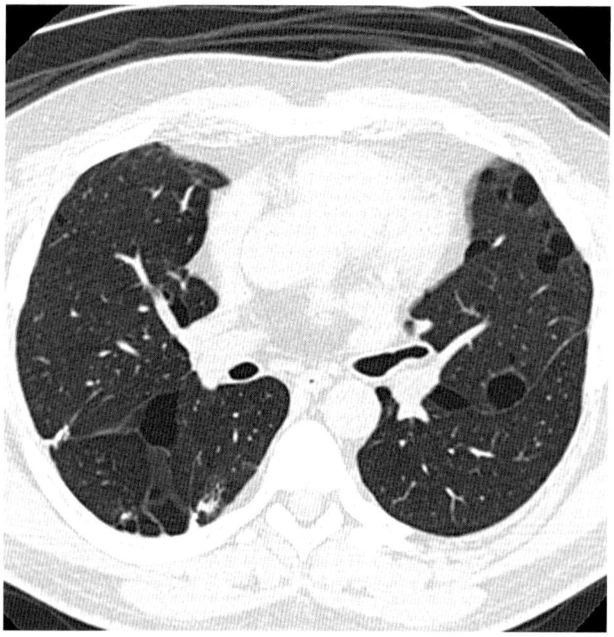

Figure 74.7. BHD syndrome. Thin-section chest CT of a 33-year-old woman with a family history of pneumothorax shows multiple well-defined cysts predominantly distributed along the pleura, some with internal septations.

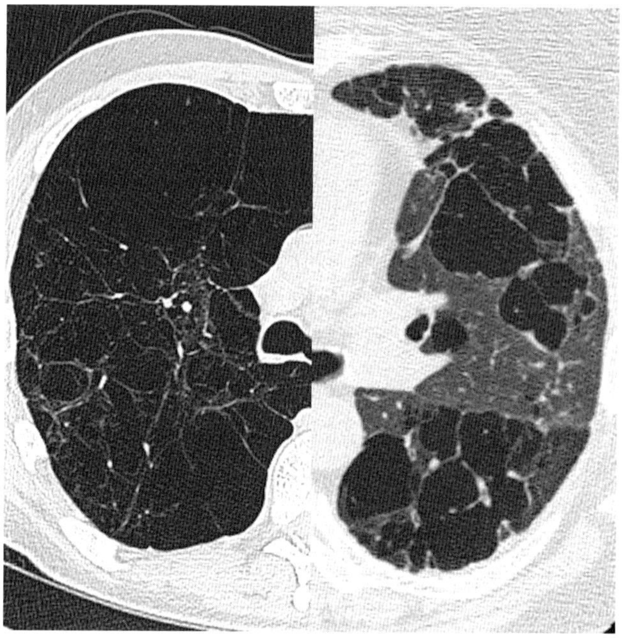

Figure 74.8. Emphysema versus late-stage PLCH. Composite image with chest CT of two different patients shows confluent emphysema (left) and end-stage PLCH (right), highlighting the difficulty in differentiating end-stage cystic lung disease from advanced emphysema.

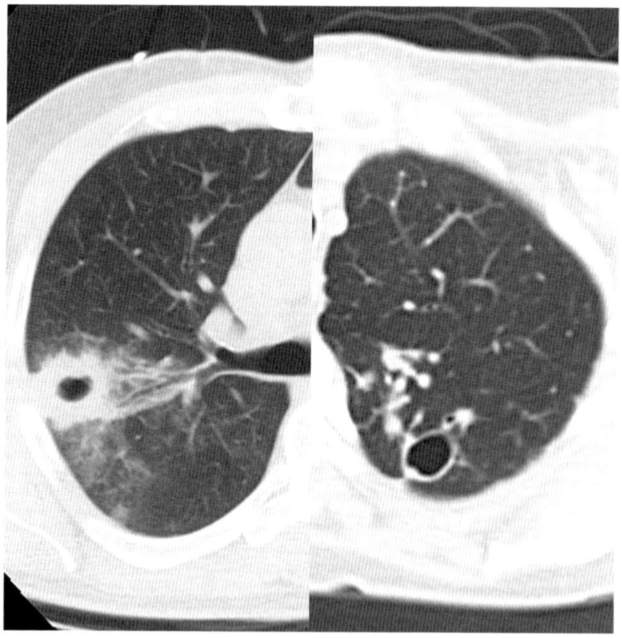

Figure 74.9. Cyst mimickers, pulmonary abscess and cavitation. Composite image with chest CT of two different patients with anaerobic aspiration pneumonia (left) and atypical mycobacterial infection (right) shows a right upper lobe nodular consolidation with intrinsic cavitation and surrounding ground-glass opacity consistent with pulmonary abscess (left) and a left upper lobe thin-walled cavity (right).

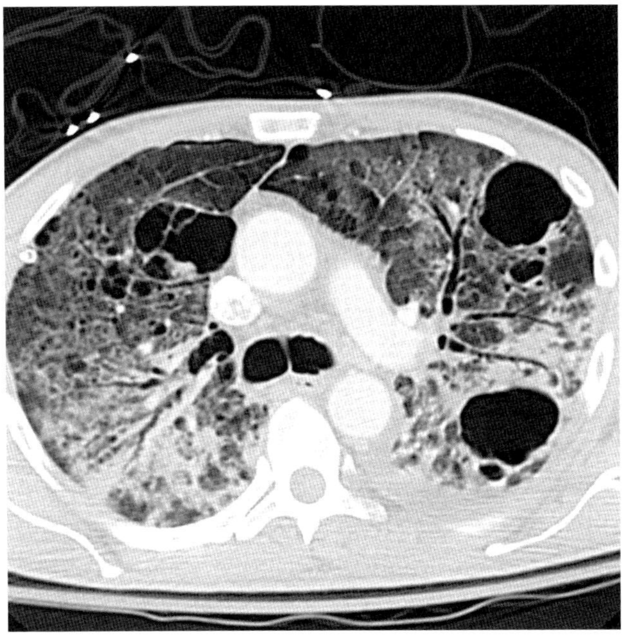

Figure 74.10. Cyst mimicker, pneumatocele. Thin-section chest CT in a patient with extensive ground-glass opacities related to pneumocystis pneumonia shows multiple pmeumatoceles within areas of airspace disease.

sclerosis is pathologically identical to LAM. The mortality of patients with LAM is variable but reaches 20% at 10 years.

- PLCH is intimately associated with cigarette smoking. Following smoking cessation, up to one-third of patients with PLCH may have regression of imaging abnormalities, but a small percentage of patients progress to end-stage pulmonary fibrosis. The extent and severity of cystic lung disease correlate with the degree of physiologic impairment.

Key Points

- The radiologist plays an important role in the diagnosis of LAM and PLCH, and typical CT findings may be considered diagnostic precluding lung biopsy.
- Spontaneous pneumothorax may be the first manifestation of cystic lung disease.
- Cavitary disease, pneumatocele formation, abscess, emphysema, and bronchiectasis may mimic cystic lung disease (Figs. 74.8–74.10).

Suggested Reading

Agarwal PP, Gross BH, Holloway BJ, Seely J, Stark P, Kazerooni EA. Thoracic CT findings in Birt–Hogg–Dube syndrome. *AJR Am J Roentgenol.* 2011 Feb;196(2):349–352.

Seaman DM, Meyer CA, Gilman MD, McCormack FX. Diffuse cystic lung disease at high-resolution CT. *AJR Am J Roentgenol.* 2011;196(6):1305–1311.

Silva CI, Flint JD, Levy RD, Müller NL. Diffuse lung cysts in lymphoid interstitial pneumonia: High-resolution CT and pathologic findings. *J Thorac Imaging.* 2006;21(3):241–244.

Tobino K, Gunji Y, Kurihara M, Kunogi M, Koike K, Tomiyama N, et al. Characteristics of pulmonary cysts in Birt–Hogg–Dubé syndrome: Thin-section CT findings of the chest in 12 patients. *Eur J Radiol.* 2011;77(3):403–409.

CHAPTER 75

Pulmonary Micronodules

Juliana Bueno

Definition

The Fleischner Society defines a micronodule as a rounded opacity that measures less than 3 mm in diameter at CT. Although micronodules are often identified in the interstitium, they may also be seen in alveolar processes such as infection. Furthermore, airspace and interstitial micronodules can coexist and may be difficult to differentiate. This chapter discusses micronodules occurring in the interstitium and distal airways.

Clinical Features

Diseases manifesting with micronodules vary widely and have variable clinical presentations. Affected patients often present with nonspecific respiratory symptoms, including dyspnea and cough.

Patients with acute infectious bronchiolitis may present with fever, cough, and sputum production. Patients with chronic infectious bronchiolitis (e.g., mycobacterial infection) may present indolent symptoms or may be asymptomatic. Hypersensitivity pneumonitis is an allergic bronchiolitis often linked to inhalation of certain organic or inorganic agents, and it has variable respiratory symptoms.

Sarcoidosis has a wide range of clinical presentations. Common nonspecific symptoms include progressive dyspnea and cough.

Patients with silicosis and coal worker's pneumoconiosis may present with dyspnea and nonproductive cough and have a history of occupational exposure to silica dust.

Finally, lymphangitic carcinomatosis and hematogenous metastasis are frequently associated with a history of malignancy.

Anatomy and Physiology

Recognizing the interstitial anatomy is fundamental when assessing micronodules (Fig. 75.1). The interstitium is defined as a continuum of connective tissue that supports

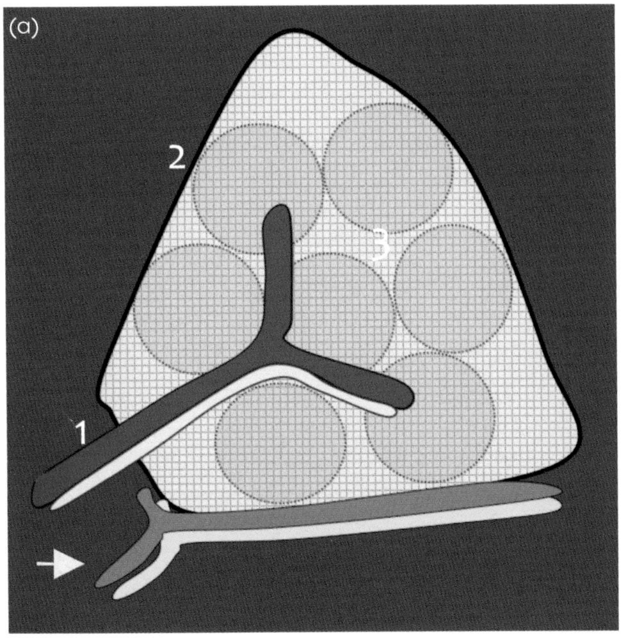

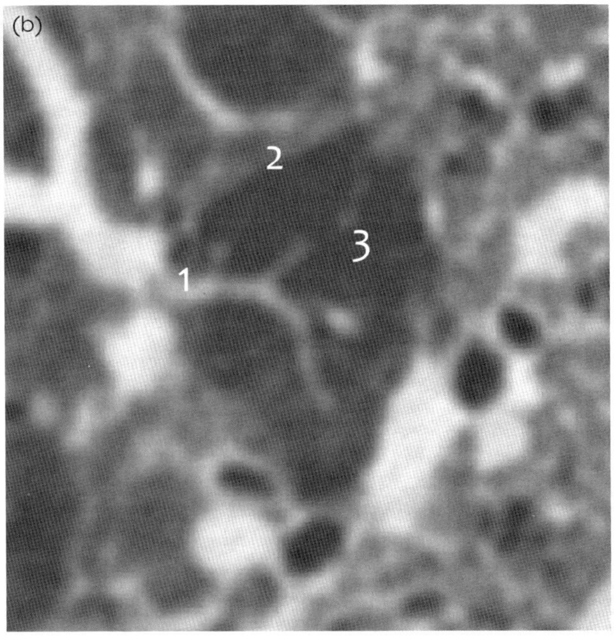

Figures 75.1. Anatomy of the SPL. (a) The anatomic components of the SPL: (1) axial interstitium (surrounds the centrilobular artery and bronchus), (2) interlobular interstitium, and (3) intralobular interstitium. (b) SPL at HRCT showing the (1) axial, (2) interlobular, and (3) intralobular interstitium. In normal cases, the centrilobular artery is the only structure visible within SPL.

the vascular, bronchial, and parenchymal structures of the lung. The axial or central interstitium arises at the hila and surrounds the bronchi and vessels and is subdivided into peribronchovascular and centrilobular interstitium. The peripheral interstitium consists of connective tissue along the periphery of the secondary pulmonary lobule (i.e., subpleural and interlobular interstitium). Both the axial and the peripheral interstitium are connected by the alveolar or intralobular interstitium. The secondary pulmonary lobule (SPL) is the smallest unit of lung surrounded by connective tissue, which can be recognized on thin-section or high-resolution chest CT (HRCT) (Fig 75.1). The pulmonary artery and accompanying bronchus course in the center of the SPL (i.e., centrilobular interstitium). Normally, only the centrilobular pulmonary artery is visible on CT. Centrilobular bronchi are visible only when abnormal. Pulmonary lymphatics course along the interlobular and centrilobular interstitium, and micronodules disposed along these areas are characterized as having a perilymphatic distribution. Thickening of the peripheral interstitium frequently manifest as fissural (subpleural) and septal (interlobular) thickening.

How to Approach the Image

Thin-section CT (and HRCT) is optimal for detection and characterization of pulmonary micronodules (Fig. 75.2):

- Micronodules are rounded opacities less than 3 mm in diameter.
- Distribution: Perifissural micronodules are often perilymphatic. Absence of fissural micronodules and involvement of the central interstitium indicate centrilobular micronodules, which often spare the subpleural regions. If there is not a clear pattern of distribution, random micronodules should be considered.
- Characterization: Centrilobular micronodules may exhibit solid or ground-glass attenuation. Solid micronodules are distinct, whereas ground-glass micronodules are hazy and ill-defined.

What Not to Miss

- Assessment of micronodules requires thin-section CT (i.e., 1 or 2 mm) and may be enhanced by using HRCT parameters such as edge-enhancing reconstruction algorithm.
- After micronodules are identified, their distribution must be determined by assessing areas less severely affected. Coronal reformations may be useful for determining upper versus lower lobe predominance.

Differential Diagnosis

Centrilobular Micronodules

- These typically occur in small airways disease; rarely relate to occlusion of centrilobular arteries (e.g., tumor emboli, cellulose, or talc granulomatosis).

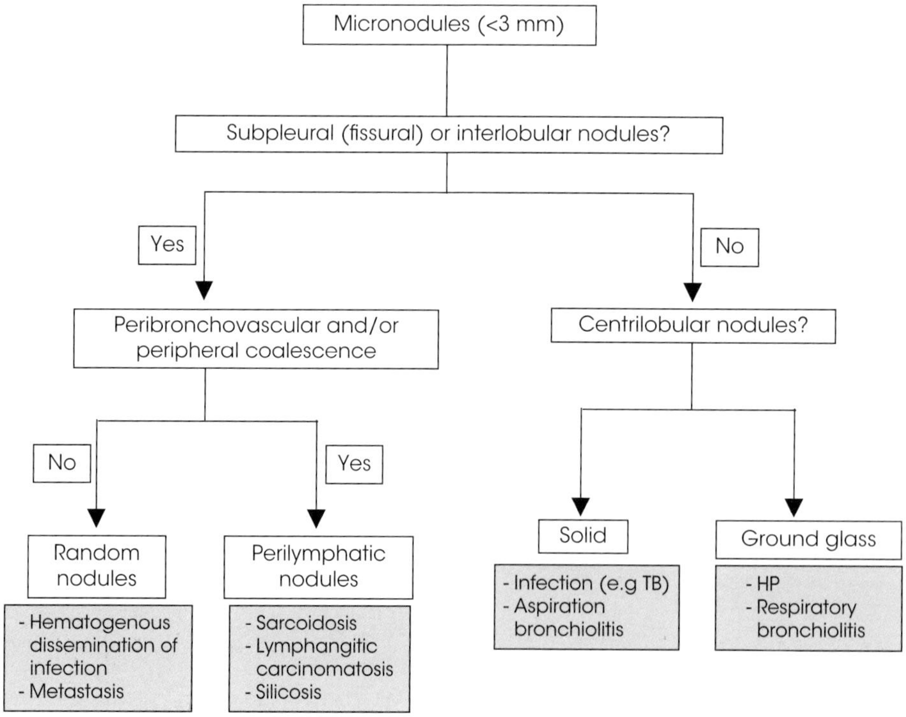

Figure 75.2. Systematic approach to pulmonary micronodules.

- Ground-glass centrilobular micronodules are typically seen in hypersensitivity pneumonitis and respiratory bronchiolitis.
- Solid micronodules are more common in infectious and aspiration bronchiolitis.
- Tree-in-bud opacities may be seen in endobronchial spread of disease (infectious/neoplastic), allergic bronchopulmonary aspergillosis, and diffuse panbronchiolitis.

Perilymphatic Micronodules

- These are characteristic of diseases affecting the pulmonary lymphatics.
- Smooth thickening of the interlobular interstitium typically indicates interstitial edema.
- Nodular interlobular or septal thickening is seen in sarcoidosis, lymphangitic carcinomatosis, and silicosis/coal worker's pneumoconiosis(CWP).

Random Micronodules

- Random micronodules are related to hematogenous spread of disease.
- Common examples include hematogenous metastatic disease (e.g., lung, breast, colon, pancreas, and prostate cancer) and miliary infection (e.g., tuberculosis and fungal infections).

Imaging Findings

Centrilobular Micronodules

- These are typically located in the axial interstitium and exhibit subpleural sparing.
- When subtle, they are better demonstrated on maximum intensity projection (MIP) reformations.
- Centrilobular solid nodules are well-defined, whereas ground-glass nodules demonstrate poorly defined contours.
- Infection and aspiration commonly exhibit solid centrilobular nodules and/or tree-in-bud opacities (coexistent centrilobular nodules and branching opacities) (Fig. 75.3). Ancillary findings include bronchial wall thickening and mucous plugging. Areas of focal fibrosis and bronchiectasis are more common in aspiration bronchiolitis.
- Respiratory bronchiolitis is characterized by centrilobular ground-glass nodules with upper lobe predominance. It often coexists with emphysema and expiratory air trapping (Fig. 75.5).
- Cluster 1 hypersensitivity pneumonitis may be characterized by centrilobular ground-glass nodules or (Fig. 75.4) diffuse ground-glass opacities often with upper lobe predominance. There may be expiratory lobular air trapping. The coexistence of ground-glass opacities and lobular air trapping is also known as the "headcheese" pattern. Emphysema can occur even in nonsmokers.

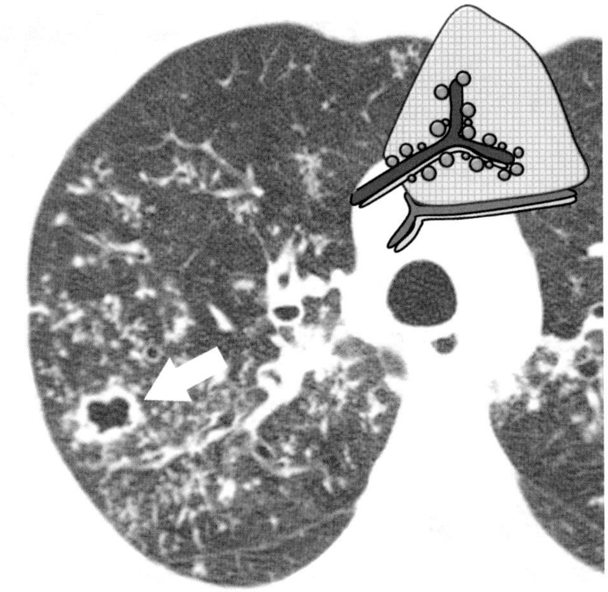

Figure 75.3. Tuberculosis, postprimary pattern. HRCT of a 42-year-old woman with cough and fever shows upper lobe predominant centrilobular and branching opacities (i.e., tree-in-bud opacities) from endobronchial spread of infection and cavitation (arrow).

Perilymphatic Micronodules

- These typically affect interlobar fissures, producing a beaded appearance.
- Silicosis and CWP are both characterized by centrilobular and subpleural micronodules (i.e., perilymphatic distribution) with upper lobe predominance.

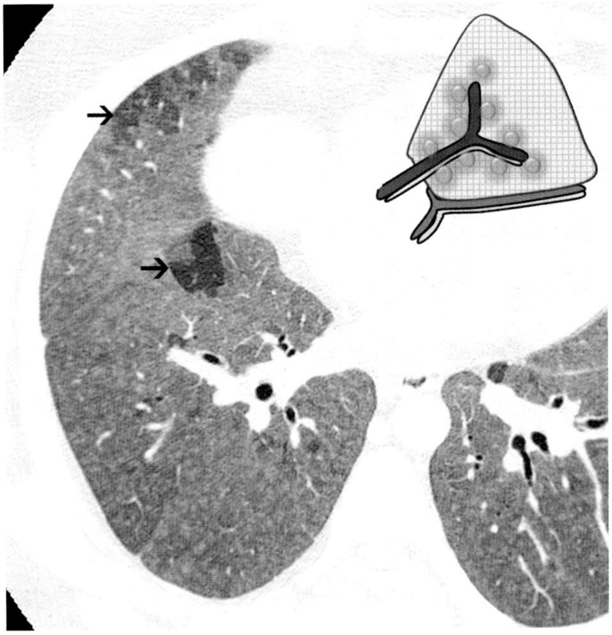

Figure 75.4. Hypersensitivity pneumonitis. HRCT of a 47-year-old man with progressive dyspnea and exposure to birds shows extensive bilateral centrilobular ground-glass micronodules and scattered areas of lobular air trapping (arrows).

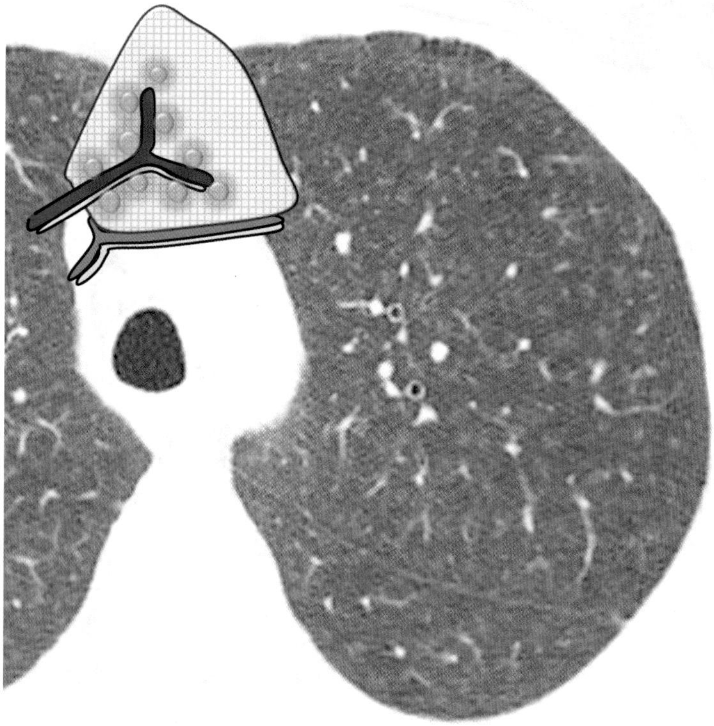

Figure 75.5. Respiratory bronchiolitis. Unenhanced chest CT of a 53-year-old man with a long history of heavy smoking shows upper lobe predominant ground-glass centrilobular micronodules with associated paraseptal emphysema.

Whereas in early stages the presence of micronodules is the predominant feature, as disease progresses, confluent parenchymal opacities with perihilar distribution and parenchymal volume loss develop—the so-called progressive massive fibrosis (Fig. 75.6).

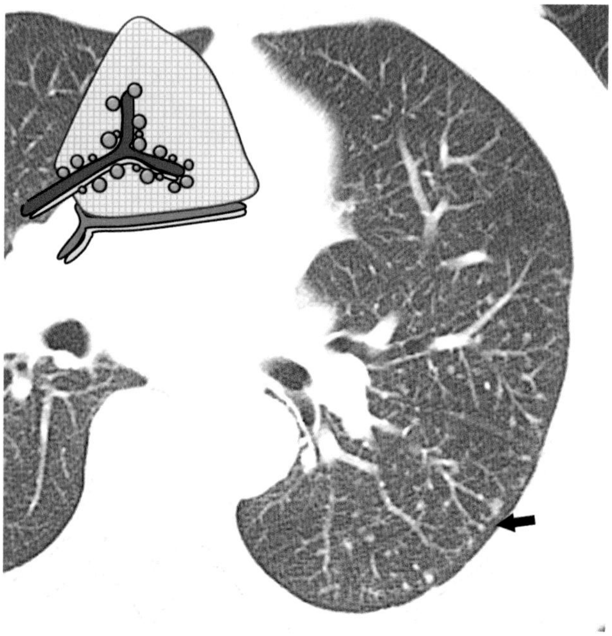

Figure 75.6. Silicosis. Chest CT of a 63-year-old man with known exposure to silica shows perilymphatic micronodules.

- Sarcoidosis classically exhibits perilymphatic micronodules that may or may not coalesce and may be associated with bilateral symmetric hilar and mediastinal lymphadenopathy Fig. 75.7).
- Lymphangitic carcinomatosis may manifest with smooth or nodular interlobular septal and fissural thickening. Peribronchovascular heterogeneous opacities and discrete solid nodules are frequently seen Fig. 75.8.
- Amyloidosis is the extracellular deposition of proteinaceous material and may have variable manifestations ranging from solitary pulmonary nodules to diffuse lung disease. In systemic amyloidosis, smooth and/or beaded interlobular septal thickening may be associated with diffuse bronchial wall thickening and parenchymal calcifications.

Random Micronodules

- Random micronodules are also known as miliary (Fig. 75.9).
- These are characteristic of hematogenous spread of diseases, primarily hematogenous metastases (e.g., melanoma, sarcoma, thyroid, colon, and breast malignancies), and hematogenous spread of infection (e.g., miliary tuberculosis and fungal infections).

Clinical Issues

- Upper lobe tree-in-bud opacities, especially if associated with cavitation and discrete nodules, should

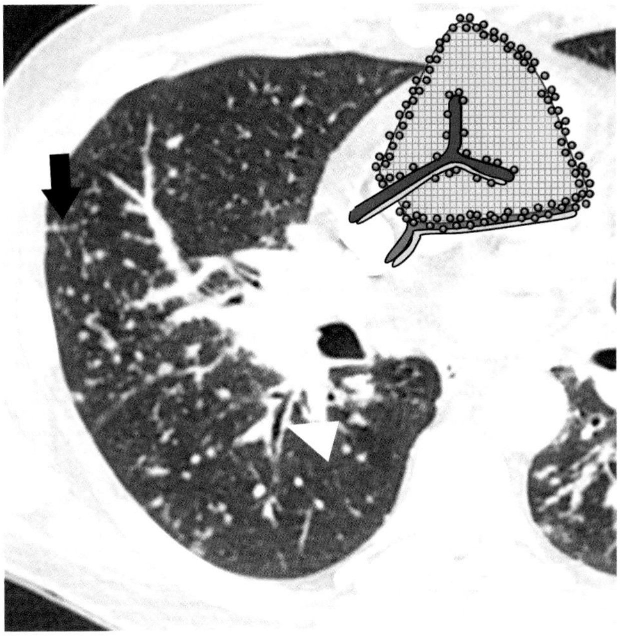

Figure 75.7. Sarcoidosis. Unenhanced chest CT of an asymptomatic 33-year-old man shows micronodules along the right oblique fissure, interlobular septa (arrow), and peribronchovascular interstitium (arrowhead).

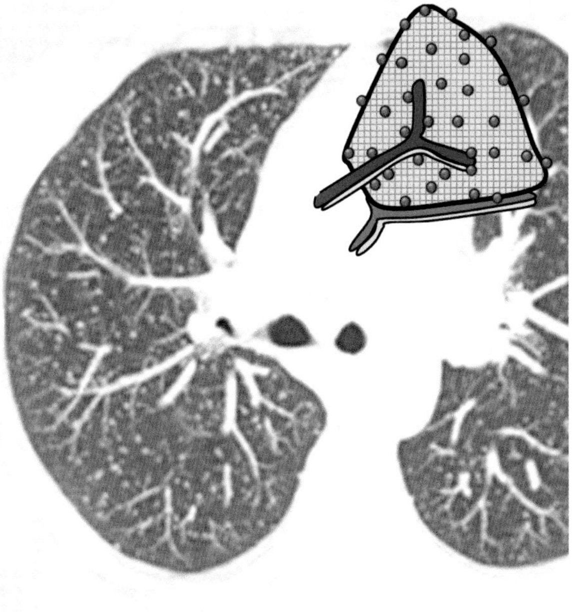

Figure 75.9. Miliary histoplasmosis. MIP reformatted unenhanced chest CT of a 42-year-old woman with dyspnea shows profuse random micronodules.

raise concern for postprimary pattern of pulmonary tuberculosis.

- Centrilobular nodules in immunosuppressed patients, even if not extensive, may represent severe infectious bronchiolitis and require immediate medical treatment.
- Extensive septal lines in the absence of heart failure should raise suspicion for lymphangitic carcinomatosis.
- Aspiration bronchiolitis is a frequently overlooked entity. The presence of hiatus hernia or dilated esophagus in association with centrilobular nodules and tree-in-bud opacities should suggest the diagnosis.

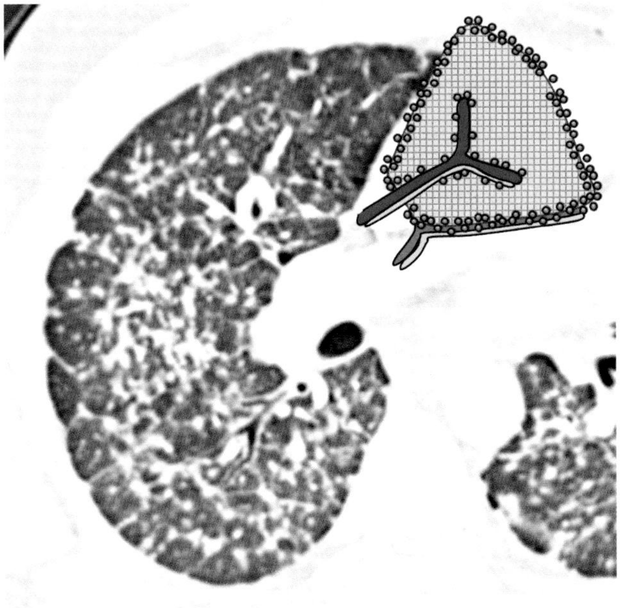

Figure 75.8. Lymphangitic carcinomatosis. Unenhanced chest CT of a 41-year-old woman with breast cancer and progressive dyspnea shows profuse perilymphatic micronodules.

Key Points

- Assessment of pulmonary micronodules is optimally achieved with thin-slice and/or high-resolution chest CT (<2-mm slice thickness).
- Differential diagnosis of micronodules mostly depends on their distribution and appearance (solid vs. ground glass).
- A pattern-based approach to micronodules allows the formulation of an appropriate differential diagnosis.
- Although sarcoidosis has variable imaging manifestations, perilymphatic micronodules are classic. However, sarcoidosis is a diagnosis of exclusion that warrants pathological confirmation.
- Tree-in-bud opacities (i.e., centrilobular nodules and branching opacities) are often associated with infectious etiology.

Suggested Reading

Boitsios G, Bankier AA, Eisenberg RL. Diffuse pulmonary nodules. *AJR Am J Roentgenol.* 2010;194(5):W354–W366.

Criado E, Sanchez M, Ramirez J, et al. Pulmonary sarcoidosis: Typical and atypical manifestations at high-resolution CT with pathologic correlation. *RadioGraphics.* 2010;30(6):1567–1586.

Kazerooni E. Perspective: High-resolution CT of the lungs. *AJR Am J Roentgenol.* 2001;177:501–518.

Rossi SE, Franquet T, Volpacchio M, et al. Tree-in-bud pattern at thin-section CT of the lungs: Radiologic–pathologic overview. *RadioGraphics.* 2005;25(3):789–801.

CHAPTER 76

Sarcoidosis

Juliana Bueno

Definition

Sarcoidosis is a systemic disease characterized by noncaseating epithelioid cell granulomas. Although its pathogenesis is unclear, it is most likely multifactorial and possibly related to an immune response triggered by antigen(s) in susceptible individuals, with consequent development of a chronic inflammatory reaction that leads to granuloma formation.

Clinical Features

Patients with sarcoidosis are frequently asymptomatic and may be diagnosed incidentally on imaging. Initial clinical manifestations in symptomatic patients usually occur in mid adulthood (<40 years). Systemic symptoms are nonspecific, including low-grade fever, fatigue, musculoskeletal symptoms, and weight loss. Commonly affected organs, such as the skin, lungs, and eyes, are responsible for most clinical manifestations, including erythema nodosum, chronic cough, nonspecific respiratory symptoms, diplopia, and uveitis. Women are slightly more frequently affected.

European countries have the highest incidence rates of sarcoidosis (~5–25 cases/100,000 persons). The incidence of sarcoidosis in African Americans is 3.5 times higher, and these patients present later in life with more severe disease.

Anatomy and Physiology

The histologic hallmark of sarcoidosis is the noncaseating granuloma, which is composed of a core of inflammatory cells such as histiocytes, epithelioid cells, and multinucleated giant cells surrounded by lymphocytes, fibroblasts, and collagen. Granulomas result from type IV or cell-mediated immunity. Over time, they may spontaneously resolve, persist for years, or evolve to interstitial fibrosis in up to 25% of patients.

The distribution of granulomas in the lungs is characteristic and correlates with imaging findings. Non-necrotizing granulomas predominantly involve the pulmonary lymphatics in the axial and peripheral interstitium, and they are characteristically found along bronchovascular bundles, interlobular septa, and in the subpleural region. This pattern of involvement is also known as perilymphatic distribution of the disease.

How to Approach the Image

In the appropriate clinical setting, the presence of bilateral hilar and right paratracheal lymphadenopathy should suggest the diagnosis. However, sarcoidosis is a diagnosis of exclusion that warrants pathological confirmation in all cases.

Screening for sarcoidosis with chest radiography has a high yield because most patients exhibit chest radiographic abnormalities, typically symmetric bilateral hilar lymphadenopathy. However, chest radiographs are normal in up to 10% of cases at presentation.

What Not to Miss

- Bilateral hilar and right paratracheal lymphadenopathy (i.e., Garland triad) should raise the suspicion of sarcoidosis, particularly in young patients.
- The absence of chest radiographic abnormalities does not exclude sarcoidosis.
- Thin-section chest CT is the imaging modality of choice for demonstrating perilymphatic pulmonary micronodules characteristic of sarcoidosis.

Differential Diagnosis

- The diagnosis of sarcoidosis is made on the basis of clinical, imaging, and histologic findings after exclusion of more common causes of granulomatous disease, such as tuberculosis, fungal infection, berylliosis, hypersensitivity pneumonitis, and Crohn disease.
- Bilateral hilar and mediastinal lymphadenopathy may be seen in tuberculosis, fungal infection, lymphoma, and metastatic disease.
- Parenchymal sarcoidosis may mimic lymphangitic carcinomatosis with subpleural, interlobular, peribronchovascular, and centrilobular nodularity.
- Sarcoid-like reactions may occur secondary to drugs or neoplasms and must also be considered.
- Irreversible perihilar fibrosis and architectural distortion may resemble tuberculosis, chronic hypersensitivity pneumonitis, or progressive massive fibrosis from silicosis.

Imaging Findings

The Siltzbach classification is based on chest radiographic manifestations of sarcoidosis and has prognostic implications:

- Stage 0 (5–10% of cases): Normal chest radiograph.
- Stage I (50% of cases) (Fig. 76.1): Bilateral, symmetric hilar lymphadenopathy, often with mediastinal lymphadenopathy, typically affecting right paratracheal, aortopulmonary window, and subcarinal nodal stations. The *Garland triad* refers to bilateral hilar and right paratracheal lymphadenopathy. Affected lymph nodes may exhibit amorphous, "eggshell" and "icing sugar" calcifications.
- Stage II (25–30% of cases): Hilar/mediastinal lymphadenopathy associated with parenchymal disease.
- Stage III (10% of cases): Lung parenchymal involvement only.
- Stage IV (<5% of cases at presentation): Advanced pulmonary fibrosis is the end result in almost 25% of cases.

The following are radiographic findings of parenchymal sarcoidosis:

- Mid and upper lung zone reticular/nodular opacities.
- Coalescent micronodules may manifest as pulmonary nodules and masses with or without air bronchograms.
- Fibrosis with architectural distortion, volume loss, and cystic bronchiectasis or bullous/honeycomb changes.
- Upper lobe cystic changes/cavitation with dependent nodular soft tissue representing saprophytic aspergillosis or mycetoma formation.

Thin-section chest CT and high-resolution CT play an important role in the diagnosis of sarcoidosis, particularly for subtle abnormalities and in the identification of fibrosis:

- 1- to 4-mm nodules with perilymphatic distribution (i.e., along peribronchovascular, interlobular, and subpleural interstitium); centrilobular micronodules and beaded peribronchovascular bundles, septal lines, fissures, and subpleural regions (Fig. 76.2).
- Coalescent micronodules may manifest as larger nodules and nodular consolidations with or without air bronchogram (i.e., "nummular" or alveolar sarcoidosis) (Fig. 76.3); the "sarcoid galaxy sign" refers to a large nodule or mass with peripheral micronodules (Fig. 76.4).
- Airway involvement may manifest with mosaic attenuation and expiratory air trapping (Fig. 76.5).
- Fibrosis manifests as upper lobe predominant peribronchovascular reticulation, honeycombing, and architectural distortion (Fig. 76.6).
- Fibrosis may also manifest with coalescent perihilar mass-like opacities often associated with calcification and posterior hilar displacement; these may

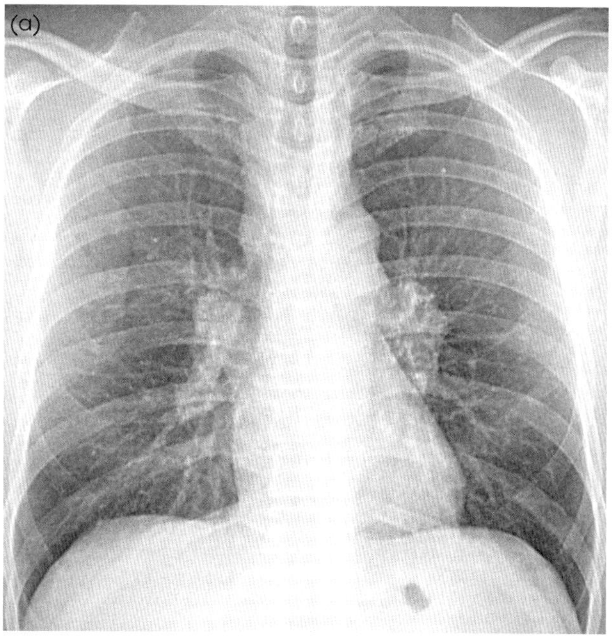

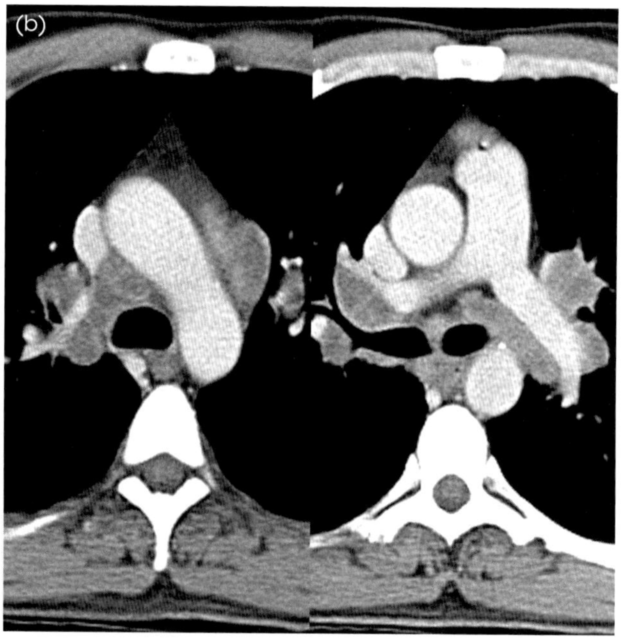

Figure 76.1. Stage I sarcoidosis. (a) Posteroanterior (PA) chest radiograph of a 39-year-old man with chronic cough shows bilateral hilar, paratracheal, and anteroposterior (AP) window lymphadenopathy. (b) Composite image from a contrast-enhanced chest CT shows symmetric bilateral hilar and mediastinal lymphadenopathy.

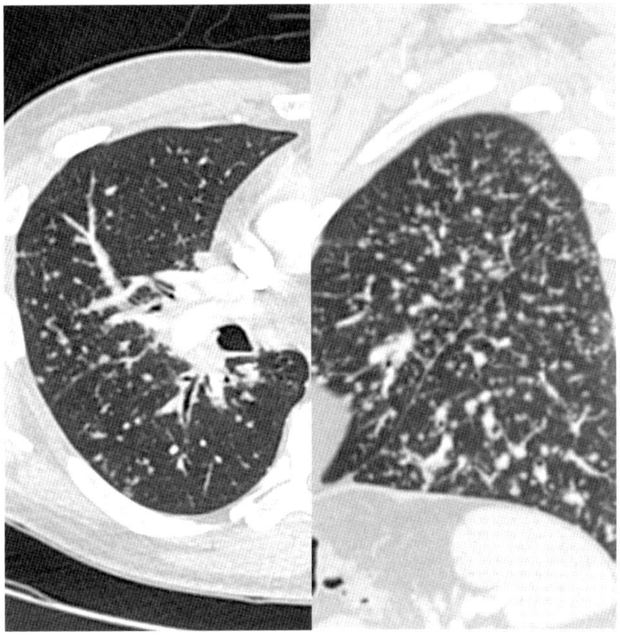

Figure 76.2. Parenchymal sarcoidosis with perilymphatic micronodules. Composite image with axial (left) and sagittal (right) unenhanced chest CT of a 37-year-old woman with sarcoidosis shows multifocal perilymphatic micronodules along bronchovascular bundles, subpleural regions, interlobar fissures, and septal lines.

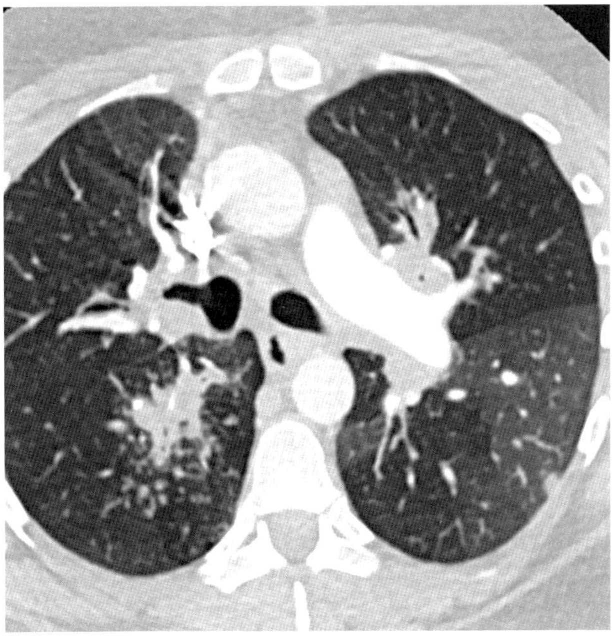

Figure 76.4. Parenchymal sarcoidosis. Chest CT of a young patient with sarcoidosis shows a right lower lobe nodule with spiculated contours and surrounding micronodules, exhibiting the so-called "sarcoid galaxy" sign. Mosaic attenuation is consistent with small airways involvement.

resemble progressive massive fibrosis secondary to pneumoconiosis and are seen in late stages of sarcoidosis (Fig. 76.7). The presence of cavitary disease with intrinsic soft tissue (mycetoma) is not uncommon (Fig. 76.8).

- Stenosis of the large airways may occasionally occur (Fig. 76.9).

Sarcoidosis in any of its forms exhibits intense FDG uptake on FDG PET. This is a common pitfall in patients with malignancy and subclinical sarcoidosis.

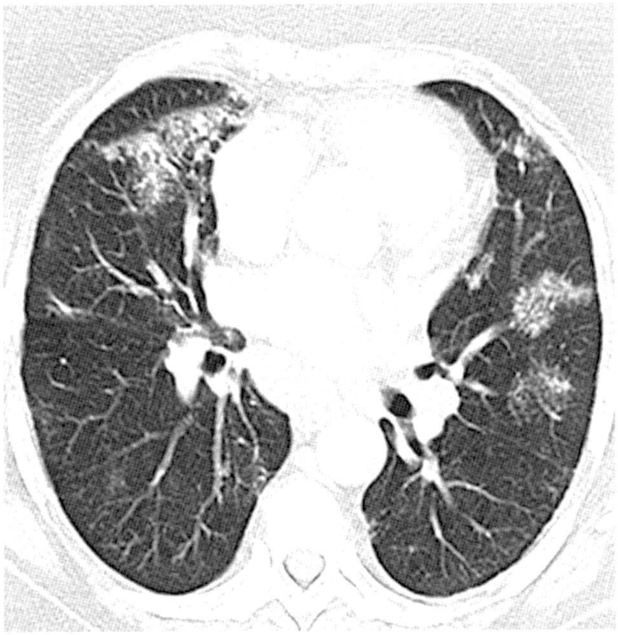

Figure 76.3. Parenchymal sarcoidosis with coalescent nodules. Chest CT of a 53-year-old woman with chronic cough shows coalescent nodular consolidations also known as "nummular" or alveolar sarcoidosis.

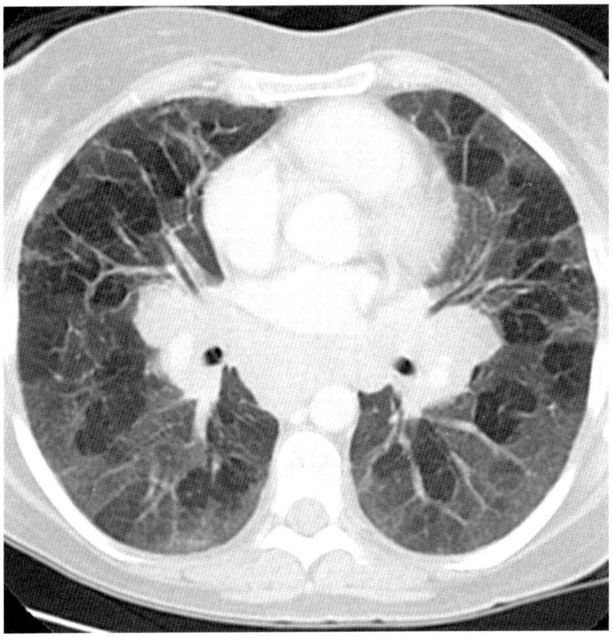

Figure 76.5. Small airway compromise in sarcoidosis. Contrast-enhanced chest CT of a 41-year-old woman with sarcoidosis shows diffuse bilateral mosaic attenuation and symmetric bilateral hilar and subcarinal lymphadenopathy.

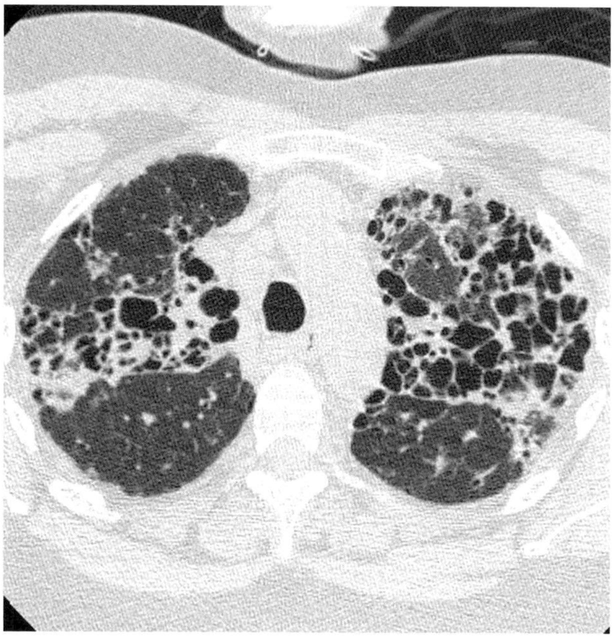

Figure 76.6. Sarcoidosis with end-stage fibrosis. Unenhanced chest CT of a 57-year-old woman with sarcoidosis shows symmetric upper lobe architectural distortion and honeycombing with associated traction bronchiectasis.

Clinical Issues

- Suggestive and even classic imaging findings of sarcoidosis warrant pathologic confirmation.
- Initial radiographic staging has prognostic implications. For example, up to 60–90% of patients in stage I sarcoidosis have spontaneous disease resolution, as opposed to 10–30% of patients with stage III sarcoidosis.
- Other diseases may exhibit histologic noncaseating granulomas and must be excluded before a final diagnosis of sarcoidosis is established.

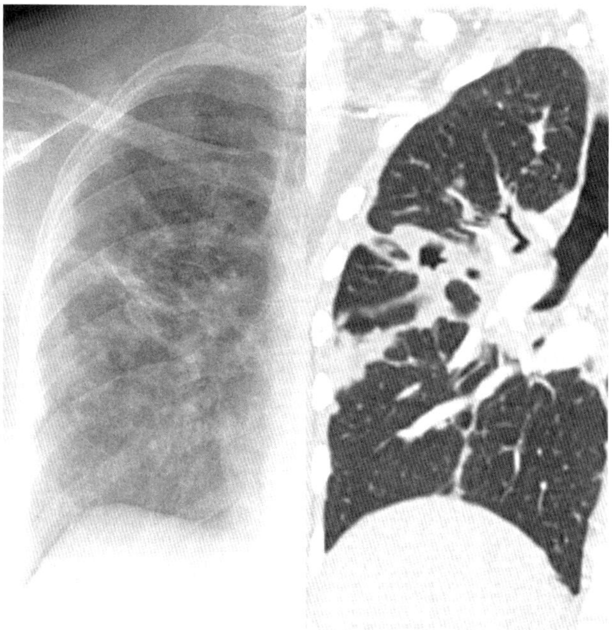

Figure 76.7. Stage IV sarcoidosis. Composite image with posteroanterior chest radiograph (left) and coronal contrast-enhanced CT (right) of a 43-year-old patient with hemoptysis shows perihilar reticular opacities and architectural distortion (left). Chest CT shows perihilar nodular fibrosis and a small, thick-walled right upper lobe cavity.

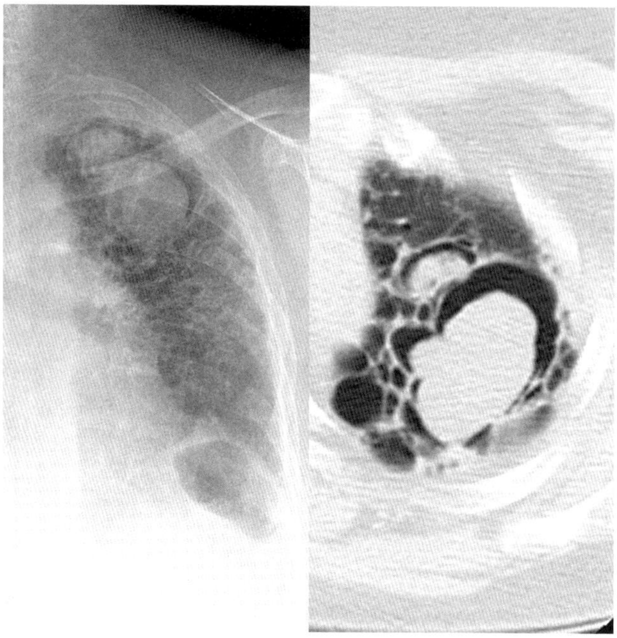

Figure 76.8. Stage IV sarcoidosis with mycetoma. Composite image with AP chest radiograph (left) and unenhanced chest CT (right) of a patient with end-stage sarcoidosis shows volume loss, diffuse reticular opacities, and a left upper lobe thin-walled cavity with dependent nodular soft tissue and a crescentic lucency superiorly. Chest CT confirms mycetoma formation within upper lobe cavities.

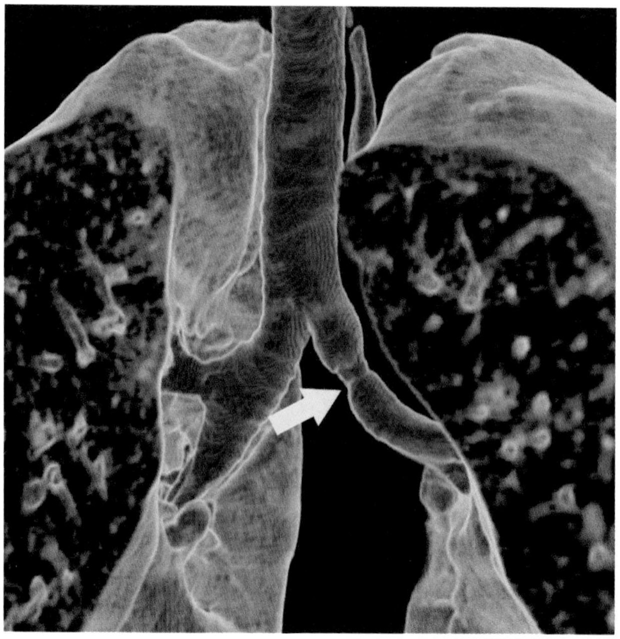

Figure 76.9. Large airway compromise in sarcoidosis. Volume-rendered coronal reformatted chest CT of a woman with known sarcoidosis shows a short segmental stenosis of the proximal left main stem bronchus (arrow).

Key Points

- The radiologist plays an important role in the initial diagnosis, staging, and follow-up of patients with sarcoidosis.
- Radiologic staging and characterization of imaging abnormalities may impact patient prognosis and guide management.
- Given nonspecific clinical manifestations, imaging findings are important in the diagnostic evaluation of patients with sarcoidosis. Definitive diagnosis warrants pathologic confirmation and exclusion of other diseases.
- On chest radiography, the presence of bilateral hilar and right paratracheal lymphadenopathy, particularly in an asymptomatic patient, should raise the possibility of sarcoidosis.
- On CT, recognition of characteristic perilymphatic distribution of parenchymal abnormalities in the appropriate clinical context is highly specific for sarcoidosis.

Suggested Reading

Al-Jahdali H, Rajiah P, Koteyar SS, Allen C, Khan AN. Atypical radiological manifestations of thoracic sarcoidosis: A review and pictorial essay. *Ann Thorac Med.* 2013 Oct;8(4):186–196.

Criado E, Sánchez M, Ramírez J, et al. Pulmonary sarcoidosis: Typical and atypical manifestations at high-resolution CT with pathologic correlation. *RadioGraphics.* 2010 Oct;30(6): 1567–1586.

Koyama T, Ueda H, Togashi K, et al. Radiologic manifestations of sarcoidosis in various organs. *RadioGraphics.* 2004;24(1): 87–104.

Section XV

Idiopathic Interstitial Pneumonias

CHAPTER 77

Idiopathic Interstitial Pneumonias

Sanjeev Bhalla

Introduction

The idiopathic interstitial pneumonias (IIPs) are a group of diffuse lung diseases that often manifest clinically with increasing dyspnea and hypoxemia. They may progress to fibrosis and in certain cases may lead to death. The advent of high-resolution CT (HRCT) and improved correlation with pathologic and clinical parameters have resulted in a better understanding of these often confusing entities. Over the past decade, diagnosis of these conditions has evolved from a purely histologic assessment to a multidisciplinary approach, relying on HRCT pattern, clinical history and physical examination, and, if performed, biopsy analysis. The multidisciplinary approach gained acceptance as a result of an American Thoracic Society/European Respiratory Society (ATS/ERS) statement in 2002. A 2013 revision of the ATS/ERS statement has built on this foundation.

Diseases Included in the Category of Idiopathic Interstitial Pneumonia

In the most recent revision of the ATS/ERS statement on IIPs, the conditions have been divided into the following three categories based on radiologic findings:

- Major IIPs: Idiopathic pulmonary fibrosis (IPF)/idiopathic usual interstitial pneumonia (UIP), idiopathic nonspecific interstitial pneumonia (NSIP), respiratory bronchiolitis–interstitial lung disease (RB-ILD), desquamative interstitial pneumonia (DIP), cryptogenic organizing pneumonia (COP), acute interstitial pneumonia (AIP)
- Rare IIPs: Idiopathic lymphoid interstitial pneumonia, idiopathic pleuroparenchymal fibroelastosis
- Unclassifiable IIPs

Although some of these patterns may be seen with other conditions (e.g., NSIP with collagen vascular disease), the term IIP refers to only the idiopathic variants. Interestingly, the smoking-related conditions (RB-ILD and DIP) are included in this idiopathic grouping despite their association with cigarette use. A fourth category of conditions with rare histologic findings was also included in the 2013 ATS/ERS statement on IIPs; it includes acute fibrinous and organizing pneumonia and interstitial pneumonias with a bronchiolocentric distribution.

The 2013 ATS/ERS statement on IIP also proposed dividing the major IIPs into three groups: chronic fibrosing conditions (IPF/UIP and NSIP), smoking-related conditions (RB-ILD and DIP), and acute/subacute IIPs (COP and AIP).

Approach to the Idiopathic Interstitial Pneumonias

The final diagnosis of an IIP rests on correlation of the HRCT findings with the clinical history and pathology (if tissue sampling has been performed). Unfortunately, as radiologists, we are not given the luxury of knowing whether the diffuse disease is truly an IIP. One helpful approach with all diffuse lung disease is the DALPO method (*d*emographic of the patient, *a*cuity of the condition, *l*ocation of the findings, *p*attern on HRCT, *o*ther findings including pleural effusion and lymphadenopathy). By evaluating these components, one can avoid confusing an acute condition such as pulmonary edema superimposed on emphysema with an IIP.

One key component of the DALPO approach is the pattern on HRCT. Generally, UIP should be diagnosed when honeycombing is present (Fig. 77.1). NSIP should have areas of reticulation (interlobular septal thickening and intralobular lines), whereas DIP should manifest with ground-glass opacities. RB-ILD is characterized by centrilobular ground-glass nodules. The use of the dominant pattern is important but should be only part of the process. Both sarcoidosis and UIP, for example, may produce honeycombing, but upper lobe predominant honeycombing in a young patient with mediastinal lymphadenopathy and splenic lesions should suggest the diagnosis of sarcoidosis.

Differential Diagnosis for the Idiopathic Interstitial Pneumonias

The diagnosis of an IIP should be based on correlation of the HRCT pattern with the clinical history and biopsy (when performed). In many instances, the radiologist has access to only the HRCT. For this reason, the radiologic report should include the predominant findings and

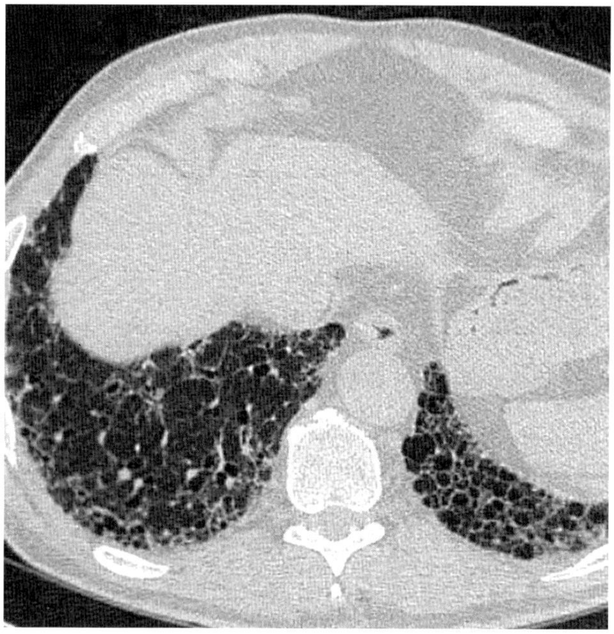

Figure 77.1. UIP. HRCT of a 65-year-old man with chronic progressive dyspnea (in the absence of collagen vascular disease or exposure to allergens) shows classic findings of basilar subpleural honeycombing. In such cases, the diagnosis of UIP/IPF can be made, and biopsy confirmation is not required.

conclude with the term *pattern*. Basilar honeycombing in a 60-year-old man might be interpreted as UIP pattern, but a history of rheumatoid arthritis should suggest the diagnosis of rheumatoid lung (not IPF). The differential diagnosis of UIP includes chronic hypersensitivity (which may exhibit upper lobe honeycombing and/or associated air trapping), collagen vascular disease (usually rheumatoid arthritis), and asbestosis (which may be associated with pleural plaques). The HRCT report in cases of idiopathic UIP should include the level of certainty or confidence in the diagnosis based on basilar honeycombing and absence of ground-glass opacity, nodules, and air trapping. The three recommended levels of certainty are inconsistent with UIP, possible UIP, and UIP. In patients with HRCT findings of UIP and a consistent history, biopsy will not be performed.

For idiopathic NSIP, the main differential diagnosis consists of collagen vascular disease (usually scleroderma or an inflammatory myopathy), subacute hypersensitivity pneumonitis (which may exhibit air trapping), and drug toxicity (Fig. 77.2). Ground-glass opacities in DIP may mimic pneumonia (most notably pneumocystis pneumonia) and drug reaction (Fig. 77.3). RB-ILD centrilobular nodules may mimic findings of subacute hypersensitivity. A history of smoking will be helpful in favoring the former condition over the latter.

Organizing pneumonia may be seen in a variety of conditions, including chronic eosinophilic pneumonia, neoplasm, infection, and vasculitis (Fig. 77.4). Before labeling it as *cryptogenic*, these other conditions must be excluded. For this reason, the term *COP* should be avoided in a radiology report because only the treating physician will truly know if all potential etiologies have been excluded.

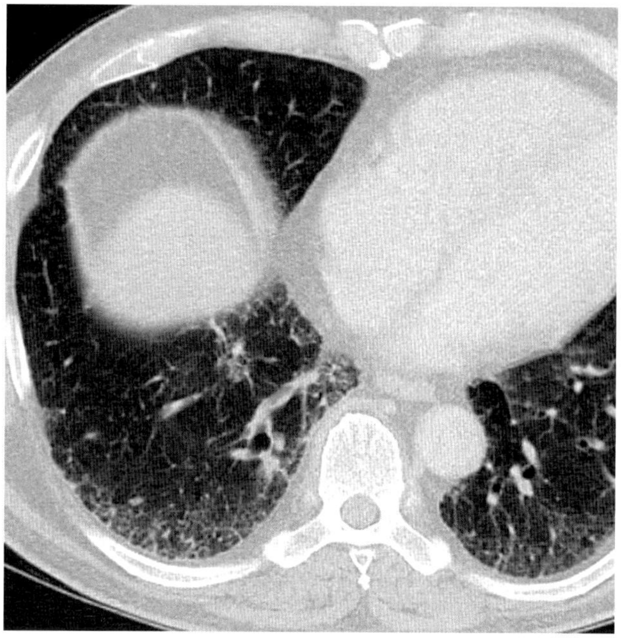

Figure 77.2. NSIP. HRCT of a 54-year-old man with a 2-year history of mild dyspnea shows basilar subpleural reticulations with interlobular septal thickening and intralobular lines with minimal ground-glass opacity in the absence of honeycombing that suggest NSIP. The patient was later diagnosed with dermatomyositis. When an HRCT NSIP pattern is found, collagen vascular disease, hypersensitivity, and drug toxicity should be excluded.

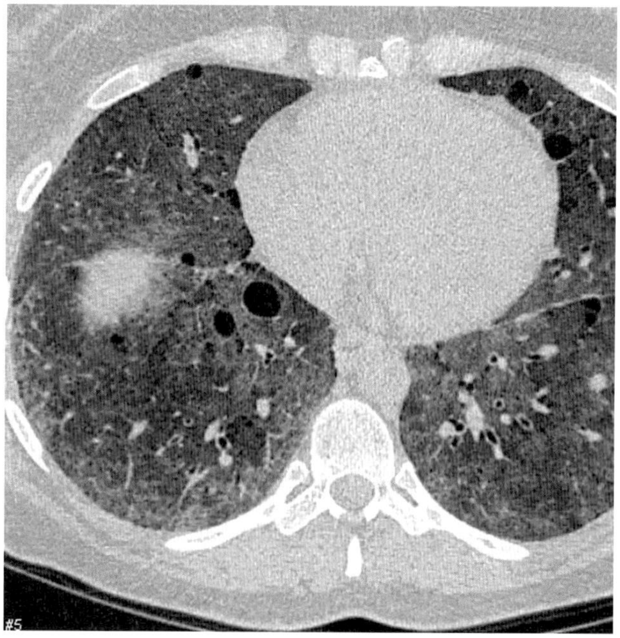

Figure 77.3. DIP. HRCT of a 38-year-old woman with a long history of cigarette smoking shows extensive ground-glass opacities with a few cysts and no honeycombing, typical of DIP.

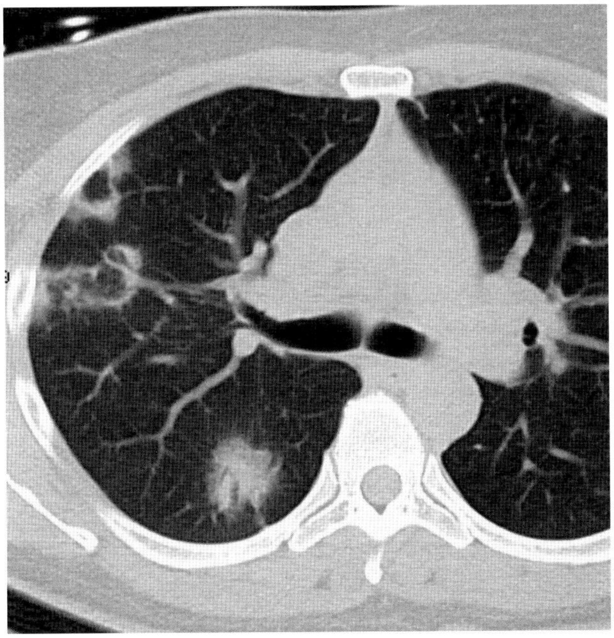

Figure 77.4. Organizing pneumonia. Thin-section CT of a 29-year-old woman with systemic lupus erythematosus shows nodular consolidations with central low attenuation (reverse halo). Biopsy showed organizing pneumonia. Given her associated collagen vascular disease, the term *cryptogenic (COP)* is not applicable.

Suggested Reading

Hobbs S, Lynch D. The idiopathic interstitial pneumonias: An update and review. *Radiol Clin North Am*. 2014 Jan;52(1):105–120.

Lynch DA, Travis WD, Müller NL, Galvin JR, Hansell DM, Grenier PA, et al. Idiopathic interstitial pneumonias: CT features. *Radiology*. 2005 Jul;236(1):10–21.

CHAPTER 78

Idiopathic Pulmonary Fibrosis

Cylen Javidan-Nejad

Definition

Idiopathic pulmonary fibrosis (IPF) is a clinical syndrome of unknown cause in which chronic progressive pulmonary fibrosis leads to severe debilitation and death. The histopathology of IPF is usual interstitial pneumonia (UIP). IPF/UIP is the most common idiopathic interstitial pneumonia, with an overall prevalence of 15–40/100,000 persons. Cryptogenic fibrosing alveolitis is a former term for UIP that is no longer favored.

Clinical Features

IPF is more common in men, and affected patients rarely present before age 50 years. The risk for IPF increases with cigarette smoking and chronic aspiration. The onset is insidious, and worsening dry cough and dyspnea are the most common symptoms. Weight loss and fatigue are also common. Physical exam reveals Velcro-like inspiratory crackles, and there is a restrictive pattern on spirometry. The median survival of patients with UIP/IPF is 3 years. Management consists of oxygen supplementation, administration of cytotoxic agents such as azathioprine on a trial basis, and, possibly, bilateral lung transplantation. Enrollment in one of the many treatment trials requires a confident diagnosis of UIP by the radiologist. Acute exacerbation of fibrosis and accelerated fibrosis are less common courses of IPF in which there are spurts of rapid deterioration of pulmonary function. Affected patients are very ill and have systemic symptoms. This rapid decline is frequently preceded by a viral infection with a prodromal period of 1 or 2 months. Treatment consists of mechanical ventilation and intravenous corticosteroids. In-hospital mortality rate approximates 50%.

Diagnosis of IPF/UIP is made by a multidisciplinary approach using a combination of typical clinical manifestations and a confident diagnosis of UIP pattern on CT, usually forgoing surgical biopsy. Pathologic diagnosis is reserved for patients in whom CT suggests a different chronic interstitial lung disease as the cause of fibrosis or if the diagnosis is suggestive but not confident for a UIP pattern.

Anatomy and Physiology

The hallmark of UIP is deposition of an extracellular matrix of collagen by clusters of fibroblasts and myofibroblasts (fibrogenic foci) in the lung interstitium (Fig. 78.1). It is associated with inflammation and honeycombing. Honeycomb cysts are enlarged airspaces surrounded by fibrosis and lined by hyperplastic alveolar epithelium. They measure from several millimeters to greater than 1 cm in diameter.

A key histologic feature of UIP is the presence of both temporal and spatial heterogeneity. Temporal heterogeneity refers to fibrosis of various ages in the same pathologic specimen. Fibrogenic foci that occur at the leading edge of fibrosis are indicative of younger fibrosis. Collagen deposition and interstitial thickening by cellular infiltration suggest intermediate fibrosis. Honeycombing with architectural distortion and traction bronchiectasis denote advanced fibrosis. Spatial heterogeneity is manifested as skipped areas of normal lung parenchyma among patchy or confluent areas of fibrosis. In UIP, the fibrosis typically extends to and abuts the visceral pleura.

How to Approach the Image

Comparison to prior imaging is critical in the assessment of patients with suspected IPF to exclude an acute process mimicking fibrosis. Interstitial edema with Kerley B lines may mimic peripheral reticulations and fibrosis, especially when superimposed on emphysema. Edema may affect relatively normal lung and spare destroyed portions of the secondary pulmonary lobule (emphysema), thus mimicking IPF. Early findings of pulmonary fibrosis are best detected in the lung bases. Superimposed reticulations and honeycomb cyst walls in severe disease may create the appearance of basilar tiny nodules or confluent opacification (Fig. 78.2).

The main goal of high-resolution CT (HRCT) evaluation of patients with suspected IPF is to establish or exclude UIP. Honeycombing with subpleural and basilar predominance is the strongest indicator of UIP. Because IPF/UIP is a multidisciplinary diagnosis, CT reporting should use the phrase "UIP pattern" rather than providing a diagnosis of UIP. Based on CT features, patients should be placed in one of the following three categories:

UIP pattern—all four features present

1. Predominant subpleural and basilar distribution
2. Honeycombing, with or without traction bronchiectasis or architectural distortion

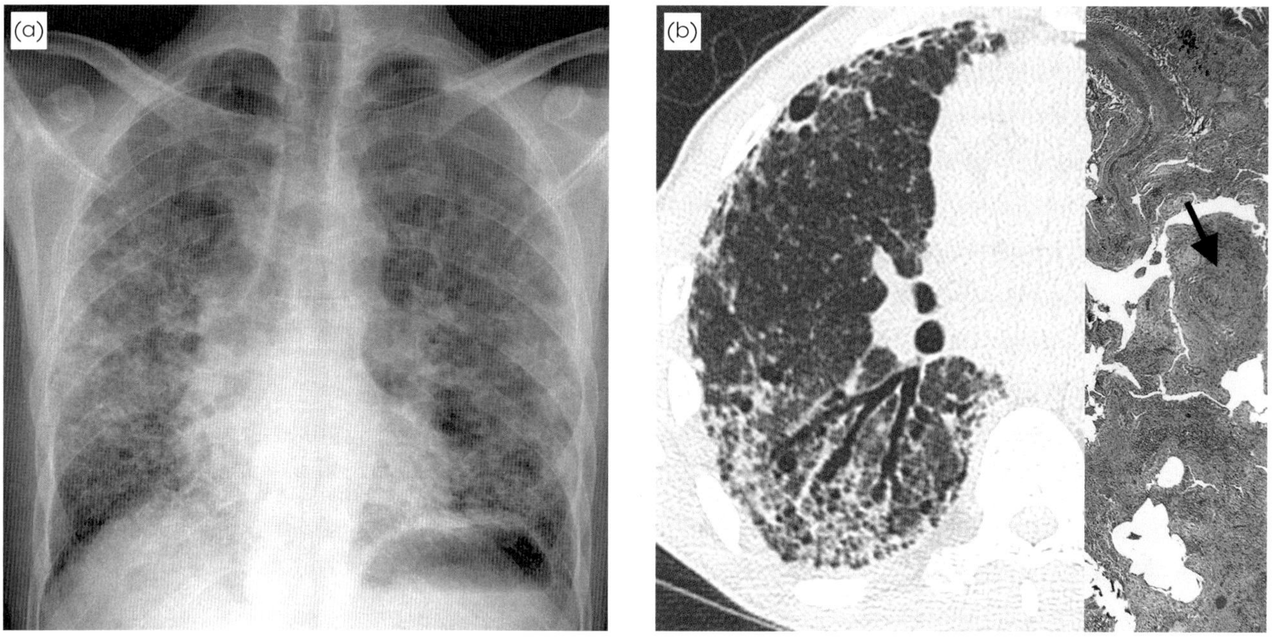

Figure 78.1. UIP pattern. (a) Posteroanterior chest radiograph of a 46-year-old man with an 8-month history of dry cough and progressive dyspnea on exertion shows basilar predominant bilateral coarse interstitial opacities. (b) Composite image with HRCT (left) and photomicrograph (right) subpleural reticulations, honeycombing, architectural distortion, and traction bronchiectasis that correlates with extensive collagen deposition, inflammation, and lung destruction by honeycombing on histopathology. Note the fibrogenic foci along the leading edge of fibrosis (arrow).

3. Reticulations and thickened interlobular septa
4. Absence of features inconsistent with UIP pattern

- A confident diagnosis by an experienced radiologist has a positive predictive value of 95% for UIP.
- Surgical biopsy is not required to establish diagnosis.

Possible UIP pattern—all three features present

1. Predominant subpleural and basilar distribution
2. Reticulations and thickened interlobular septa
3. Absence of features inconsistent with UIP pattern

- Wedge biopsy may be performed to establish diagnosis.

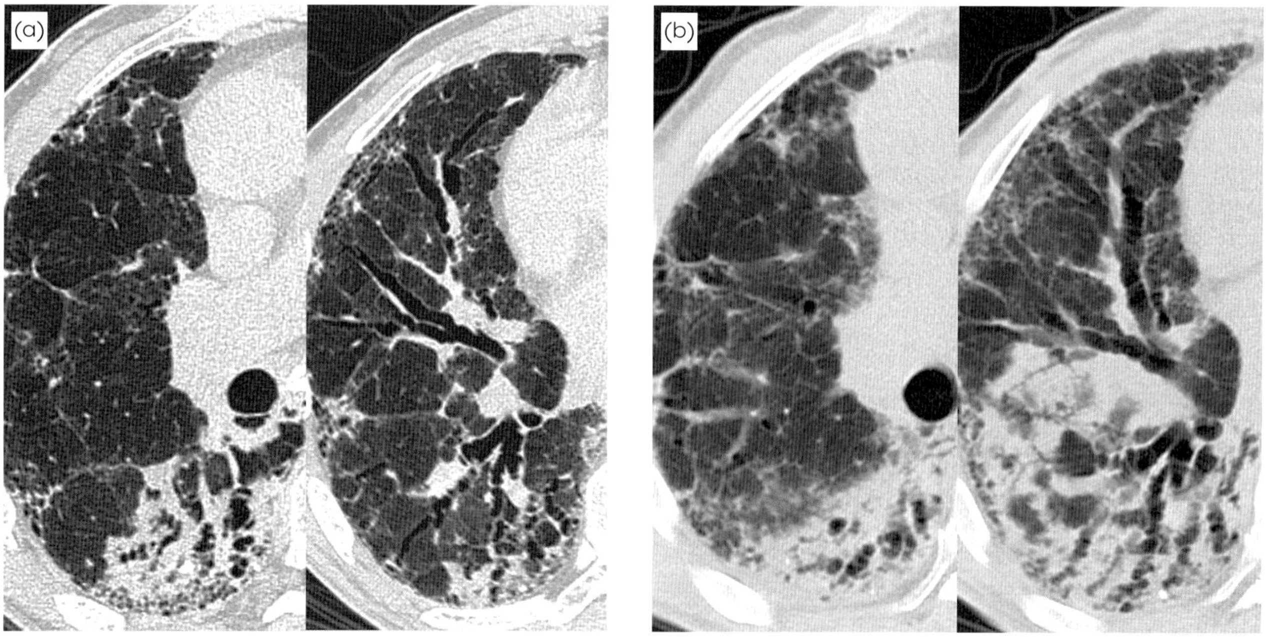

Figure 78.2. Progressive IPF/UIP. (a) Composite image with HRCT of a 65-year-old man with known IPF and respiratory decline after failing immunotherapy shows bilateral peripheral subpleural honeycombing with irregular nodular consolidations with intrinsic traction bronchiectasis indicating fibrosis. (b) Follow-up composite image with HRCT of the same patient performed 10 months later shows progressive lower lobe fibrosis with increasing large confluent consolidative fibrosis with increasing traction bronchiectasis. Pneumonia, chronic aspiration, and lung cancer should be excluded in such cases.

Inconsistent with UIP—any of the following seven features present

1. Upper or mid lung predominance
2. A predominantly peribronchovascular distribution
3. Extensive ground-glass opacities, out of proportion to the reticular opacities
4. Diffuse micronodules, especially when bilateral and upper lobe predominant
5. Discrete cysts separate from the honeycombing
6. Mosaic attenuation due to air trapping
7. Consolidations

- CT suggests an alternative cause for fibrosis, such as sarcoidosis, hypersensitivity pneumonitis, and desquamative interstitial pneumonia. The alternative diagnosis should be suggested in the CT report.
- Biopsy (commonly transbronchial) is required to establish or confirm the diagnosis.

What Not to Miss

Lung cancer has a higher incidence in UIP. Diagnosis can be a challenge because of the potential for severe architectural distortion. Care must be taken to assess for nodules and, on follow-up imaging, any growth. Another potentially lethal finding is an accelerated phase of fibrosis that may manifest with areas of confluent ground glass or consolidation (Figs. 78.3 and 78.4). Finally, an acute change should be placed into context because a community-acquired pneumonia can easily be overlooked in the setting of diffuse lung disease.

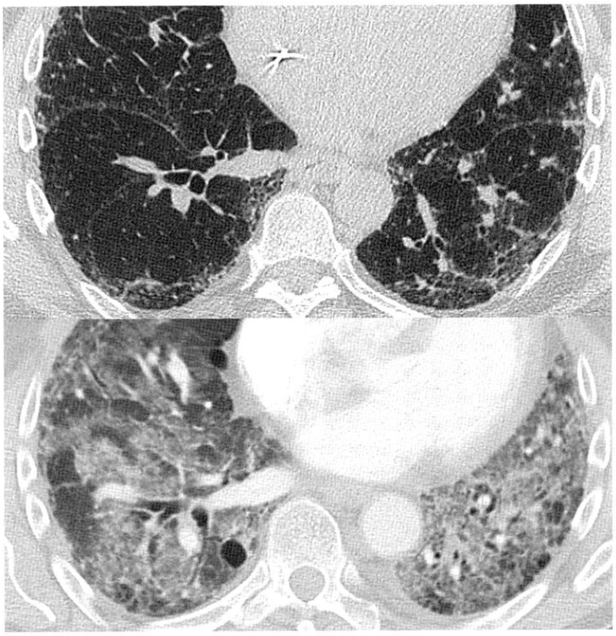

Figure 78.3. Acute exacerbation of pulmonary fibrosis. Composite image with HRCT of a patient with IPF (top) and 2 years later (bottom) after the patient was admitted with severe dyspnea, deterioration of oxygenation, fever, chills, and nasal congestion shows progression from basilar predominant subpleural reticulation (top) to new confluent ground-glass opacities superimposed on preexisting fibrosis (bottom). Extensive clinical workup for infection was negative.

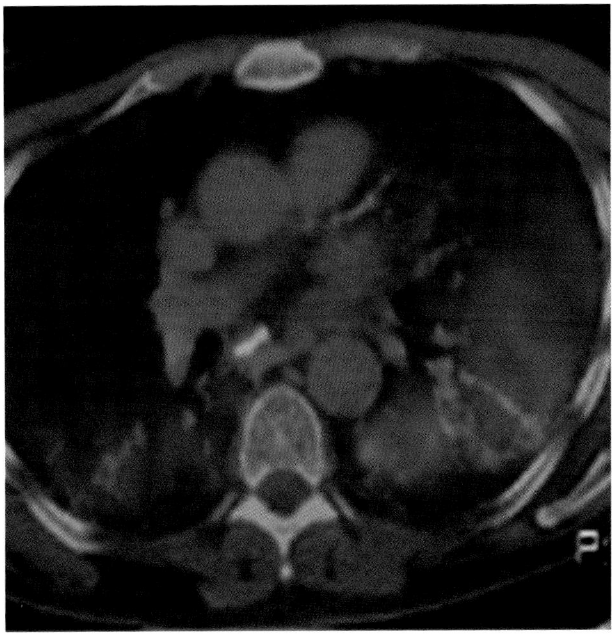

Figure 78.4. Acute exacerbation of IPF. Fused FDG PET of a patient with known IPF and new progressive dyspnea and clinical deterioration shows extensive FDG uptake by the affected lung parenchyma.

Differential Diagnosis

Honeycombing can be seen with end-stage fibrosis of various causes. In addition, UIP is not always idiopathic. Other causes of UIP include drug toxicities (bleomycin, nitrofurantoin, and amiodarone), asbestosis, chronic hypersensitivity pneumonitis, and connective tissue diseases, especially rheumatoid arthritis. The diagnosis of IPF must be made after exclusion of these entities.

Imaging Findings

IPF/UIP

- On radiography, UIP presents as a basilar and peripheral interstitial process with small lung volumes. Often, the trachea will appear large from the traction and will buckle. Diagnosis can be suggested on radiography but must be confirmed on HRCT.
- HRCT findings
  - Honeycombing manifests as multiple rows of small cysts.
  - Subpleural reticulations and irregular septal thickening.
  - Beaded dilation of the bronchi and bronchioles in areas of fibrosis representing traction bronchiectasis and indicative of advanced fibrosis.
  - Ground-glass opacification is absent or minimal.

- Skipped areas of involvement correlate with spatial heterogeneity of disease.
- Progression of severity and extent of fibrosis on serial CT imaging is typical with gradual increase of honeycomb cyst size and progression of volume loss. Disease progresses from the periphery toward the central parenchyma and in a cephalad direction.

- The accelerated phase of UIP/IPF may present with increased areas of ground glass that correspond to areas of alveolar damage. These may have increased uptake on FDG PET (Fig. 78.4).

Asbestosis

- Peripheral reticulations, subpleural bands, and sometimes honeycombing with subpleural and basilar predominance
- Bilateral calcified or noncalcified pleural plaques consistent with asbestos exposure; should suggest asbestosis as the cause of fibrosis

Rheumatoid Arthritis

- CT findings identical to IPF/UIP

Chronic Hypersensitivity Pneumonitis

- Early fibrosis, reticulation, and honeycombing in hypersensitivity pneumonitis (HP) begin about the bronchovascular bundles, but chronic HP may exhibit a subpleural predominance very similar to IPF.
- Upper and mid lung predominance or with greater upper lung involvement than expected with IPF/UIP.
- Diffuse mosaic attenuation with extensive air trapping is a key feature of HP.

Familial Interstitial Pneumonia

- When two or more close family members develop IPF, a genetic mutation may be the cause.
- Clinical presentation, CT findings, and pathology are indistinguishable from IPF/UIP. A genetic mutation should be considered when the fibrosis has an equal or upper lobe predominance or when the patient presents at a relatively younger age.
- Various genes have been implicated. The *Muc5B* gene is a common mutation.

Clinical Issues

- Patients with IPF have a marked risk of developing lung cancer, usually in areas of severe fibrosis.
- Combined pulmonary fibrosis and emphysema (CPFE) is defined as emphysema involving greater than 10% of the lung parenchyma, superimposed on IPF/UIP. Spirometry of patients with CPFE reveals a less restrictive pattern and a lower CO_2 diffusion capacity than expected. These patients have higher oxygen requirements and pulmonary arterial pressures than those with pure IPF. However, CPFE does not hasten the fibrotic process.
- The presence of severe pulmonary hypertension is associated with a higher mortality. The presence of pericardial effusion, moderate to severe right ventricle (RV) dysfunction, and RV chamber dilation greater than that of the left ventricle are associated with earlier death in patients with IPF.
- Fibrosis related to rheumatoid arthritis has a slower progression than in IPF and a better prognosis.
- Chronic HP can mimic UIP radiologically, but in 60% of patients an underlying antigen may be uncovered (by history or laboratory testing) to help confirm the diagnosis.

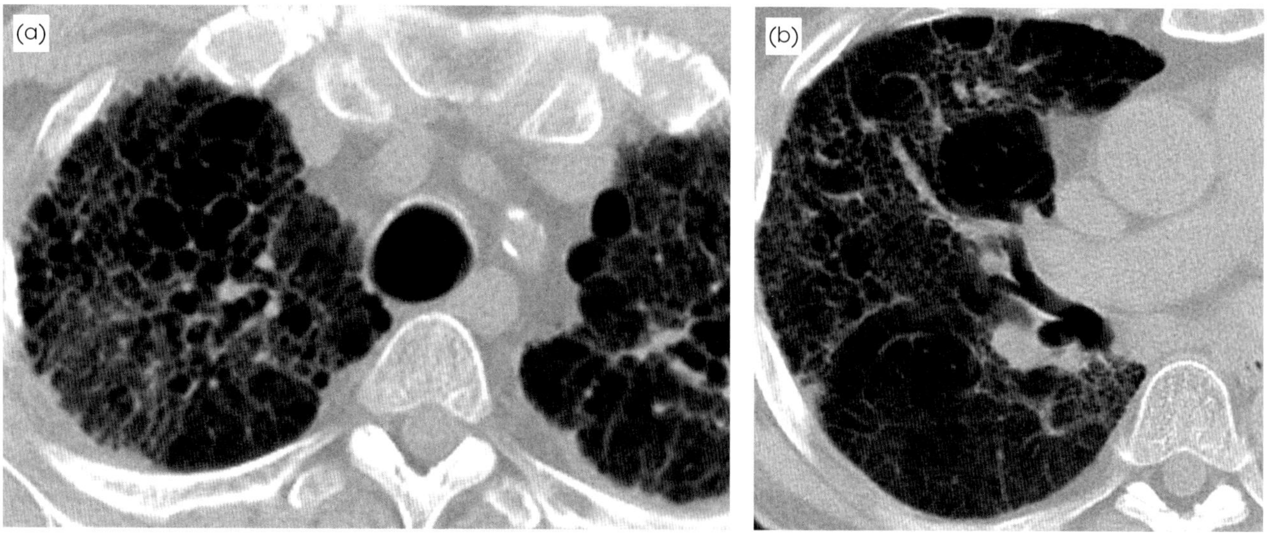

Figure 78.5. Pattern inconsistent with UIP. (a) HRCT of a 63-year-old man with progressive shortness of breath unresponsive to steroid and immunosuppressive therapy shows honeycombing and traction bronchiectasis with an upper lobe predominance. (b) Mosaic attenuation suggestive of air trapping is evident in areas where the fibrosis is not as severe. These findings are inconsistent with a UIP pattern. Biopsy suggested end-stage fibrosis due to hypersensitivity pneumonitis.

Key Points

- Serial imaging with HRCT is used to evaluate progression of disease and response to immunosuppressive therapy. It is also used to identify potential complications, including lung cancer, pulmonary infection, and acute exacerbation of fibrosis.
- A multidisciplinary approach is used to diagnose IPF/UIP. CT reports should include one of the following three categories: UIP pattern, possible UIP pattern, or pattern inconsistent with UIP.
- A CT diagnosis of UIP pattern precludes biopsy. Biopsy is reserved for the other two categories (Fig. 78.5).
- Subpleural and basilar predominant honeycombing is the most reliable CT finding to diagnose IPF/UIP.
- Follow-up imaging in patients with IPF should be interpreted with a high level of suspicion for lung cancer, particularly in areas of advanced fibrosis in which detection may be difficult.

Suggested Reading

Hobbs S, Lynch D. The idiopathic interstitial pneumonias: An update and review. *Radiol Clin North Am.* 2014 Jan;52(1): 105–120.

Meltzer EB, Noble PW. Idiopathic pulmonary fibrosis. *Orphanet J Rare Dis.* 2008 Mar 26;3:8.

Raghu G, Collard HR, Egan JJ, et al.; ATS/ERS/JRS/ALAT Committee on Idiopathic Pulmonary Fibrosis. An official ATS/ERS/JRS/ALAT statement: Idiopathic pulmonary fibrosis: Evidence-based guidelines for diagnosis and management. *Am J Respir Crit Care Med.* 2011 Mar 15;183(6):788–824.

CHAPTER 79

Nonspecific Interstitial Pneumonia

Cylen Javidan-Nejad

Definition

Nonspecific interstitial pneumonia (NSIP) is an idiopathic interstitial pneumonia (IIP) with a clinical presentation similar to that of idiopathic pulmonary fibrosis/usual interstitial pneumonia (IPF/UIP) but with a much better prognosis.

A patient is considered to have idiopathic NSIP when pathology reveals an NSIP pattern, but only after all other conditions associated with NSIP have been excluded, such as collagen vascular disease, drug-induced lung disease (e.g., methotrexate), and hypersensitivity pneumonitis (HP). In these situations, NSIP represents the parenchymal response to the particular insult.

Clinical Features

Patients with idiopathic NSIP usually present between ages 40 and 50 years, typically with insidious onset of dyspnea. Other symptoms include cough, weight loss, fever, and malaise. Physical exam reveals inspiratory bibasilar crackles. Spirometry shows decreased volumes and diminished CO_2 diffusion capacity.

Both systemic corticosteroid and cytotoxic therapy are used to treat NSIP with variable success. In more than 75% of affected patients, the outcome is favorable, with stable or improved disease or even complete resolution. Relapse occasionally occurs. Disease progression despite therapy and death are unusual outcomes. The greater the amount of interstitial fibrosis identified on initial biopsy, the worse the outcome.

Anatomy and Physiology

The main histologic features of NSIP are alveolar wall infiltration by lymphocytes and plasma cells (chronic inflammatory cells) associated with fibrosis (Fig. 79.1). Fibrosis is characteristically of uniform age (temporal homogeneity) without skipped areas of normal lung between the areas of fibrosis (spatial homogeneity).

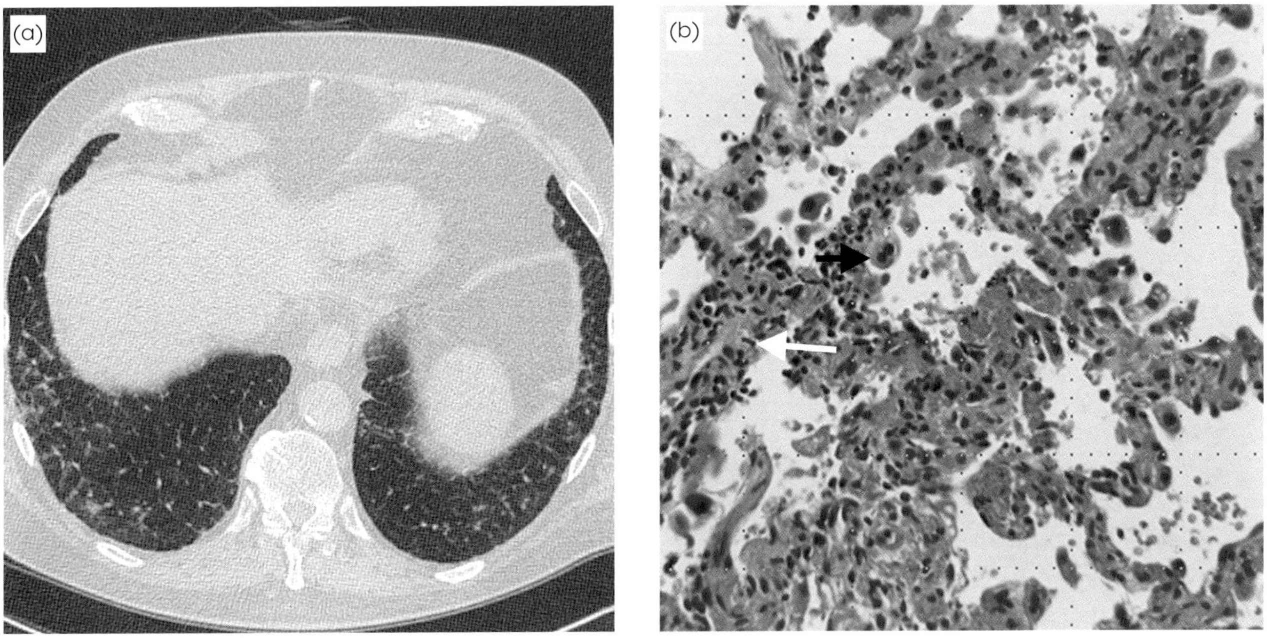

Figure 79.1. Nonspecific interstitial pneumonia. (a) HRCT of a 76-year-old man on long-term medical therapy for paroxysmal atrial fibrillation who had mild basilar crackles on auscultation shows mild bilateral subpleural lower lobe irregular septal thickening that developed since the onset of antiarrhythmogenic therapy. (b) High-power photomicrograph (hematoxylin and eosin stain) shows alveolar septal thickening due to lymphocyte infiltration (white arrow), hyperplasia of type II pneumocytes (black arrow), and the absence of fibroblastic foci.

Relative to UIP, the amount of collagen deposition is less, with few or no honeycomb cysts. Fibrogenic foci are either absent or sparse. Secondary expansion of the airspaces and bronchioles occurs but is less severe than that in UIP.

Two pathologic subtypes have been described—cellular and fibrosing NSIP—based on the relative predominance of chronic inflammation to fibrosis. Most specimens reveal a combination of both types.

Although small clusters of organizing pneumonia (OP) may be seen in NSIP, the amount of OP should not exceed 10% of the abnormal area. Histologic diagnosis requires an open-lung biopsy or video-assisted thoracic surgery biopsy of more than one site. Areas of honeycombing (if present) or end-stage lung should be avoided because these areas rarely help lead to a specific diagnosis.

How to Approach the Image

The current recommended method for diagnosing an IIP is through a multidisciplinary discussion involving the pulmonologist, radiologist, and pathologist. When evaluating the CT or HRCT of a patient with suspected NSIP, the radiologist must strive to differentiate the disease process from UIP and should determine the following:

- Is there a diagnostic or highly suggestive pattern?
  - UIP pattern: Mixed reticulation and honeycombing with basilar predominance with minimal or absent ground-glass opacity
    - Considered diagnostic and no need for pathologic confirmation
  - NSIP pattern: Ground-glass opacity with or without reticulation with basilar predominance (Fig. 79.2)
    - Considered highly suggestive, but pathologic confirmation is required in the absence of a history of collagen vascular disease, HP, or drug therapy associated with fibrosis
- In the absence of a diagnostic or highly suggestive pattern:
  - What is the predominant imaging finding?
    - Ground-glass opacity: Often seen with NSIP, but often a finding of desquamative interstitial pneumonia (DIP) (Fig. 79.3)
    - Reticulation: Common in NSIP
    - Honeycombing: The most reliable indicator of UIP
    - Consolidation: Unlikely in NSIP; occasionally seen in UIP; highly suggestive of a different disease such as OP when it is the predominant finding
  - What is the axial distribution?
    - Peripheral with no subpleural sparing: Either UIP or NSIP
    - Peripheral with subpleural sparing: Suggestive of NSIP
    - Diffuse: More common with NSIP
    - Peribronchovascular (nodular): Not seen with UIP; more likely NSIP, sarcoidosis, or OP (Fig. 79.4)
  - What is the craniocaudal distribution?
    - Downward gradient (worse at the bases): Both UIP and NSIP
    - Upward or equal gradient: Can be seen with NSIP and occasionally UIP

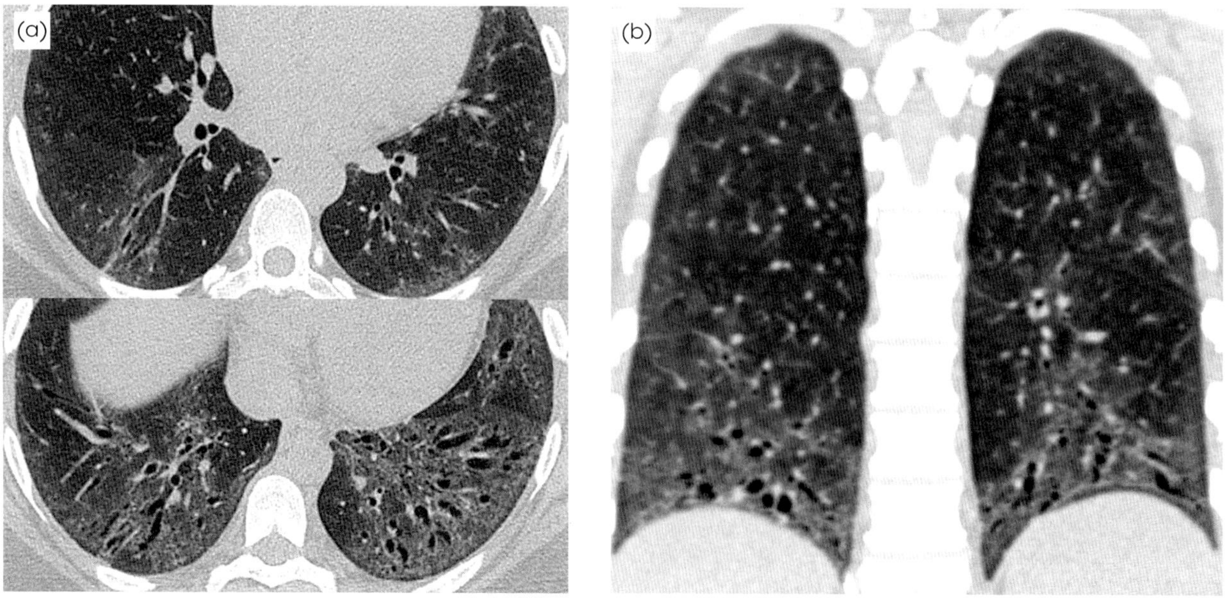

Figure 79.2. NSIP associated with systemic sclerosis. (a) Composite image with HRCT of a 37-year-old woman with chronic dyspnea shows peripheral confluent ground-glass opacities and fine reticulation in both lower lobes with extensive bronchiectasis that is out of proportion to the degree of fibrosis. (b) Coronal reformatted image of the same patient confirms the lower lobe predominance of fibrosis, subpleural sparing, and extensive bronchiectasis.

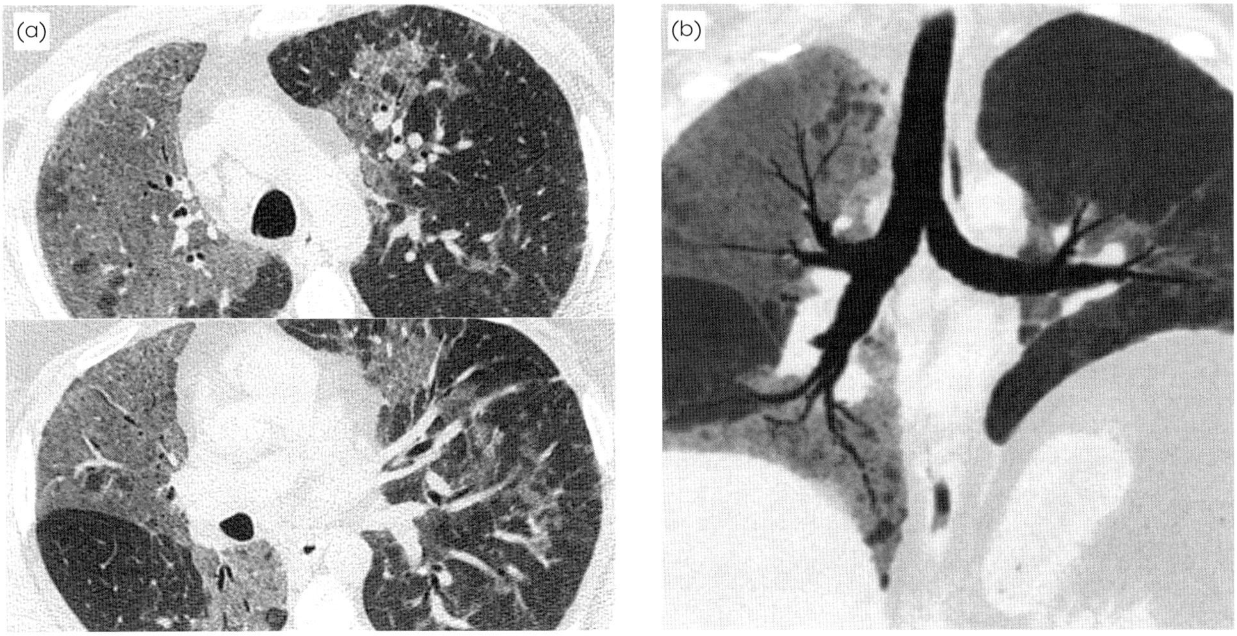

Figure 79.3. DIP. (a) Composite image with HRCT of a 67-year-old heavy smoker with gradual onset of progressive dyspnea shows asymmetric confluent ground-glass opacities with predominant involvement of the right lung and the peribronchovascular left lung. (b) Coronal minimum intensity projection image shows asymmetric distribution of ground-glass opacities. Such asymmetry is not typical of NSIP. Biopsy revealed DIP.

- Is the process contiguous or patchy with skip areas?
  - Contiguous: Both UIP and NSIP
  - Patchy with skip areas: Less likely NSIP
- Regarding traction bronchiectasis
  - If out of proportion to the degree of parenchymal fibrosis: Highly suggestive of collagen vascular disease-related interstitial lung disease (CVD-ILD) (usually scleroderma), and bronchiectasis likely caused by chronic microaspiration

What Not to Miss

As with UIP, NSIP has a higher incidence of lung cancer, especially in the setting of collagen vascular disease. The diagnosis

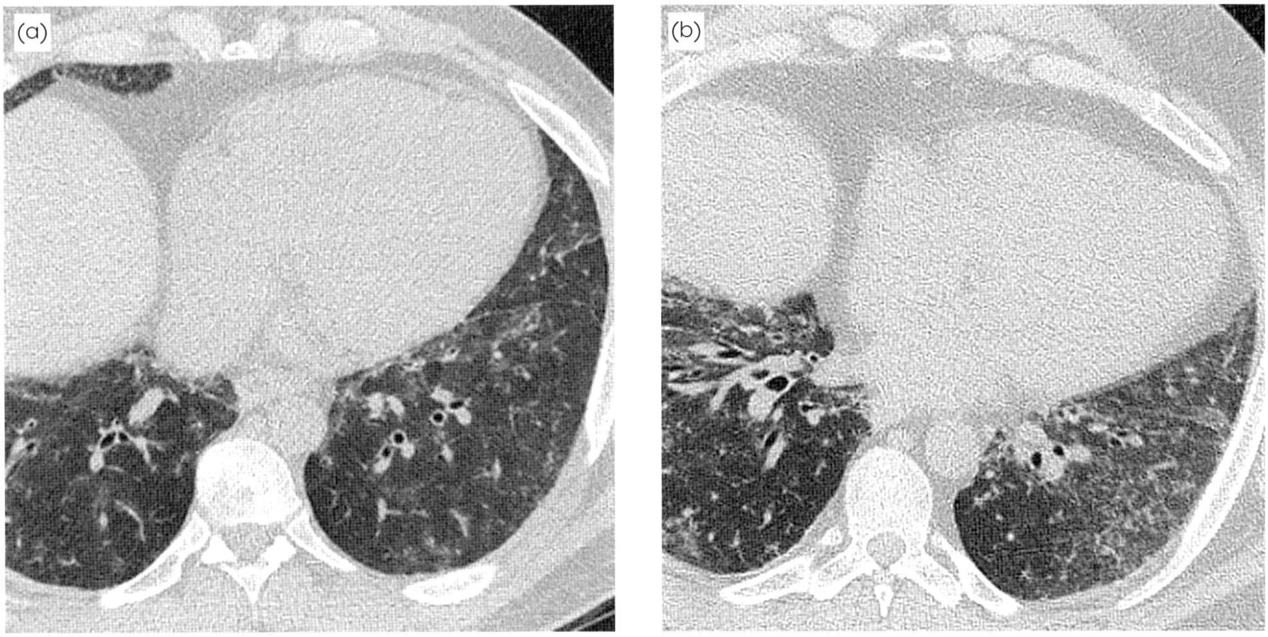

Figure 79.4. Idiopathic NSIP with gradual progression of fibrosis. (a) HRCT of a 43-year-old man with a 3-month history of chest pain, shortness of breath, and cough shows peripheral confluent ground-glass opacities with superimposed peribronchovascular ground-glass nodules. Surgical wedge biopsy of the right middle and lower lobes was performed, which revealed fibrotic NSIP. (b) HRCT performed 4 years later shows progressive fibrosis that developed despite immunosuppressive therapy.

can be challenging given the underlying reticulation and fibrosis. Comparison with prior examinations can be very helpful. Often, follow-up imaging is required to determine whether a nodule is malignant. Focal airspace opacities or consolidation are concerning for pneumonia and should also be carefully compared with prior images. Infectious pneumonia is common in patients who are immunocompromised in the setting of either collagen vascular disease or chemotherapy. Organizing pneumonia is also fairly common in these patient groups and is frequently quite responsive to corticosteroids.

Differential Diagnosis

As previously described, an NSIP pattern may be idiopathic or secondary to HP, collagen vascular disease, or drug toxicity. Certain CT features may suggest a secondary cause. Another IIP (DIP) may overlap with NSIP given its propensity for ground-glass opacity on CT. Distinction from UIP is discussed in Chapter 80. OP may also overlap with NSIP and is discussed in Chapter 82.

Desquamative Interstitial Pneumonia

- Confluent areas of ground-glass opacity on CT
- Usually exhibits a basilar predominant distribution
- Contrary to NSIP, progression from ground-glass opacities to reticulation uncommon
- May have cysts and often has underlying emphysema

Hypersensitivity Pneumonitis

- Bronchocentric fibrosis leads to air trapping. When an NSIP pattern is seen in association with extensive air trapping, HP should be considered.
- Occasionally, centrilobular nodules are also seen, which can help support the diagnosis of HP.

Imaging Findings

NSIP

- Chest radiographs may appear normal or show hazy basilar opacities that may extend to the mid lung zone when severe.
- Ground-glass opacity is the salient CT feature.
- Irregular reticulation can be present in up to half of cases and becomes more conspicuous as fibrosis progresses, whereas ground-glass opacities are the first to resolve in response to treatment.
- Typically absent or minimal honeycombing.
- Axial distribution of NSIP is more variable than that of UIP. NSIP may exhibit subpleural sparing and a peribronchovascular distribution, but neither is a requirement for diagnosis.

CVD-ILD

- In up to 25% of patients with CVD, the ILD may precede the clinical diagnosis by months or years.
- Scleroderma and polymyositis/dermatomyositis tend to present with an NSIP pattern on imaging. The latter tends to also have a higher incidence of superimposed OP. Rheumatoid arthritis (as discussed in Chapter 80) is more likely to present with a UIP pattern.

Clinical Issues

- NSIP may overlap DIP on imaging, but DIP has a much closer association with smoking and has characteristic histologic features based on accumulation of alveolar macrophages.
- HP may result in an NSIP pattern on imaging. The presence of loosely formed granulomas on a histologic specimen can establish the diagnosis of HP. Such microscopic granulomata are never visible by HRCT.
- NSIP may be seen with many collagen vascular diseases, most commonly scleroderma.
- NSIP may be complicated by atypical infections and acute accelerated fibrosis similar to UIP.
- Idiopathic NSIP is much less common than NSIP associated with CVD, drug reaction, or HP. If an NSIP pattern is identified on CT or histology, a thorough search for other underlying causes should be made. Serologic testing for autoimmune antibodies and sensitivity testing for exposure and reaction to various allergens are commonly performed.

Key Points

- The histologic and imaging findings of NSIP are common in patients with collagen vascular disease, hypersensitivity pneumonitis, and drug-induced lung disease. Recognition of an NSIP imaging pattern should prompt a search for an underlying cause.
- A diagnosis of NSIP on HRCT warrants a surgical biopsy for definitive diagnosis. The absence of honeycombing as a predominant CT feature has a high negative predictive value for NSIP (90%).

Suggested Reading

Elliot TL, Lynch DA, Newell JDJr, et al. High-resolution computed tomography features of nonspecific interstitial pneumonia and usual interstitial pneumonia. *J Comput Assist Tomogr.* 2005 May–Jun;29(3):339–345.

Mueller-Mang C, Grosse C, Schmid K, et al. What every radiologist should know about idiopathic interstitial pneumonias. *RadioGraphics.* 2007 May–Jun;27(3):595–615.

Travis WD, Costabel U, Hansell DM, et al.; ATS/ERS Committee on Idiopathic Interstitial Pneumonias. An official American Thoracic Society/European Respiratory Society statement: Update of the international multidisciplinary classification of the idiopathic interstitial pneumonias. *Am J Respir Crit Care Med.* 2013;188(6):733–748.

CHAPTER 80

Organizing Pneumonia

Cylen Javidan-Nejad

Definition

Organizing pneumonia (OP) is considered a nonfibrotic idiopathic interstitial pneumonia (IIP) characterized by a nonspecific reparative response of the parenchyma to acute alveolar injury. It commonly occurs in the setting of collagen vascular disease and in response to drug therapy. The term *OP* is best used for the typical histologic and radiologic pattern. The term *cryptogenic organizing pneumonia* (*COP*) is reserved for the idiopathic form of OP.

Bronchiolitis obliterans organizing pneumonia (BOOP) is a former name of OP that has fallen out of favor because it may be confused with obliterative or constrictive bronchiolitis, an unrelated small airway disease that does not share pathologic, imaging, or clinical features with OP.

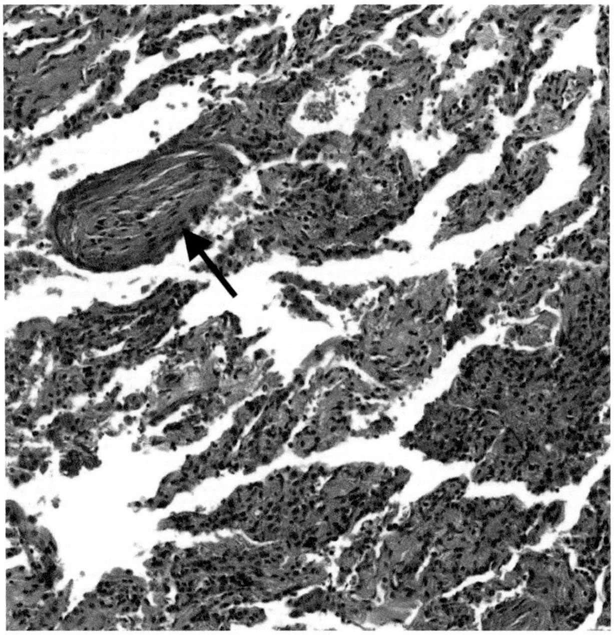

Figure 80.1. Histologic pattern of organizing pneumonia. High-power photomicrograph (hematoxylin and eosin stain) shows a polypoid plug of organizing fibrosis in the alveolar space (arrow) representing a Masson body. There is also an inflammatory interstitial infiltrate.

Clinical Features

COP is a subacute disease of indolent onset that can be confused clinically with community-acquired pneumonia or chronic eosinophilic pneumonia. Peak incidence is in the sixth decade of life. There is no gender predilection or known risk factor for COP; however, nonsmokers are twice as likely to develop COP.

Affected patients present with cough, dyspnea, intermittent fever, chills, myalgia, and weight loss lasting for weeks or months, with no response to antibiotics. Physical exam reveals mid inspiratory crackles or squeaks, laboratory abnormalities include leukocytosis, and there may be a restrictive ventilatory pattern with decreased diffusion capacity on spirometry.

Patients with COP have a very good prognosis, and two-thirds completely recover with corticosteroid therapy. Recurrence is common, especially when corticosteroids are tapered too quickly.

Anatomy and Physiology

The hallmark histologic feature of OP is polypoid masses or plugs (Masson bodies) composed of loosely formed immature fibroblasts and organizing connective tissue, located in the distal airspaces, namely the alveolar spaces and the lumina of the alveolar ducts and terminal bronchioles (Fig. 80.1).

Another histologic feature is the presence of varying degrees of interstitial infiltration by neutrophils, eosinophils, plasma cells, and macrophages. The alveolar walls and lung architecture are preserved. Occasionally and with time, collagen deposition occurs, leading to scarring and architectural distortion.

Because of the non-uniform involvement of the lung by OP, transbronchial biopsy can be subject to sampling error. For this reason, wedge resection is a preferred method for biopsy. Tissue sampling from multiple locations may be needed to determine if OP is present in isolation, as in COP, or if it is a minor histologic finding superimposed on another disease process, such as nonspecific interstitial pneumonia, vasculitis, or infection.

How to Approach the Image

There are diverse imaging manifestations of OP. Although the classic pattern is most common, there are various other "nonclassic" manifestations. The latter include focal, crescentic, linear or band-like, multinodular, bronchocentric, perilobular, and progressive fibrotic patterns. Often, a mixed pattern of imaging abnormalities exists. Biopsy is commonly needed for definitive diagnosis. When an image with possible OP is encountered, one must look for any signs of fibrosis, most notably traction bronchiectasis and any underlying process that may result in OP.

What Not to Miss

The most challenging aspect of imaging OP is that the pathologic diagnosis can be seen in the setting of another clinical diagnosis. Two of the more common entities are lung cancer and infectious pneumonia. If the lung adjacent to the neoplasm or on the periphery of the infection is sampled, the pathologic specimen may return as OP. The role of the radiologist, then, is to ensure that the imaging findings are concordant with OP and not with these other conditions. The presence of a pleural effusion or lymphadenopathy would be atypical for OP and is more suggestive of one of the other conditions.

Differential Diagnosis

- In the acute setting, single or multiple pulmonary consolidations with a peripheral distribution suggest pulmonary infarctions. Acute or subacute fungal infections may follow an indolent course similar to that of OP and should also be considered.
- When findings are chronic, the differential diagnosis of classic and focal OP includes chronic eosinophilic pneumonia, mucinous invasive adenocarcinoma of the lung (formerly bronchioloalveolar carcinoma), sarcoidosis, vasculitis, and pulmonary lymphoma.

Chronic Eosinophilic Pneumonia

- Multiple subsegmental consolidations in the lung periphery are the most common imaging finding. In contrast to OP, the upper lobes are more commonly involved and nodules are not common.
- Subpleural bands, linear opacities, and "crazy paving" are less common imaging manifestations, but these findings can also be seen in OP.

Invasive Mucinous Adenocarcinoma

- Formerly called bronchioloalveolar carcinoma, this malignancy mimics both classic and focal imaging manifestations of OP.
- Imaging features
  - Localized or multifocal
  - Solid or subsolid bronchiolocentric nodules
  - Consolidations with air bronchograms, usually involving more than one lung segment

Sarcoidosis

- Sarcoidosis may mimic both the classic and the multinodular patterns of OP.
- Multiple consolidations and nodules with an upper and mid lung zone predominance rather than the lower lung zone predominance seen in most cases of OP.
- Lymphadenopathy is common in sarcoidosis, but it is usually absent with OP.

Vasculitis—Granulomatosis with Polyangitis

- Formerly called Wegener's granulomatosis.
- Multiple wedge-shaped consolidations and peribronchovascular nodules and masses are common findings and can mimic the classic form of OP.
- Small "Cheerio nodules" may be present and are much smaller than the atoll findings of OP.

Imaging Findings

Classic

- This pattern is present in the majority of patients with OP and is characterized by multiple bilateral patchy airspace consolidations and confluent ground-glass opacities, typically in the lung periphery abutting the pleura, similar to lung infarction, or around the bronchovascular bundles.
- The lower lung zones are more commonly affected. The lung volume is usually preserved. Bronchial dilation within the consolidation is a common feature (Fig. 80.2).
- CT may demonstrate sparing of the subpleural parenchyma and commonly reveals much more extensive lung involvement by ground-glass opacity.
- The presence of reticulation denotes development of fibrosis.
- Serial imaging shows progression, spontaneous regression, or change in location of the consolidations over time. This form typically responds well to steroid therapy, often with complete resolution of CT abnormalities.

Focal

- Single or multiple mass-like consolidations.
- Cavitation is rare and may be associated with hemoptysis.
- Distribution is different from that of the classic pattern in that it is more common in the upper lobes.
- Helpful (but not definitive) identifying CT features center on the shape of the consolidation, which tends to be flat (rather than spherical) and trapezoidal or polygonal (Fig. 80.3).

Crescentic

- Curvilinear consolidations or nodular opacities surrounding a central area of ground-glass opacity, known as the reverse halo or atoll sign. The ground-glass opacity centers correlate with alveolar

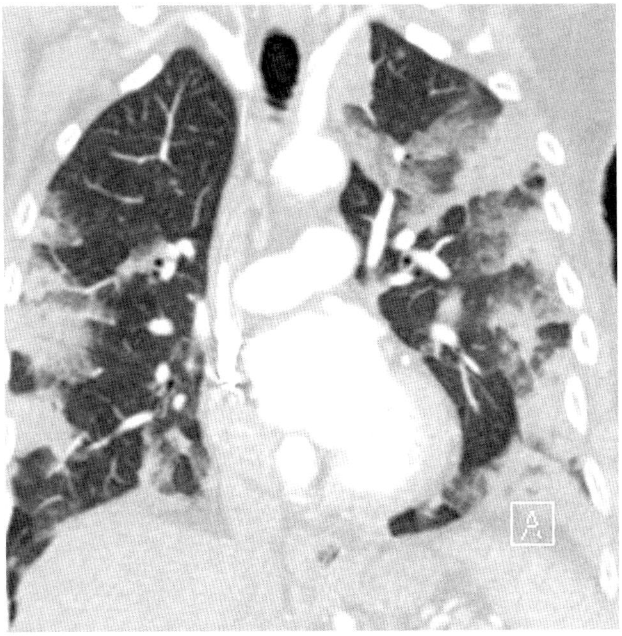

Figure 80.2. Classic pattern of organizing pneumonia. Coronal contrast-enhanced chest CT of an 80-year-old woman on chemotherapy for metastatic cancer who presented with gradual onset of dyspnea and hypoxemia shows multiple bilateral peripheral subpleural consolidations and ground-glass opacities related to drug reaction-related OP. No pulmonary emboli were found.

septal inflammation and cellular debris on pathology (Fig. 80.4).

- Lesions are usually multiple and exhibit the same peripheral or peribronchovascular distribution as the classic pattern.

Multinodular

- Bronchocentric OP pattern characterized by either acinar opacities (8–10 mm) or micronodules (<5 mm) in a tree-in-bud or centrilobular distribution.
- Micronodules tend to be ill-defined.
- This pattern most commonly occurs when OP is associated with polymyositis or dermatomyositis, and it is rare in patients with COP (Fig. 80.5).

Progressive Fibrotic

- Reticulations and architectural distortion with paucity of consolidations or confluent ground-glass opacities.
- Mild honeycombing and traction bronchiectasis may develop.
- This pattern is more common with OP due to connective tissue disease and denotes an unfavorable outcome.

Clinical Issues

- The consolidative or classic form of OP/COP responds better to corticosteroid therapy with fewer recurrences compared to the micronodular pattern. Recurrence is most commonly due to inadequate treatment duration or fast tapering of corticosteroids.
- Reticular opacities on CT in a patient with OP suggest a poor response to steroid therapy.
- OP can occur in association with collagen vascular diseases (CVDs) and may coexist with nonspecific interstitial pneumonia in such patients. The two CVDs most likely to be associated with OP are dermatomyositis and polymyositis.

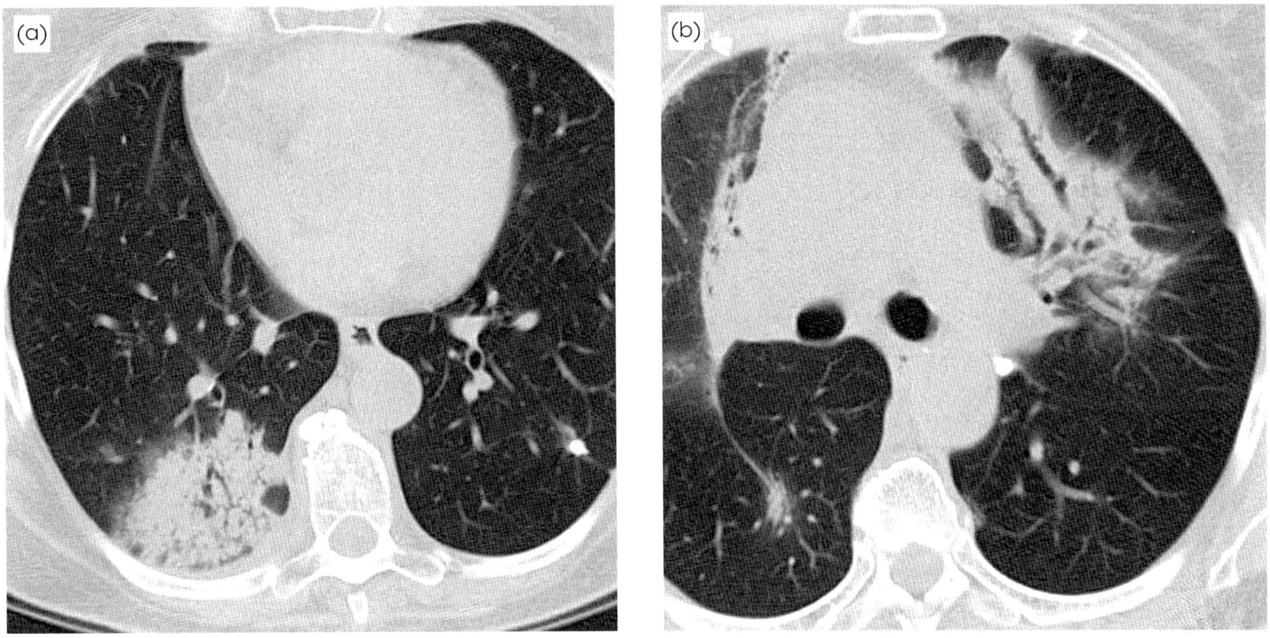

Figure 80.3. Focal pattern of OP. Unenhanced chest CT of a 64-year-old woman with breast cancer treated with lumpectomy and radiation shows multiple mass-like consolidations. (a) The right lower lobe lesion is surrounded by mild ground-glass opacity, is adjacent to the pleura, and exhibits minimal sparing of the subpleural lung. (b) The left upper lobe lesion is a polygonal-shaped, sharply marginated consolidation centered about the bronchovascular bundles. Wedge biopsy revealed OP. Note right paramediastinal radiation fibrosis.

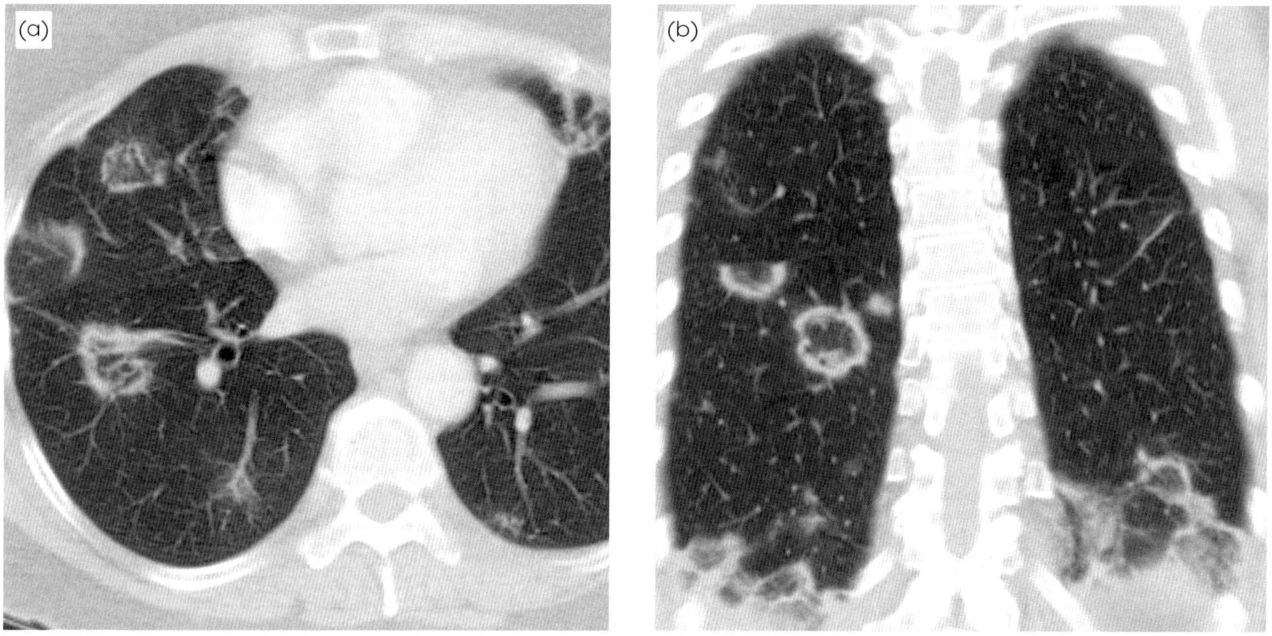

Figure 80.4. Atoll sign in OP. (a) Axial and (b) coronal contrast-enhanced chest CT of a 59-year-old woman with known OP undergoing immunosuppressive therapy shows multiple bilateral rounded curvilinear consolidations with central ground-glass opacity exhibiting the reverse halo or atoll signs of OP.

- Chronic eosinophilic pneumonia can mimic OP on imaging. A history of asthma may suggest the former as well as peripheral eosinophilia.
- Although mucinous adenocarcinoma can also mimic OP, a history of bronchorrhea or malignant cytology from bronchoalveolar lavage fluid are typical of neoplasm.
- Usually a surgical biopsy is needed to establish the diagnosis of OP. This is performed after a complete workup for alternate causes of the imaging findings has been exhausted.
- Serologic testing (usually cytoplasmic anti-neutrophil cytoplasmic antibody) is useful in distinguishing granulomatosis with polyangitis from COP.

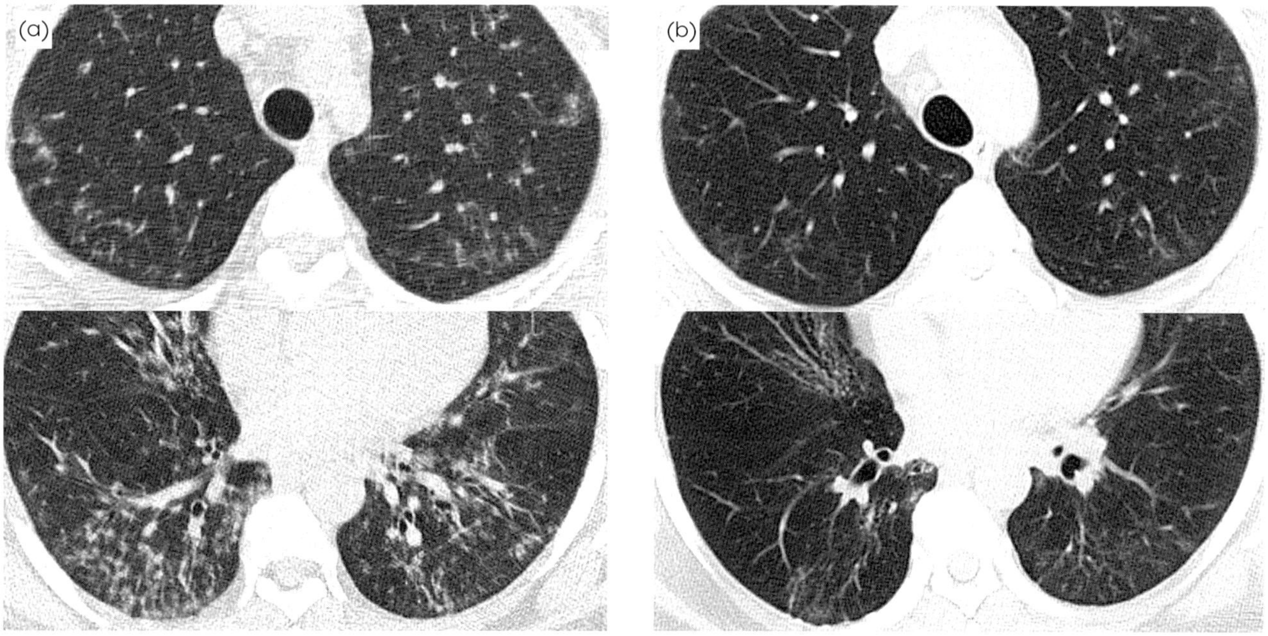

Figure 80.5. Micronodular pattern of OP. (a) Composite image with HRCT of a 41-year-old woman with polymyositis with nonproductive cough and dyspnea shows multiple basilar predominant tree-in-bud nodules. Open surgical biopsy showed typical histology of OP. Treatment required steroids and additional immunosuppression with azathioprine. (b) Composite image with HRCT obtained 4 years later shows marked improvement with residual faint ground-glass opacities and reticulations, mild architectural distortion, and traction bronchiectasis in the middle lobe due to fibrosis.

Key Points

- OP is a nonspecific pathologic entity that occurs with various causes of lung injury, the most common of which is drug reaction.
- Idiopathic OP (clinically called COP) exhibits imaging and pathologic characteristics similar to those of OP caused by a known insult. The diagnosis of COP can be made only after exclusion of known causes, such as infection, neoplasm, or vasculitis.
- Consolidations are the most common imaging features of OP and tend to have a peripheral or peribronchovascular distribution.

Suggested Reading

Ferguson EC, Berkowitz EA. Lung CT: Part 2. The interstitial pneumonias—Clinical, histologic, and CT manifestations. *AJR Am J Roentgenol*. 2012 Oct;199(4):W464–W476.

Lynch DA, Travis WD, Müller NL, et al. Idiopathic interstitial pneumonias: CT features. *Radiology*. 2005 Jul;236(1):10–21.

Oikonomou A, Hansell DM. Organizing pneumonia: The many morphological faces. *Eur Radiol*. 2002 Jun;12(6):1486–1496.

Travis WD, Costabel U, Hansell DM, et al.; ATS/ERS Committee on Idiopathic Interstitial Pneumonias. An official American Thoracic Society/European Respiratory Society statement: Update of the international multidisciplinary classification of the idiopathic interstitial pneumonias. *Am J Respir Crit Care Med*. 2013;188(6):733–748.

Zhao F, Yan SX, Wang GF, et al. CT features of focal organizing pneumonia: An analysis of consecutive histopathologically confirmed 45 cases. *Eur J Radiol*. 2014 Jan;83(1):73–78.

Section XVI

Mediastinal Abnormalities

CHAPTER 81

Introduction to Mediastinal Abnormalities

Melissa L. Rosado-de-Christenson

Introduction

The mediastinum is the space between the pleura and lungs. It extends from the thoracic inlet to the diaphragm and is bound anteriorly by the sternum and posteriorly by the vertebral bodies. The mediastinum contains the heart and pericardium, the great vessels of the thorax, the trachea and central tracheobronchial tree, the thymus, the esophagus, and the thoracic duct. The mediastinum also contains fat, nerves, and lymph nodes.

Diseases of the Mediastinum

Several disease processes may affect the mediastinum, including primary neoplasms, metastatic lymphadenopathy, various congenital cysts, enlarged mediastinal and extramediastinal organs such as the thymus and the thyroid, and vascular lesions including vascular proliferations and aneurysms. Lesions of cardiovascular origin, herniation of abdominal structures into the chest through the various diaphragmatic foramina, and unencapsulated mediastinal fat deposition such as lipomatosis may all produce mediastinal enlargement or contour abnormalities. Unusual non-neoplastic lesions may produce mediastinal masses, including entities such as extramedullary hematopoiesis.

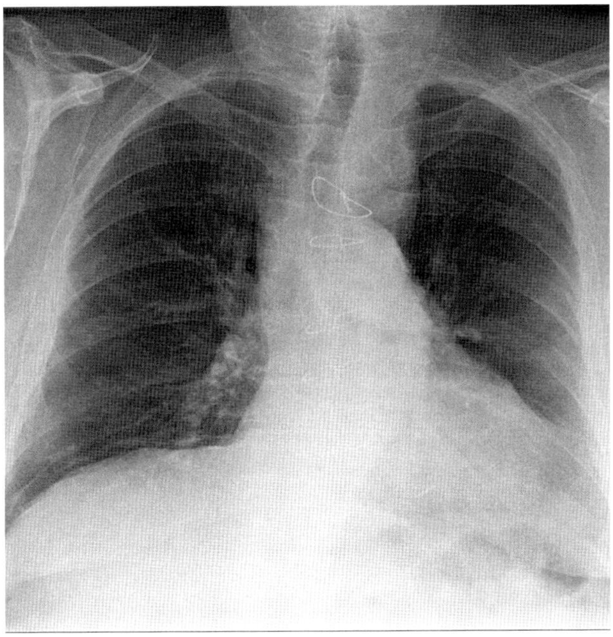

Figure 81.1. Mediastinal contour abnormality: Vascular. Posteroanterior chest radiograph of an asymptomatic 59-year-old man shows a left superior mediastinal contour abnormality that follows the course of the thoracic aorta. A cervical aortic arch with pseudocoarctation was identified on chest CT. Vascular lesions account for approximately 10% of mediastinal abnormalities.

Approach to Mediastinal Abnormalities

Mediastinal abnormalities are usually identified on chest radiography because these lesions cause alterations of the normal mediastinal contours with focal or diffuse mediastinal enlargement. Aggressive malignancies and lymphadenopathies characteristically produce diffuse mediastinal enlargement. Focal lesions typically represent primary mediastinal neoplasms and congenital cysts. Approximately 10% of mediastinal contour abnormalities are of vascular origin and may represent acquired or congenital abnormalities (Fig. 81.1).

Once a mediastinal lesion is identified and evaluated on the frontal chest radiograph, it is further localized in a mediastinal compartment on the lateral chest radiograph. The radiographic mediastinal compartments are not bound by tissue planes, and mediastinal lesions may affect more than one compartment. However, localization of a given abnormality within a specific compartment is helpful in formulating a focused differential diagnosis. Cross-sectional imaging evaluation usually follows, typically chest CT. Contrast administration is useful in identifying vascular lesions and evaluating locally invasive behavior.

Radiographic Mediastinal Compartments

Radiographic mediastinal compartments do not necessarily follow tissue planes and are based on a series of imaginary lines drawn along various structures seen on the lateral chest radiograph (Fig. 81.2).

The Felson classification divides the mediastinum into anterior, middle, and posterior compartments. The anterior mediastinum is located anterior to a line drawn along the anterior trachea and continued behind the posterior cardiac border. The posterior mediastinum is located posterior to a

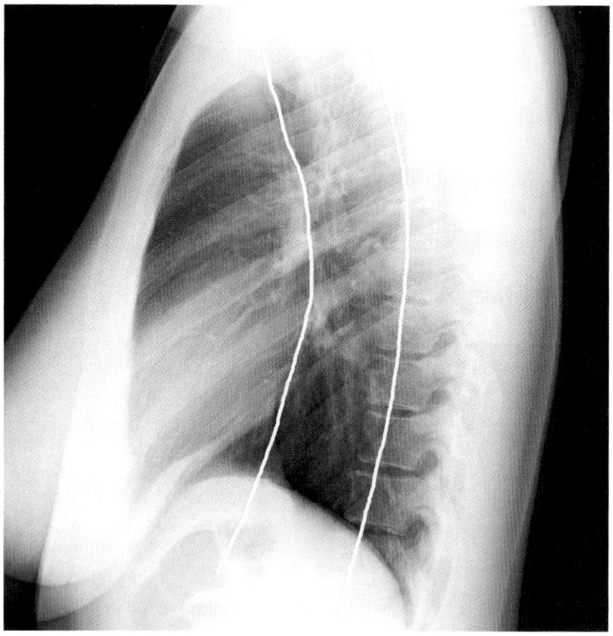

Figure 81.2. Mediastinal compartments according to Felson. Imaginary lines divide the mediastinum on the lateral chest radiograph. The anterior mediastinum is located anterior to a line drawn along the anterior trachea and posterior cardiac border. The posterior mediastinum is located posterior to a line drawn 1 cm behind the anterior vertebral margins. The middle mediastinum is between the anterior and posterior compartments.

line drawn 1 cm behind the anterior vertebral margins. The middle mediastinum is located between the anterior and posterior mediastinal compartments. Note that the Felson mediastinal divisions include the paravertebral regions that are not part of the mediastinum proper. In addition, large lesions may occupy more than one mediastinal compartment. However, in most cases, the radiologist is able to formulate a focused differential diagnosis and recommend the next management step that typically includes further imaging.

CT Mediastinal Compartments

Cross-sectional imaging with CT or MRI allows direct visualization of a mediastinal lesion and accurate localization in one of 3 CT mediastinal compartments: prevascular, visceral and paravertebral (Fig. 81.3). The prevascular mediastinal compartment is bound anteriorly by the sternum, posteriorly by the pericardium, and laterally by the mediastinal parietal pleura. The visceral compartment is bound anteriorly by the pericardium, the proximal ascending aorta, lateral rim of the aortic arch and the intrapericardial pulmonary arteries and posteriorly by an imaginary vertical line connecting a point on the thoracic vertebral bodies 1 cm posterior to the anterior thoracic spine, called the visceral-paravertebral compartment boundary line. The paravertebral compartment is bound anteriorly by the visceral-paravertebral compartment boundary line and posteriorly and laterally by an imaginary vertical line that courses along the posterior margin of the chest wall at the lateral rim of the transverse processes.

Cross-sectional imaging allows characterization of a lesion's tissue components and identification of associated findings including lymphadenopathy and local invasion (Fig. 81.4). In the case of lesions related to glandular enlargement, cross-sectional imaging allows localization of the lesion in the anatomic location of the thymus or thyroid or establishment of anatomic continuity between the lesion

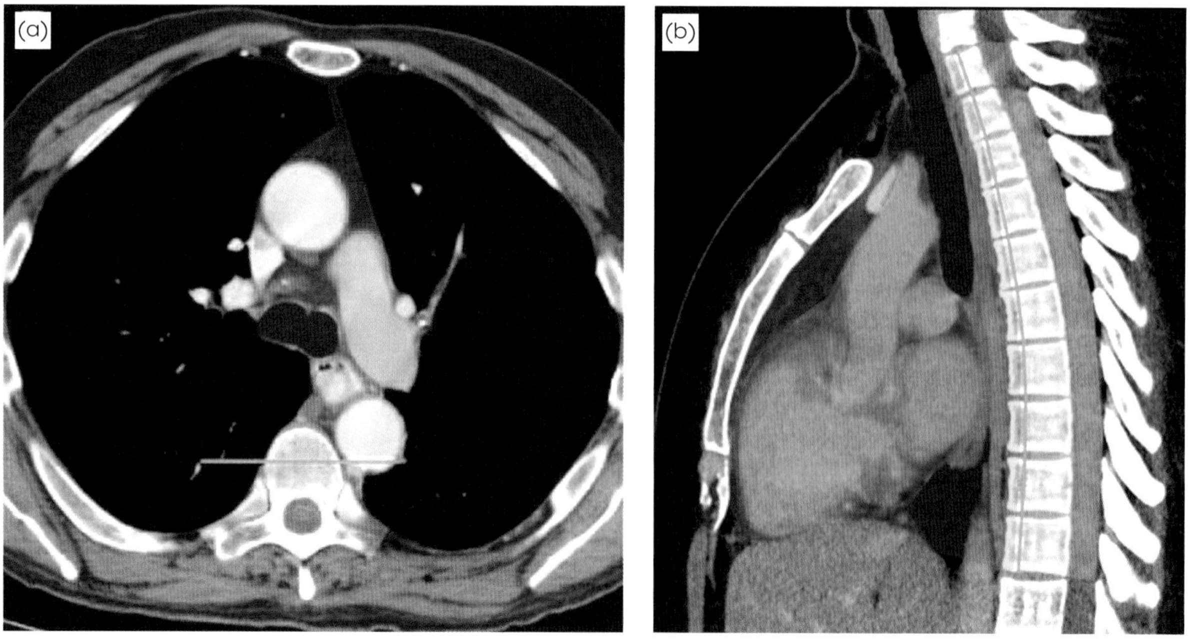

Figure 81.3. CT mediastinal compartments.

A, B. Axial and sagittal contrast-enhanced chest CT images are used to illustrate the prevascular (red), visceral (green) and paravertebral (yellow) mediastinal compartments. Note the location of the visceral-paravertebral compartment boundary line (blue).

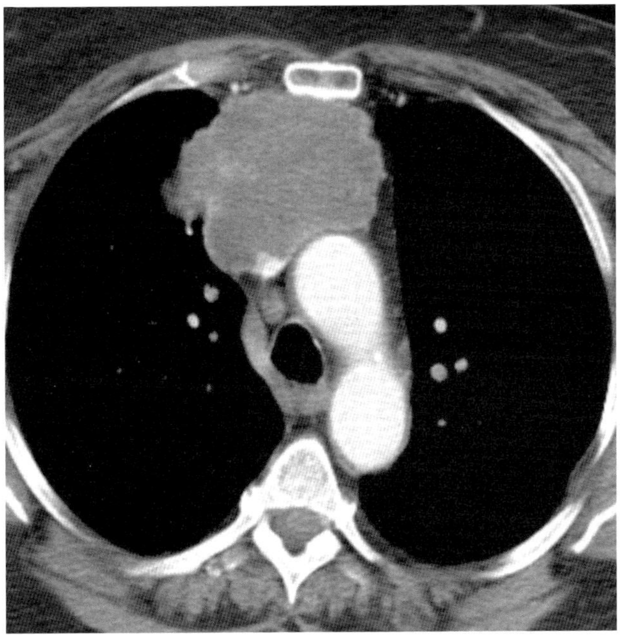

Figure 81.4 Mediastinal mass: Local invasion. Contrast-enhanced chest CT of an 80-year-old woman shows a heterogeneously enhancing prevascular mediastinal mass which directly invades the superior vena cava. Low-attenuation areas in the lesion correspond to tumor necrosis. Thymic carcinoma was diagnosed at surgery.

and the gland of origin. In the case of vascular lesions, cross-sectional imaging allows accurate diagnosis and identification of the vessel or cardiac chamber of origin.

Differential Diagnosis

The majority of mediastinal abnormalities seen in clinical practice are related to mediastinal lymphadenopathy and often result from secondary mediastinal involvement by an intra- or extrathoracic malignancy. Many of these represent metastatic lung cancer, metastases from another malignant neoplasm, and/or lymphoma. In many cases, the diagnosis of malignancy is known, and the radiologist can confidently diagnose metastatic disease.

Many incidentally discovered focal mediastinal masses in asymptomatic patients are benign. Anterior (prevascular) mediastinal abnormalities often originate in the thymus and include thymomas, thymic malignancies, and mature teratomas. Congenital mediastinal cysts and vascular lesions characteristically affect the middle (visceral) mediastinum. Lesions in the paravertebral region (Felson's posterior mediastinum) are typically related to neurogenic neoplasms, which are usually benign in adult subjects.

Mediastinal lesions that extend into the neck and produce mass effect on the suprasternal trachea are often of thyroid origin. Cardiophrenic angle lesions often relate to mediastinal fat, Morgagni hernias, or pericardial cysts. Hiatus hernia is a common mediastinal mass that characteristically produces lateral displacement of the inferior aspect of the azygoesophageal recess and is readily diagnosed when the herniated stomach contains air or an air–fluid level.

Radiologists must be familiar with the various etiologies of mediastinal abnormalities and their treatment, and they should be able to differentiate surgical lesions from those in which the diagnosis requires biopsy. Pericardial cyst and mediastinal lipomatosis should be confidently identified to prevent unnecessary intervention in affected patients.

Suggested Reading

Benveniste MFK, Rosado-de-Christenson ML, Sabloff BS, Moran CA, Swisher SG, Marom EM. Role of imaging in the diagnosis, staging, and treatment of thymoma. *RadioGraphics.* 2011;31:1847–1861.

Carter BW, Tomiyama N, Bhora FY, Rosado-de-Christenson ML, Nakajima J, Boiselle PM, Detterbeck FC, Marom EM. A modern definition of mediastinal compartments. *J Thorac Oncol.* 2014; 9: S97–S101.

Shaham D, Skilakaki MG, Goitein O. Imaging of the mediastinum: Applications for thoracic surgery. *Thorac Surg Clin.* 2004;14:25–42.

CHAPTER 82

Primary Mediastinal Neoplasms

Melissa L. Rosado-de-Christenson

Definition

Primary mediastinal neoplasms are rare and include benign and malignant lesions. Thymoma, mediastinal germ cell neoplasms, and lymphoma typically affect the anterior mediastinum. Neurogenic neoplasms from peripheral nerves and sympathetic ganglia often affect the paravertebral region.

Clinical Features

Although patients with benign primary mediastinal neoplasms are often asymptomatic, they may present with symptoms related to mass effect on adjacent structures. Malignant neoplasms may produce symptoms related to local invasion or metastatic disease. Patients with primary thymic neoplasms (typically thymoma) may present with parathymic syndromes, including myasthenia gravis, hypogammaglobulinemia, or pure red cell aplasia. Patients with mature teratoma may be diagnosed because of an incidental abnormality or because of mass effect by or rupture of the tumor. Patients with malignant germ cell neoplasm are nearly always males who are typically severely symptomatic. The latter may benefit from evaluation of serologic markers because α-fetoprotein may be elevated in embryonal carcinoma and endodermal sinus tumor and β-human chorionic gonadotropin may be elevated in choriocarcinoma. Serum lactate dehydrogenase may be an important marker in the evaluation and management of patients with primary malignant germ cell neoplasms because it is considered a marker of tumor burden.

Anatomy and Physiology

Radiographic diagnosis of primary mediastinal neoplasms relies on knowledge of normal radiographic anatomy, particularly for the identification of early neoplasms. Small neoplasms may not be border-forming on frontal radiography, and may manifest as subtle abnormalities on lateral radiographs. Primary mediastinal neoplasms are usually focal, unilateral lesions that abut the mediastinum, precluding radiographic visualization of a medial lesion border. These neoplasms typically displace the normal mediastinal interfaces and manifest as mediastinal contour abnormalities. For example, a small thymic neoplasm may produce subtle thickening of the anterior junction line. Thus, evaluation of this anatomic landmark on serial images may allow early diagnosis.

How to Approach the Image

The first step in the imaging diagnosis of a primary mediastinal neoplasm is the identification of a mediastinal contour abnormality on radiography. Evaluation of the lateral chest radiograph allows localization of the lesion within a radiographic mediastinal compartment and the formulation of a focused differential diagnosis. Most lesions are then evaluated with contrast-enhanced chest CT, which allows specific localization of the lesion, assessment of its various tissue elements, and identification of associated abnormalities including lymphadenopathy and invasion of local structures. MRI may be useful in selected cases.

What Not to Miss

Patients with primary mediastinal neoplasms are often asymptomatic. Therefore, the mediastinum has to be thoroughly evaluated in every chest radiograph. Comparison to prior chest radiographs is very helpful in the identification of early mediastinal neoplasms that may produce subtle findings. The radiologist should always

- assess the normal mediastinal contours and identify any contour abnormality;
- correlate mediastinal abnormalities with corresponding abnormalities on the lateral chest radiograph to localize the lesion to a specific radiographic mediastinal compartment;
- use contrast-enhanced CT for evaluation to exclude local invasion (including invasion of vascular structures); and
- identify associated abnormalities such as lymphadenopathy, calcification, and skeletal erosion.

Differential Diagnosis

Differential diagnosis of mediastinal lesions is highly influenced by lesion location within the mediastinum, demographic information, and clinical history.

Anterior (Prevascular) Mediastinum

- Thymoma: Men and women older than age 40 years; may be asymptomatic, may have symptoms related to mass effect or local invasion, or may exhibit an association with a parathymic syndrome such as myasthenia gravis
- Mature teratoma: Men and women younger than age 40 years, including children, often asymptomatic
- Malignant germ cell neoplasm: Men in third and fourth decades, typically symptomatic
- Primary mediastinal lymphoma: Young women, typically symptomatic
- Thymolipoma: Young adult or child, typically asymptomatic

Middle (Visceral) Mediastinum

- Rare location for primary mediastinal neoplasm
- Common location for lymphadenopathies, cysts, and vascular lesions

Posterior (Paravertebral) Mediastinum

- Schwannoma and neurofibroma: Young adults in third and fourth decades, may be asymptomatic
- Ganglioneuroma: Older children and young adults, may be asymptomatic
- Ganglioneuroblastoma and neuroblastoma: Infants and children younger than age 5 years, may be congenital

Imaging Findings

Thymoma

- Roughly spherical, unilateral, anterior (prevascular) mediastinal soft tissue mass; may be subtle on radiography (Fig. 82.1)
- May exhibit cystic change (mural nodules are typical), local invasion, calcification on cross-sectional imaging
- Evaluate contours, determine size in three dimensions, describe degree of contact with adjacent structures, exclude vascular invasion/encasement, identify associated pleural nodules that may represent drop metastases (Figs. 82.2 and 82.3)

Mature Teratoma

- Roughly spherical, unilateral anterior (prevascular) mediastinal soft tissue mass
- Heterogeneous attenuation with high frequency of multilocular cystic change (89%), fat attenuation (75%), calcification (50%) (Fig. 82.4)
- No lymphadenopathy or local invasion

Malignant Germ Cell Neoplasm

- Large anterior (prevascular) mediastinal mass (Fig. 82.5)
- May mimic lymphoma with nodal coalescence, may exhibit local invasion and lymphadenopathy
- Seminoma often exhibits homogeneous soft tissue attenuation with rare cystic change (Fig 82.5).

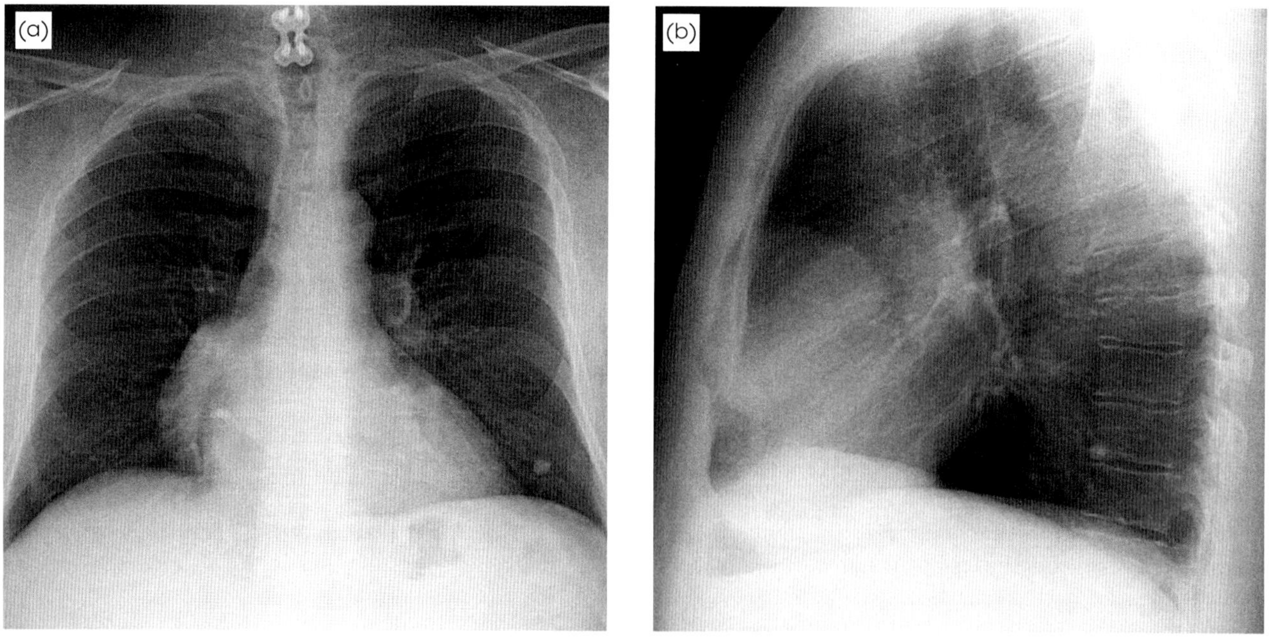

Figure 82.1. Mediastinal mass: Thymoma. (a) Posteroanterior (PA) and (b) lateral chest radiographs of an asymptomatic 58-year-old man with thymoma demonstrate a focal unilateral lobular mass located in the right anterior mediastinum. The lesion produces an abnormal contour of the right cardiac silhouette and projects over the heart on the lateral chest radiograph. The lesion borders are incompletely visualized in both projections, confirming its extrapulmonary location. Thymoma is the most likely diagnosis in this age group given the imaging findings.

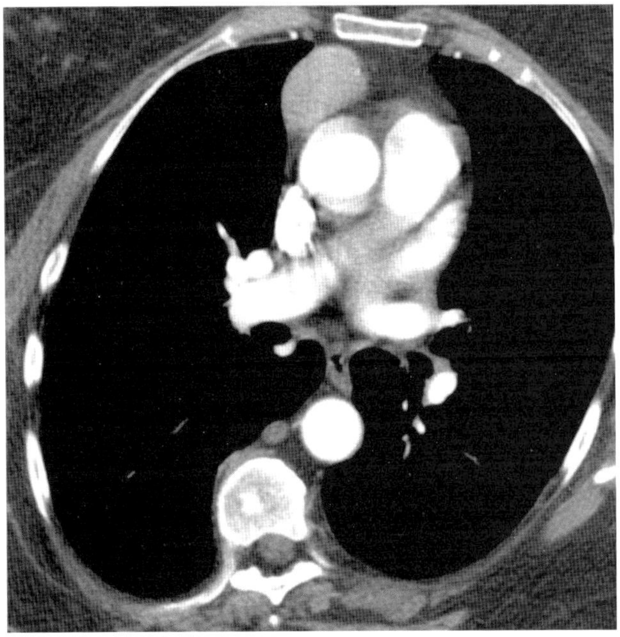

Figure 82.2. Thymoma. Contrast-enhanced chest CT of a 69-year-old woman with an incidentally discovered encapsulated thymoma shows a well-defined homogeneous ovoid prevascular mediastinal mass with an intact tissue plane between it and the adjacent ascending aorta.

- Non-seminomatous malignant germ cell neoplasms often exhibit heterogeneous attenuation with large areas of central necrosis and frond-like (enhancing) peripheral soft tissue.

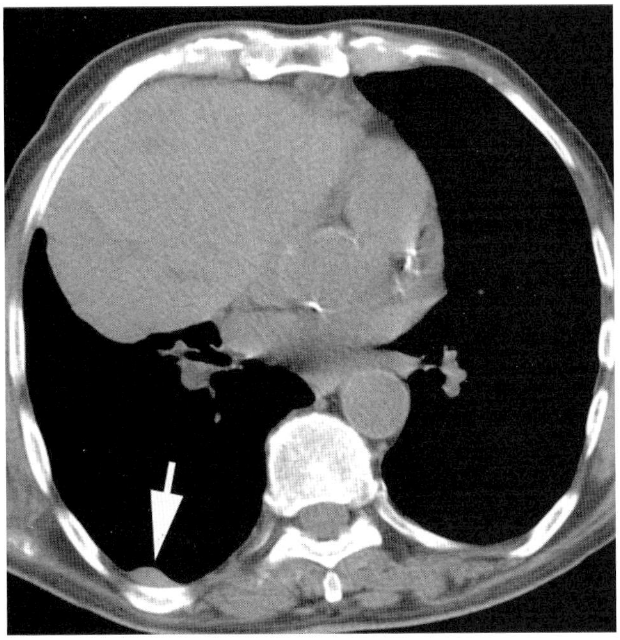

Figure 82.3. Invasive thymoma. Unenhanced chest CT of a 76-year-old man with chest pain shows a large polylobular right prevascular mediastinal mass with poor visualization of tissue planes between the lesion and the adjacent mediastinum. A right posterior pleural soft tissue nodule (arrow) represents a drop metastasis consistent with a stage III thymoma.

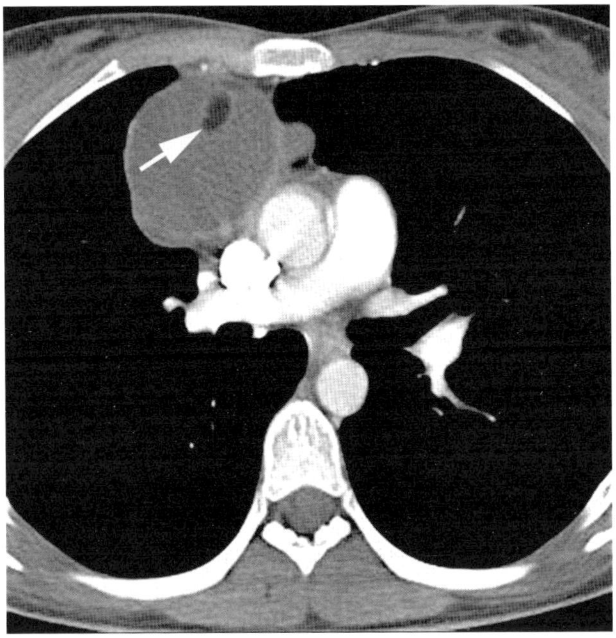

Figure 82.4. Mature teratoma. Contrast-enhanced chest CT of an asymptomatic 24-year-old woman with mature teratoma shows a spherical right prevascular mediastinal mass with predominant fluid attenuation, a soft tissue capsule, and internal fat (arrow), diagnostic of mature teratoma.

Primary Mediastinal Lymphoma

- Large locally invasive anterior (prevascular) mediastinal soft tissue mass

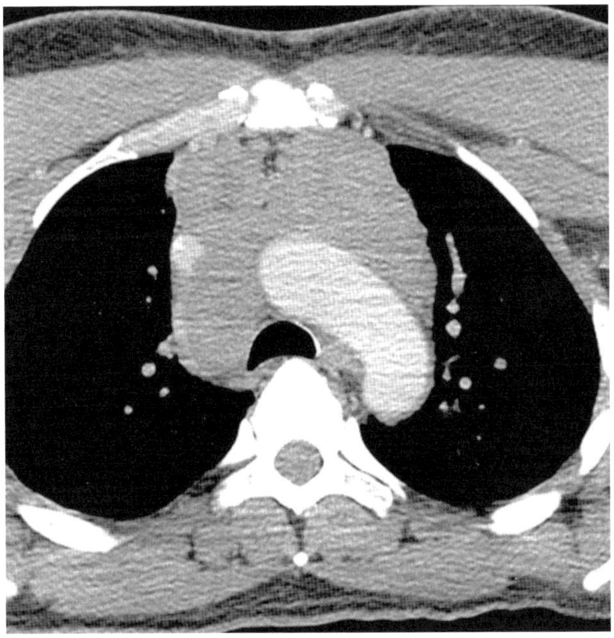

Figure 82.5. Seminoma. Contrast-enhanced chest CT of a 47-year-old man with chest pain shows a primary mediastinal seminoma that manifests as a homogeneous, bilateral, locally invasive predominantly prevascular mediastinal mass that encases adjacent vascular structures. The differential diagnosis also includes lymphoma.

- Frequent superior vena cava encasement/obstruction and lymphadenopathy or involvement of multiple lymph node stations

Thymolipoma

- Heterogeneous anterior (prevascular) mediastinal mass
- May be bilateral and exhibit a predilection for the inferior aspect of the mediastinum
- Admixture of soft tissue and fat attenuation/signal in a mediastinal mass with an anatomic connection to the thymus

Neurogenic Neoplasm (Schwannoma, Neurofibroma)

- Paravertebral, roughly spherical soft tissue mass (Fig. 82.6a)
- No associated lymphadenopathy
- Associated benign skeletal erosion or displacement of adjacent ribs and/or vertebral bodies; may exhibit enlargement of adjacent neuroforamen
- MRI evaluation for assessment of intraspinal extension (Fig. 82.6b)

Neurogenic Neoplasm (Ganglioneuroma, Ganglioneuroblastoma, Neuroblastoma)

- Paravertebral, elongate soft tissue mass, may span several thoracic vertebral bodies
- No associated lymphadenopathy
- Benign pressure erosion or displacement of adjacent ribs, vertebral erosion, enlarged neuroforamina
- *Neuroblastoma*: May exhibit calcification on radiography, may produce local invasion
- MRI for evaluation of intraspinal growth

Clinical Issues

- Thymomas are currently considered primary malignant thymic neoplasms because of their unpredictable biological behavior. The radiologist plays an important role in preoperative staging and patient management. Patients with locally invasive potentially resectable lesions generally require neoadjuvant chemotherapy.
- Thymomas may be indistinguishable from thymic carcinomas and thymic carcinoids. Both thymic carcinomas and carcinoids often exhibit lymphadenopathy. Thymic carcinoids may produce a clinical hormone syndrome.
- Mature teratomas are benign neoplasms that are typically cured by surgical excision. Preoperative diagnosis allows prompt surgical management and prediction of an excellent prognosis. Malignant germ cell neoplasms are not treated surgically, and affected patients often benefit from image-guided biopsy for diagnosis. These patients typically undergo cisplatin-based chemotherapy. Patients with non-seminomatous malignant germ cell neoplasms may require resection of residual tumor following chemotherapy. Radiologists play an important role in identifying residual abnormal mediastinal soft tissue to help guide surgical planning.

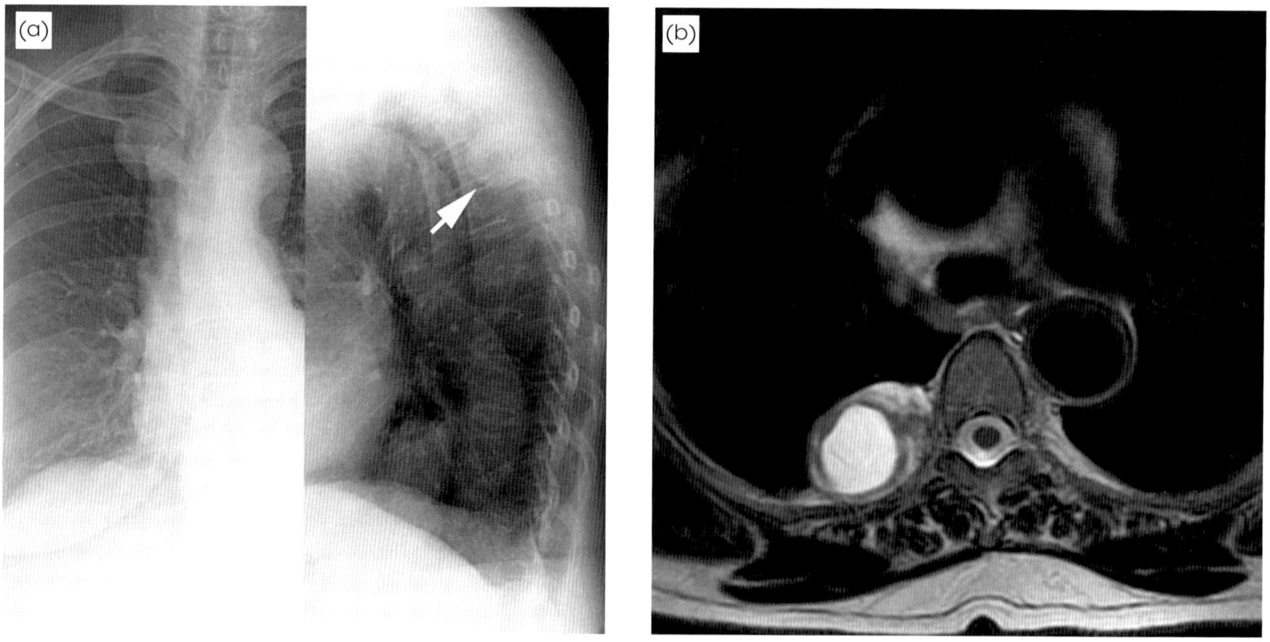

Figure 82.6. Neurogenic neoplasm: Schwannoma. (a) Composite image with PA (left) and lateral (right) chest radiographs of an asymptomatic 78-year-old woman with Schwannoma shows a spherical right posterior mediastinal mass (arrow) with well-defined lesion borders and no associated skeletal abnormalities. Note incidental hiatus hernia. (b) Axial T2-weighted MR of the same patient shows a cystic right paravertebral lesion without involvement of the neuroforamina or spinal canal.

- Primary mediastinal lymphoma (often a large B-cell non-Hodgkin lymphoma) may mimic a malignant germ cell neoplasm but typically affects young women. These lesions are not managed surgically and are usually accessible to image-guided biopsy for diagnosis.
- Thymolipomas are benign mediastinal neoplasms, and affected patients have an excellent prognosis. Although small asymptomatic lesions may be observed, growing lesions are typically excised.
- Neurogenic neoplasms in adults (Schwannoma and neurofibroma) are surgical lesions. MRI is required for surgical planning to identify intraspinal and neuroforaminal involvement. Malignant degeneration is reported, but is uncommon. These lesions may occur as single lesions or may be multifocal in the setting of neurofibromatosis 1.
- Neurogenic neoplasms in children may be benign (ganglioneuroma) or highly malignant (ganglioneuroblastoma and neuroblastoma).

Key Points

- Primary mediastinal neoplasms predominantly affect the anterior (prevascular) mediastinum and the paravertebral regions.
- Lesion localization in a radiographic mediastinal compartment together with knowledge of clinical and demographic information allow the formulation of a focused differential diagnosis and optimal planning of further imaging studies.
- Primary mediastinal neoplasms are typically focal and unilateral, but primary malignant neoplasms may produce diffuse and bilateral mediastinal involvement.
- Primary mediastinal neoplasms are optimally evaluated with contrast-enhanced chest CT. Neurogenic neoplasms should be evaluated with MRI to exclude intraspinal growth.
- Chest CT allows identification of invasive behavior and prediction of malignant histology. It also allows optimal management planning with regard to whether the lesion should be excised or biopsied.
- Lymphoma and malignant germ cell neoplasms are not surgical lesions and are often accessible to image-guided biopsy for diagnosis.

Suggested Reading

Benveniste MFK, Rosado-de-Christenson ML, Sabloff BS, Moran CA, Swisher SG, Marom EM. Role of imaging in the diagnosis, staging, and treatment of thymoma. *RadioGraphics.* 2011;31:1847–1861.

Shaham D, Skilakaki MG, Goitein O. Imaging of the mediastinum: Applications for thoracic surgery. *Thorac Surg Clin.* 2004;14:25–42.

CHAPTER 83

Mediastinal Lymphadenopathy

Brett W. Carter

Definition

Lymphadenopathy is the pathologic enlargement of lymph nodes. Intrathoracic lymphadenopathy complicates many malignancies, infections, and inflammatory processes, and the mediastinum is the most commonly affected region of the chest. Specific size criteria on CT are typically used to determine whether lymph nodes are enlarged. Additional features of mediastinal lymph nodes, such as attenuation, enhancement, and the presence of calcification, may be used to narrow the differential diagnosis regarding possible etiologies of lymphadenopathy. Note that enlarged lymph nodes may coalesce into a single mass that may mimic a primary neoplasm of the mediastinum.

Clinical Features

Patients with mediastinal lymphadenopathy may be entirely asymptomatic. However, some patients may present with symptoms that are typically related to the specific disease process producing the lymphadenopathy. For instance, patients with mediastinal lymphadenopathy secondary to sarcoidosis may present with respiratory symptoms such as dry cough, dyspnea, and bronchial hyperreactivity. Nonspecific symptoms and signs such as fatigue, night sweats, fever, and weight loss may occur in several diseases, including lymphoma, tuberculosis, fungal infection, and sarcoidosis. Mediastinal lymph nodes may become coalescent soft tissue masses and may exert mass effect on adjacent structures such as the trachea or esophagus with resultant dyspnea or dysphagia, respectively.

Anatomy and Physiology

Radiographic diagnosis of mediastinal lymphadenopathy relies on knowledge of the normal and abnormal appearance of the mediastinum, including its interfaces, lines, and stripes. Isolated borderline enlarged lymph nodes are usually not visible on radiography, but marked lymph node enlargement, involvement of multiple lymph node groups, and/or nodal coalescence may be evident on radiography and may produce thickening of mediastinal lines and stripes and mediastinal contour abnormalities.

How to Approach the Image

Detection of mediastinal lymphadenopathy on chest radiography relies on careful evaluation of frontal and lateral chest radiographs and knowledge of normal mediastinal contours. Once the abnormality is identified and localized to a mediastinal compartment, further evaluation with cross-sectional imaging such as contrast-enhanced chest CT is typically performed. CT effectively demonstrates the size of mediastinal lymph nodes; the number of compartments and/or lymph node stations involved; and the imaging characteristics of the abnormal lymph nodes, such as attenuation, enhancement, and calcification. MRI is not used routinely to evaluate lymphadenopathy, but its accuracy is comparable to that of CT. The administration of intravenous contrast material greatly enhances the detection and characterization of mediastinal lymphadenopathy. FDG PET/CT is useful in evaluating the metabolic activity of lymph nodes, and it is superior to CT for staging lymphoma and other malignancies. However, FDG uptake may be present in benign diseases such as sarcoidosis and infections, and PET/CT cannot reliably distinguish between lymphadenopathy due to malignancies and lymphadenopathy due to benign processes.

What Not to Miss

- Lymphadenopathy is suggested when lymph nodes measure above a specific short-axis diameter. Most lymph nodes measuring more than 1 cm are considered enlarged.
- Visualization of certain lymph nodes, such as internal mammary nodes, is considered abnormal regardless of size.
- Lymph node attenuation should be described because hypodense lymph nodes may occur in certain conditions.
- Following the administration of intravenous contrast, most lymph nodes enhance homogeneously. Intense enhancement may suggest a specific diagnosis. Heterogeneous enhancement or absence of enhancement suggest necrosis.

Differential Diagnosis

The differential diagnosis of mediastinal lymphadenopathy is highly influenced by the clinical history and the imaging characteristics of the lymph nodes.

Metastatic Disease

- Affected lymph nodes may or may not enhance (Fig. 83.1).
- Lymph node metastases from vascular malignancies such as renal and thyroid cancers may result in hyperenhancing lymph nodes (Fig. 83.2).
- Lymph node metastases from mucinous colon and ovarian cancers, osteosarcoma, and chondrosarcoma may calcify or ossify (Fig. 83.3).

Lymphoma

- Affected lymph nodes may or may not enhance.
- Lymph nodes may coalesce into mediastinal masses.
- Untreated lymphoma does not calcify, but treated lymphoma may calcify (Fig. 83.4).

Infection

- Lymph node infection or reaction to infection elsewhere in the chest may produce lymphadenopathy.
- Typical bacterial organisms and atypical organisms such as fungi, viruses, and mycobacteria may produce lymphadenopathy.
- Tuberculosis may result in necrotic lymph nodes (Fig. 83.5).
- Lymph node calcification commonly occurs in granulomatous infections such as tuberculosis and histoplasmosis.

Sarcoidosis

- Sarcoidosis is a multisystem disorder characterized by noncaseating granulomas.
- The most common pattern of lymph node involvement is right paratracheal and bilateral hilar lymphadenopathy (Fig. 83.6).
- Lymph node calcification may occur and increases in frequency with increasing chronicity of lymph node involvement.

Imaging Findings

Radiography

- Chest radiographs may be normal.
- The most common abnormalities include abnormal mediastinal contours, loss of interfaces, and thickening of lines and stripes.
- Thickening of the right paratracheal stripe or convexity of the superior vena cava interface may represent right paratracheal lymphadenopathy.
- Thickening of the left paratracheal stripe or convexity of the left subclavian artery interface may represent left paratracheal lymphadenopathy.
- Prevascular lymphadenopathy may manifest as an anterior mediastinal mass or thickening of the anterior junction line.
- Subcarinal lymphadenopathy may produce convexity of the upper azygoesophageal recess.
- Hilar enlargement and lobulation are typical of hilar lymphadenopathy.
- Aortopulmonary lymphadenopathy may produce convexity of the aortopulmonary window.

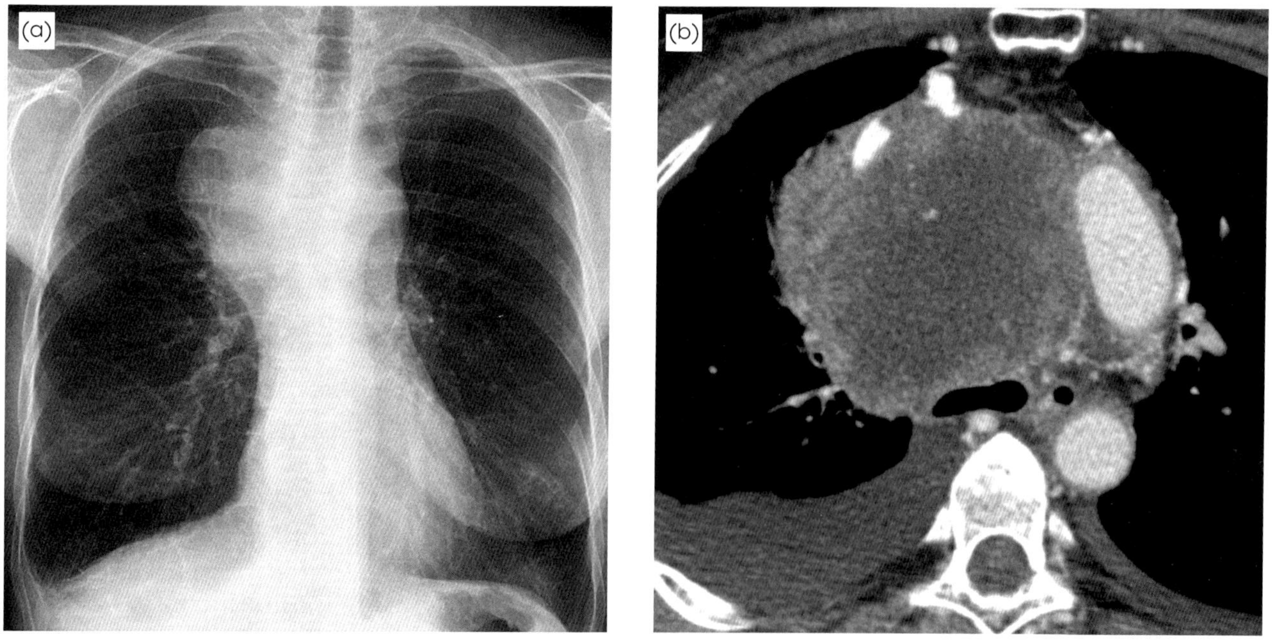

Figure 83.1. Metastatic disease. (a) PA chest radiograph of a 53-year-old woman with metastatic melanoma shows a lobulated mass in the right superior mediastinum producing marked thickening of the right paratracheal stripe. (b) Contrast-enhanced chest CT of the same patient shows a large heterogeneously enhancing visceral mediastinal mass that produces mass effect on the trachea and great vessels. Central low attenuation relates to necrosis from rapid tumor growth.

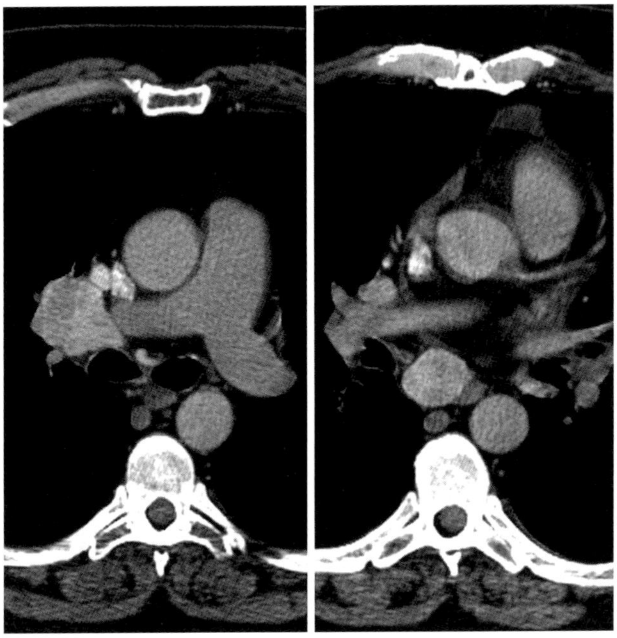

Figure 83.2. Metastatic disease. Composite image with contrast-enhanced chest CT of a 47-year-old woman with metastatic thyroid cancer shows hyperenhancing right hilar and subcarinal lymph nodes consistent with the vascular nature of the primary malignancy.

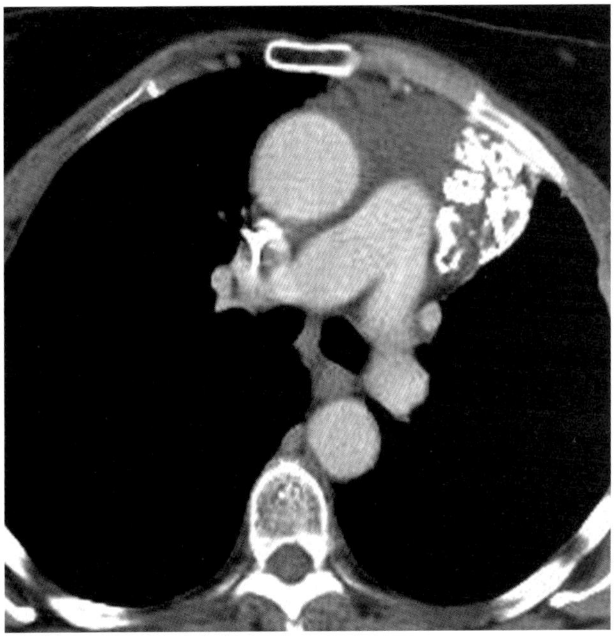

Figure 83.4. Treated lymphoma. Contrast-enhanced chest CT of a 38-year-old woman with prior radiation therapy for mediastinal lymphoma shows a partially calcified prevascular mediastinal soft tissue mass. Treated lymphoma may exhibit calcification.

Computed Tomography

- The most reliable method for diagnosing lymphadenopathy is identification of lymph node enlargement based on short-axis measurements on CT.
- Mediastinal lymph nodes measuring more than 1 cm in short axis are considered enlarged. However, for some lymph node groups such as the subcarinal station, lymph nodes measuring more than 1.5 cm are considered enlarged.
- There are no specific size criteria for internal mammary, retrocrural, and extrapleural lymph nodes,

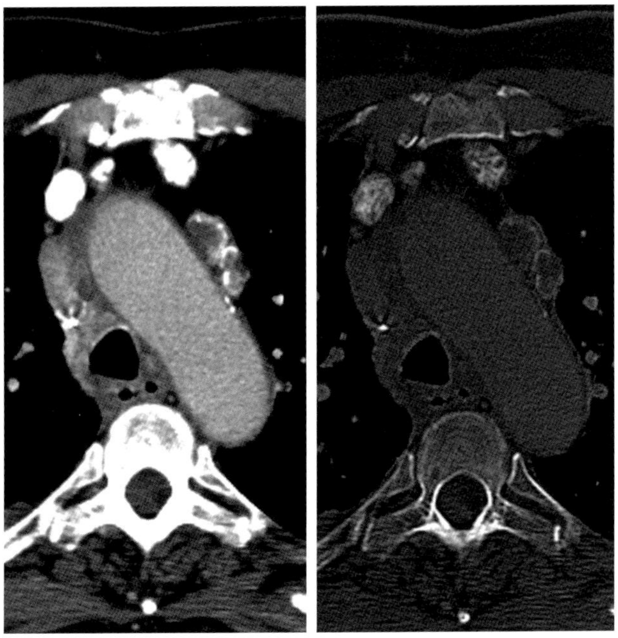

Figure 83.3. Metastatic disease. Composite image with contrast-enhanced chest CT of a 54-year-old man with metastatic chondrosarcoma shows multiple calcified mediastinal lymph node metastases.

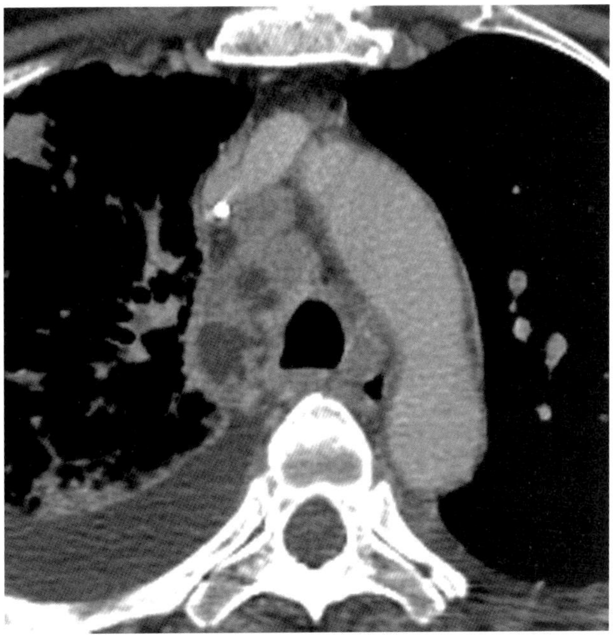

Figure 83.5. Tuberculosis. Contrast-enhanced chest CT of a 61-year-old woman with leukemia shows enlarged right paratracheal lymph nodes with central low-attenuation foci indicative of necrosis, small bilateral pleural effusions, and right pulmonary opacities from active tuberculosis infection.

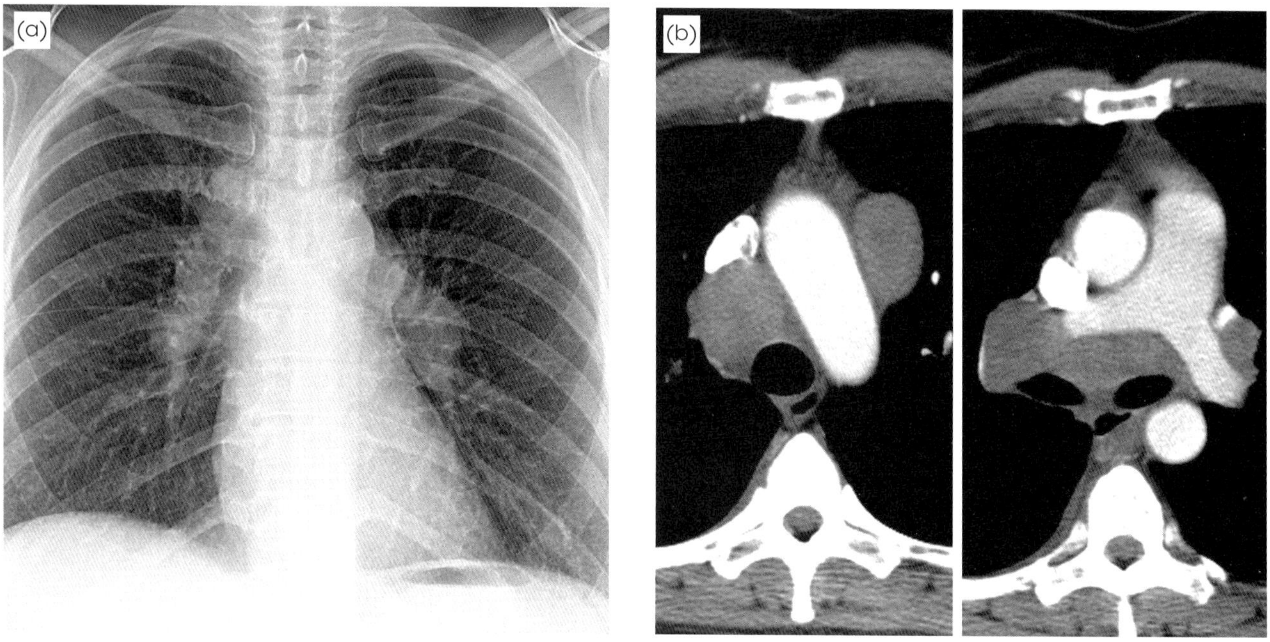

Figure 83.6. Sarcoidosis. (a) Posteroanterior chest radiograph of a 37-year-old man with sarcoidosis shows bilateral hilar and right paratracheal lymphadenopathy manifesting with hilar enlargement and lobulation and thickening of the right paratracheal stripe. (b) Composite image with contrast-enhanced chest CT of the same patient shows right paratracheal and prevascular lymphadenopathy (left) and bilateral hilar and subcarinal lymphadenopathy (right). The most specific pattern of lymphadenopathy in sarcoidosis is right paratracheal and bilateral hilar lymphadenopathy.

and visualization of these lymph nodes is considered abnormal regardless of size.

- Specific features of lymph nodes on CT, such as location, attenuation, enhancement characteristics, and calcification, should be noted because they may help narrow the differential diagnosis of possible etiologies of lymphadenopathy.
- Hypoattenuating lymph nodes may be present in lung cancer, seminoma, ovarian cancer, gastric cancer, and infections.
- Enhancing lymph nodes may be present in lung cancer, renal cell cancer, thyroid cancer, melanoma, and sarcoma.
- Intrathoracic malignancies typically spread along specific lymph node pathways, and the pattern of mediastinal lymphadenopathy can be predicted based on the location of the primary tumor.

FDG PET/CT

- CT is not always reliable in identifying pathologic lymphadenopathy because normal sized lymph nodes and those that demonstrate benign features such as fatty hila may contain metastatic foci. In addition, enlarged lymph nodes may be reactive rather than neoplastic.
- PET/CT evaluates the metabolic activity within lymph nodes and other structures, and higher levels of FDG uptake reflect greater metabolic activity.
- PET/CT is more accurate than CT at detecting lymph node involvement in lymphoma, with a sensitivity of 94% and a specificity of 100%, respectively, compared with 88% and 86% for CT.
- PET/CT is also effective in evaluating treatment response because FDG uptake in treated lymph nodes typically decreases or completely resolves.
- However, FDG uptake may be present in benign diseases such as infections and sarcoidosis, and PET/CT cannot reliably distinguish between lymphadenopathy due to malignancy and lymphadenopathy due to these benign processes.

Clinical Issues

- Treatment of mediastinal lymphadenopathy is related to the underlying disease process.
- The presence of lymphadenopathy in intrathoracic malignancies such as lung cancer, malignant pleural mesothelioma, and breast cancer impacts the overall stage of disease and the treatment options available.
- Internal mammary lymphadenopathy ipsilateral to the primary breast cancer without axillary lymphadenopathy is typically treated with a combination of surgery, chemotherapy, and radiation. Ipsilateral internal mammary and axillary lymphadenopathy necessitates preoperative chemotherapy.
- Lymphadenopathy secondary to lymphoma may demonstrate calcification after treatment.
- In the setting of metastatic disease, treatment of the primary tumor may result in improvement or resolution of the pathologic lymphadenopathy. Following treatment, characteristic features of involved lymph

nodes such as hyperenhancement due to tumor vascularity may decrease or resolve.

- Mediastinal lymphadenopathy due to infectious etiologies may improve or resolve with treatment specific to the causative organism. Granulomatous infections such as tuberculosis and histoplasmosis may result in calcified lymph nodes.
- The treatment of sarcoidosis is typically guided by a combination of clinical, functional, and radiologic findings, and corticosteroids are the mainstay of therapy.

Key Points

- Intrathoracic lymphadenopathy complicates many malignancies, infections, and inflammatory processes, and the mediastinum is the most commonly affected region.
- The most common abnormalities on radiography include abnormal mediastinal contours, loss of normal interfaces, and thickening of lines and stripes.
- Enlargement of mediastinal lymph nodes is the most reliable method of diagnosing lymphadenopathy on CT.
- Specific lymph node characteristics on CT, such as attenuation, enhancement, calcification, and distribution, may be used to narrow the differential diagnosis of possible etiologies.
- PET/CT is more accurate than CT at detecting lymph node involvement in lymphoma and other malignancies, but it cannot reliably distinguish between lymphadenopathy due to malignancies and lymphadenopathy due to benign processes such as infection and sarcoidosis.

Suggested Reading

Prabhakar HB, Rabinowitz CB, Gibbons FK, O'Donnell WJ, Shepard JA, Aquino SL. Imaging features of sarcoidosis on MDCT, FDG PET, and PET/CT. *AJR Am J Roentgenol.* 2008;190(3 Suppl):S1–S6.

Sharma A, Fidias P, Hayman LA, Loomis SL, Taber KH, Aquino SL. Patterns of lymphadenopathy in thoracic malignancies. *RadioGraphics.* 2004;24(2):419–434.

CHAPTER 84

Cysts of the Mediastinum

Brett W. Carter

Definition

A cyst is a closed fluid-filled sac bound by a thin cyst wall that is lined by an epithelium. Mediastinal cysts are typically congenital, account for approximately 15–20% of all mediastinal masses, and can be found in all mediastinal compartments. The most common mediastinal cysts are bronchogenic and pericardial cysts.

Clinical Features

The majority of mediastinal cysts are congenital. Affected patients are usually asymptomatic, and these lesions are often incidentally discovered on imaging studies performed for other reasons. Some affected patients may present with symptoms of mass effect on adjacent structures related to growth of the mediastinal cyst or its anatomic location.

Bronchogenic cysts are the most common congenital mediastinal cysts and result from abnormal budding from the ventral foregut or anomalous branching of the tracheobronchial tree. Bronchogenic cysts may compress the airway, leading to respiratory symptoms, or may become complicated by hemorrhage and produce chest pain. Esophageal duplication cysts may be of foregut or neurenteric origin. They may exert mass effect on adjacent structures such as the airway and esophagus and produce respiratory symptoms and dysphagia, respectively, or lead to chest pain secondary to cyst rupture. Esophageal duplication cysts may contain ectopic gastric mucosa and may become complicated by hemorrhage or perforation. Bronchogenic and esophageal duplication cysts rarely become infected with resultant associated signs and symptoms.

Although thymic cysts may be congenital, they are more commonly acquired and may be related to inflammatory or degenerative processes, neoplasms such as Hodgkin lymphoma, thymic malignancies such as thymoma and thymic carcinoma, and germ cell neoplasms such as seminoma.

Meningoceles represent herniation of cerebrospinal fluid-filled leptomeninges through an intervertebral foramen or a vertebral defect, and they may mimic true mediastinal cysts. Pericardial cysts result from anomalous outpouchings of the parietal pericardium.

Anatomy and Pathology

Mediastinal cysts are fluid-filled lesions surrounded by a thin wall with an epithelial lining, are typically well-circumscribed, and often exhibit a spherical morphology. The pathologic diagnosis relies on the identification of specific tissues within the cyst wall (e.g., a bronchogenic cyst has bronchial elements in its wall, including cartilage, submucosal glands, and smooth muscle). Congenital cysts may exhibit variable fluid content including serous, mucoid, purulent, or hemorrhagic fluid.

How to Approach the Image

Mediastinal cysts may be initially visualized on chest radiography, and detection relies on knowledge of the normal mediastinal contours and interfaces. Mediastinal cyst should not be the first consideration in the case of an anterior mediastinal mass because mediastinal neoplasms are more common. However, mediastinal cyst should be strongly considered in patients with spherical middle mediastinal masses, particularly masses in the subcarinal region (typically bronchogenic or other foregut-derived cysts) and well-defined cardiophrenic angle masses (typically pericardial cysts).

Once a mediastinal cyst is considered in the differential diagnosis, further evaluation with contrast-enhanced chest CT typically follows. MRI may be necessary in specific situations to document fluid content in high-attenuation mediastinal cysts and to evaluate the cyst wall for exclusion of mural nodules, which would suggest a cystic neoplasm.

What Not to Miss

The radiographic diagnosis of mediastinal cyst requires a thorough evaluation of the mediastinal contours on chest radiography. Although comparison to prior radiographs may facilitate determination of stability, most mediastinal cysts do not significantly change in size over time unless complicated by infection or hemorrhage. CT is the modality of choice for evaluating mediastinal abnormalities and distinguishing cysts from neoplasms and other lesions.

Characteristic imaging features include the following:

- Smooth, spherical, ovoid, or tubular unilocular cystic lesion with a thin wall that may enhance with contrast
- Homogeneous water attenuation contents, typically measuring 0–20 HU
- No internal enhancement
- No lymphadenopathy or locally invasive behavior

Differential Diagnosis

Mediastinal cysts may mimic solid primary mediastinal masses and mediastinal lymphadenopathy. Cross-sectional imaging is valuable in demonstrating their fluid content and excluding a cystic neoplasm.

Anterior (Prevascular) Mediastinum

- Thymic cyst: Represents 1% of all mediastinal masses; may be multilocular or unilocular; multilocular cysts associated with inflammatory processes and more common in men; mural nodules should suggest cystic neoplasm rather than congenital cyst (Fig. 84.1)

Middle (Visceral) Mediastinum

- Bronchogenic cyst: Unilocular cyst that may exhibit water, soft tissue, or heterogeneous attenuation and/or milk of calcium; typically subcarinal
- Esophageal duplication cyst: Unilocular cyst that typically affects children; may exhibit soft tissue or heterogeneous attenuation; typically located adjacent to the esophagus (Fig. 84.2)

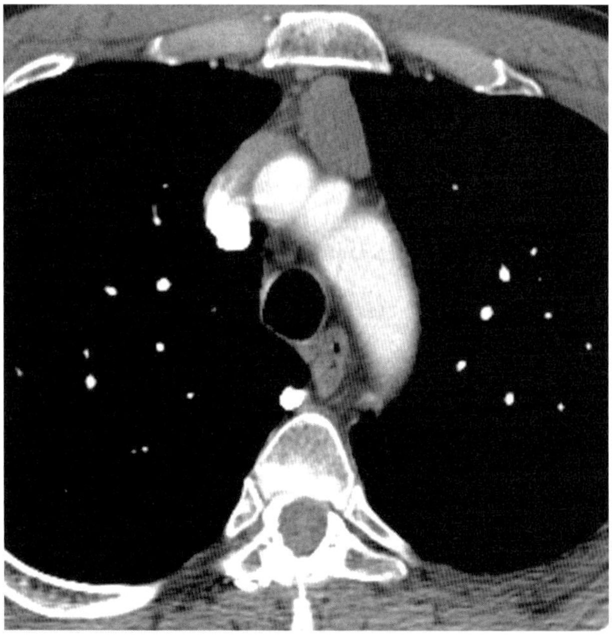

Figure 84.1. Thymic cyst. Contrast-enhanced chest CT of a 39-year-old asymptomatic woman shows a well-circumscribed, ovoid homogeneous low-attenuation thymic lesion. Despite the homogeneous water attenuation content of the lesion suggestive of a thymic cyst, the lesion was resected because of a history of prior thymoma.

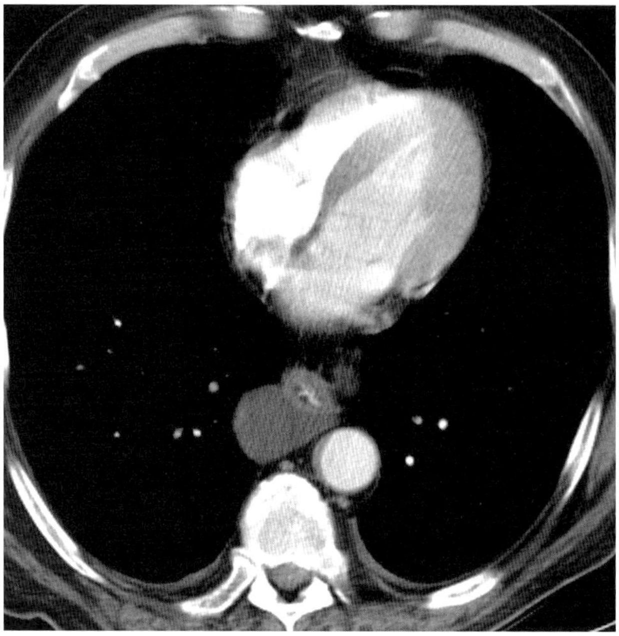

Figure 84.2. Esophageal duplication cyst. Contrast-enhanced chest CT of a 45-year-old man with an esophageal duplication cyst shows a well-circumscribed, hypodense lesion of water attenuation in the visceral mediastinum abutting the posterolateral distal esophagus.

Posterior (Paravertebral) Mediastinum

- Meningocele: Low-attenuation paravertebral "cystic" lesion that communicates with the spinal canal with associated abnormalities of the spine and other osseous structures (not a true mediastinal cyst); adults are most commonly affected; frequent association with neurofibromatosis
- Neurenteric cyst: Unilocular homogeneous cystic lesion; associated with spinal anomalies located cephalad to the cyst

Cardiophrenic Angle

- Pericardial cyst: Unilocular (80%) or multilocular (20%) cyst; found in either cardiophrenic angle but much more common on the right than the left

Imaging Findings

Thymic Cyst

- Spherical or ovoid well-defined anterior (prevascular) mediastinal cyst; may reach large sizes (Fig. 84.1)
- Thin or imperceptible wall; unilocular or multilocular—the latter may exhibit internal soft tissue septa
- Well-defined, homogeneous lesion of water attenuation (0–20 HU) contents on CT; infected/hemorrhagic cysts may exhibit high-attenuation contents

- Low signal intensity on T1-weighted MRI; hemorrhage or infection may result in intermediate or high signal intensity; high signal intensity on T2-weighted MRI and thin wall of low signal intensity

Bronchogenic Cyst

- Spherical middle (visceral) mediastinal mass, typically subcarinal on chest radiography, produces lateral displacement of the upper azygoesophageal recess (Fig. 84.3); may produce mass effect on the medial wall of the bronchus intermedius; may be paratracheal
- Well-defined borders and homogeneous water attenuation (0–20 HU) on CT (Fig. 84.3c); frequent soft tissue attenuation (44%) content due to proteinaceous fluid, hemorrhage, or infection; may exhibit milk of calcium

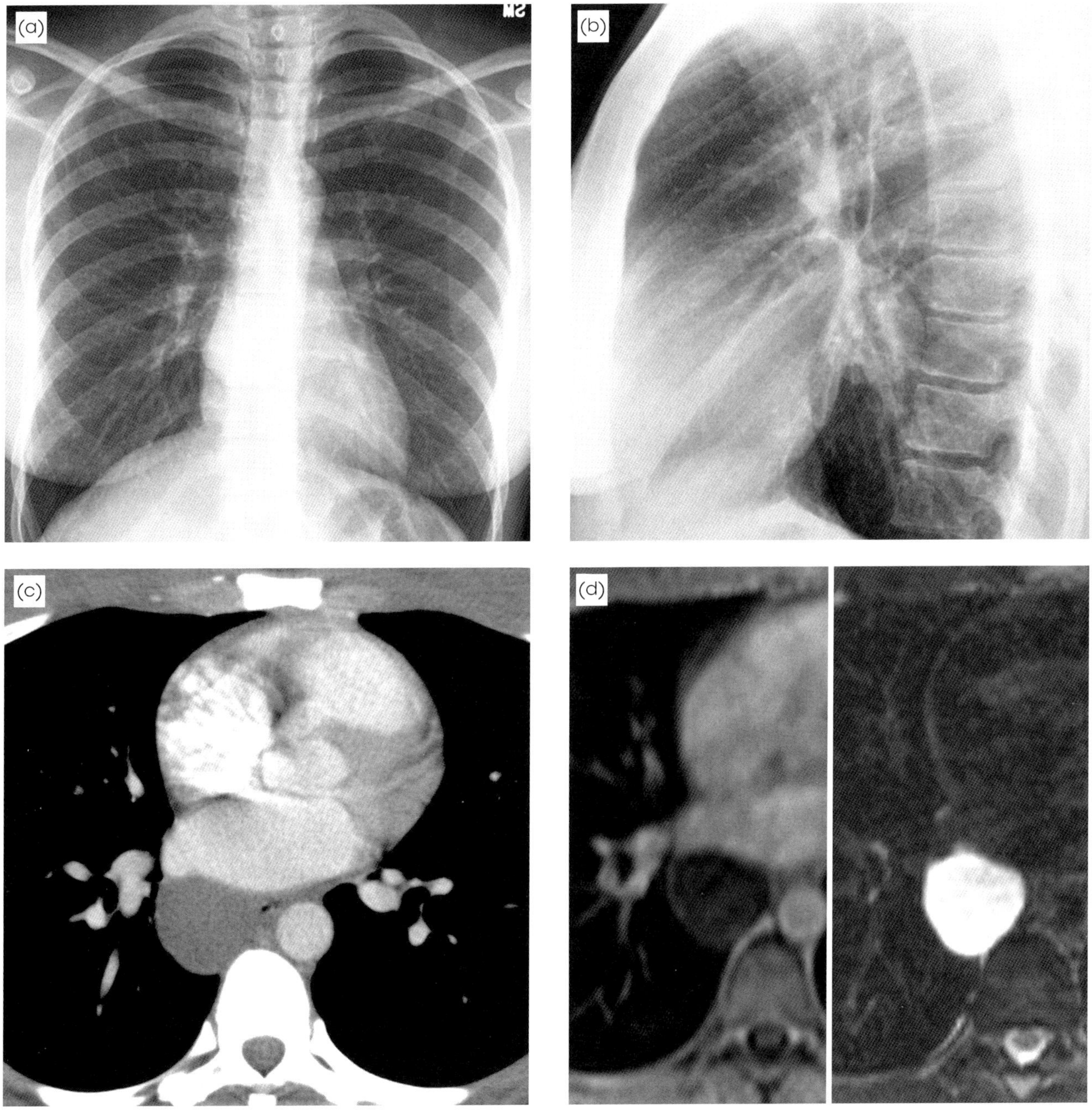

Figure 84.3. Bronchogenic cyst. (a, b) Posteroanterior and lateral chest radiographs of an asymptomatic 34-year-old woman show a well-circumscribed rounded middle mediastinal mass in the subcarinal region that produces a contour abnormality of the upper azygoesophageal recess. The lateral chest radiograph shows a spherical retrocardiac middle mediastinal lesion. Based on location and morphology, the differential diagnosis should include bronchogenic and esophageal duplication cysts. (c) Contrast-enhanced chest CT of the same patient shows a well-defined water attenuation visceral mediastinal mass located to the right of the esophagus and posterior to the left atrium. Hounsfield units measured slightly greater than water attenuation. (d) Composite image with contrast-enhanced T1-weighted (left) and T2-weighted (right) MR images of the same patient shows a nonenhancing spherical lesion with a thin perceptible wall. The lesion exhibits high signal intensity on the T2-weighted image consistent with fluid.

- Unilocular; thin wall may exhibit calcification and contrast enhancement
- Low signal intensity on T1-weighted MRI, although hemorrhage or infection may result in intermediate or high signal intensity; high signal intensity on T2-weighted MRI and visualization of low-signal-intensity thin cyst wall (Fig. 84.3d)

Esophageal Duplication Cyst

- Round or spherical middle (visceral) mediastinal lesion, most commonly in a paraesophageal location
- Well-defined homogeneous mass of water attenuation (0–20 HU), closely associated with the esophagus
- Internal hyperattenuation may be present in cysts complicated by hemorrhage or infection
- Thin wall that may be thicker than that of bronchogenic cyst
- Low signal intensity on T1-weighted MRI, although hemorrhage or infection may result in intermediate or high signal intensity; high signal intensity on T2-weighted MRI

Meningocele

- Spherical, smooth, or lobulated posterior mediastinal/paravertebral mass
- Well-defined, homogeneous lesion of water attenuation on CT and communication with spinal canal (Fig. 84.4)
- Association with enlarged intervertebral foramina, vertebral defects, scoliosis, and rib anomalies

Neurenteric Cyst

- Round or spherical posterior mediastinal/paravertebral region lesion
- Well-defined, homogeneous cyst with water attenuation (0–20 HU) contents on CT; internal hyperattenuation may occur in cysts complicated by hemorrhage or infection
- Low signal intensity on T1-weighted MRI, although hemorrhage or infection may result in intermediate or high signal intensity; high signal intensity on T2-weighted MRI

Pericardial Cyst

- Cardiophrenic angle mass on frontal radiography, overlies the anterior–inferior cardiac silhouette on lateral radiography
- Abuts the pericardium
- Smoothly marginated, homogeneous water attenuation (0–20 HU) cyst with imperceptible wall (Fig. 84.5)
- Low signal intensity on T1-weighted MRI; high signal intensity on T2-weighted MRI

Clinical Issues

- Most mediastinal cysts are asymptomatic. However, affected patients may develop symptoms, typically related to compression of adjacent structures.

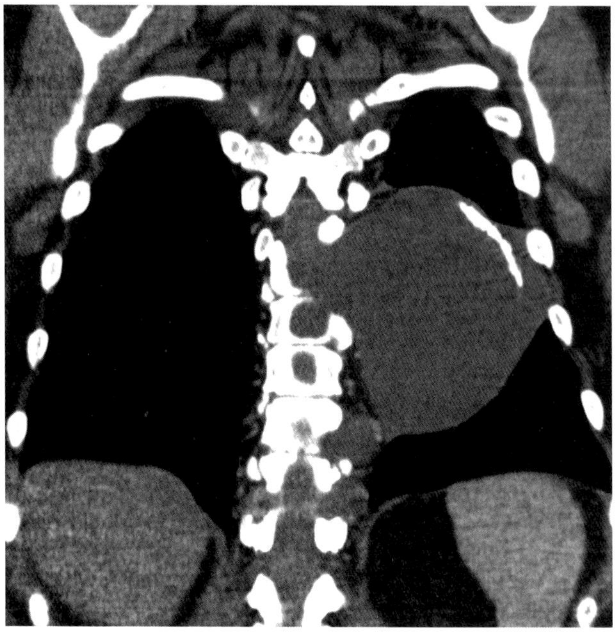

Figure 84.4. Meningocele. Coronal contrast-enhanced chest CT of a 37-year-old woman with neurofibromatosis shows large water attenuation left paravertebral mass with peripheral linear calcification, communication with the spinal canal, and marked enlargement of the adjacent neuroforamina.

- Appropriate management of mediastinal cysts is controversial and ranges from observation to surgical resection. Some clinicians recommend resection of all mediastinal cysts, even in asymptomatic patients, in order to establish the diagnosis and prevent complications.

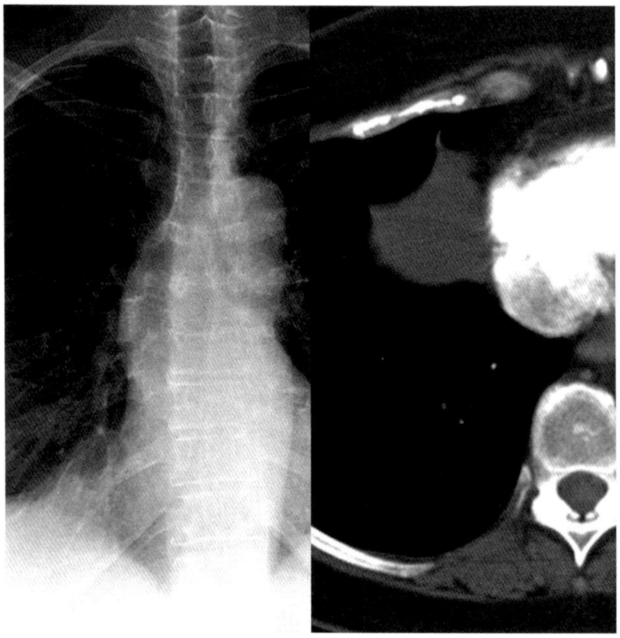

Figure 84.5. Pericardial cyst. Composite image with PA chest radiograph (left) and contrast-enhanced chest CT (right) shows a right cardiophrenic opacity that corresponds to a water attenuation lesion with imperceptible walls on CT consistent with pericardial cyst.

- Most thymic cysts are observed, although drainage or resection may be performed in symptomatic patients.
- Small bronchogenic cysts may be observed. However, surgical resection, drainage, or ablation should be performed for symptomatic lesions and should be considered in young, asymptomatic patients with low surgical risk.
- Esophageal duplication cysts may be observed or surgically resected.
- Pericardial cysts usually require no further follow-up or management.

Key Points

- Cysts may affect any mediastinal compartment but are typically located in the middle (visceral) mediastinum.
- Bronchogenic and pericardial cysts are the most commonly diagnosed mediastinal cysts.
- Although mediastinal cysts may first be identified on chest radiographs, the lesions are optimally evaluated on CT.
- Mediastinal cysts are typically well-circumscribed, homogeneous, low-attenuation masses on CT. However, they may be heterogeneous or of high attenuation in cases with proteinaceous, hemorrhagic, or infected fluid.
- Identification of a mural nodule(s) should suggest a cystic neoplasm rather than a congenital cyst.
- MRI may be useful in specific circumstances, such as characterization of the cyst wall, identification of soft tissue septa and mural nodules, and evaluation of cyst content.

Suggested Reading

Jeung MY, Gasser B, Gangi A, Bogorin A, Charneau D, Wihlm JM, et al. Imaging of cystic masses of the mediastinum. *RadioGraphics*. 2002;22(Spec No):S79–S93.

Takeda S, Miyoshi S, Minami M, Ohta M, Masaoka A, Matsuda H. Clinical spectrum of mediastinal cysts. *Chest*. 2003;124(1):125–132.

Zambudio AR, Lanzas JT, Calvo MJ, Fernandez PJ, Paricio PP. Non-neoplastic mediastinal cysts. *Eur J Cardiothorac Surg*. 2002;22(5):712–716.

CHAPTER 85

Glandular Enlargement

Brett W. Carter

Definition

Glandular enlargement due to hyperplasia may affect the thymus in the anterior mediastinum or the thyroid. The latter may be localized to the neck, originate in the lower neck and extend inferiorly into the mediastinum, or be ectopic and located in the mediastinum.

Clinical Features

Patients with glandular enlargement are typically asymptomatic. However, mediastinal goiter may produce symptoms related to mass effect on the trachea and other structures.

Thymic enlargement typically relates to rebound hyperplasia and, less frequently, to lymphoid hyperplasia. Rebound thymic hyperplasia is typically secondary to chemotherapy, radiation therapy, corticosteroid therapy, and stresses such as burns and injuries. It may be associated with other conditions, such as hyperthyroidism and sarcoidosis. Lymphoid hyperplasia is typically due to myasthenia gravis, although it is also associated with other autoimmune diseases, including systemic lupus erythematosus, rheumatoid arthritis, and scleroderma.

Mediastinal goiters represent enlarged thyroid tissue and may be classified as primary or secondary. Primary mediastinal goiters originate in ectopic thyroid tissue located in the mediastinum and are supplied by intrathoracic vessels. Secondary mediastinal goiters originate in the cervical thyroid but extend into the mediastinum and are supplied by vessels in the lower neck. Most goiters are secondary and arise from thyroid tissue in the lower neck. Mediastinal extension is common and occurs in approximately 35% of cases. Retrosternal goiters extend into the anterior mediastinum, and retrotracheal and retroesophageal goiters involve the middle and posterior mediastinum.

Anatomy and Physiology

Radiologic diagnosis of thymic enlargement relies on knowledge of the normal appearance of the thymus on both radiography and CT. Whereas the normal thymus may manifest as a large anterior mediastinal mass on chest radiographs of neonates and infants, it is not visible radiographically in normal adults. On CT of patients younger than age 20 years, the normal thymus manifests as homogeneous soft tissue in the prevascular mediastinum. Patients 20–50 years of age exhibit progressive fatty infiltration of the thymus, which shows a mixture of soft tissue and fatty elements. In patients older than age 50 years, the normal thymus is almost completely replaced by fat. Although the normal thymus is highly variable in size and shape, it usually exhibits straight or concave margins.

The normal thyroid is located in the lower neck and does not extend into the mediastinum. Thyroid goiters vary in size and morphology, and they may be localized to the neck or involve one or more mediastinal compartments as a primary or secondary process.

How to Approach the Image

Although thymic abnormalities are not usually visible on chest radiography, nonspecific mediastinal widening may be identified on frontal radiography and subtle anterior mediastinal opacity may be present on lateral radiography. Thymic enlargement may produce thickening of the anterior junction line. Therefore, careful evaluation of the mediastinal contours and the retrosternal region on radiography is important for detection of subtle thymic abnormalities.

Thyroid goiters typically manifest as mediastinal masses that exhibit continuity with an enlarged cervical thyroid gland and produce mass effect on the trachea. These lesions may demonstrate the radiographic cervicothoracic sign. Cross-sectional imaging with CT or MRI is often used to document continuity between the cervical and mediastinal components of the goiter and to exclude lymphadenopathy as the etiology of the mediastinal abnormality. Intravenous contrast may be withheld to avoid thyrotoxicosis in patients with hyperthyroidism and in patients who are candidates for radioiodine therapy.

What Not to Miss

Thymic hyperplasia should be considered in patients with abnormal anterior or prevascular mediastinal soft tissue. The enlarged thymus should be similar in attenuation and enhancement characteristics to the normal thymus on CT, and it should not demonstrate lobular contours or heterogeneous enhancement, which suggest neoplastic involvement.

Identification of secondary mediastinal goiter relies on recognition of mediastinal enlargement associated with enlargement of the cervical thyroid and associated tracheal displacement. Although the latter is almost always present on radiography, the extent of tracheal compression cannot be ascertained on radiography alone, and CT is required for delineating the extent of tracheal narrowing. Multiplanar imaging is also useful in documenting continuity between the cervical and mediastinal components of the mass.

Differential Diagnosis

The differential diagnosis of glandular enlargement is influenced by lesion location within the mediastinum, demographic information, and clinical history.

Thymic Hyperplasia

- Normal thymus: Homogeneous prevascular mediastinal soft tissue in patients younger than age 20 years; progressive fatty infiltration of the thymus occurs after the age of 20 years, resulting in greater heterogeneity with complete fatty replacement after age 50 years; loss of signal on opposed-phase T1-weighted MRI
- Thymoma: Men and women older than age 40 years; may be asymptomatic; may produce symptoms related to mass effect, local invasion, or metastases or may be associated with a paraneoplastic syndrome such as myasthenia gravis; no signal loss on opposed-phase T1-weighted MRI
- Lymphoma: Mediastinal lymphadenopathy that may coalesce as a dominant mass; homogeneous thymic enlargement; no signal loss on opposed-phase T1-weighted MRI
- Thymic cyst: Multilocular or unilocular cystic lesion in the prevascular mediastinum; may be associated with neoplasms such as lymphoma and thymoma
- Metastatic disease: Nodular soft tissue in the prevascular mediastinum (and/or other compartments); heterogeneous enhancement, necrosis; no signal loss on opposed-phase T1-weighted MRI

Thyroid Goiter

- Thymoma: Men and women older than age 40 years; may be asymptomatic; may have symptoms related to mass effect, local invasion, or metastases or may be associated with a paraneoplastic syndrome such as myasthenia gravis; absence of continuity with cervical thyroid tissue
- Lymphoma: Mediastinal lymphadenopathy may coalesce to form a dominant mass; no continuity with thyroid tissue
- Mediastinal cysts: Multilocular or unilocular cystic lesions that are typically well circumscribed, homogeneous, and low attenuation; may be heterogeneous due to hemorrhage or infection
- Lymphangioma: May exhibit macroscopic cystic changes; may displace or insinuate itself around adjacent mediastinal structures; calcification uncommon

Imaging Findings

Thymic Hyperplasia

- Chest radiographs are usually normal, but nonspecific mediastinal widening or retrosternal opacity may be identified.
- True thymic hyperplasia most commonly manifests with diffuse, symmetric enlargement of the thymus on CT (Fig. 85.1).
- Lymphoid hyperplasia may manifest as normal thymus (45% of patients), thymic enlargement (35%), or focal thymic mass (20%). Rebound and lymphoid hyperplasia demonstrate the same attenuation and enhancement characteristics as normal thymus.
- MRI may be used to differentiate normal thymus and thymic hyperplasia from mediastinal neoplasms using chemical shift imaging. Normal thymus and thymic hyperplasia lose signal on opposed-phase T1-weighted MRI (Fig. 85.2).

Thyroid Goiter

- The most common imaging appearance is a mediastinal mass with extension into the neck on chest radiography exhibiting the cervicothoracic sign (Figs. 85.3 and 85.4).
- Lateral chest radiographs may demonstrate abnormal soft tissue in the retrosternal clear space. Retrotracheal goiters may produce mass effect on the posterior trachea.
- Although tracheal displacement is almost always present on radiography, the extent of tracheal compression and narrowing cannot be ascertained on radiography alone. CT optimally demonstrates the size and extent of the goiter and allows delineation of the degree of tracheal compression (Figs. 85.3 and 85.4).
- The most common finding of a secondary mediastinal goiter on CT is a heterogeneous soft tissue mass that demonstrates contiguity with the cervical thyroid gland (Figs. 85.3 and 85.4).
- The typical CT appearance of a primary mediastinal goiter is a solitary, heterogeneous soft tissue focus localized to one of the mediastinal compartments.
- Goiters are hyperdense on unenhanced CT due to the presence of iodine within the thyroid tissue, and they measure 70–85 HU.
- Calcification and cystic change are common.
- On contrast-enhanced CT, goiters demonstrate intense and sustained enhancement. However, cystic areas do not demonstrate enhancement.

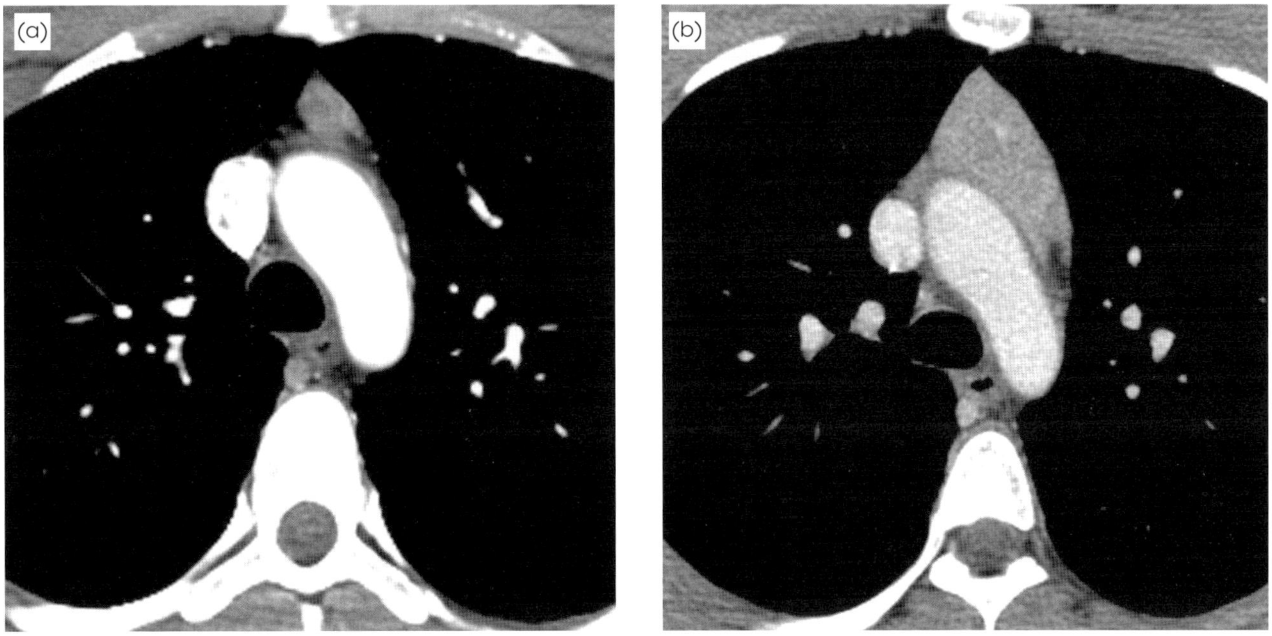

Figure 85.1. Thymic hyperplasia. (a) Contrast-enhanced chest CT of a 33-year-old woman with lymphoma shows a round prevascular mediastinal soft tissue nodule in the region of the thymus, representing normal thymic tissue in a patient of this age. (b) Contrast-enhanced chest CT of the same patient 3 months after chemotherapy shows diffuse thymic enlargement with attenuation and enhancement characteristics similar to those of normal thymus. Thymic hyperplasia commonly occurs following chemotherapy, radiation, and corticosteroids.

- Intravenous contrast should be avoided in patients with hyperthyroidism to prevent thyrotoxicosis and also in potential candidates for radioactive iodine therapy.
- Goiters demonstrate intermediate signal intensity on T1-weighted MRI. Cystic foci may demonstrate high signal intensity on T1-weighted MRI due to hemorrhagic or proteinaceous content. Although goiters are typically heterogeneous on T2-weighted MRI, they usually demonstrate high signal intensity relative to surrounding structures.

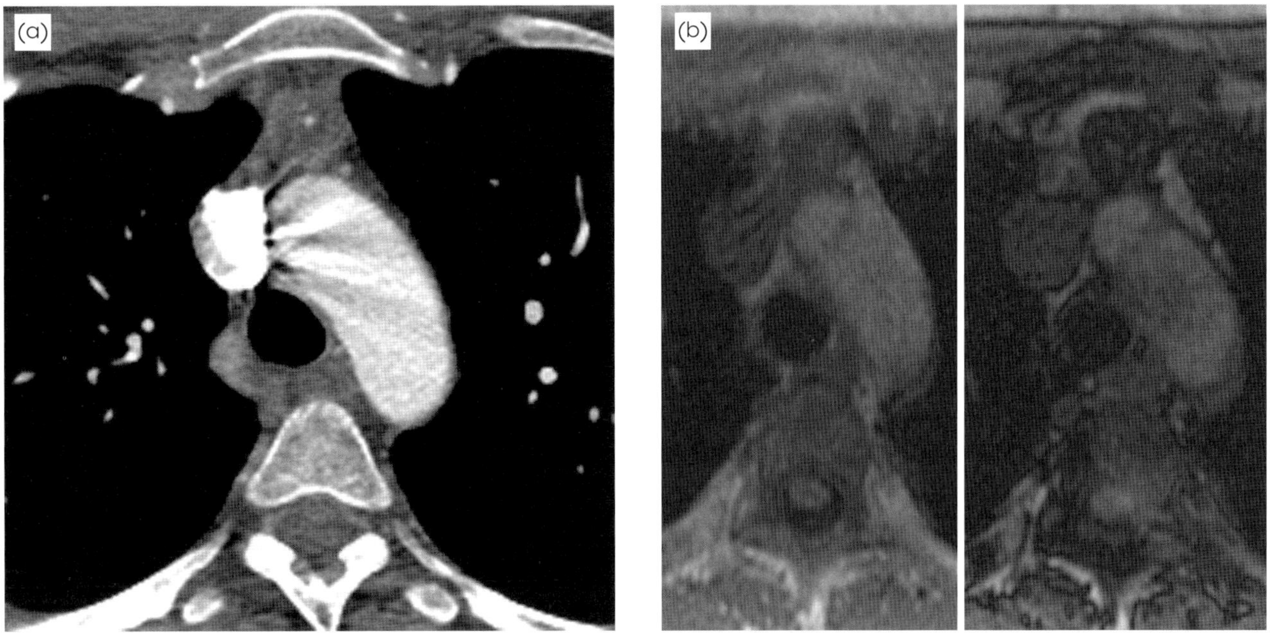

Figure 85.2. Thymic hyperplasia. (a) Contrast-enhanced chest CT of an asymptomatic 41-year-old woman shows a prevascular mediastinal soft tissue nodule in the region of the thymus. Central enhancement and slight heterogeneity were concerning for malignancy. (b) Composite image with in-phase (left) and opposed-phase (right) T1-weighted MRI of the same patient shows a nodule of homogeneous low signal intensity that exhibits near complete loss of signal on opposed-phase imaging consistent with microscopic fat within thymic tissue.

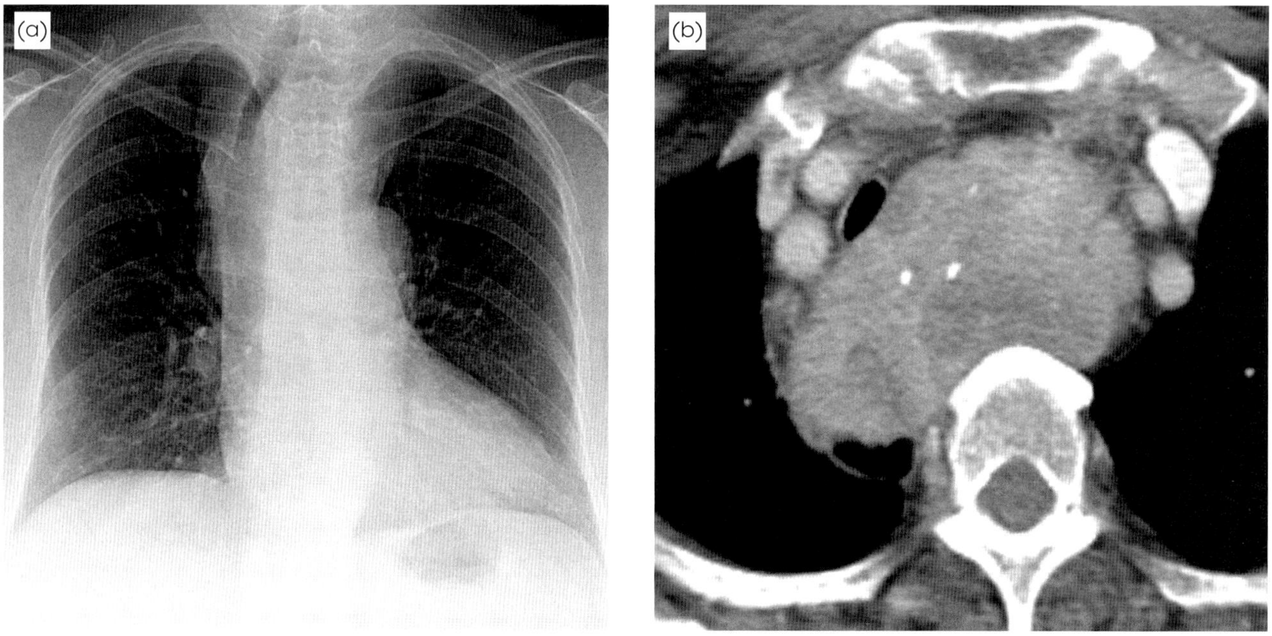

Figure 85.3. Thyroid goiter. (a) PA chest radiograph shows a large left superior mediastinal mass extending into the neck, narrowing the suprasternal trachea, which is deviated to the right, and exhibiting the cervicothoracic sign with loss of the lesion's borders as it traverses cephalad through the thoracic inlet into the neck. (b) Contrast-enhanced chest CT of the same patient shows a large, heterogeneous visceral mediastinal mass with punctate calcifications that produces mass effect on the trachea and esophagus. The lesion enhances intensely with contrast, consistent with thyroid tissue.

Clinical Issues

- Thymic hyperplasia typically does not require treatment.
- Lymphoid thymic hyperplasia should prompt clinical assessment to identify associated autoimmune conditions.
- Thymic hyperplasia may decrease in size or resolve over time following completion of chemotherapy or radiation therapy or as thyroid function normalizes in cases due to hyperthyroidism.

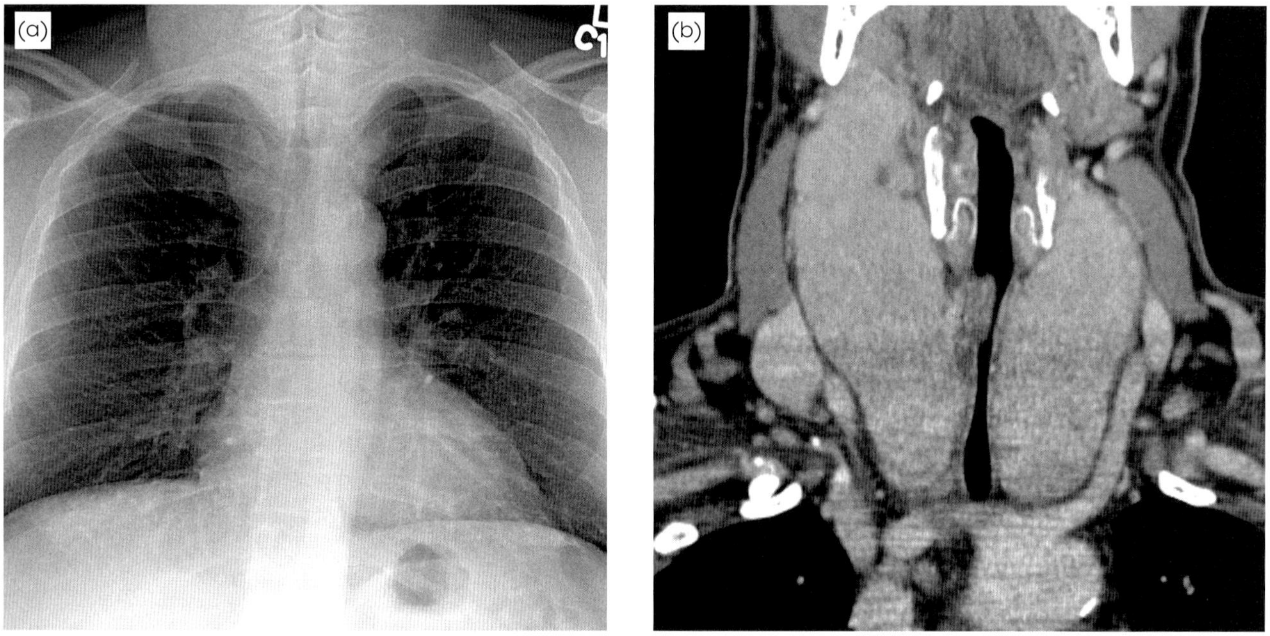

Figure 85.4. Thyroid goiter. (a) PA chest radiograph of a 44-year-old man with dyspnea and wheezing shows increased opacity in the thoracic inlet and marked tracheal narrowing. Note that the borders of the cervical component of the mass are poorly defined on radiography. (b) Coronal contrast-enhanced neck CT of the same patient shows diffuse bilateral thyroid enlargement with extension of the goiter inferiorly into the superior mediastinum and marked tracheal narrowing.

- Small goiters and those affecting elderly patients may be observed. The only definitive treatment for symptomatic thyroid goiter is surgical resection.

Key Points

- Thymic enlargement may represent thymic or lymphoid hyperplasia.
- Thymic hyperplasia is typically due to rebound thymic enlargement. It may be secondary to chemotherapy, radiation therapy, or corticosteroids; stresses such as burns and severe injuries; as well as hyperthyroidism and sarcoidosis.
- The most common manifestation of thymic hyperplasia on CT is homogeneous soft tissue in the prevascular mediastinum that demonstrates similar attenuation and enhancement characteristics as normal thymus.
- MRI can be used to differentiate normal thymus and thymic hyperplasia, which demonstrate signal loss on opposed-phase T1-weighted MRI, from other prevascular mediastinal neoplasms, which do not exhibit signal loss.
- Thyroid goiters may be primary when located in the mediastinum or secondary when originating in the lower neck and extending inferiorly into the mediastinum.
- Secondary mediastinal goiters manifest as mediastinal masses that exhibit continuity with the cervical thyroid, typically displace the trachea, and may result in airway compression.
- CT of goiter demonstrates a heterogeneous mass with intense and sustained contrast enhancement with frequent intrinsic calcification.
- CT and MRI are useful in documenting continuity between the cervical and mediastinal components of the goiters.

Suggested Reading

Ackman JB, Wu CC. MRI of the thymus. *AJR Am J Roentgenol.* 2011;197(1):W15–W20.

Nasseri F, Eftekhari F. Clinical and radiologic review of the normal and abnormal thymus: Pearls and pitfalls. *RadioGraphics.* 2010;30(2):413–428.

Nishino M, Ashiku SK, Kocher ON, Thurer RL, Boiselle PM, Hatabu H. The thymus: A comprehensive review. *RadioGraphics.* 2006;26(2):335–348.

Pollard DB, Weber CW, Hudgins PA. Preoperative imaging of thyroid goiter: How imaging technique can influence anatomic appearance and create a potential for inaccurate interpretation. *Am J Neuroradiol.* 2005;26(5):1215–1217.

CHAPTER 86

Vascular Lesions of the Mediastinum

Brett W. Carter

Definition

Vascular lesions of the mediastinum include abnormalities of the systemic and pulmonary arteries and veins and the aortic arch, as well as benign neoplasms such as hemangiomas and lymphangiomas. These lesions may be found in any compartment, but anomalies of the great vessels are most commonly encountered in the middle and posterior mediastinum, and hemangiomas and lymphangiomas are most common in the anterior mediastinum. Vascular lesions represent approximately 10% of mediastinal masses detected on chest radiography and may be mistaken for solid tumors.

Clinical Features

Mediastinal vascular lesions may be congenital or acquired. Congenital lesions may be associated with congenital heart disease in the pediatric population. Degenerative, post-traumatic, and neoplastic etiologies are the most common causes of acquired lesions. Hemangiomas are benign lesions composed of vascular spaces, and lymphangiomas are malformations of the lymphatic system. The latter typically affect children. Although many patients with vascular masses are often asymptomatic, and the abnormalities are incidentally discovered on radiologic studies performed for other reasons, some affected patients may present with symptoms.

Anatomy and Physiology

The radiographic identification of mediastinal vascular masses relies on knowledge of normal mediastinal anatomy and a high index of suspicion. Although these lesions may involve any mediastinal compartment, they are most common in the middle and posterior mediastinum.

How to Approach the Image

Although chest radiography may be normal in patients with vascular masses, careful evaluation of the frontal and lateral radiographs may allow identification of subtle radiographic abnormalities. Alterations of the normal mediastinal contours are the most common feature of vascular lesions. For example, aneurysms of the ascending and descending thoracic aorta may result in abnormal convexity of the right cardiomediastinal silhouette and obscuration of the left para-aortic interface, respectively. Vascular lesions may also manifest as nonspecific mediastinal widening or sharply marginated opacities localized to specific mediastinal compartments. Once the precise location of the abnormality has been determined, a focused differential diagnosis may be generated, and further evaluation with cross-sectional imaging such as contrast-enhanced CT or CT angiography (CTA) is usually performed. MRI may be necessary in situations in which intravenous contrast is contraindicated due to allergy or renal failure.

What Not to Miss

- Although CT allows optimal evaluation of mediastinal masses, the utilization of intravenous contrast material greatly improves detection of vascular lesions, which may manifest as hypodense masses on unenhanced CT.
- A high index of suspicion is required for the evaluation of masses that abut adjacent vascular structures and lesions that exhibit peripheral rim or intrinsic punctate calcification.

Differential Diagnosis

The differential diagnosis of mediastinal vascular masses is highly influenced by history, lesion location within the mediastinum, and morphologic features.

- Metastatic disease: Enlarged enhancing mediastinal lymph nodes or masses; typically from renal and thyroid cancers, melanoma, and sarcoma
- Hematoma: Typically seen in the postoperative or post-traumatic setting; may be heterogeneous due to blood products of different ages

Imaging Findings

Radiography

Systemic Arteries

- Aortic aneurysms and pseudoaneurysms (Fig. 86.1): Abnormal convexity of the right cardiomediastinal

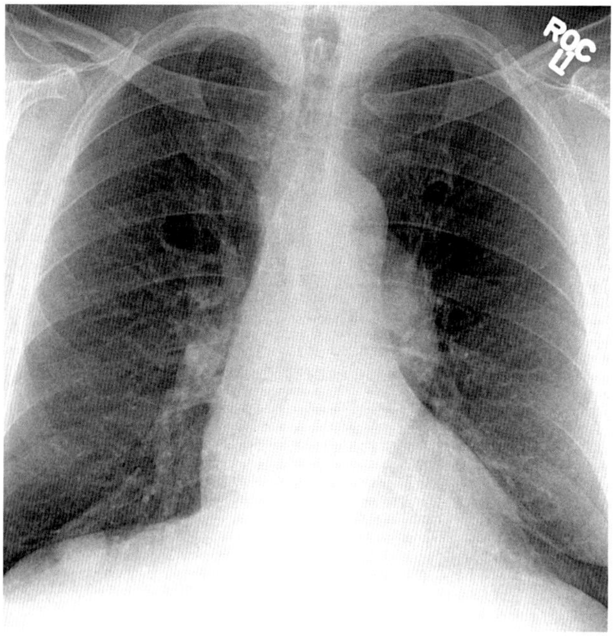

Figure 86.1. Aortic aneurysm. Posteroanterior (PA) chest radiograph of an asymptomatic 53-year-old man shows enlargement of the descending thoracic aorta consistent with aortic aneurysm.

silhouette with involvement of ascending aorta; obscuration or enlargement of the left para-aortic interface with involvement of the descending aorta. Saccular aneurysms may mimic primary mediastinal neoplasms and may exhibit peripheral calcification

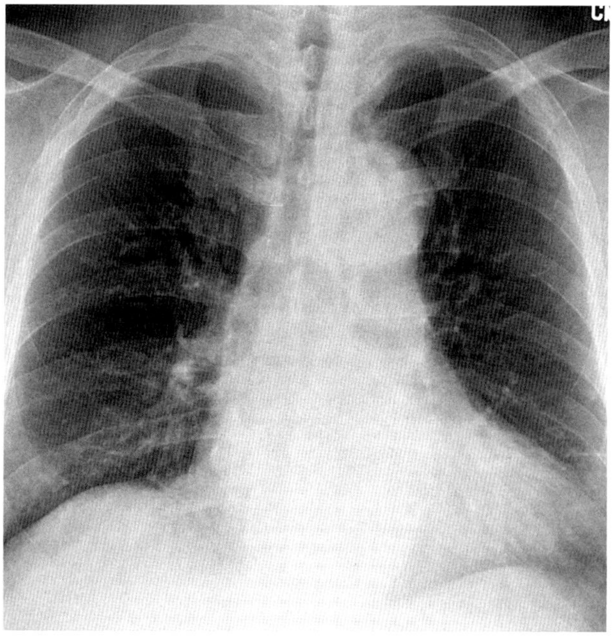

Figure 86.2. Aortic dissection. PA chest radiograph of a 59-year-old man with chest pain shows marked enlargement of the aortic arch, a wide descending thoracic aorta, thickened bilateral paratracheal stripes, and tracheal narrowing near the thoracic inlet. CT (not shown) confirmed aortic dissection and mediastinal hemorrhage that extended along the trachea.

- Aortic dissection (Fig. 86.2): Mediastinal widening; size discrepancy between ascending and descending aorta; displacement of intimal calcification from the aortic wall by approximately 1 cm (the most specific sign on chest radiography)
- Brachiocephalic artery aneurysm: Left or right superior mediastinal mass
- Left ventricular aneurysm: Paracardiac mass that may demonstrate calcification

Systemic Veins

- Persistent left superior vena cava (Fig. 86.3): Radiography may be normal; wide left superior mediastinum, lateral displacement of aortopulmonary interface
- Right superior vena cava aneurysm: Wide right superior mediastinum
- Venous graft aneurysm (Fig. 86.4): Left mediastinal/perihilar mass
- Left superior intercostal vein: Aortic nipple
- Paraesophageal varices (Fig. 86.5): Radiography often normal; middle or posterior mediastinal mass

Pulmonary Arteries

- Pulmonary artery enlargement: Typically from pulmonary hypertension; enlarged pulmonary trunk
- Aberrant left pulmonary artery (pulmonary sling): Opacity between the trachea anteriorly and the esophagus posteriorly

Pulmonary Veins

- Partial anomalous pulmonary venous return: Radiography may be normal; wide left superior mediastinum; lateral displacement of the aortopulmonary interface
- Pulmonary venous confluence: Retrocardiac mediastinal mass

Aortic Arch

- Right aortic arch (Fig. 86.6): Right paratracheal or superior mediastinal mass
- Double aortic arch: Left aortic arch in expected position with associated right paratracheal mass formed by the right arch
- Coarctation: Characteristic "figure 3" sign, which describes a mediastinal contour abnormality produced by the dilated left subclavian artery proximal to the coarctation and the descending aorta distal to the coarctation

Computed Tomography

- Vascular lesions may mimic solid masses on unenhanced CT.
- Although communication with parent and/or branch vessels may be evident on unenhanced CT, contrast-enhanced CT and CTA optimally demonstrate opacification of the vascular lesion and similar opacification of parent and/or branch vessels.

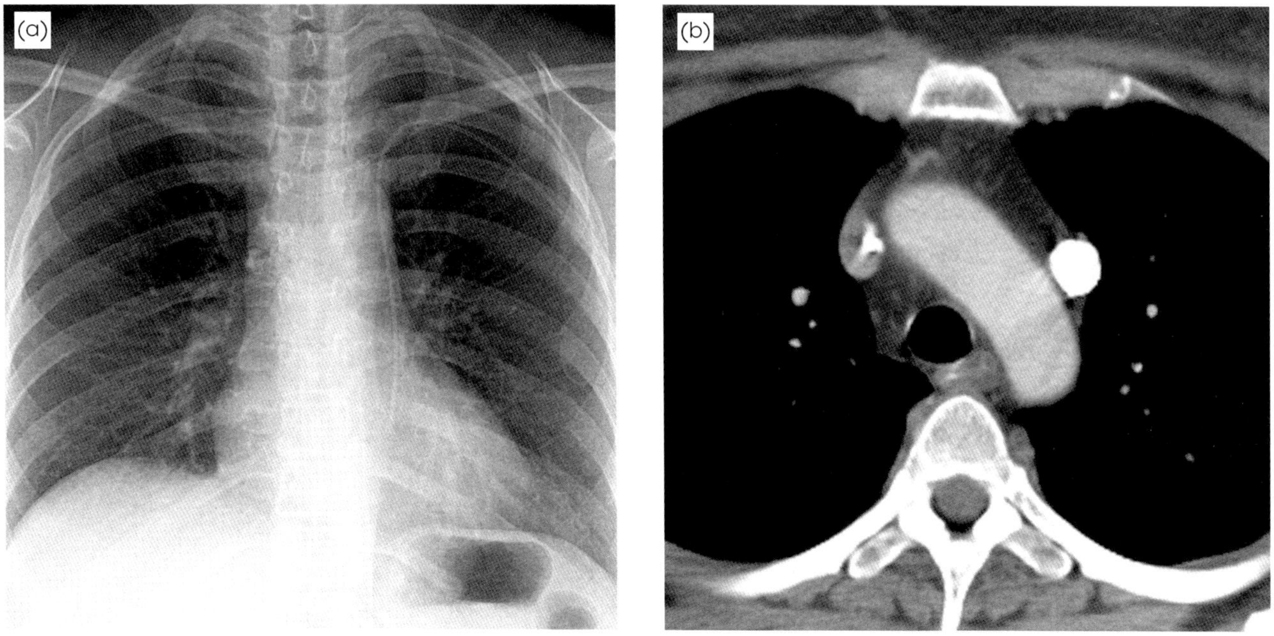

Figure 86.3. Persistent left superior vena cava. (a) PA chest radiograph of a 36-year-old man with a history of lymphoma shows a left subclavian central venous catheter extending vertically along the left aspect of the mediastinum. (b) Contrast-enhanced CT of the same patient demonstrates a contrast-filled vessel in the left prevascular mediastinum, consistent with a persistent left superior vena cava.

- Opacification of vascular masses depends on appropriate timing of the contrast bolus. Abnormalities of the systemic arteries are optimally evaluated on studies timed for evaluation of the aorta, whereas anomalies of the pulmonary arteries are best visualized on studies timed for evaluation of the pulmonary arteries. Systemic venous lesions are optimally characterized on routine contrast-enhanced chest CT.
- Although they are vascular lesions, lymphangiomas do not typically enhance with contrast.

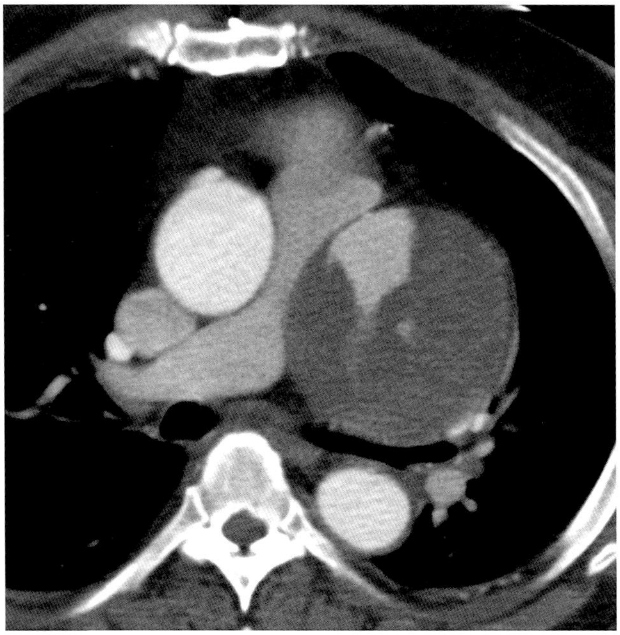

Figure 86.4. Saphenous vein graft aneurysm. Contrast-enhanced chest CT of a 65-year-old man with a history of coronary artery bypass grafting shows a round left visceral mediastinal mass with internal enhancement and thrombus.

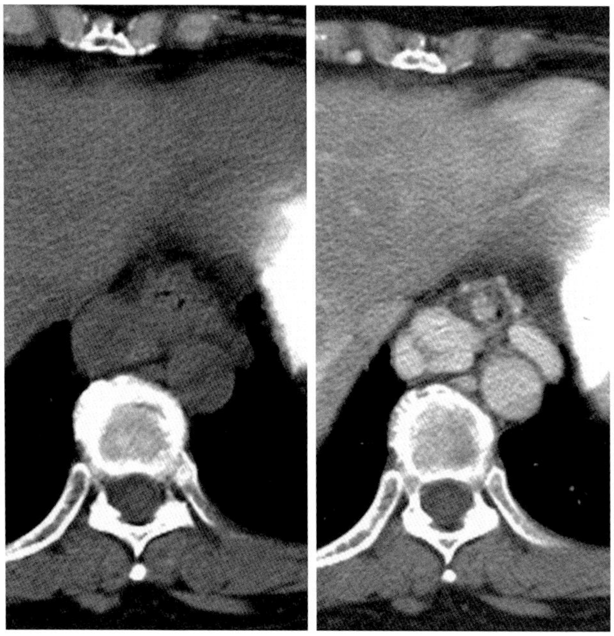

Figure 86.5. Paraesophageal varices. Composite image with unenhanced (left) and contrast-enhanced (right) chest CT of a 58-year-old man with cirrhosis and portal hypertension shows intense enhancement of paraesophageal soft tissue confirming large varices.

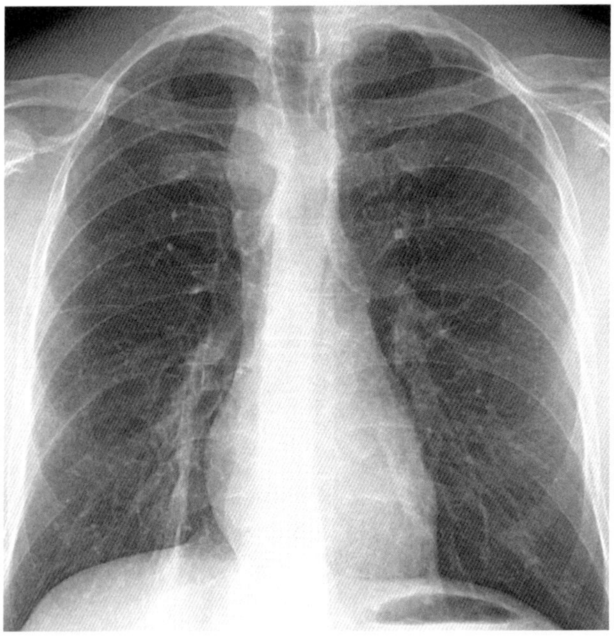

Figure 86.6. Right aortic arch. PA chest radiograph of a 42-year-old man shows absence of a normal left aortic arch and an ovoid opacity in the right paratracheal middle mediastinum that indents the right trachea consistent with a right aortic arch.

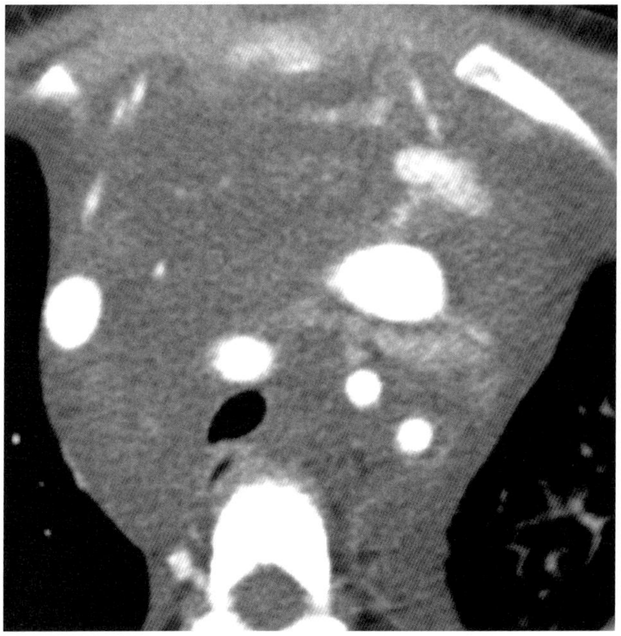

Figure 86.7. Lymphangioma. Contrast-enhanced chest CT of a child with dyspnea shows a large low-attenuation mass involving the prevascular and visceral mediastinal compartments and encasing the mediastinal vessels without evidence of obstruction. Enhancing foci within the lesion corresponded to foci of hemangioma within the lesion.

Hemangioma

- Radiography typically shows a well-defined mediastinal soft tissue mass. Intralesional phleboliths are rarely seen on radiography.
- Most lesions are heterogeneous on CT, with regions of intratumoral thrombus and vessels. Phleboliths are present in 30% of cases.
- Following the administration of intravenous contrast, enhancement may be central, peripheral, or mixed. Progressive enhancement on dynamic CT is typical.
- Heterogeneous signal intensity on T1-weighted MRI secondary to intratumoral fat and hemorrhage and on T2-weighted MRI secondary to vascular and myxoid components are typical.

Lymphangioma

- Radiography typically shows a well-defined mediastinal soft tissue mass that may exhibit smooth or lobulated margins. Extramediastinal extension into the chest wall or neck may be evident.
- Lymphangiomas are uniformly cystic masses that may displace adjacent mediastinal structures or insinuate themselves around these structures (Fig. 86.7).
- Attenuation on CT is typically greater than water, reflecting the presence of proteinaceous components.
- Most lymphangiomas do not demonstrate enhancement, although intrinsic hemangiomatous elements may enhance (Fig. 86.7).
- Lymphangiomas demonstrate high signal intensity relative to muscle on T1-weighted MRI and high signal intensity on T2-weighted MRI.

Clinical Issues

- Congenital vascular lesions may be associated with congenital heart disease in the pediatric population.
- Degenerative, post-traumatic and neoplastic etiologies are the most common causes of acquired lesions and are typically encountered in the adult population.
- Many patients with mediastinal vascular lesions are asymptomatic, but some patients may present with acute symptoms in emergent situations. Patients with rapidly enlarging or ruptured aortic aneurysms and those with aortic dissection may present emergently with chest pain, dyspnea, and hemodynamic instability. Aneurysm rupture and aortic dissection involving the ascending thoracic aorta are surgical emergencies. Some of these lesions may be managed with endovascular therapy with stent grafts.
- Mediastinal hemangiomas are associated with peripheral hemangiomas and hereditary hemorrhagic telangiectasia. Surgical resection of hemangiomas is typically necessary for diagnosis but carries the risk of significant blood loss.

- Lymphangiomas typically affect the pediatric population and may be diagnosed in utero. Surgical resection or ablation may be required to manage continued growth.

Key Points

- Vascular lesions represent approximately 10% of mediastinal masses and contour abnormalities detected on chest radiography.
- The most common mediastinal vascular masses are aneurysms of the aorta and great vessels. Graft aneurysms and pseudoaneurysms are important considerations in patients with a history of prior coronary bypass. Hemangiomas and lymphangiomas are rare.
- Vascular lesions may simulate soft tissue masses on unenhanced CT. Therefore, contrast-enhanced CT and CTA are the optimal modalities to evaluate these abnormalities for demonstration of opacification of vascular lesions and connections with parent and/or branch vessels.
- Optimal visualization of vascular abnormalities is dependent on correct timing of the contrast bolus.
- Hemangiomas are heterogeneous on CT, with regions of intratumoral thrombus and vascularity, heterogeneous enhancement, and phleboliths.
- Lymphangiomas are uniformly cystic masses that may displace or insinuate themselves around adjacent mediastinal structures and typically do not enhance.

Suggested Reading

Boateng P, Anjum W, Wechsler AS. Vascular lesions of the mediastinum. *Thorac Surg Clin*. 2009;19(1):91–105.

Demos TC, Posniak HV, Pierce KL, Olson MC, Muscato M. Venous anomalies of the thorax. *AJR Am J Roentgenol.* 2004;182(5):1139–1150.

CHAPTER 87

Miscellaneous Lesions of the Mediastinum

Brett W. Carter

Definition

Several types of lesions distinct from benign or malignant neoplasms, cysts, lymphadenopathy, and vascular lesions may affect the mediastinum. Extramedullary hematopoiesis affects the paravertebral regions. Herniations into the mediastinum can also occur, including hiatal, paraesophageal, and Morgagni hernias, and they may affect one or more mediastinal compartments. Hiatal hernias may be classified as sliding type, in which the gastroesophageal junction and gastric cardia herniate through the esophageal hiatus into the thorax, and paraesophageal type, in which the stomach herniates into the thorax alongside the esophagus. A Morgagni hernia is an anteromedial herniation through a retrosternal diaphragmatic defect and typically contains fat, but it may also include various abdominal organs.

Clinical Features

Extramedullary hematopoiesis is characterized by the proliferation of hematopoietic cells outside of the bone marrow and is commonly associated with myelofibrosis, ß-thalassemia, sickle cell anemia, and hereditary spherocytosis. Hiatal, paraesophageal, and Morgagni hernias increase in frequency with age and obesity. Although these hernias are typically asymptomatic, affected patients may present with symptoms.

Anatomy and Physiology

The radiologic diagnosis of extramedullary hematopoiesis and herniations relies on knowledge of normal chest radiographic anatomy. These lesions are most common in the posterior and middle mediastinum, respectively. Although small lesions may not be visible on radiography, large lesions manifest as distinct masses and often produce an abnormal mediastinal interface such as thickening of the paravertebral stripes in extramedullary hematopoiesis and lateral displacement of the azygoesophageal recess in herniations through the esophageal hiatus.

How to Approach the Image

Because many mediastinal lesions are initially identified on chest radiography, careful radiographic analysis is important for identification of abnormal opacities or alteration of mediastinal contours. Extramedullary hematopoiesis may manifest as a paravertebral mass and may exhibit associated skeletal abnormalities. Hiatus and paraesophageal hernias are often diagnosed on radiography. Once the precise location of the abnormality has been determined and associated findings are identified, a focused differential diagnosis can be generated, and further evaluation with cross-sectional imaging such as contrast-enhanced chest CT may be performed.

What Not to Miss

- Mediastinal abnormalities are optimally evaluated with CT.
- Extramedullary hematopoiesis should be included in the differential diagnosis of a posterior mediastinal or paravertebral mass and must be distinguished from neurogenic neoplasms. The relationship between the lesion and the spinal canal should be ascertained because intraspinal extension may occur.
- Widening of the esophageal hiatus is seen in hiatal and paraesophageal hernias.
- Diaphragmatic defects can be identified in Morgagni hernias. Multiplanar imaging allows confident identification of herniated abdominal structures through the hernia defect.
- Hernias may contain abdominal fat, bowel, liver, and other organs, and careful assessment of hernia contents is important to exclude complications of herniation.

Differential Diagnosis

Extramedullary Hematopoiesis

- Neurogenic neoplasm: Spherical or elongated paravertebral mass; may produce erosion or displacement of adjacent osseous structures; intraspinal extension/growth may be present; no associated lymphadenopathy
- Meningocele: Spherical water attenuation paravertebral lesion; frequently associated with neurofibromatosis; associated with abnormalities of the spine and other osseous structures

- Neurenteric cyst: Rare unilocular cyst with water attenuation or heterogeneous cyst content; associated with abnormalities of the spine occurring cephalad to the cyst
- Lymphadenopathy: Enlarged posterior mediastinal (paravertebral) lymph nodes may coalesce to form masses; no associated skeletal abnormalities

Hiatal and Paraesophageal Hernia
- Bronchogenic cyst: Unilocular cyst that may exhibit heterogeneous contents; typically identified in the subcarinal region displacing the upper aspect of the azygoesophageal recess
- Esophageal duplication cyst: Unilocular cyst that may exhibit heterogeneous content; typically identified adjacent to the esophagus

Morgagni Hernia
- Mediastinal fat pad: Homogeneous fat attenuation; no abdominal contents; intact adjacent diaphragm; found in cardiophrenic angles
- Pericardial cyst: Unilocular or multilocular cyst of water attenuation with imperceptible wall; represents a noncommunicating outpouching of pericardium; found in either cardiophrenic angle but much more common on the right; intact diaphragm

Imaging Findings

Extramedullary Hematopoiesis
- Chest radiographs may be normal if lesions are small.
- Abnormal chest radiographs typically show a well-circumscribed posterior mediastinal or paravertebral mass that produces thickening of the ipsilateral paravertebral stripe.
- May be unilateral or bilateral, symmetric or asymmetric (Fig. 87.1).
- CT usually shows a well-marginated soft tissue mass in the paravertebral region, specifically along the costovertebral junctions.
- Fat attenuation may be identified in old, burned-out lesions.
- Mild enhancement may be seen following the administration of intravenous contrast.
- MRI effectively demonstrates the presence and extent of intraspinal extension in symptomatic patients (Fig. 87.2).
- Lesions may demonstrate high signal intensity on T1- and T2-weighted MRI in cases with fatty replacement, and they may demonstrate low signal intensity on T1- and T2-weighted MRI in cases with iron deposition.

Hiatal and Paraesophageal Hernia
- Well-circumscribed retrocardiac opacity; may be homogeneous or contain air and/or air–fluid levels (Fig. 87.3).
- Lateral displacement of the lower aspect of the azygoesophageal recess (Fig. 87.3a).
- CT enables characterization of hernias and differentiation between sliding and paraesophageal types (Fig. 87.4).

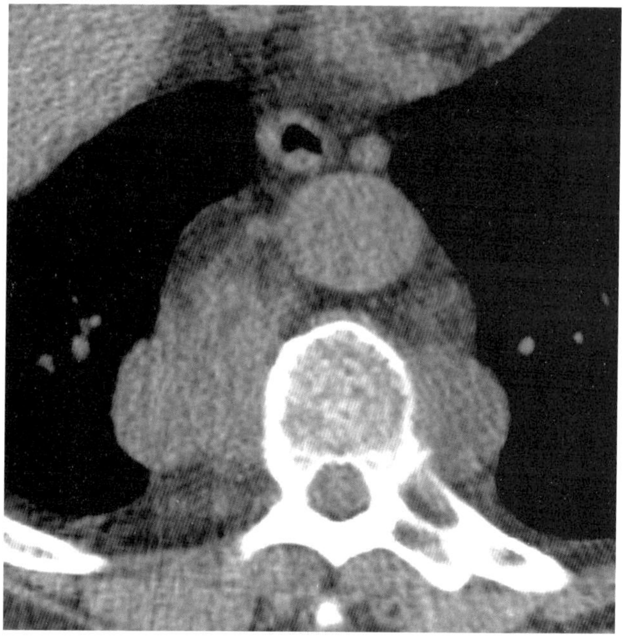

Figure 87.1. Extramedullary hematopoiesis. Unenhanced chest CT of a 41-year-old woman with hereditary spherocytosis shows bilateral lobulated paravertebral soft tissue masses consistent with extramedullary hematopoiesis.

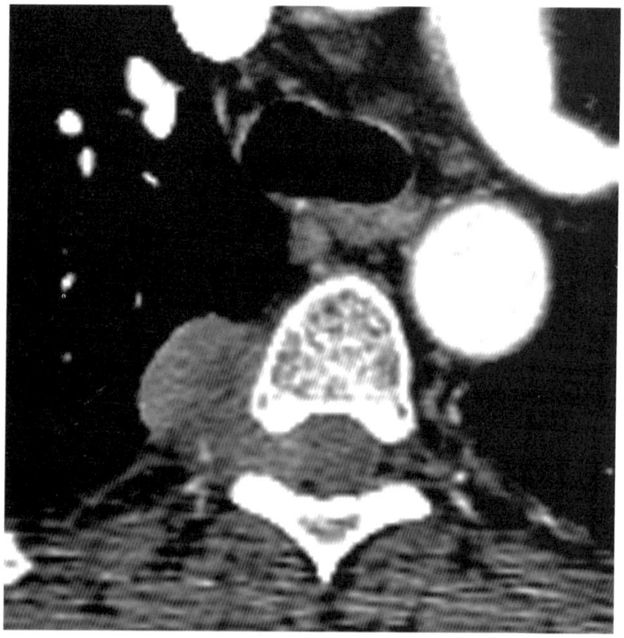

Figure 87.2. Extramedullary hematopoiesis. Contrast-enhanced chest CT of a 34-year-old man with sickle cell anemia shows a lobular heterogeneous right paravertebral mass extending through the neural foramen into the spinal canal and abutting the spinal cord.

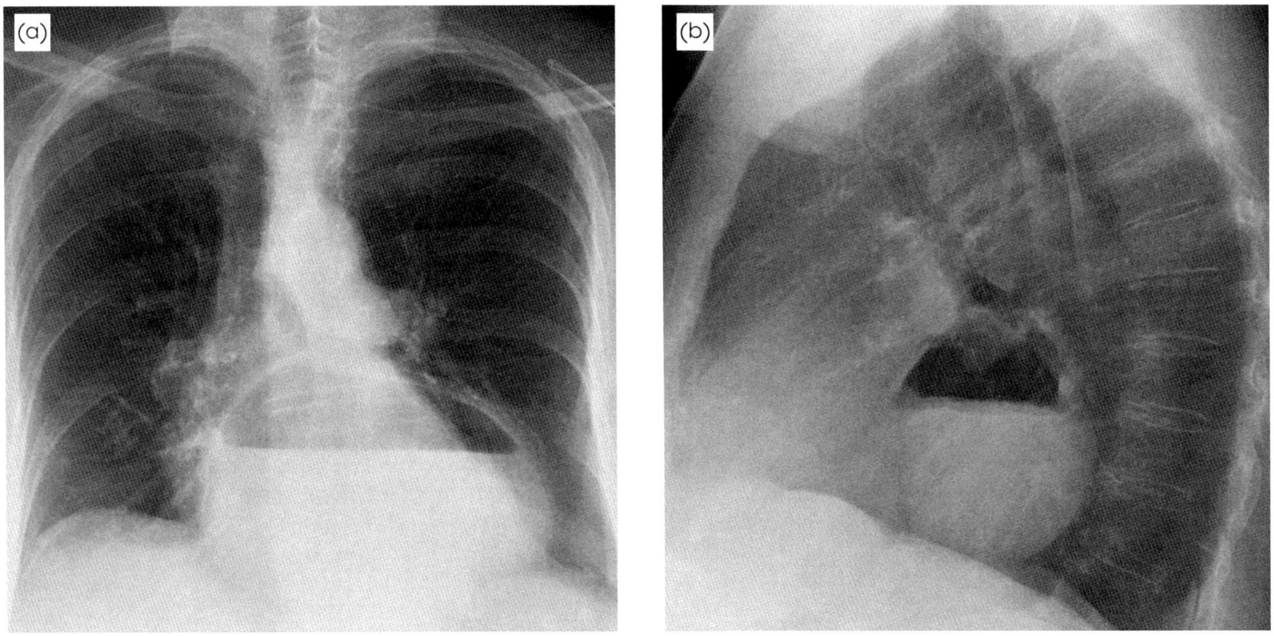

Figure 87.3. Hiatal hernia. (a) Posteroanterior and (b) lateral chest radiographs of a 53-year-old man with gastroesophageal reflux disease show a large middle mediastinal mass with an intrinsic air–fluid level. The mass displaces the mid and inferior aspects of the azygoesophageal recess (a), which together with the intrinsic air–fluid level is virtually diagnostic of hiatal hernia.

- CT optimally demonstrates widening of the esophageal hiatus and identifies the contents of the hernia.
- Hernias may contain stomach, fat, omentum, and other abdominal structures.
- Sliding type: Herniation of the gastroesophageal junction and gastric cardia through the esophageal hiatus into the chest.

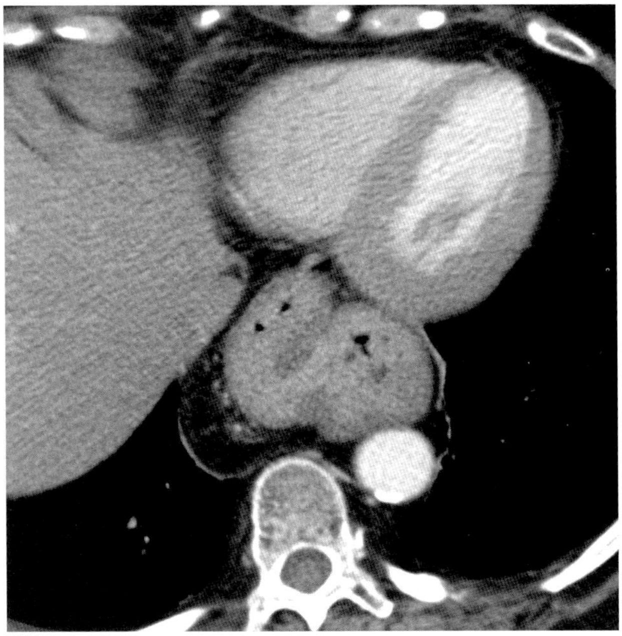

Figure 87.4. Hiatal hernia. Contrast-enhanced chest CT of an asymptomatic 37-year-old man shows herniation of a portion of the stomach through the esophageal hiatus consistent with a hiatal hernia.

- Paraesophageal type: Herniation of stomach through the esophageal hiatus into the chest alongside the esophagus; normal position of the gastroesophageal junction.

Morgagni Hernia

- Well-marginated opacity obscuring the heart border; most commonly in the right cardiophrenic angle (Figs. 87.5 and 87.6).
- CT with coronal and sagittal multiplanar reformatted images is useful for visualization of the retrosternal diaphragmatic defect and identification of the hernia contents as they course through the diaphragmatic defect.
- Typically contains omental fat identified as abdominal by visualization of accompanying omental vessels.
- May contain organs such as transverse colon, liver, small bowel, and stomach.
- With associated pericardial defects, the hernia may extend into the pericardial space.

Clinical Issues

Extramedullary Hematopoiesis

- Extramedullary hematopoiesis is typically asymptomatic, but it may be complicated by hemothorax.
- Spinal cord compression may result from extension of the paravertebral mass into the spinal canal or intraspinal hematopoiesis.

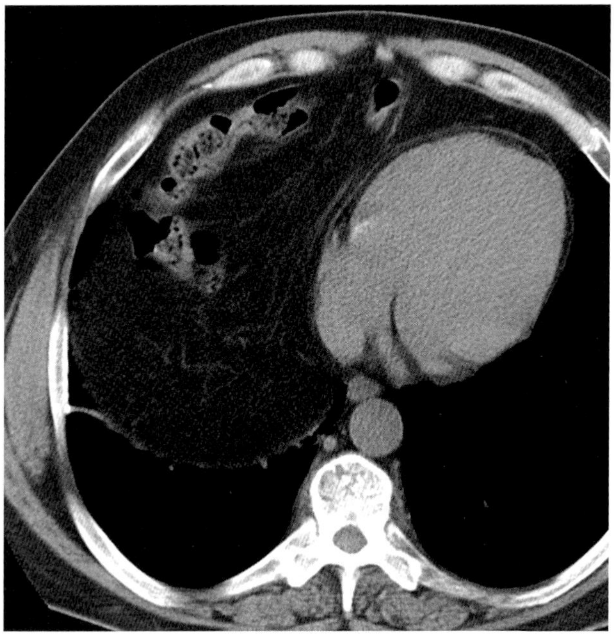

Figure 87.5. Morgagni hernia. Unenhanced CT shows a large herniation in the anterior right hemithorax containing abdominal fat and a segment of transverse colon. Morgagni hernias often contain fat, but they may also contain organs such as the liver, colon, small bowel, and/or stomach, which must be carefully evaluated for incarceration or strangulation.

- No treatment is necessary for asymptomatic patients with extramedullary hematopoiesis. Splenectomy may be performed in cases resulting from hereditary spherocytosis. Small doses of radiation may be administered in the setting of spinal cord compression.

Hiatal Hernia

- Many patients with hiatal hernias are asymptomatic, and the lesions are incidentally discovered on imaging.
- Patients with sliding hiatal hernias may develop gastroesophageal reflux disease, for which medical therapy is typically sufficient. However, surgery may be performed in cases refractory to medical therapy or in cases of recurrent aspiration or chronic cough.
- Paraesophageal hiatal hernias may be complicated by gastric volvulus, resulting in severe epigastric pain. For this reason, paraesophageal hernias may be surgically corrected prophylactically. Gastric volvulus, which carries a mortality rate of 50%, is surgically treated and involves fixation of the stomach in its normal anatomic position. Partial or total gastrectomy may be performed in cases of necrosis.

Morgagni Hernia

- Morgagni hernias are typically asymptomatic, although epigastric and retrosternal chest pain may be present.
- Incarceration and strangulation may result in infarction of hernia contents. Therefore, hernias containing loops of bowel may be surgically repaired.
- Morgagni hernias containing loops of herniated bowel may be associated with malrotation.

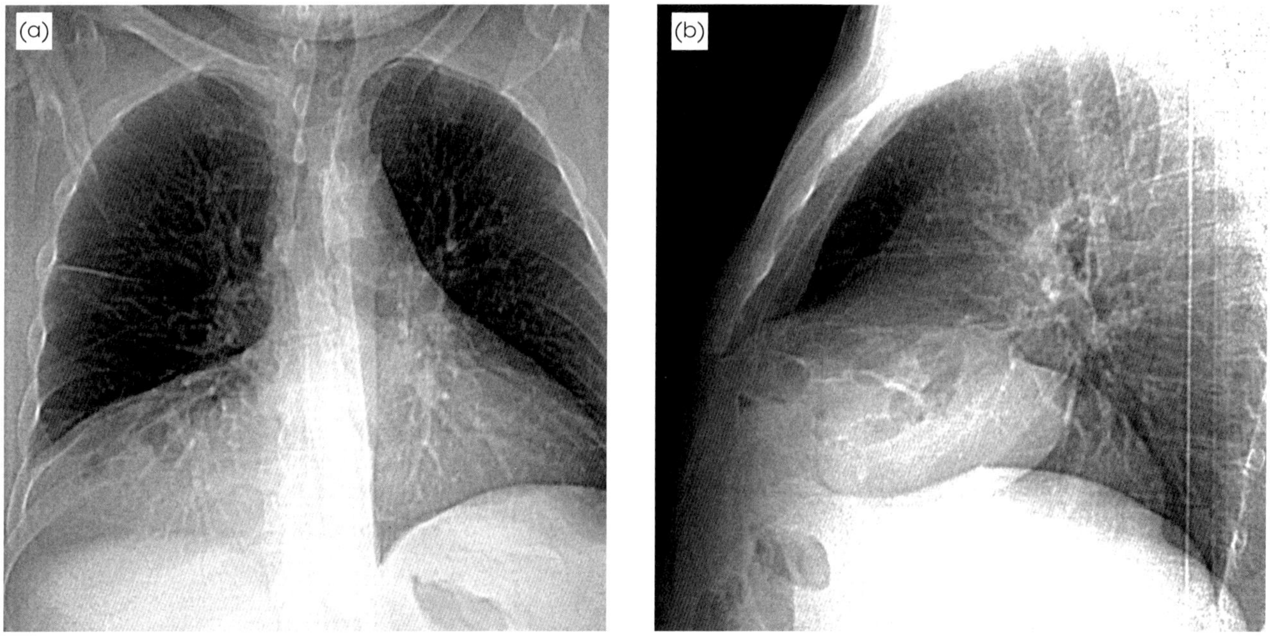

Figure 87.6. Morgagni hernia. (a) Frontal and (b) lateral CT scout images of a patient with a Morgagni hernia show a large right anterior mediastinal opacity that obscures the right heart border and contains air-filled loops of herniated bowel.

Key Points

- Extramedullary hematopoiesis may develop in patients with hematologic disorders such as myelofibrosis, ß-thalassemia, sickle cell anemia, and hereditary spherocytosis.
- The most common imaging appearance of extramedullary hematopoiesis is a paravertebral mass. Fat attenuation may be present in old, burned-out lesions.
- CT allows differentiation between the types of hiatal hernias and identification of the hernia contents.
- Hiatal hernias are the most common herniations to involve the mediastinum, and they may be sliding type or paraesophageal type.
- Morgagni hernias are secondary to defects in the retrosternal hemidiaphragm that typically contain omental fat but may also include organs such as transverse colon, liver, small bowel, or stomach.

Suggested Reading

Gaerte SC, Meyer CA, Winer-Muram HT, Tarver RD, Conces DJJr. Fat-containing lesions of the chest. *RadioGraphics.* 2002;22(Spec No):S61–S78.

Georgiades CS, Neyman EG, Francis IR, Sneider MB, Fishman EK. Typical and atypical presentations of extramedullary hemopoiesis. *AJR Am J Roentgenol.* 2002;179(5):1239–1243.

Kahrilas PJ, Kim HC, Pandolfino JE. Approaches to the diagnosis and grading of hiatal hernia. *Best Pract Res Clin Gastroenterol.* 2008;22(4):601–616.

Sirmali M, Türüt H, Gezer S, et al. Clinical and radiologic evaluation of foramen of Morgagni hernias and the transthoracic approach. *World J Surg.* 2005;29(11):1520–1524.

Section XVII

Developmental Abnormalities

CHAPTER 88

Introduction to Developmental Abnormalities

Melissa L. Rosado-de-Christenson

Introduction

Thoracic developmental abnormalities are often diagnosed in infancy and childhood, but they may also be discovered and evaluated *in utero*. However, a number of developmental disorders are diagnosed in adulthood. An understanding of the most frequent developmental abnormalities that affect adult patients allows the radiologist to accurately identify and assess such conditions and contribute to the appropriate management of affected patients.

Developmental Abnormalities

Developmental abnormalities that manifest in adulthood may or may not produce symptoms. Many so-called developmental conditions are really anatomic variants and have little or no clinical significance. These can be classified based on the affected organ(s) and include anatomic variants and anomalies of the airways, lungs, pleura, heart, blood vessels, mediastinum, diaphragm, and chest wall. A select number of developmental conditions and anatomic variants are discussed in this section.

Approach to Developmental Abnormalities

Many adults with developmental anomalies are asymptomatic and diagnosed incidentally because of a chest imaging study obtained for other reasons. A systematic assessment of all thoracic structures allows the radiologist to identify and correctly diagnose these conditions. Knowledge of the widely variable conditions is important because many of these anomalies and variants require no further imaging or management.

Airways

Evaluation of the chest radiograph should always include a thorough assessment of the central tracheobronchial tree. In fact, assessment of the morphologic features of the tracheobronchial tree is an important step in the prediction of visceroatrial situs. The right upper lobe bronchus exhibits an eparterial morphology because it originates above the ipsilateral pulmonary artery. The left upper lobe bronchus exhibits a hyparterial morphology because it originates below the ipsilateral pulmonary artery. Patients with normal situs have a right eparterial and a left hyparterial bronchus. Situs inversus (right hyparterial and left eparterial bronchi) and left isomerism or polysplenia (bilateral hyparterial bronchi) are congenital anomalies typically diagnosed in the adult. Identification of such abnormalities is important because affected patients may have significant associated anomalies (Fig. 88.1).

The branching pattern of the lobar bronchi is highly variable. Displaced or supernumerary bronchi are not unusual findings on CT. Although tracheal bronchi occur and arise from the right lateral tracheal wall, a more common variant of bronchial branching is the displaced pre-eparterial bronchus in which the apical segmental right upper lobe bronchus arises as a separate branch of the right upper lobe bronchus (Fig. 88.2).

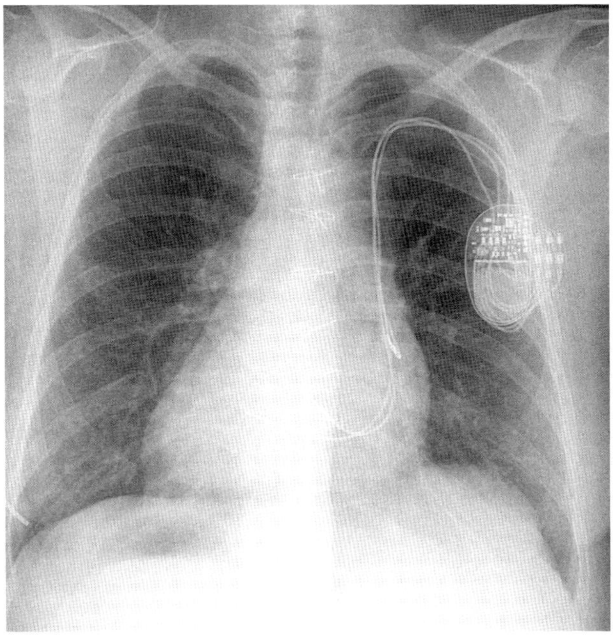

Figure 88.1. Airway situs abnormalities. Posteroanterior chest radiograph of a patient with previous repair of complex heart disease shows abnormal situs with left superior vena cava, right-sided cardiac apex, and right-sided gastric bubble. Note symmetric central bronchi with hyparterial morphology consistent with situs ambiguous (polysplenia) or left isomerism.

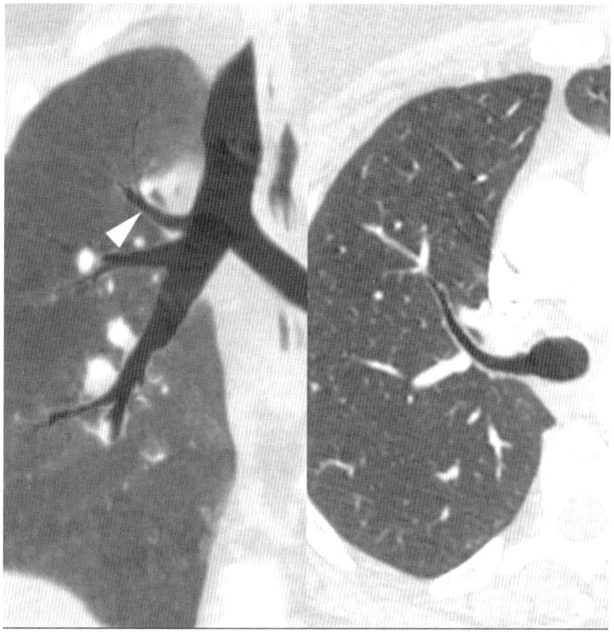

Figure 88.2. Airway anatomic variants. Composite chest CT with coronal minimum intensity projection (left) and axial contrast-enhanced chest CT (right) shows a right upper lobe displaced apical segmental pre-eparterial bronchus (left; arrowhead) and a tracheal bronchus (right) arising from the right tracheal wall.

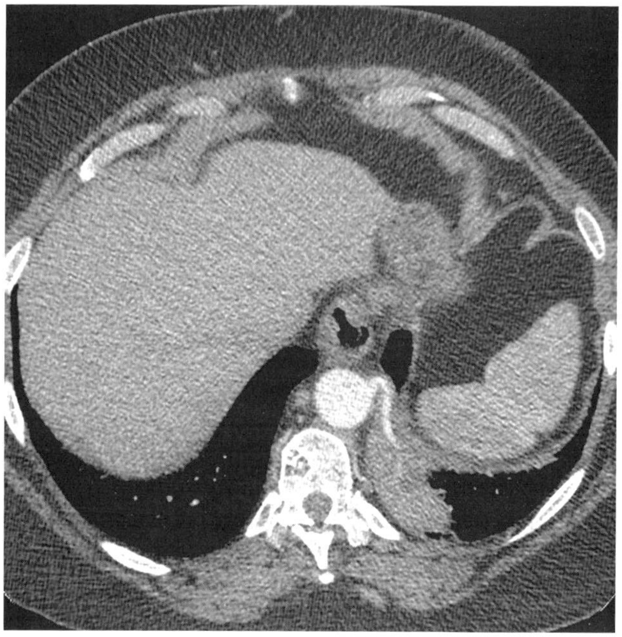

Figure 88.3. Intralobar sequestration. Contrast-enhanced chest CT of a patient with a persistent left basilar consolidation shows a systemic artery arising from the descending thoracic aorta and supplying the consolidated left basilar lung, confirming an intralobar sequestration.

Bronchial atresia is the result of in utero interruption of a bronchus with relatively normal development of the distal airway and surrounding lung. It is characterized by the formation of a bronchocele or mucocele distal to the atretic bronchial segment, which is often surrounded by hyperlucent lung.

Lungs and Pleura

Cross-sectional imaging with CT frequently demonstrates incomplete and accessory fissures. The accessory azygos fissure is often visualized on chest radiography, and it contains four layers of pleura as well as the azygos arch, which may exhibit a characteristic teardrop shape. Superior accessory and left minor fissures are also common. The right major fissure is more often incomplete compared to the left. Description of incomplete fissures may be relevant in the treatment planning of patients with lung cancer who are surgical candidates.

Intralobar sequestration is a pulmonary anomaly that is often diagnosed in older children, adolescents, and adults. This lesion exhibits highly variable imaging findings, but a confident diagnosis can be made when systemic blood supply to the lung is identified. The latter often arises from the distal descending thoracic aorta, but it may also originate in branches of the abdominal aorta (Fig. 88.3).

Mediastinum

Congenital foregut cysts are the most common nonvascular developmental anomalies of the mediastinum and are secondary to anomalous foregut budding. Bronchogenic cyst is the most common foregut cyst. Pericardial cysts are also frequent. They arise from the pericardium but do not communicate with the pericardial space. These lesions are discussed in Section XVI.

Cardiovascular System

A wide variety of developmental abnormalities affect the cardiovascular system. Although many of these lesions manifest initially in symptomatic infants and children, many are first diagnosed in adult patients. Cardiovascular anomalies may be categorized as those affecting the heart, the systemic circulation, and the pulmonary circulation (Fig. 88.4). The latter may consist of anomalous venous return that drains into systemic veins or right cardiac chambers and may be associated with additional cardiovascular anomalies. Adult patients may present with intracardiac shunts. Abnormalities of the vascular structures include anomalies of the thoracic aorta and its branches and abnormalities of the vena cava and the azygos venous system. Extracardiac vascular shunts may also occur, typically in the form of arteriovenous malformations. CT is helpful in documenting the direct communication between a pulmonary artery or arteries and the pulmonary venous system.

Diaphragm

Diaphragmatic congenital anomalies that manifest in adulthood are usually Morgagni hernias, which may manifest as diaphragmatic contour abnormalities. These diaphragmatic defects may allow herniation of abdominal contents. Although the diagnosis can be suggested on radiography, it

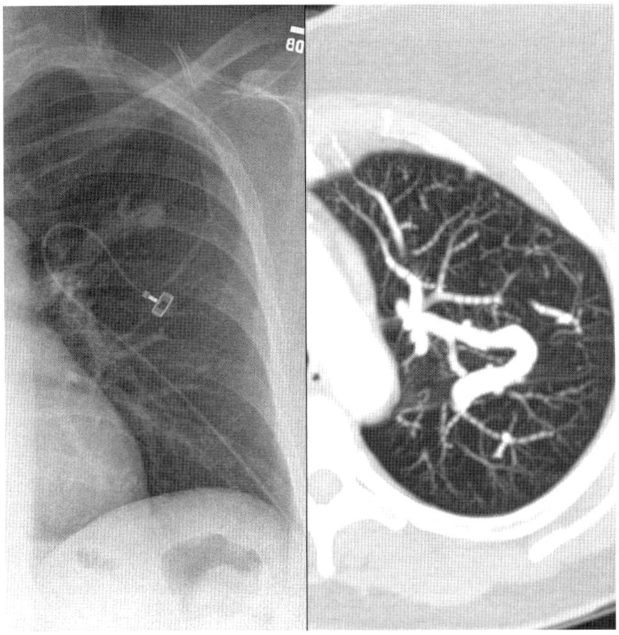

Figure 88.4. Meandering pulmonary vein. Composite image with anteroposterior chest radiograph (left) and axial contrast-enhanced maximum intensity projection image (right) shows a conspicuous tubular structure in the left upper lung zone initially thought to represent an arteriovenous malformation. Chest CT confirmed a normal connection to the left atrium for this meandering pulmonary vein and excluded the possibility of an extracardiac shunt lesion.

is typically confirmed on chest CT with multiplanar reformatted images.

Chest Wall

Congenital chest wall lesions may affect the spine, ribs, sternum, and chest wall soft tissues. Pectus excavatum deformity is the most common developmental lesion of the chest wall. The diagnosis is typically made on radiography.

Suggested Reading

Asiz A, Ashizawa K, Nagaoki K, Hayashi K. High resolution CT anatomy of the pulmonary fissures. *J Thorac Imaging.* 2004;19:186–191.

Berrocal T, Madrid C, Novo S, Gutiérrez J, Arjonilla A, Gómez-León N. Congenital anomalies of the tracheobronchial tree, lung, and mediastinum: Embryology, radiology and pathology. *RadioGraphics.* 2004;24:e17.

Davies M, Guest PJ. Developmental abnormalities of the great vessels of the thorax and their embryological basis. *Br J Radiol.* 2003;76:491–502.

Desir A, Ghaye B. Congenital abnormalities of intrathoracic airways. *Radiol Clin North Am.* 2009;47:203–225.

CHAPTER 89

Congenital Bronchial Atresia

Ryo E. C. Benson

Definition

Congenital bronchial atresia (CBA) is a benign congenital abnormality that is postulated to occur after the 16th gestational week and characterized by focal atresia of a bronchus. The bronchial interruption results in the formation of a mucocele or bronchocele distal to the atresia, with hyperinflation of the surrounding lung.

The finger-in-glove sign is the radiographic appearance of finger-like branching opacities that represent dilated bronchi filled with water or soft tissue density content. In most cases, this represents endoluminal mucus, but endoluminal tumor may rarely produce the same imaging findings.

Clinical Features

Patients with CBA usually present in the second or third decade of life, and men are more frequently affected, with a male-to-female ratio of 2:1. Affected patients are usually asymptomatic (60%) and are often diagnosed incidentally because of an abnormal chest imaging study (Fig. 89.1). Approximately one-fifth of affected patients have a history of recurrent infection or cough. Dyspnea, chest pain, wheezing, and hemoptysis may also occur.

Anatomy and Physiology

CBA typically affects the apicoposterior segment of the left upper lobe. However, any lobe may be affected (Fig. 89.2). Segmental bronchi are most commonly involved, and lobar and subsegmental bronchi are rarely affected. The atresia is postulated to result from focal intrauterine ischemia or abnormal bronchial budding. A mucocele distal to the atretic focus results from endoluminal debris propelled centrally by the mucociliary escalator. Surrounding hyperlucent lung results from oligemia secondary to hypoxic vasoconstriction and air trapping (Fig. 89.3). Collateral air drift through canals of Lambert and pores of Kohn may also play a role.

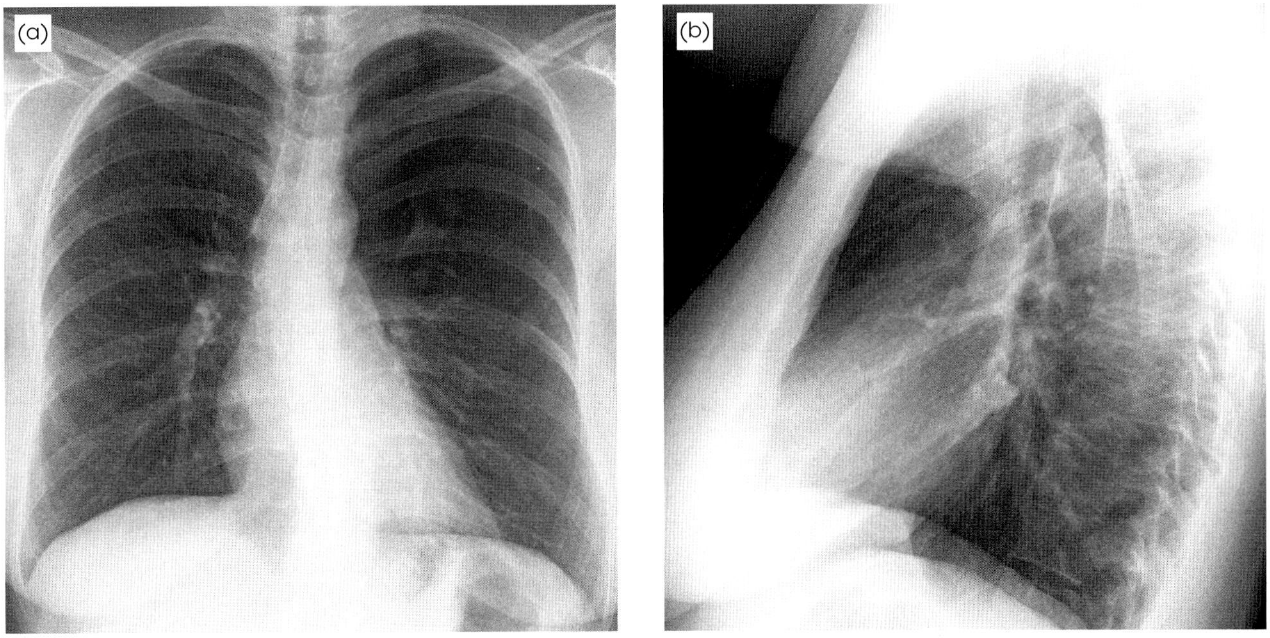

Figure 89.1. Left upper lobe bronchial atresia. (a) Posteroanterior (PA) and (b) lateral chest radiographs of an asymptomatic 32-year-old woman show a left upper lobe perihilar branching tubular opacity with surrounding hyperlucency and paucity of vascular markings.

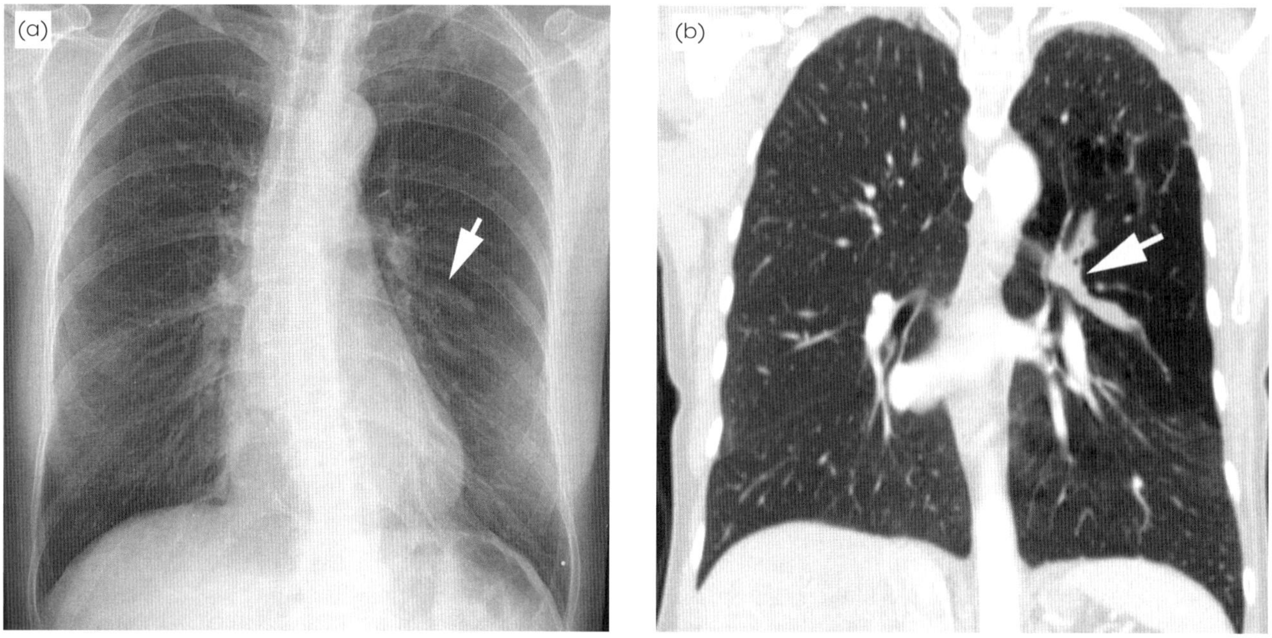

Figure 89.2. Left lower lobe bronchial atresia. (a) PA chest radiograph of an asymptomatic 51-year-old woman shows branching opacities (arrow) pointing toward the left hilum and subtle surrounding pulmonary hyperlucency. (b) Coronal contrast-enhanced chest CT of the same patient shows that the perihilar branching opacities (arrow) correspond to a nonenhancing left lower lobe branching mucocele with surrounding hyperlucent lung parenchyma.

How to Approach the Image

The radiographic diagnosis is made by recognition of a well-circumscribed nodule (mucocele) that may exhibit elongate or branching morphology with surrounding lung hyperlucency. The morphology of the mucocele and the pulmonary hyperlucency may not be recognized prospectively. Additional imaging with chest CT usually follows and allows definitive diagnosis. Intravenous contrast is useful in excluding a vascular etiology for the branching opacity (Figs. 89.4 and 89.5). Gas within the mucocele should suggest superimposed infection (Fig. 89.6). Expiratory CT, MRI, and ventilation/perfusion scintigraphy have been reported but are usually not necessary.

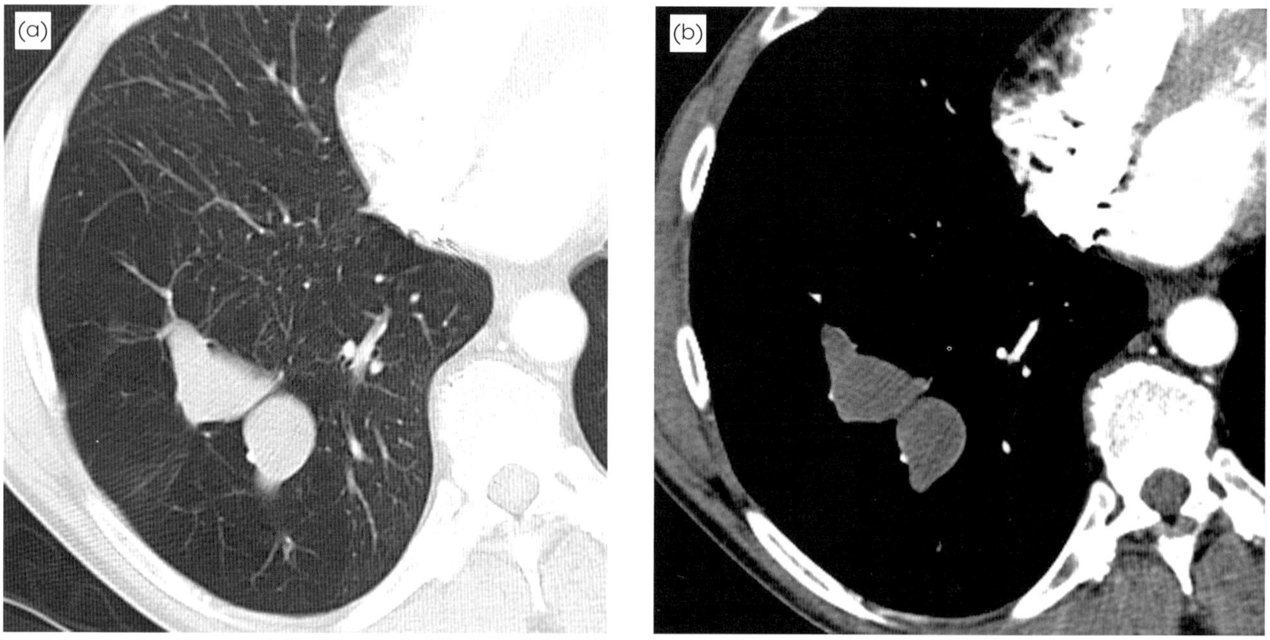

Figure 89.3. Right lower lobe bronchial atresia. (a, b) Contrast-enhanced chest CT of an asymptomatic 39-year-old man shows a branching opacity surrounded by hyperlucent lung. The branching mucocele exhibits low attenuation and absence of contrast enhancement (b).

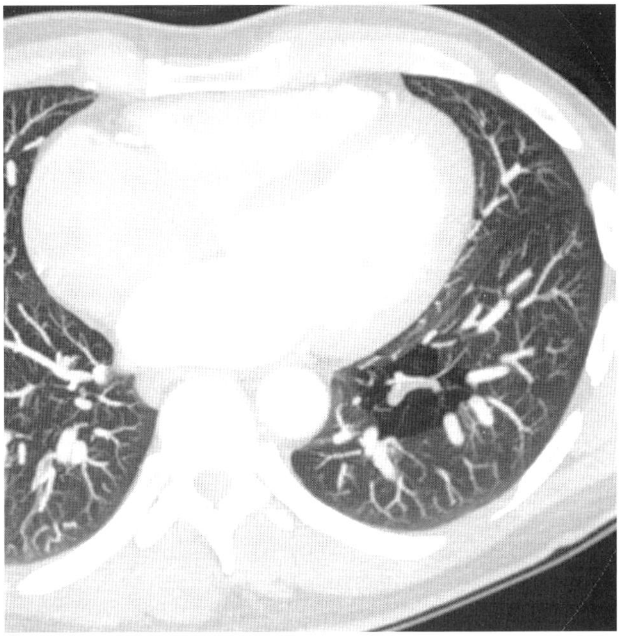

Figure 89.4. Small left lower lobe bronchial atresia. Contrast-enhanced chest CT maximum intensity projection image shows a tiny left lower lobe mucocele with surrounding hyperlucency. Note that the mucocele does not enhance, unlike the adjacent pulmonary arteries.

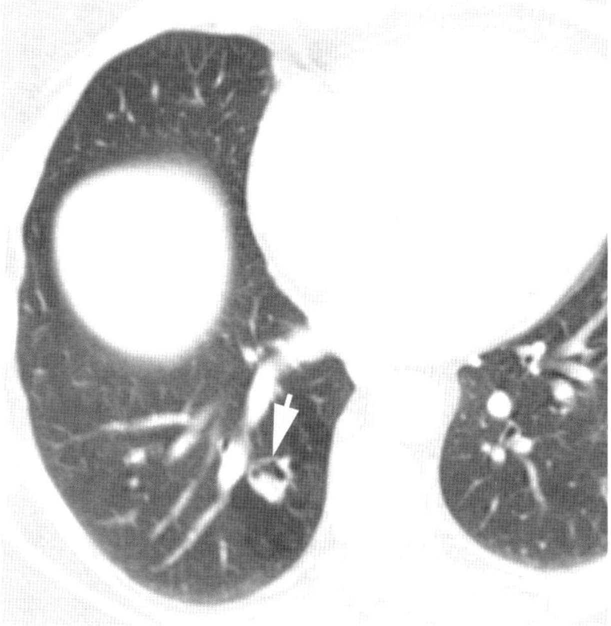

Figure 89.6. Infected bronchial atresia. Unenhanced chest CT of a patient with cough and fever shows a right lower lobe mucocele surrounded by hyperlucent hypovascular lung. Gas within the mucocele (arrow) is an atypical finding consistent with superimposed infection.

What Not to Miss

- Careful analysis of pulmonary opacities is required for identification of tubular or branching morphology.
- Visualization of tubular or branching opacities should suggest vascular or airway abnormalities.

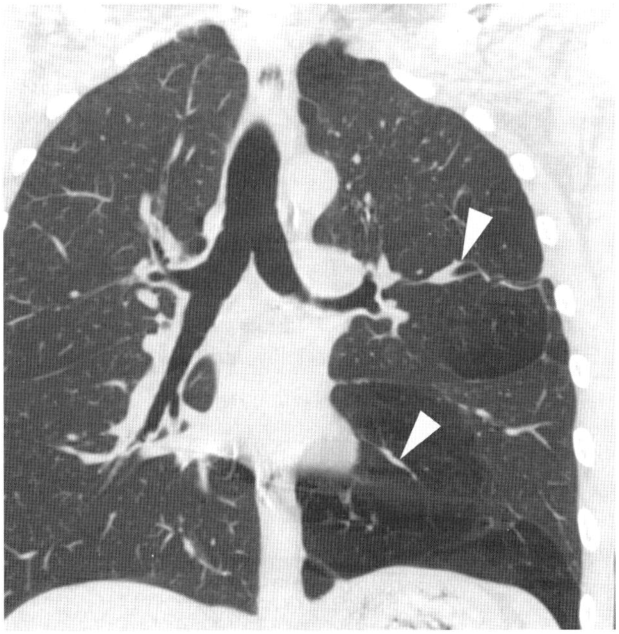

Figure 89.5. Multisegmental bronchial atresia. Unenhanced coronal chest CT of a 44-year-old man with left lung hyperlucency noted on radiography shows multifocal left upper and left lower lobe branching mucoceles (arrowheads) and surrounding hyperlucency.

- Characteristic CT imaging features often allow a confident prospective diagnosis of CBA.
- Endobronchial obstructing lesions such as carcinoid tumor or lung cancer may exhibit distal mucus plugs and must be differentiated from CBA.

Differential Diagnosis

Endobronchial Neoplasm

- Carcinoid tumor and mucoepidermoid carcinoma in younger patients; lung cancer in older patients; rarely endoluminal lipoma, neurogenic neoplasm, or hamartoma.
- May produce peripheral mucoid impaction and air trapping that may mimic CBA (Fig. 89.7).
- Enhancement and/or calcification of the endobronchial tumor may allow distinction from adjacent peripheral mucus plugs.

Broncholithiasis

- Erosion of calcified lymph node into adjacent bronchial lumen
- Typically completely calcified nodule with evidence of other adjacent calcified lymph nodes and granulomas

Allergic Bronchopulmonary Aspergillosis

- Asthma, peripheral eosinophilia, allergy to *Aspergillus* antigens
- Acute transient consolidations and mucoid impaction or chronic central bronchiectasis

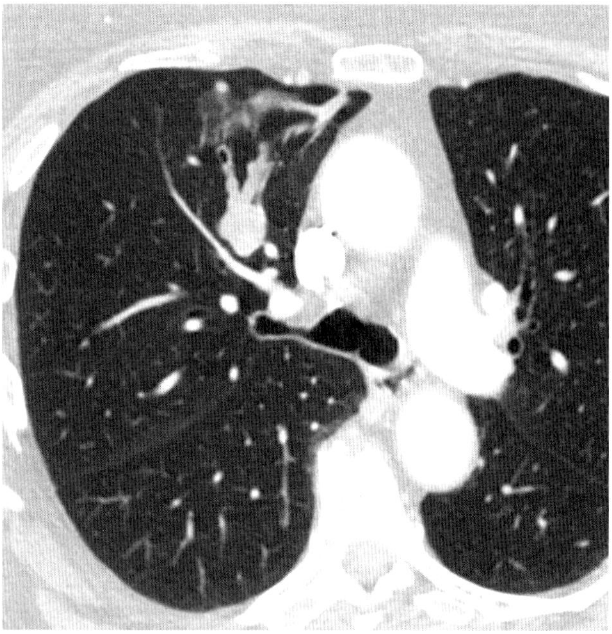

Figure 89.7. Bronchial carcinoid with mucus plugs. Contrast-enhanced chest CT shows a carcinoid tumor manifesting as a right upper lobe anterior segment polylobular nodule with distal branching mucus plugs and surrounding subsegmental atelectasis and hyperlucency mimicking bronchial atresia.

- CT: Central, thin-walled, varicoid or cystic bronchiectasis of first- and second-order bronchi (highly specific for allergic bronchopulmonary aspergillosis), multifocal mucous plugs, mucoceles (may exhibit high attenuation from calcium or metallic ions), and tree-in-bud and centrilobular nodules

Intralobar Sequestration
- More common in the lower lobes
- May exhibit hyperlucent lung and bronchiectasis
- Systemic blood supply

Foreign Body
- Typically radiolucent, rarely radiopaque
- May result in mucocele formation distal to obstruction

Intrapulmonary Bronchogenic Cyst
- May be fluid-filled, air-filled, or both without surrounding hyperlucency
- Typically affects the lower lobes in the medial one-third of the lung

Congenital Lobar Emphysema (or Overinflation)
- Affects symptomatic neonates and infants
- Most commonly in the left upper lobe and typically lobar, not segmental
- Progressive lobar hyperinflation due to check valve bronchial obstruction
- Atelectasis of adjacent uninvolved normal lung

Arteriovenous Malformation
- May exhibit branching morphology without surrounding hyperinflation
- Enhances with contrast; mucocele does not

Imaging Findings

Radiography
- Well-circumscribed rounded, ovoid, or tubular opacity (representing the mucocele) near the hilum; may exhibit branching morphology (finger-in-glove sign)
- Often located in the left upper lobe (Fig. 89.1)
- Mucocele may exhibit intrinsic air or air–fluid level
- Longitudinal axis of mucocele often directed toward the hilum (Fig. 89.2)
- Hyperlucency surrounding the mucocele may be visible
- Combined findings of mucocele and hyperinflation identified in approximately 57–83% of cases.

CT
- Round, ovoid, tubular, or branching, nonenhancing, low-attenuation mucocele (Figs. 89.3 and 89.4)
- Surrounding wedge-shaped hyperlucent lung with paucity of vasculature
- Combination of mucocele and surrounding hyperlucency considered diagnostic (Fig. 89.5)
- Air or air–fluid levels within mucocele in patients with superimposed infection (Fig. 89.6)

MRI
- Mucocele exhibits high signal intensity on T1- and T2-weighted images in 86% of cases.

Scintigraphy
- Ventilation segmental defect with delayed clearance

Clinical Issues
- Affected patients are typically asymptomatic.
- No treatment is required for asymptomatic patients.
- Patients with repeated pulmonary infections may require conservative surgical resection of the affected lung.

Key Points
- Tubular or branching opacities are not specific for CBA.
- Upper lobe focal branching or tubular opacity surrounded by hyperlucent lung on radiography and confirmed on CT in a young asymptomatic patient is diagnostic of CBA.
- CBA is a radiologic diagnosis, and asymptomatic affected patients require no further evaluation or treatment.
- Exclusion of obstructing endobronchial neoplasm with peripheral mucoid impaction.

Suggested Reading

Biyyam DR, Chapman T, Ferguson MR, Deutsch G, Dighe MK. Congenital lung abnormalities: Embryologic features, prenatal diagnosis and postnatal radiologic–pathologic correlation. *RadioGraphics*. 2010;30:1721–1738.

Desir A, Ghaye B: Congenital abnormalities of intrathoracic airways. *Radiol Clin North Am*. 2009;4:203–225.

Gipson MG, Cummings KW, Hurth KM. Bronchial atresia. *RadioGraphics*. 2009;29:1531–1535.

Martínez S, Heyneman LE, McAdams HP, Rossi SE, Restrepo CS, Eraso A. Mucoid impactions: Finger-in-glove sign and other CT and radiographic features. *RadioGraphics*. 2008;28 :1369–1382.

CHAPTER 90

Sequestration

Kristopher W. Cummings

Definition

Sequestration refers to nonfunctioning pulmonary tissue isolated from the tracheobronchial tree with systemic arterial supply. Sequestrations are sometimes referred to as *bronchopulmonary sequestrations*. Lesions can be divided into extralobar or intralobar types depending on whether they occur as supernumerary pulmonary tissue (typically covered by pleura) or as a lesion within an otherwise non-sequestered pulmonary lobe.

Clinical Features

Extralobar sequestrations are commonly diagnosed in newborns or early childhood and rarely in adults. With the increased utilization of prenatal ultrasound, the diagnosis may be made antenatally. These lesions are often detected incidentally as a mass on chest radiograph or rarely on abdominal ultrasound. Affected newborns may present with respiratory distress due to large lesions associated with secondary pulmonary hypoplasia or associated congenital diaphragmatic defects. Unlike intralobar sequestrations, extralobar sequestrations rarely become superinfected because they have no communication with normal lung or tracheobronchial tree. In adults, their detection is almost always incidental, although torsion and subsequent infarction have been reported.

Intralobar sequestrations are more commonly discovered in late childhood, adolescence, and adulthood in patients who characteristically present with recurrent or nonresolving pneumonia isolated to one region of the lung (Fig. 90.1). The absence of a separate pleural covering may predispose to spread of infection from the adjacent lung, which is not adequately cleared due to the lack of a normal tracheobronchial communication. Although superinfection may bring these lesions to attention in adults, intralobar sequestrations are also frequently encountered incidentally and must not be mistaken for other pathology, especially malignancy.

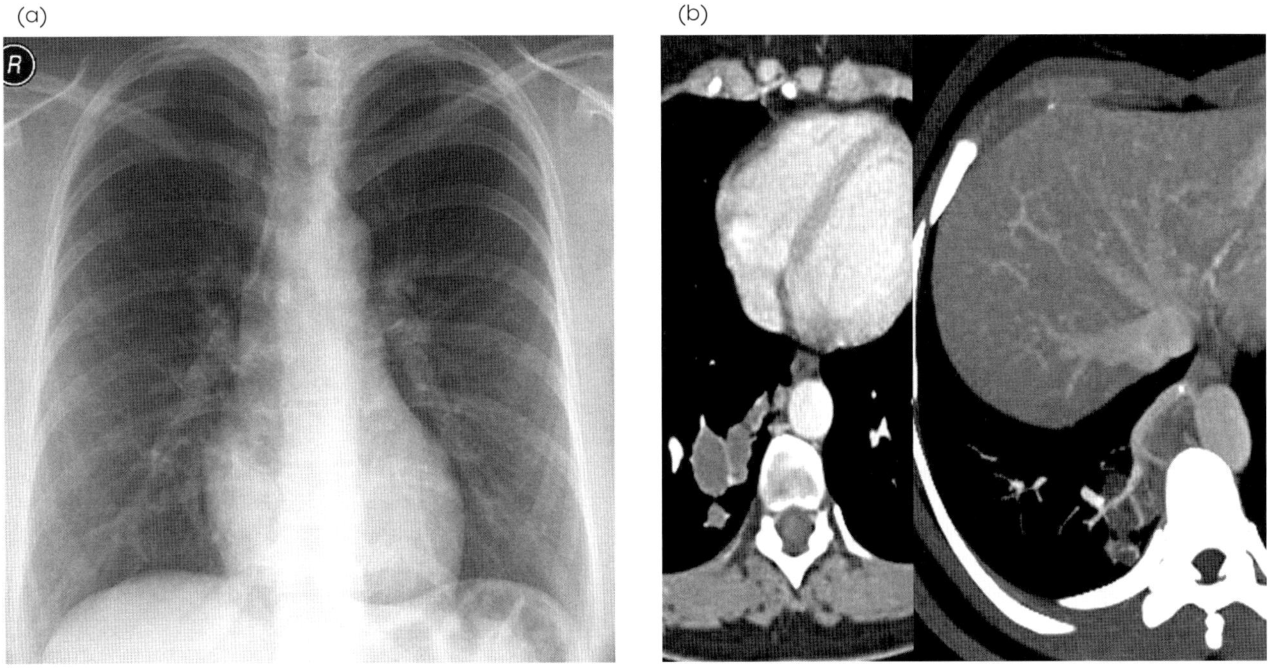

Figure 90.1. Intralobar sequestration. (a) Posteroanterior chest radiograph shows a retrocardiac consolidation in the right lower lobe initially diagnosed as pneumonia. (b) Composite image with contrast-enhanced chest CT axial (left) and oblique axial maximum intensity projection images (right) performed due to persistence of the abnormality shows a multicystic right lower lobe lesion (left) supplied by a systemic descending thoracic aorta branch. Venous drainage (not shown) was to the right inferior pulmonary vein.

Anatomy and Physiology

Extralobar sequestration is a congenital lesion thought to result from maldevelopment of a portion of lung isolated from the normal tracheobronchial tree and may share similar histopathologic features with cystic pulmonary airway malformations. Arterial supply is systemic, and although the descending thoracic aorta is often the source, there is a higher incidence of feeding arteries arising from the abdominal aorta or celiac axis. Venous drainage is more commonly systemic than pulmonary and may be to the inferior vena cava or azygous system.

Some intralobar sequestrations are likely congenital in nature given histopathologic features similar to those seen in bronchial atresia and the presence of elastic feeding arteries (Fig. 90.2). However, an acquired pathway is also thought to result from recurrent infections or inflammation and may explain the later clinical presentation. In these acquired sequestrations, the feeding artery is believed to represent a hypertrophied systemic artery. The systemic arterial supply most commonly originates from the descending thoracic aorta but also may be derive from intercostal, internal mammary, or abdominal arterial sources. Unlike extralobar sequestrations, venous drainage is more commonly to the pulmonary venous system.

How to Approach the Image

Sequestration typically manifests on radiography as a focal mass or consolidation, nearly always in the lower lobes. Occasionally, it may be detected in infancy or in the neonatal or antenatal period as a mass lesion. In an adult patient with nonresolving consolidation or recurrent infections isolated to one region of the lung, suspicion for malignancy (manifesting as either consolidation or secondary to a centrally obstructive endobronchial lesion) should be a primary concern. Therefore, further evaluation with cross-sectional imaging such as CT should be performed. CT and occasionally MRI should be performed to clearly identify the systemic feeding artery. This is key for diagnosis. Usually, contrast material and multiplanar images are used to optimize systemic artery visualization.

What Not to Miss

When dealing with a potential sequestration, the feeding artery must be clearly delineated for surgical excision. Occasionally, more than one feeding artery is present, and each must be described for optimal surgical treatment. Another potential pitfall is that the feeding artery may arise from the abdominal aorta or celiac axis. This is more typical of extralobar sequestrations. To avoid this trap, one should try to scan through the celiac axis on an initial scan of a potential sequestration.

Differential Diagnosis

- A focal parenchymal pulmonary abnormality with systemic arterial supply should raise the possibility of a pulmonary sequestration as the primary diagnostic consideration.

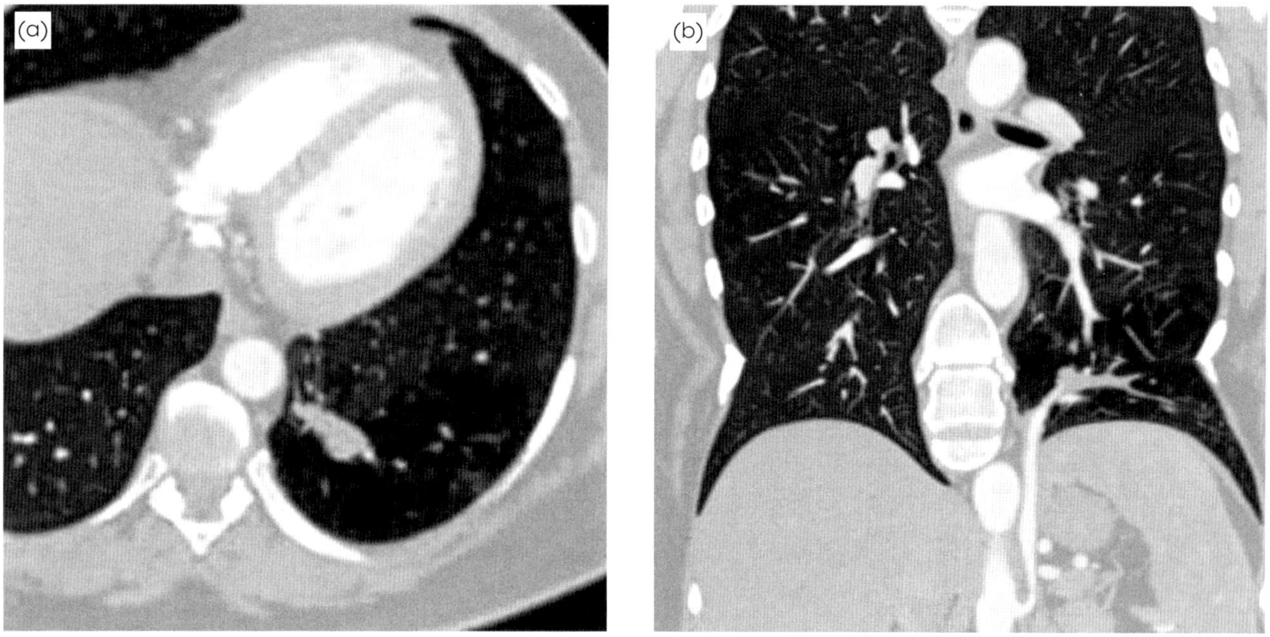

Figure 90.2. Intralobar sequestration. (a) Contrast-enhanced chest CT of a patient with a persistent left lower lobe lesion shows a left lower lobe nonenhancing tubular lesion with an appearance of mucoid impaction surrounded by hyperlucent lung parenchyma and suggestive of bronchial atresia. (b) Curved multiplanar CT of the same patient demonstrates arterial supply to the lesion arising from the abdominal aorta. Venous drainage was to the left inferior pulmonary vein (not shown). Absence of a defined margin between the lesion and the adjacent lung is consistent with intralobar sequestration. This lesion exhibits features of both bronchial atresia and sequestration.

- In the commonly encountered scenario of nonresolving or recurrent consolidation, the following must be considered:
  - Post-obstructive causes of pneumonia, including centrally obstructing neoplasm (especially malignancy) and foreign body
  - Malignancy manifesting as consolidation or mass-like lesion, such as pulmonary adenocarcinoma
  - Aspiration pneumonia, particularly lipoid pneumonia
  - Inflammatory pneumonia, including nummular sarcoidosis and organizing pneumonia
  - Other structural lung abnormalities, such as bronchiectasis and congenital pulmonary airway malformations

Imaging Findings

Extralobar Sequestration

Radiography

- Focal unilateral soft tissue mass or mass-like consolidation on radiography

CT

- On CT looks like a mass
- Affecting basilar segments of the lower lobes, closely associated with diaphragm
- Systemic feeding artery, especially from celiac axis or abdominal aorta
- Feeding vessel usually more difficult to see than with an intralobar sequestration and occasionally may not be discovered until surgery
- Typically, systemic venous drainage to inferior vena cava or azygous/hemiazygous system
- Associated congenital abnormalities including diaphragmatic defects or hernias
- Usually homogeneous but internal cysts may be seen because up to 40% may have associated congenital pulmonary airway malformations (usually type 2)

MRI

- Higher signal intensity than the adjacent lung on both T1- and T2-weighted images
- Separate pleural envelope in thoracic lesions usually difficult to see on CT or MRI but may be appreciated in setting of pleural effusion (Fig. 90.3)

Intralobar Sequestration

Radiography

- Unilateral, soft tissue or mass-like consolidation on radiography
- Usually in the left lower lobe
- May mimic an unresolving pneumonia

CT

- On CT, may look like an area of consolidation; lack of separate pleural envelope explains why the interface

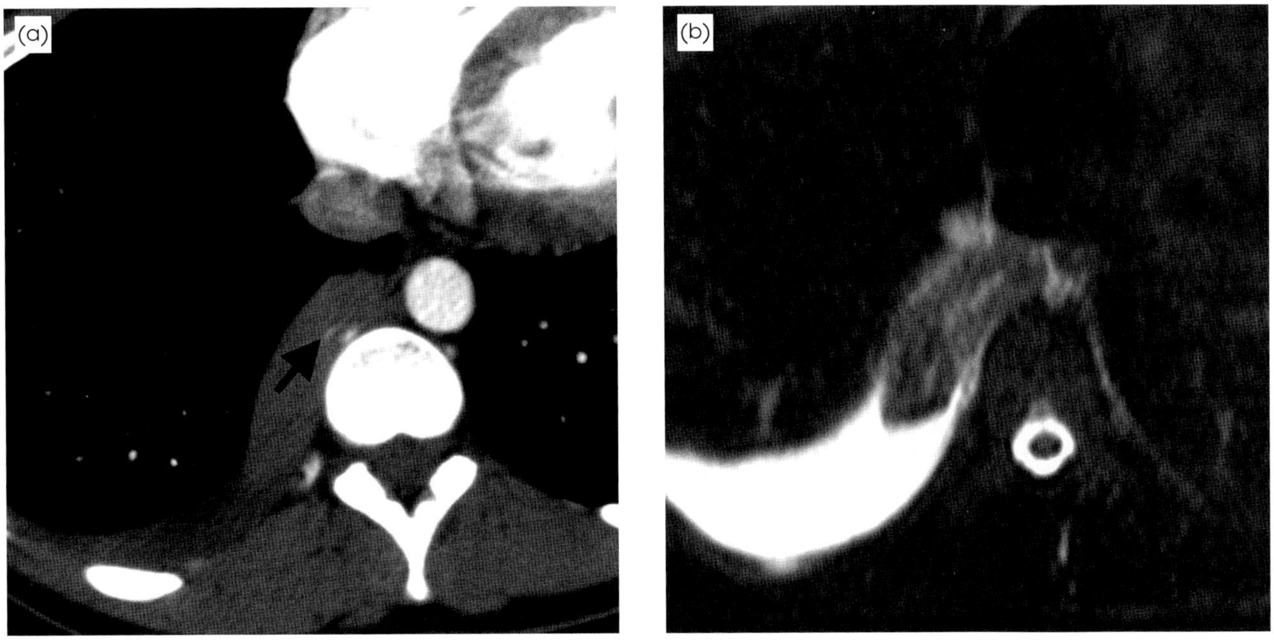

Figure 90.3. Extralobar sequestration. (a) Contrast-enhanced chest CT of a patient with right pleuritic chest pain shows a paravertebral soft tissue mass in the right lower hemithorax and a small right pleural effusion. A tiny feeding artery (arrow) seen just anterior to the intercostal artery arose from the descending thoracic aorta. (b) Axial T2-weighted MR image of the same patient shows the soft tissue mass in the right pleural space separate from the right lower lobe consistent with extralobar sequestration. Increased T2 signal within the mass is in keeping with infarction due to torsion found at the time of operative resection.

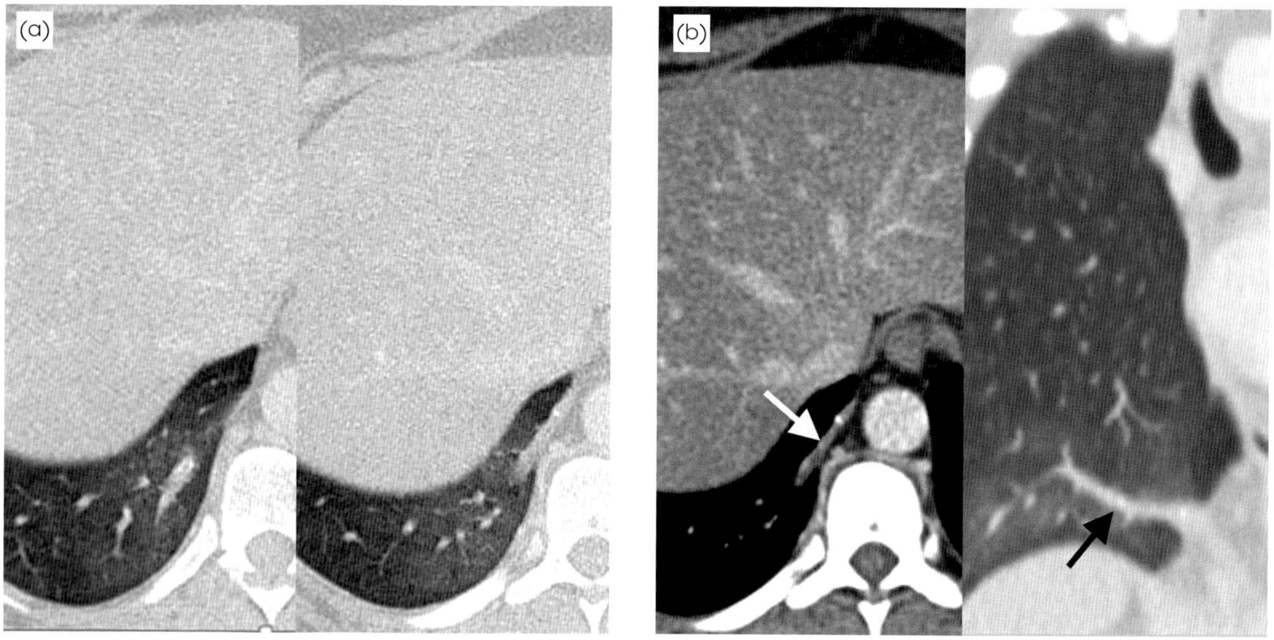

Figure 90.4. Sequestration with thrombosed feeding artery. (a) Composite CT in a 25-year-old woman who presented with chest pain and hemoptysis. The lung windows showed right lower lobe ground glass in keeping with hemorrhage. (b) Composite of a soft tissue image and coronal reconstruction shows a tubular structure (arrows) with lack of enhancement and a faint calcification. This corresponded to a thrombosed feeding artery. Because of her symptoms, the patient underwent resection, and this area was found to correspond to an intralobar sequestration.

with the remainder of the lung is irregular and not well-defined

- Cystic areas usually from bronchiectasis but may also arise rarely from a fistulous communication with airway
- Surrounding air trapping common due to collateral air drift from adjacent lung
- Systemic feeding artery, most commonly from descending thoracic aorta
- More frequently normal pulmonary venous drainage

MRI

- Higher signal intensity than the adjacent lung on both T1- and T2-weighted images

Clinical Issues

- In adults, sequestrations are often asymptomatic incidental findings on studies performed for other reasons and may not require further intervention in the absence of recurrent infection.
- Sequestrations should be in the differential diagnosis for a persistent opacity on a chest radiograph, especially in the left lower lobe.
- Superinfected intralobar sequestrations may form a nidus for recurrent infection, and surgical resection may be required.
- Rarely, a sequestration may present with hemoptysis (Fig. 90.4).
- Intralobar sequestrations may be mass-like and may not be easy to differentiate from other soft tissue masses, including neoplasms. In these cases, surgical resection may be needed.
- Extralobar sequestrations are generally easier to resect because they are isolated from the adjacent lung.
- Intralobar sequestrations often require lobectomy.

Key Points

- Identification of a systemic feeding artery to a parenchymal lung abnormality is key in establishing the diagnosis of sequestration.
- Intralobar sequestration is more commonly encountered in adults than extralobar sequestration.
- Both types are considered congenital lesions, although a mechanism for acquired development of intralobar sequestration is thought to exist.
- If asymptomatic and otherwise incidentally discovered, no further treatment is needed in an adult. Symptomatic lesions are surgically resected.

Suggested Reading

Frazier AA, Rosado de Christenson ML, Stocker JT, Templeton PA. Intralobar sequestration: Radiologic–pathologic correlation. *RadioGraphics*. 1997 May–Jun;17(3):725–745.

Langston C. New concepts in the pathology of congenital lung malformations. *Semin Pediatr Surg*. 2003 Feb;12(1):17–37.

CHAPTER 91

Abnormal Aorta and Aortic Branching

Kristopher W. Cummings

Definition

Congenital anomalies of the aortic arch result in deviation from the normal left aortic arch, which usually gives rise to the right brachiocephalic, left common carotid, and left subclavian arteries in a proximal-to-distal manner. In adults, the more commonly encountered anomalies include left aortic arch with aberrant right subclavian artery, right aortic arch with aberrant left subclavian artery, double aortic arch, and aortic coarctation.

Clinical Features

In the vast majority of adult patients, congenital anomalies of the aortic arch are asymptomatic and discovered incidentally on studies performed for other reasons. However, lesions resulting in complete vascular rings or aortic coarctation may become symptomatic.

A vascular ring is the result of complete encirclement of the trachea and esophagus by vascular structures or their remnants (most notably a ligamentum arteriosum). Although airway compromise is more commonly encountered in children, chronic extrinsic compression can lead to tracheomalacia and respiratory symptoms. More commonly, vascular rings present with esophageal symptoms, usually dysphagia. Double aortic arch is the most common form of vascular ring, followed by right aortic arch and aberrant left subclavian artery (Fig. 91.1). Although left aortic arch with aberrant right subclavian artery is not typically a vascular ring, occasionally patients present with dysphagia from extrinsic compression on the esophagus, referred to as *dysphagia lusoria* (Fig. 91.2).

Unlike right aortic arch with mirror-image branching, which is most commonly diagnosed in childhood, double aortic arch and left aortic arch with aberrant right subclavian artery are not associated with an increased incidence of congenital heart disease, and right aortic arch with aberrant left subclavian artery has only a very low incidence.

Aortic coarctation typically presents with upper extremity systemic arterial hypertension and weak lower extremity pulses. Patients may present with chest pain,

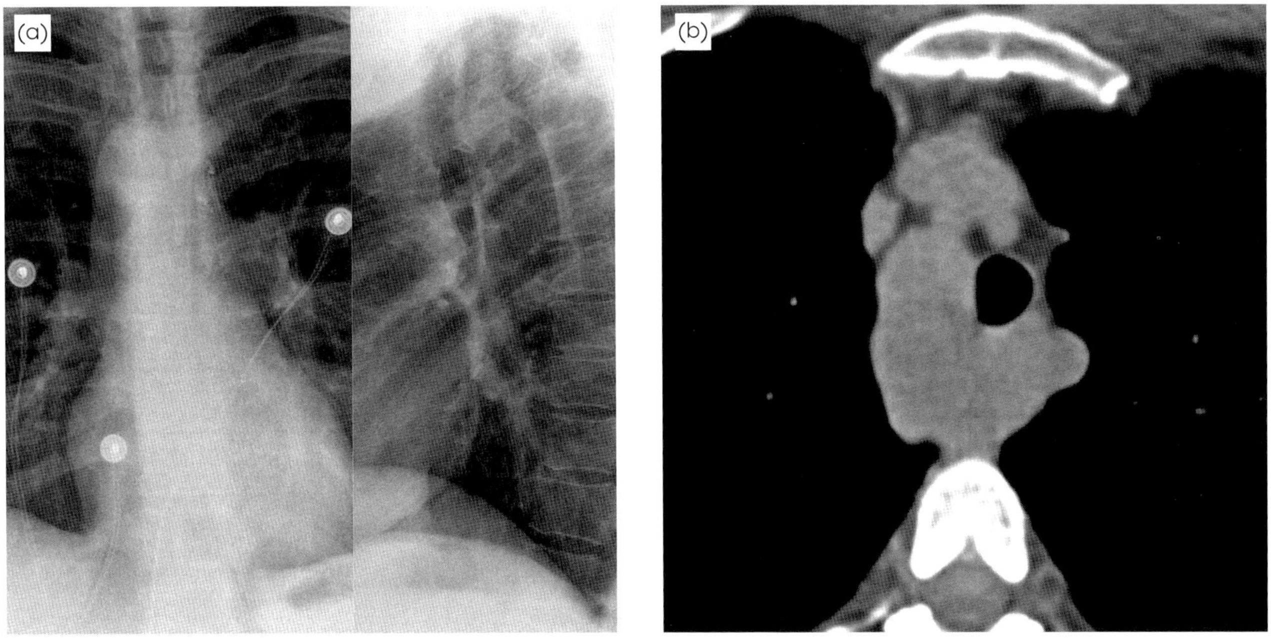

Figure 91.1. Right aortic arch with aberrant left subclavian artery. (a) Frontal and lateral radiographs of the chest demonstrate a right-sided aortic knob as well as a retrotracheal opacity on the lateral that slightly bows the trachea anteriorly. (b) Non-contrast CT axial image reveals the retrotracheal opacity to be an aberrant left subclavian artery coursing posterior to the esophagus and trachea. The left-sided ligamentum arteriosum (not shown) completed a vascular ring.

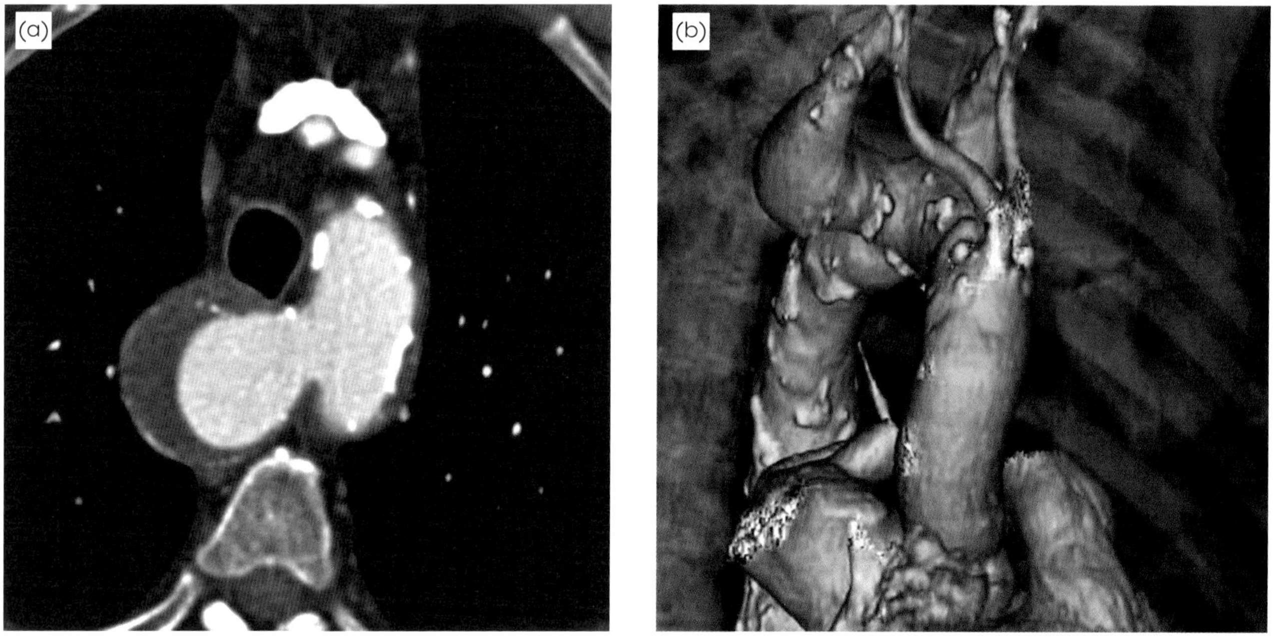

Figure 91.2. Left aortic arch with aberrant right subclavian artery aneurysm. (a) Axial contrast-enhanced CT image demonstrates a left-sided aortic arch with an aberrant right subclavian artery coursing posterior to the esophagus and trachea. There is aneurysmal dilatation of the proximal aberrant subclavian artery with associated mural thrombus. (b) Three-dimensional volume-rendered image demonstrates the abnormal course of the right subclavian artery that arises from the proximal descending thoracic aorta and the aneurysmal dilatation of this vessel. Note that this is not a vascular ring because the trachea and esophagus are not enclosed along their right anterolateral margins.

syncope, or lower extremity claudication. Coarctation is more common in men and has many associations, including bicuspid aortic valve, intracranial aneurysm, Turner syndrome, and ventricular and atrial septal defects.

Anatomy and Physiology

The aortic arch and its branches develop embryologically from development and regression of various portions of six paired aortic arches. A normal left aortic arch and branching pattern occurs when the left fourth arch persists with regression of the right fourth and bilateral first, second, and fifth arches. The third arches give rise to the common carotid arteries, and the sixth arches give rise to the pulmonary arteries and ductus arteriosus.

Persistence of the right fourth arch and regression of the left fourth arch results in a right aortic arch, whereas persistence of both fourth arches results in a double aortic arch. Various abnormalities of regression, segmentation, and interruption result in the remaining congenital arch variants.

Aortic coarctation is a focal narrowing that occurs just distal to the takeoff of the left subclavian artery in the region where the ductus arteriosus/ligamentum arteriosum inserts. In adults, this is usually at or just distal to the insertion, whereas in children it more commonly occurs just proximal to this site. As a result of the restriction to flow, there is elevated afterload in the proximal aorta that leads to upper body systemic arterial hypertension and may lead to left ventricular hypertrophy. In an attempt to maintain arterial perfusion to the abdomen and lower body, collateral arterial pathways develop with enlargement of inter-costal, internal mammary, and thyrocervical trunk arteries.

Aortic pseudo-coarctation results from elongation and tortuosity of the proximal descending thoracic aorta, giving rise to areas of apparent narrowing. Atherosclerosis may also be present in the affected segment. However, unlike true coarctation, no pressure gradient exists. Therefore, collateral vessel formation does not occur, and craniocaudal blood pressure gradients do not exist.

How to Approach the Image

Whereas some congenital arch variants may be difficult to identify on radiographs, others are readily apparent in adults. First, the laterality of the aortic arch should be determined. Normally, the left-sided aortic knob causes mild rightward deviation of the airway in the mid left paratracheal stripe. A right-sided aortic knob presents with a focal leftward deviation of the trachea in the same region with absence of the normal left aortic knob. In double aortic arch, the right-sided arch is usually larger and more superior than the left arch. Radiographic evidence of an aberrant subclavian artery is frequently subtle but can be seen as a posterior indentation along the upper trachea on the lateral radiograph.

In young patients presenting with hypertension, close attention should be paid to the inferior margins of the fourth through eighth ribs because intercostal artery hypertrophy in the setting of aortic coarctation most commonly manifests as bilateral inferior rib notching. The first and second ribs do not display notching because their intercostal arteries arise from the costocervical trunk and therefore are not collateral pathways to the descending thoracic aorta. Unilateral inferior rib notching can be encountered in patients with ipsilateral upper extremity vascular shunt lesions or aortic coarctation with contralateral aberrant subclavian arteries. Attention should also be paid to the left paratracheal stripe because dilatation of the left subclavian artery and post-stenotic aorta can cause a pair of convex bulges at the aortic knob, resulting in the "figure 3" sign. Rarely, hypertrophy of the internal mammary vessels may manifest with an undulating soft tissue stripe posterior to the sternum on lateral view. Cross-sectional imaging better characterizes these abnormalities.

Differential Diagnosis

Because congenital arch variants result in abnormal paratracheal opacities, other lesions known to occur in these locations include lymphadenopathy, bronchogenic cysts, and vascular aneurysms. Retrotracheal opacities created by aberrant subclavian arteries also have esophageal neoplasms, foregut duplication cysts, and tracheal tumors in their differential diagnosis.

Aortic coarctation on radiographs may be confused with mediastinal lymphadenopathy or masses. On cross-sectional imaging, aortic coarctation must be differentiated from pseudo-coarctation. Bilateral inferior rib notching is most commonly seen in aortic coarctation or neurofibromatosis.

Imaging Findings

Congenital Arch Variants

- Left aortic arch with aberrant right subclavian artery results in a retrotracheal opacity on radiographs. On CT, the right subclavian artery arises distal to the isthmus and travels posterior to the trachea and esophagus before coursing superiorly into the subclavian fossa.
- Focal ectasia or aneurysmal dilatation may be seen at the origin of an aberrant subclavian artery and is referred to as a diverticulum of Kommerell.
- Right aortic arch with aberrant left subclavian artery will demonstrate absence of the normal left aortic knob and a right paratracheal opacity on radiography. A retrotracheal opacity may be encountered due to the course of the aberrant left subclavian artery. In most cases, the descending aorta retains its normal left-sided location. The esophagus and trachea are usually encircled by the right aortic arch, posterior aberrant left subclavian artery, and left-sided ligamentum arteriosum (from subclavian artery to pulmonary artery). Look for evidence of proximal esophageal dilatation or tracheomalacia.

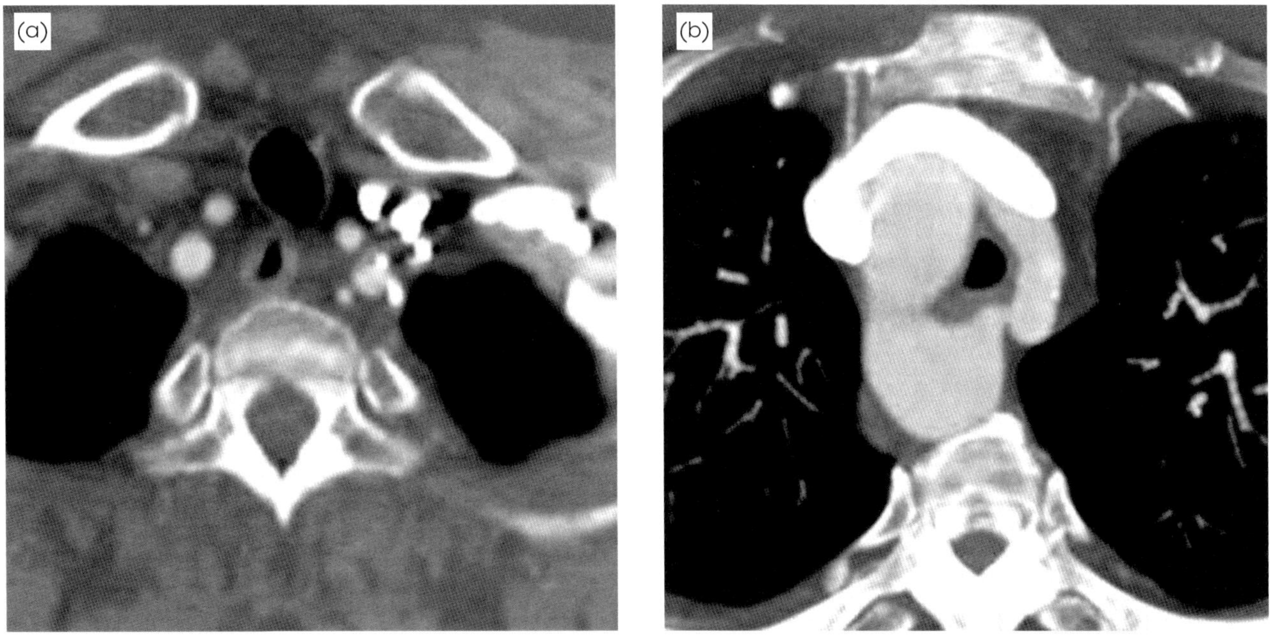

Figure 91.3. Double aortic arch. (a) Axial contrast-enhanced CT image near the thoracic inlet demonstrates symmetric arrangement of the bilateral common carotid and subclavian arteries, all of which lie orthogonal to the image plane ("four vessel" sign). (b) Axial maximum intensity projection image demonstrates a slightly more superior and larger right aortic arch that communicates posterior to the esophagus and trachea with a smaller left aortic arch. This is the most common form of vascular ring. Note the mild dilatation and hypertrophy of the esophagus (a) as a result of the tight vascular ring.

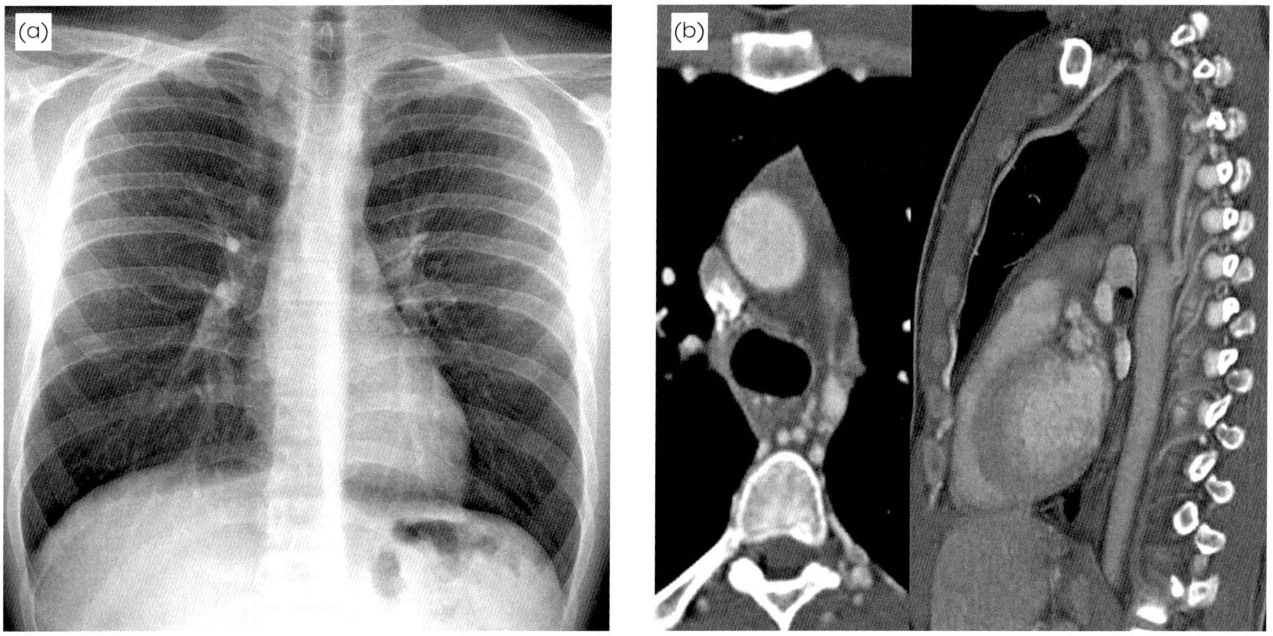

Figure 91.4. Aortic coarctation. (a) Frontal chest radiograph demonstrates bilateral inferior rib notching most prominent in the third through sixth ribs. (b) Contrast-enhanced axial and sagittal oblique volume-rendered images demonstrate focal severe narrowing of the proximal descending thorax aorta near the isthmus with enlargement of the internal mammary and intercostal arteries in keeping with.

- Double aortic arch most commonly has a larger and more superior right aortic knob and a smaller left aortic knob on radiography. On CT, in the upper mediastinum, the carotid and subclavian vessels are seen in cross section symmetrically distributed about the airway and esophagus ("four vessel" sign) (Fig. 91.3). The left-sided moiety may be diminutive or even atretic, leaving only a thin fibrous cord between the proximal left arch and the descending aorta that is usually left-sided. This cord is often difficult to see even on thin-section CT or high-resolution MRI.

Aortic Coarctation

- On radiography, bilateral inferior rib notching along the posterior ribs (especially the fourth through eighth) and convex outward left paratracheal opacity above the aortic knob (figure 3 sign) may be seen (Fig. 91.4).
- On CT and MRI, focal narrowing of the aorta in the region of the ductus is seen and often best demonstrated on sagittal oblique views.
- Enlarged bilateral intercostal, internal mammary, and descending scapular arteries, as well as enlargement of the thyrocervical and thoracoacromial trunks, are indicative of significant pressure gradient when encountered on CT or MRI.
- On MRI, dark dephasing jets from elevated velocities across the area of narrowing are seen on cine steady-state free precession sequences. Flow quantification sequences performed perpendicular to the dephasing jet allow calculation of peak velocity and estimation of gradient pressure.
- On CT and MRI, left ventricular hypertrophy can be seen, as can as frequently encountered associated anomalies such as bicuspid aortic valve and septal defects.
- Pseudo-coarctation is manifest by a tortuous or kinked proximal descending thoracic aorta without collateral arterial vessel recruitment because there is usually no significant gradient across the narrowing.

Clinical Issues

Left aortic arch with aberrant right subclavian artery is almost always an incidental finding. Although there are reports of dysphagia (dysphagia lusoria) occurring with this lesion, it is best managed conservatively.

Double aortic arch and right aortic arch with aberrant left subclavian artery are vascular rings. In asymptomatic adults, no intervention is necessary. In patients with dysphagia, respiratory complaints, or tracheomalacia, surgical intervention with ligation of the nondominant (usually) left aortic arch or ligation of the ligamentous arteriosum may be performed.

In adults, aortic coarctation is most commonly managed with percutaneous angioplasty followed by endovascular stent placement. Refractory, or otherwise complex with arch hypoplasia, cases may be treated with surgical resection and composite graft placement.

Key Points

- Left-sided aortic arch with aberrant right subclavian artery, double aortic arch, and right-sided aortic arch with aberrant left subclavian artery are the most commonly encountered arch variants in adults and are rarely associated with congenital heart disease.
- Double aortic arch and right aortic arch with aberrant left subclavian artery are the most common causes of a vascular ring. Only symptomatic adults are treated with ligation of the nondominant arch or ligamentum arteriosum.
- Symmetric bilateral inferior fourth through eighth rib notching is commonly seen in long-standing aortic coarctation, although neurofibromatosis is a well-known mimic and can also cause bilateral inferior rib notching.
- In the evaluation of aortic coarctation, MRI can assess both the anatomic characteristics and collateral vascularity, as well as provide quantitative pressure gradient estimates.
- Pseudo-coarctation of the aorta is differentiated from true coarctation by lack of arterial collaterals and the absence of a pressure gradient across the area of apparent narrowing.

Suggested Reading

Kanne JP, Godwin JD. Right aortic arch and its variants. *J Cardiovasc Comput Tomogr*. 2010 Sep–Oct;4(5):293–300.

Kimura-Hayama ET, Melendez G, Mendizabal AL, Meave-Gonzalez A, Zambrana GF, Corona-Villalobos CP. Uncommon congenital and acquired aortic disease: Role of multidetector CT angiography. *RadioGraphics*. 2010 Jan;30(1):79–98.

CHAPTER 92

Abnormalities of Pulmonary Venous Return

Kristopher W. Cummings

Definition

In adults, partial anomalous pulmonary venous return (PAPVR) is the most commonly encountered abnormality of pulmonary venous drainage and is present when one or more pulmonary veins drains into the systemic venous system. Total anomalous pulmonary venous return results when all pulmonary veins drain to the systemic circulation, an anomaly diagnosed in infancy or early childhood.

Clinical Features

PAPVR in adults is usually diagnosed incidentally on imaging studies performed for other reasons. However, due to the presence of a chronic left-to-right shunt, a minority of patients present with signs and symptoms of pulmonary hypertension. Affected patients are usually acyanotic but may complain of dyspnea, particularly on exertion. If the volume of shunted blood is large, right heart failure develops over time, resulting in lower extremity edema and hepatic congestion. Rarely, irreversible pulmonary hypertension develops.

Due to the high frequency of associated sinus venosus atrial septal defect (ASD), patients with right upper PAPVR often present earlier with symptoms of dyspnea and shunt physiology (Fig. 92.1). Also, paradoxical embolic events may occur across the ASD, resulting in transient ischemic attack or stroke. The presence of an ASD also increases the risk of endocarditis. A cardiac murmur related to the ASD may be heard along the right cardiac border.

Right lower PAPVR is usually seen with a hypoplastic right lung in a condition known as scimitar syndrome or hypogenetic venolobar syndrome. This condition may be seen with an ASD and present with a murmur. Rarely, the hypoplastic lung will be symptomatic.

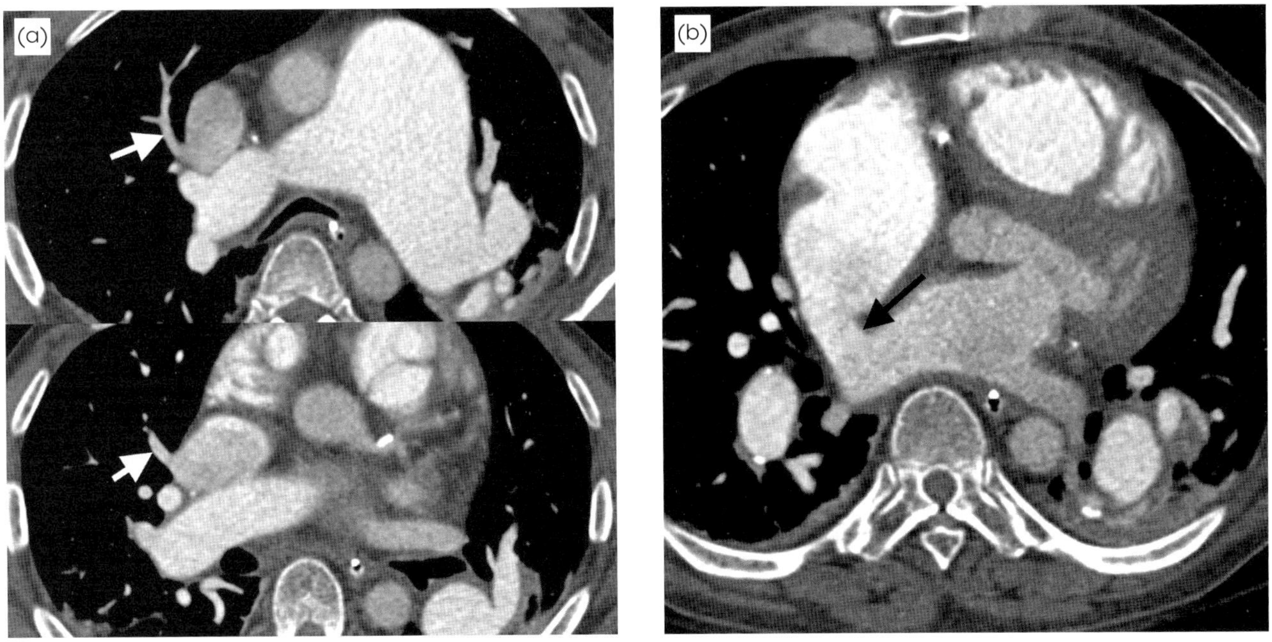

Figure 92.1. Right upper partial anomalous pulmonary venous return with sinus venosus ASD: CT in a 60-year-old man with pulmonary hypertension. (a) Composite CT with contrast shows two right upper anomalous pulmonary veins (arrows). (b) CT at the level of the heart confirms the presence of the sinus venosus ASD (arrow). Note the right ventricle hypertrophy and enlargement in keeping with marked pulmonary hypertension.

Anatomy and Physiology

During embryological development, the pulmonary venous system is in continuity with the splanchnic venous system. A common pulmonary vein develops and merges with the pulmonary venous system as regression of the splanchnic connection occurs. As the common pulmonary vein merges with the primordial left atrium, two right and two left pulmonary veins—superior and inferior, respectively—drain to the left atrium. Anomalies occurring during this process result in persistent venous connections with the splanchnic circulation allowing pulmonary veins to drain to systemic venous structures such as the superior vena cava, inferior vena cava, left brachiocephalic vein, coronary sinus, or azygous/hemiazygous system.

In PAPVR, oxygenated pulmonary venous blood is admixed with deoxygenated systemic venous blood, resulting in a left-to-right shunt. Generally, 50% or more of the total pulmonary venous return must be abnormally shunted to produce symptoms or pulmonary hypertension. Therefore, most adult patients are asymptomatic at diagnosis. If associated lesions such as ASD coexist, patients are more likely to be symptomatic from the larger shunt fraction.

PAPVR is more common in the upper than the lower lobes and is exceedingly rare as an isolated entity in the left lower lobe. Although right upper PAPVR is frequently reported as the most common form, in the age of multidetector CT, left upper PAPVR is likely slightly more common.

In left upper PAPVR, the left superior pulmonary vein drains to a vertical vein that courses superiorly along the lateral aspect of the aortic arch before draining into the left brachiocephalic vein. Associated lesions are uncommon. This anomalous vessel may or may not drain the lingula.

In right upper PAPVR, the right upper lobe, frequently the right middle lobe, and occasionally the superior segment of the right lower lobe drain into the superior vena cava either separately or after converging. The anomalous vein or veins drain into the superior vena cava very close to its junction with the right atrium. Right upper PAPVR is very frequently associated with a sinus venosus ASD that lies high in the atrial septum in the same region where the superior vena cava joins the right atrium.

Right lower PAPVR is most frequently encountered as part of congenital venolobar or scimitar syndrome, in which there are various degrees of right lung hypoplasia, right pulmonary artery hypoplasia, and frequently bronchial and fissural anomalies (Fig. 92.2). A systemic feeding artery may also supply the affected lung without a structural abnormality to suggest sequestration. Drainage from the right lower lobe, middle lobe, and/or the entire right lung occurs via a vertically and inferiorly oriented vein (scimitar vein) into the infra- or supradiaphragmatic inferior vena cava, hepatic veins, or, rarely, the portal vein. Meandering pulmonary veins can occasionally mimic right lower PAPVR as they follow a circuitous path through the lung before emptying normally into the left atrium. Meandering pulmonary veins are frequently seen in conjunction with the other abnormalities of scimitar syndrome and are believed to represent scimitar variants.

Isolated left lower PAPVR is exceedingly rare and may be seen with congenital heart disease, most notably tetralogy of Fallot.

How to Approach the Image

Isolated PAPVR is rarely detectable on radiography. The vertical vein in left upper PAPVR may be seen as widening of the left mediastinal border or, in the event of cannulation by a left internal jugular central venous catheter, abnormal course of the catheter along the left paratracheal stripe before deviating laterally into the lung. Right lower PAPVR in the setting of scimitar syndrome is the most readily detected venous anomaly on radiography due to the tubular anomalous vein draining inferiorly along the right heart border in association with various degrees of right lung volume loss. If significant shunting or pulmonary hypertension has developed, enlargement of the pulmonary trunk and central pulmonary arteries, right atrial and ventricular enlargement, pulmonary artery pruning, and shunt vascularity may be seen as with other atrial or ventricular septal defects.

On cross-sectional images, enlargement of the right atrium or pulmonary arteries should prompt interrogation for an underlying etiology, particularly in younger patients. Although many entities can produce these findings, such as parenchymal lung and chronic thromboembolic disease, left-to-right shunt lesions should always be considered. Careful assessment for atrial and ventricular septal defects or a patent ductus arteriosus should be performed. The pulmonary veins should be individually assessed because anomalous pulmonary veins can be difficult to detect, particularly in the case of right upper PAPVR.

Right lower PAPVR is seen in the setting of scimitar syndrome, which also includes right pulmonary artery hypoplasia, right hemithorax volume loss, and often systemic feeding artery without parenchymal changes of a sequestration.

What Not to Miss

The key with PAPVR is to be mindful of the associations with the various locations. Whereas left upper PAPVR is almost always an isolated phenomenon, right upper PAPVR is not. In 50% of cases, right upper PAPVR will be associated with a sinus venosus ASD. These defects are easily overlooked if they are not specifically searched for. Conversely, when a sinus venosus ASD is encountered, one

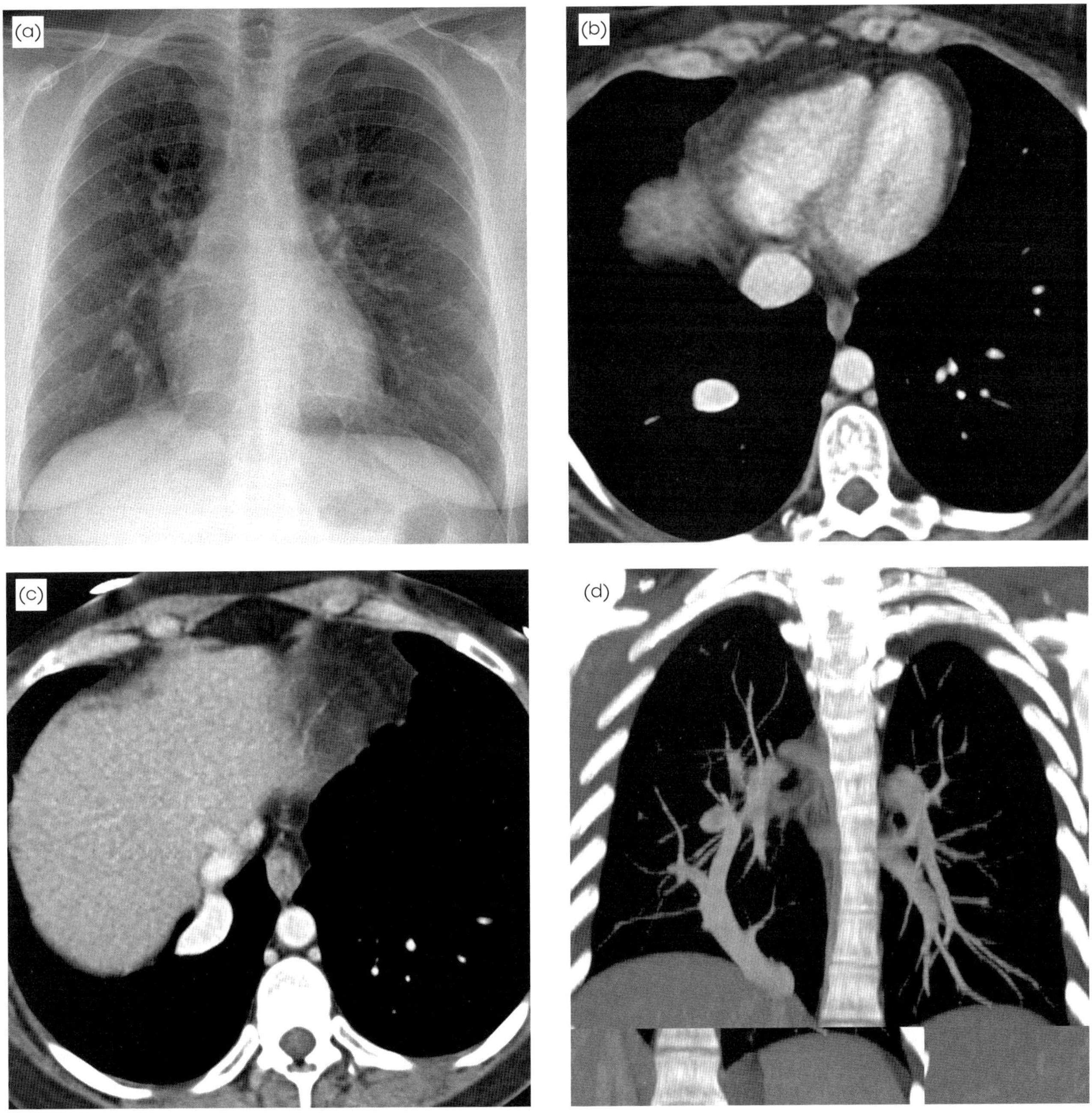

Figure 92.2. Scimitar syndrome. (a) Posteroanterior chest radiograph shows low right lung volume, subtle mediastinal shift to the right, and a vertically oriented tubular opacity adjacent to the right heart border coursing toward the diaphragm. (b, c) Contrast-enhanced chest CT show an enhancing tubular structure representing the right inferior pulmonary vein that drains into the inferior vena cava. (d) Coronal maximum intensity projection image lays out the course of the right lower lobe anomalous pulmonary vein.

must search for right upper PAPVR. Right lower PAPVR does not usually provide a diagnostic challenge because the vertical vein can often be seen on radiography, but a systemic feeding artery to the lower lobe can often be missed. The reader must remember that these frequently arise from the upper abdominal aorta or celiac axis. One also must be careful not to confuse scimitar with a meandering pulmonary vein that exhibits features similar to those of scimitar syndrome but the tortuous right inferior pulmonary vein eventually drains normally into the left atrium (and a shunt is not present).

Differential Diagnosis

- Right cardiac chamber and pulmonary artery enlargement, consider chronic causes of pulmonary hypertension
  - Parenchymal lung disease
  - Chronic thromboembolic disease
  - Left-to-right shunts (ASD, ventricular septal defect, and patent ductus arteriosus)
  - Idiopathic or familial pulmonary hypertension
- Vascular structures located lateral and to the left of the aortic arch
  - Persistent left superior vena cava

- Left superior intercostal vein
- Vertical vein of left upper PAPVR.
- Right hemithorax volume loss in a young patient
  - Swyer–James syndrome
  - Atelectasis
  - Pulmonary artery hypoplasia
  - Scimitar syndrome

Imaging Findings

All forms of PAPVR may present with enlargement of the right heart and main pulmonary artery. The degree of enlargement will be based on the size of the shunt (ratio of pulmonary to systemic blood flow (Q_p:Q_s)). If it is a large enough shunt, it may lead to pulmonary hypertension.

Right Upper PAPVR

- Direct drainage of right upper lobe, middle lobe, and/or superior segment of the right lower lobe venous tributaries into the superior vena cava
- Superior vena below the entry point of the PAPVR will be enlarged
- Associated sinus venosus ASD that is located at the junction of the superior vena cava and right atrium

Right Lower PAPVR (Scimitar Syndrome)

- Drainage of right inferior pulmonary vein (or potentially entire right lung) into inferior vena cava, hepatic vein, or, rarely, portal vein
- Radiography: Right-sided volume loss, tubular vertically oriented scimitar vein in the right lung base
- CT: Right pulmonary artery hypoplasia, right hemithorax volume loss (hypoplasia), anomalous draining vein (scimitar vein), potentially isolated systemic feeding artery from descending thoracic aorta to otherwise normal lung parenchyma

Left Upper PAPVR

- Tubular vascular structure lateral to the aortic arch in the left superior mediastinum coursing between the left brachiocephalic vein and left upper lobe (Fig. 92.3)
- Absence of the normal left superior pulmonary vein in its typical location anterior to the left main bronchus

Left Lower PAPVR

- Exceedingly rare; systemic venous drainage more commonly seen in setting of sequestration

Clinical Issues

- Although PAPVR is often an incidental finding, affected patients may present with dyspnea on exertion or right heart failure.
- Determination of the degree of shunting (Q_p:Q_s) is important in guiding management and can be determined with cardiac catheterization or, more commonly, with flow quantification cardiac MRI sequences run above the aortic and pulmonic valves orthogonal to the long axis of each vessel. Q_p:Q_s of 1.5:1 or greater is considered a hemodynamically significant shunt

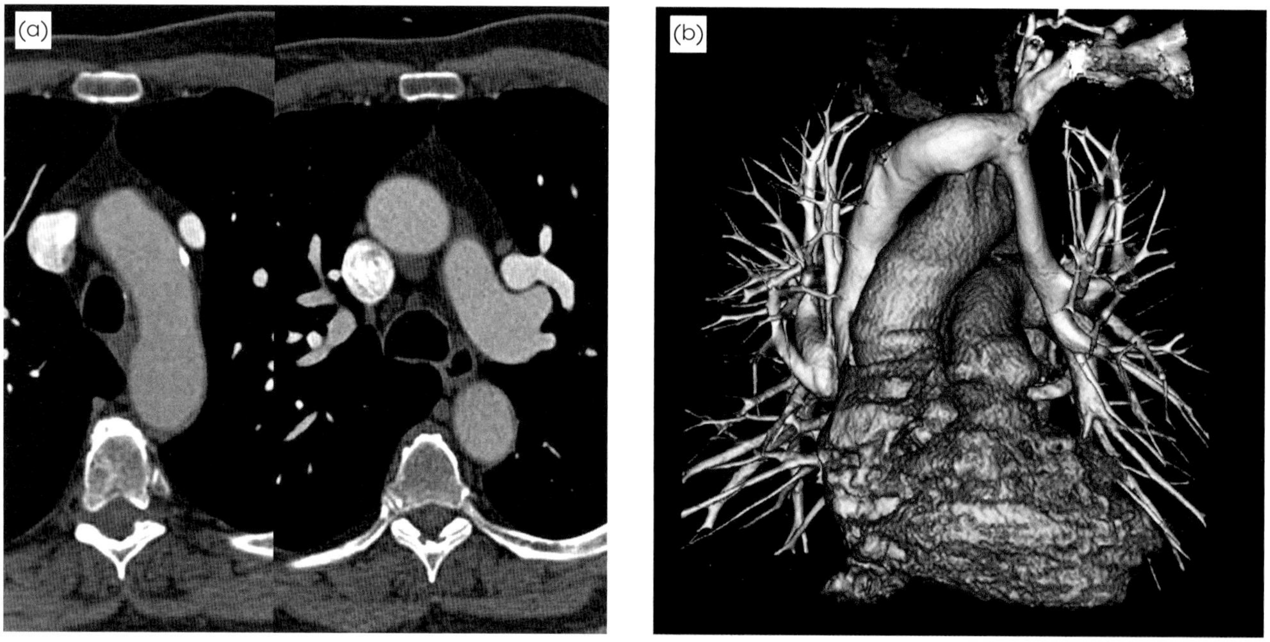

Figure 92.3. Left upper partial anomalous pulmonary venous return. (a) Composite image with contrast-enhanced chest CT shows an enhancing vessel located lateral to the aortic arch that receives tributaries from the left superior pulmonary vein. (b) Three-dimensional volume rendered image shows left upper lobe venous drainage into a vertical left superior mediastinal vein that drains into the left brachiocephalic vein.

and places the patient at risk for development of pulmonary hypertension. In such cases, surgical repair with baffling of the anomalous pulmonary vein back to the left atrium would be indicated.

- Patients with right upper PAPVR and associated sinus venosus ASD often come to clinical attention earlier and often require surgical closure of the ASD at the time of repair.

Key Points

- PAPVR is a left-to-right shunt that is most commonly diagnosed incidentally in asymptomatic adults.
- Right upper PAPVR has a strong association with sinus venosus ASDs, which lie high in the atrial septum near the superior vena cava and right atrial junction.
- Left upper PAPVR is usually an isolated anomaly and drains via a vertical vein coursing lateral to the aortic arch to drain into the left brachiocephalic vein.
- Left lower PAPVR is extremely rare.
- Q_p:Q_s ratio of 1.5:1 or greater is indicative of a clinically significant shunt and places the patient at risk of developing pulmonary hypertension. This can be assessed with cardiac catheterization or flow quantification cardiac MRI.

Suggested Reading

Dillman JR, Yarram SG, Hernandez RJ. Imaging of pulmonary venous development anomalies. *AJR Am J Roentgenol.* 2009 May;192(5):1272–1285.

Ho ML, Bhalla S, Bierhals A, Gutierrez F. MDCT of partial anomalous pulmonary venous return (PAPVR) in adults. *J Thorac Imaging.* 2009 May;24(2):89–95.

CHAPTER 93

Mediastinal Veins and Anomalies

Sanjeev Bhalla

Definition

Mediastinal venous anomalies and normal venous tributaries may result in confusing imaging findings, especially when a chest radiograph shows a catheter or device within one of these vessels. The more commonly encountered variants are left superior vena cava (SVC) and azygous continuation of an interrupted inferior vena cava (IVC), in which the normal connection of right-sided vena cava to right atrium may be altered. Commonly encountered venous tributaries include the left superior intercostal vein and systemic-to-pulmonary vein collaterals.

Clinical Features

Most patients with left SVC or azygous continuation of an interrupted IVC are asymptomatic (Fig. 93.1) because neither represents a shunt lesion. When a left superior intercostal vein is visible on radiography, it is often referred to as an aortic nipple. The left superior intercostal vein may be seen normally on CT, but it is usually dilated as a result of venous stenosis. Clinical symptoms and signs from venous occlusion include edema of the neck and upper extremities and/or cutaneous vascular collaterals. The left superior intercostal vein is often more distended in patients with end-stage renal disease and indwelling catheters. Occasionally, SVC obstruction results in mediastinal venous collaterals that drain directly into the pulmonary veins. These vessels can serve as a right-to-left shunt and may produce cyanosis.

Anatomy and Physiology

The vena cavae develop from the cardinal venous system. Normally, the SVC and the IVC drain into the right atrium. When the left anterior cardinal vein persists, a left-sided SVC is present. This vessel drains into the right atrium via the coronary sinus (Fig. 93.2). When the suprarenal IVC does not develop normally, the IVC drains into the right

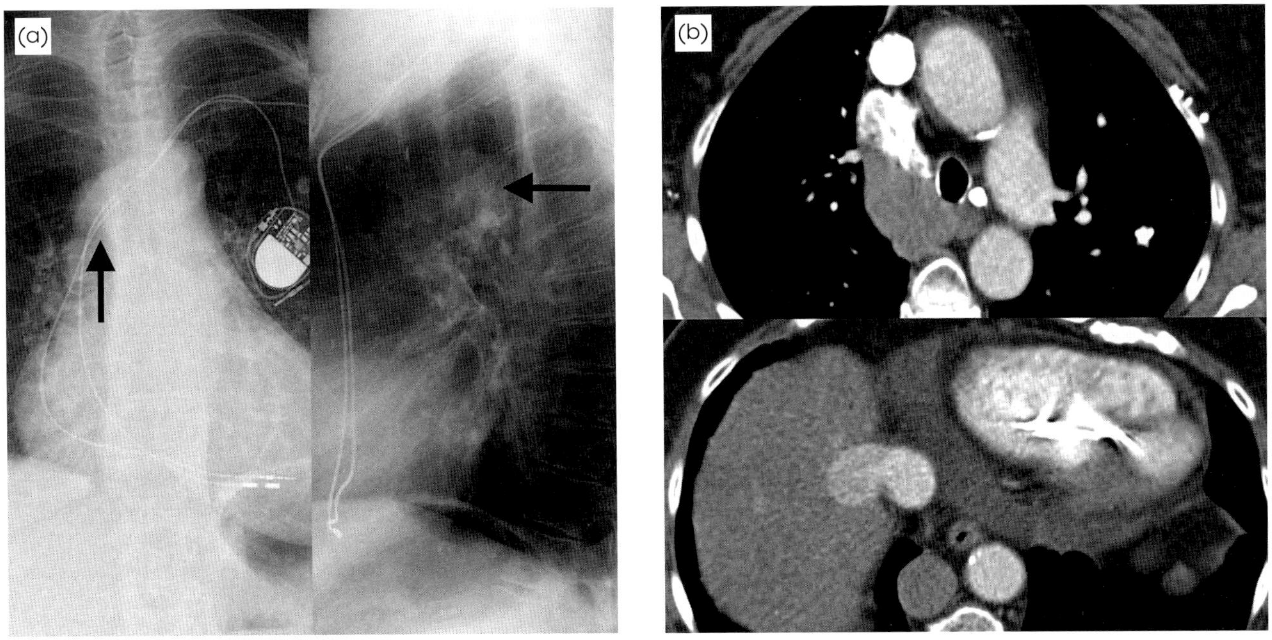

Figure 93.1. Azygous continuation of an interrupted inferior vena cava. (a) Composite image with posteroanterior (left) and lateral (right) chest radiographs of an asymptomatic 72-year-old woman imaged after pacemaker placement shows a wide right paratracheal opacity (arrows). Note that the opacity is posterior to the trachea on the lateral radiograph, suggesting an enlarged azygous vein instead of lymphadenopathy. (b) Composite image with contrast-enhanced chest CT shows the large azygos arch (top) and enlargement of the azygos vein coursing parallel to the descending aorta (bottom). The hepatic veins drain separately into the right atrium.

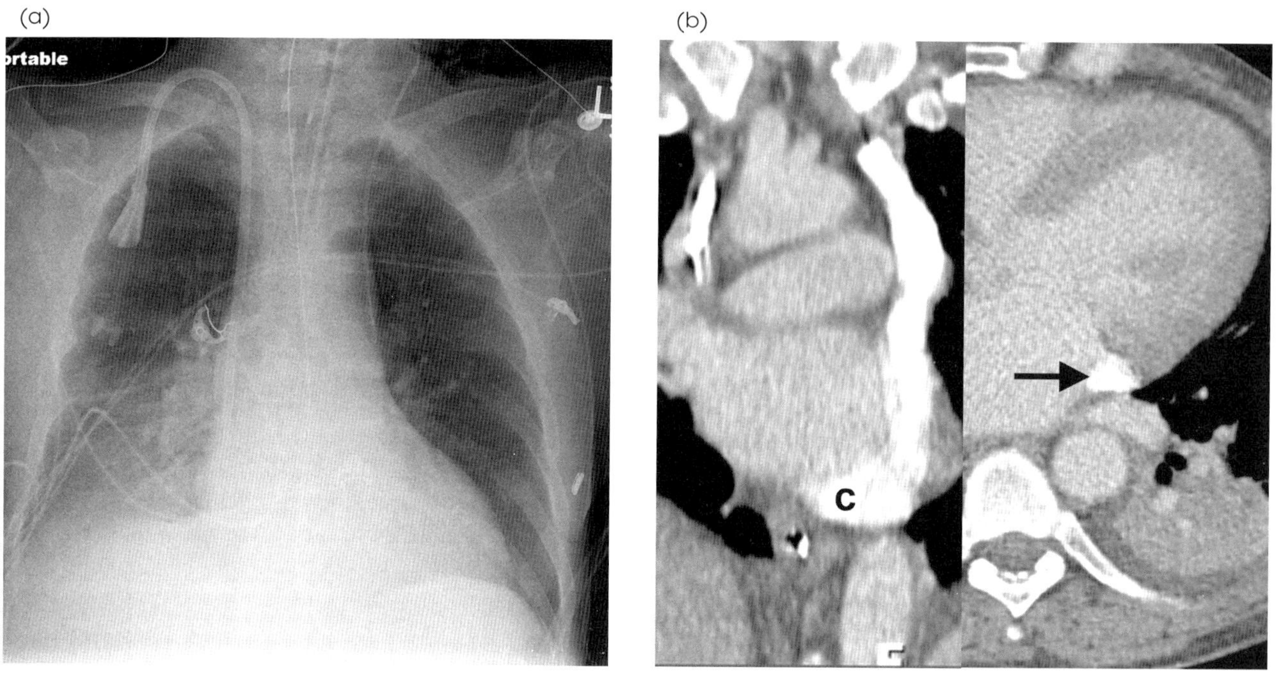

Figure 93.2. Left SVC. (a) Anteroposterior (AP) chest radiograph of a 52-year-old intensive care unit patient shows a left-sided catheter coursing vertically along the left mediastinal border. (b) Contrast-enhanced chest CT performed with a left arm injection revealed a left SVC that is well seen on the coronal maximum intensity projection (MIP) ending in the coronary sinus (C). The transverse image (right; arrow) shows the course of the left SVC through the ligament of Marshall.

SVC via the azygous system (azygous continuation of an interrupted IVC), which can occur in isolation or as part of the polysplenia syndrome.

The left superior intercostal vein drains the upper part of the left hemithorax and represents a connection between the left brachiocephalic vein and hemiazygous system (Fig. 93.3). Note that this vein does not course into the lungs like anomalous pulmonary venous drainage or drain into the coronary sinus like left SVC. Other tributaries that may be visualized on imaging include the pericardiophrenic veins, which travel along the pericardium (Fig. 93.4) and anastomose with inferior phrenic veins, and the internal mammary veins, which are located anteriorly adjacent to the sternum.

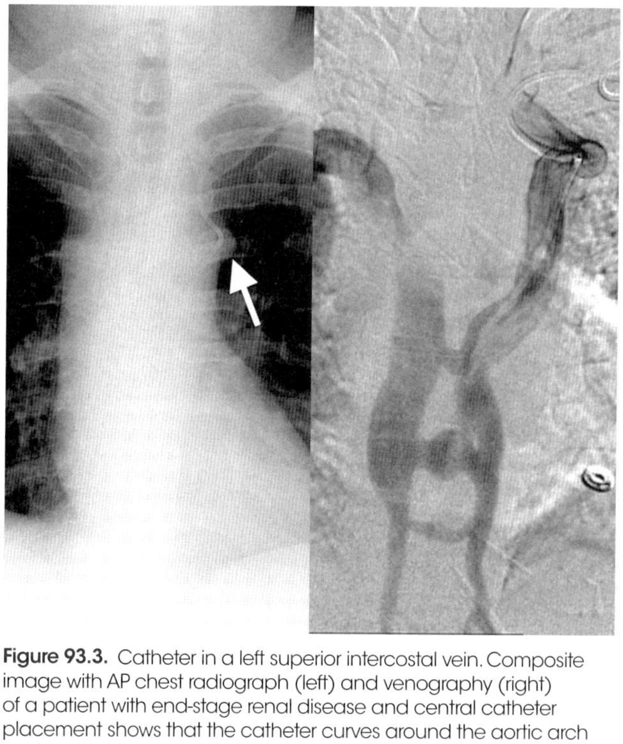

Figure 93.3. Catheter in a left superior intercostal vein. Composite image with AP chest radiograph (left) and venography (right) of a patient with end-stage renal disease and central catheter placement shows that the catheter curves around the aortic arch and terminates medial to the left mediastinal border, a course typical for the left superior intercostal vein, termed aortic nipple when dilated on radiography (arrow). Venography confirmed a dilated left superior intercostal vein secondary to left brachiocephalic vein thrombosis from multiple prior central catheter placements.

How to Approach the Image

Anomalous veins or enlarged venous tributaries are often encountered when a chest radiograph shows a central catheter in an unusual location. Analysis of the catheter course and the location of the catheter tip often allows a confident diagnosis of the anomaly or dilated tributary. When in doubt, a lateral radiograph can be very helpful for further assessment. When such vessels are visualized on CT, the vessel course can be followed to allow accurate identification of the vessel in question.

What Not to Miss

It is important to decide when the condition is simply an anatomic variant or an abnormality that requires intervention. On radiography, the issue often centers on an abnormal catheter course. Extravascular and extra-arterial catheter courses must be diagnosed. When in doubt, connection to a pressure transducer is a reliable means of clarification. Another option is to obtain an

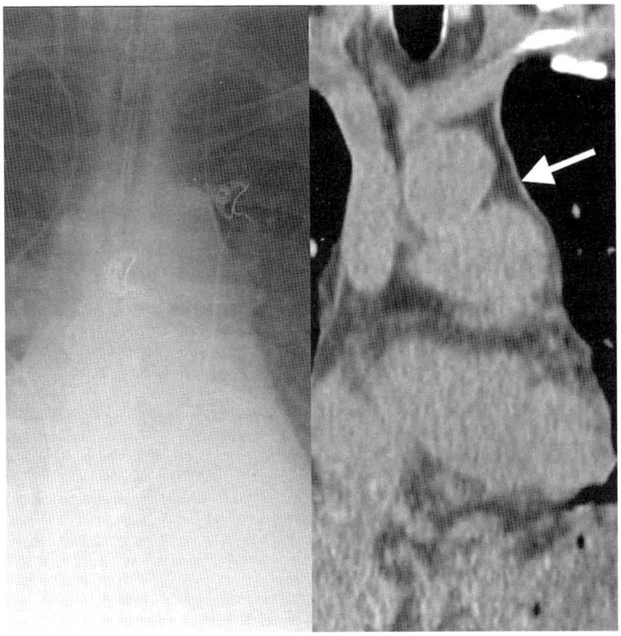

Figure 93.4. Catheter in left pericardiophrenic vein. Composite image with AP chest radiograph (left) and coronal unenhanced chest CT (right) shows an abnormal vertical left central catheter course into a pericardiophrenic vein (arrow). Because of the need for rapid infusion of fluid, the catheter was repositioned.

arterial blood gas, although interpretation of this blood test may be equivocal. In select cases, CT imaging is performed to determine the exact catheter course or to confidently identify the vascular structure in question.

Differential Diagnosis

The differential diagnosis for the various entities is determined by the location of the vascular structure.

Left Mediastinum

- Left SVC
- Left superior intercostal vein
- Left internal mammary vein
- Left pericardiophrenic vein
- Left superior anomalous venous return

Right Mediastinum

- Right pericardiophrenic vein
- Azygous vein
- Right paratracheal lymphadenopathy
- Duplication cyst

Bilateral

- Venovenous collaterals

Imaging Findings

Left SVC

- Left para-aortic vessel that takes a vertical course
- Travels through ligament of Marshall (between left superior and inferior pulmonary veins) and drains into the coronary sinus
- Direct connection to left atrium should be excluded
- Right SVC may or may not be present
- Left brachiocephalic vein or bridging vein may be present

Left Superior Intercostal Vein

- Normal structure that connects the left brachiocephalic vein with the hemiazygous system
- May dilate with stenoses and become apparent on chest radiography as a focal protrusion off the lateral aspect of the aortic arch, sometimes called the aortic nipple
- When there is a left SVC, the left superior intercostal vein may drain into that structure and may continue as a hemiazygous vein
- Rarely, hemiazygous vein will be distended from hemiazygous continuation of an interrupted IVC—a condition also seen in isolation or with polysplenia

Azygous Continuation of an Interrupted IVC

- Radiography
  - Enlarged right paratracheal opacity. A vascular interface coursing inferiorly toward the abdomen akin to the left para-aortic interface formed by the descending thoracic aorta may be seen.
  - Unlike lymphadenopathy, a distended azygous vein changes in size between an upright and a supine radiography. On supine radiography, venous return increases, and the opacity is larger than that on an upright radiograph.
  - On a lateral radiograph, it can be seen posterior to the trachea (unlike lymphadenopathy which will be seen anterior to the trachea).
- CT
  - Azygous continuation of an interrupted IVC may be seen with polysplenia (which may exhibit bilateral hyparterial bronchi or two left lungs sometimes known as left homoisomerism).
  - The intrahepatic veins drain normally into the right atrium in azygous continuation of an interrupted IVC.
  - Rarely, the hemiazygous vein will serve as the continuation of an interrupted IVC. In this condition, the hemiazygous vein dilates and results in a markedly enlarged left superior intercostal vein.

Systemic Venous Collaterals to the Pulmonary Veins

- Rarely detected on radiography
- CT/MRI: Collateral veins that can be followed to a pulmonary vein or directly to the left atrium
- One clue might be a pulmonary vein that enhances much more than the others (Fig. 93.5)

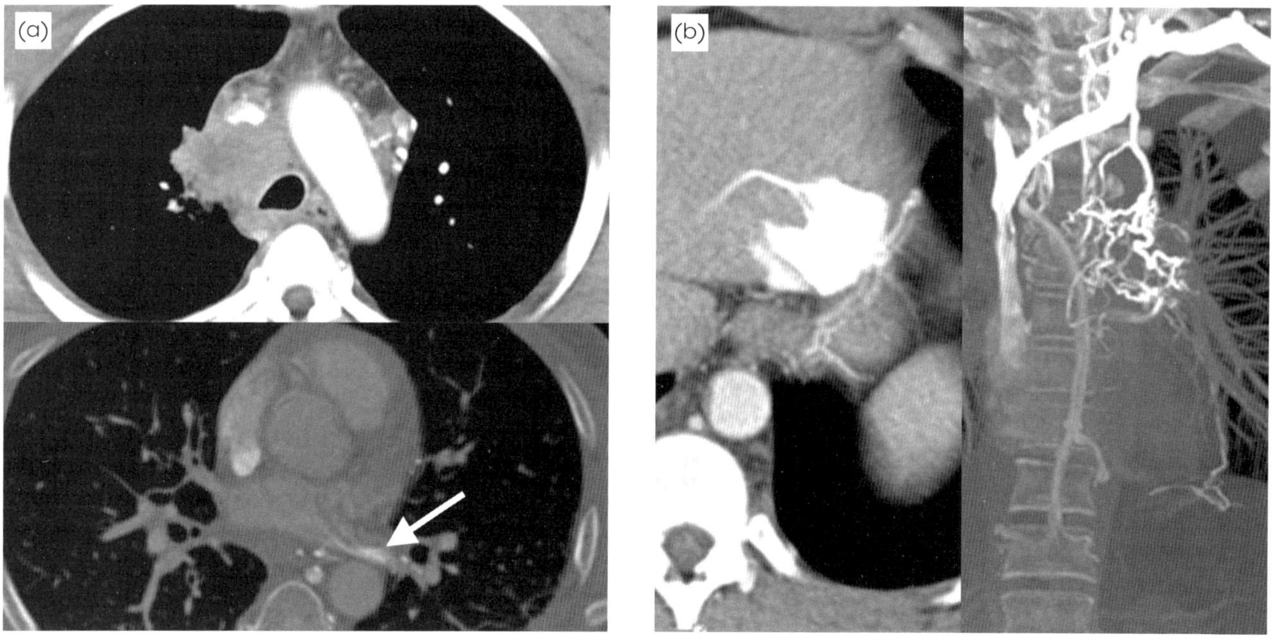

Figure 93.5. Systemic venous collaterals to the pulmonary veins. (a) Composite image with contrast-enhanced chest CT of a 60-year-old man with small cell lung cancer shows a large right paratracheal lymph node mass with SVC obstruction and multiple mediastinal vascular collaterals that drain into the pulmonary veins (arrow) and may produce cyanosis from right-to-left shunting. (b) Composite image with axial (left) and coronal MIP image (right) shows brisk enhancement of a portion of the liver from venous collaterals that are well delineated on the MIP image.

Pericardiophrenic Veins

- Whether on the right or left, they tend to course vertically along the pericardium in the mid axillary line.
- These veins become apparent on cross-sectional imaging in the setting of superior vena caval obstruction.
- These veins anastamose with inferior phrenic veins and may result in a focal area of increased attenuation of the liver. This is sometimes referred to as the "hot quadrate" sign in reference to the appearance on technetium sulfur colloid scans.

Internal Mammary Veins

- Paired anterior chest wall vertically oriented vessels in a parasternal location

Clinical Issues

- A left SVC is an interesting anatomic variant in most cases. However, it become important when it communicates directly with the left atrium, resulting in a right-to-left shunt that can produce cyanosis.
- A left SVC may also become important in patients with recurrent atrial fibrillation being considered for ablation. If pulmonary venous ablation fails, the ligament of Marshall may be targeted next. Knowledge of a left SVC coursing through this ligament can be important because targeted ablation may damage the coursing vein.
- Anomalous veins become significant in the setting of a catheter taking an unusual course.
- Venous collateral may be seen when small venous networks develop in the mediastinum. If they drain from one systemic vein to another, they tend to be asymptomatic. Such collaterals may be seen in the post congenital heart surgery patient and in patients with fibrosing mediastinitis.

Key Points

- Persistent left SVC drains into the coronary sinus and is not a shunt lesion.
- Azygous continuation of an interrupted IVC may be suggested on radiography because of an enlarged right paratracheal opacity that changes size with changes in patient position. Visualization of the interface of the dilated azygos vein as it courses toward the abdomen is confirmatory.
- Unlike lymphadenopathy, an enlarged azygous vein appears posterior to the trachea on the lateral projection.
- In SVC or brachiocephalic vein stenosis/occlusion, collateral veins may drain directly into the pulmonary veins and result in right-to-left shunting.
- Enlarged pericardiophrenic veins may result in vigorous enhancement of the medial segment of the left hemiliver (the hot quadrate sign).
- A central catheter that takes an unusual course within the mediastinum on radiography may be within one of many venous tributaries or within an anomalous vessel. Careful radiographic analysis of both posteroanterior and lateral radiographs often reveals the diagnosis.

Suggested Reading

Burney K, Young H, Barnard SA, McCoubrie P, Darby M. CT appearances of congential and acquired abnormalities of the superior vena cava. *Clin Radiol.* 2007 Sep;62(9):837–842.

Gilkeson RC, Nyberg EM, Sachs PB, Wiant AM, Zahka KG, Siwik ES. Systemic to pulmonary venous shunt: Imaging findings and clinical presentations. *J Thorac Imaging.* 2008 Aug;23(3):170–177.

Kamel IR, Lawler LP, Corl FM, Fishman EK. Patterns of collateral pathways in extrahepatic portal hypertension as demonstrated by multidetector row computed tomography and advanced image processing. *J Comput Assist Tomogr.* 2004 Jul–Aug;28(4):469–477.

CHAPTER 94

Shunts, Intracardiac and Intrapulmonary

Kristopher W. Cummings

Definition

Shunting refers to abnormal mixture of deoxygenated systemic venous blood and oxygenated systemic arterial blood. This can occur across cardiac chambers, as in atrial septal defect (ASD) and ventricular septal defect (VSD), or across a patent ductus arteriosus (PDA). Pulmonary shunting most commonly occurs across vascular abnormalities such as pulmonary arteriovenous malformations (PAVMs).

Clinical Features

Most intracardiac shunts diagnosed in adults result in a left-to-right shunt with oxygenated blood from the systemic circulation (left) mixing with deoxygenated blood from the pulmonary circulation (right). In this scenario, no hypoxia occurs and many patients remain asymptomatic, especially if the lesion is small and thus restrictive to flow. However, even small ASDs or VSDs place the patient at risk for endocarditis and paradoxical embolic events. Larger defects that are nonrestrictive to flow can cause volume overload of the right heart and pulmonary overcirculation that place the patient at risk for developing pulmonary hypertension that may become irreversible (Eisenmenger physiology). Elevation of pulmonary vascular resistance may lead to reversal of shunt direction, with deoxygenated pulmonic circulation blood admixing with oxygenated systemic circulation blood resulting in hypoxia.

PAVMs can occur in isolation, but the majority of patients with incidentally discovered AVMs have hereditary hemorrhagic telangiectasia (HHT) or Osler–Weber–Rendu syndrome, an autosomal dominant genetic condition with variable penetrance. These AVMs are direct communications of small arterioles and venules without an intervening capillary bed. Affected patients may present with paradoxical embolic events (stroke and brain abscess), hypoxia, or spontaneous hemorrhage, especially during pregnancy. The Curacao criteria are used to establish the diagnosis of HHT and include spontaneous recurrent epistaxis, multiple cutaneous or mucocutaneous telangiectasias, visceral arteriovenous malformations (most commonly in the lung, liver, and brain), and first-degree family history of the syndrome. Recurrent nosebleeds and gastrointenstinal bleeding are common nonpulmonary presentations of patients with HHT. The second most common association with PAVMs is from prior congenital heart disease surgery (usually a superior vena cava-to-pulmonary conduit known as a Glenn shunt).

Anatomy and Physiology

ASD is the most common intracardiac shunt detected in adulthood. Ostium secundum defects are the most common type of ASD and occur at the fossa ovalis due to overresorption or underdevelopment of the septum primum or septum secundum. Sinus venosus ASD occurs high within the atrial septum at the junction of the superior vena cava and the right atrium, and it has a strong association with right upper partial anomalous pulmonary venous return. Rarely, an inferior type of sinus venosus defect may occur at the junction of the inferior vena cava and the right atrium. Ostium primum defects occur in the portion of the atrial septum just above the atrioventricular valve plane, which is formed from the endocardial cushions, and primum ASD is almost always seen in association with endocardial cushion or atrioventricular canal defect. Patent foramen ovale occurs in approximately 25% of adults when the septum primum and septum secundum fail to anatomically fuse, depending solely on left greater than right atrial pressures to keep the membranes apposed.

The most common VSD in adults is a perimembranous defect in the membranous portion of the interventricular septum, immediately beneath the aortic valve in the left ventricular outflow tract. The second most common type of VSD in adults is within the muscular portion of the septum. Myocardial infarction and trauma are common causes of acquired muscular defects in adults, whereas the majority of congenital muscular defects either regress spontaneously or are surgically corrected in childhood. Outlet-type VSD occurs high in the portion of the septum that separates the right ventricular outflow tract and proximal pulmonary trunk from the aorta. It is commonly seen in association with conotruncal abnormalities such as tetralogy of Fallot, truncus arteriosus, and transposition. The crista supraventricularis is a muscular band in the right ventricle that marks the beginning of the right ventricular outflow tract or infundibulum, above which lies the outlet portion of the ventricular septum. Thus, this type of VSD is often called a supracristal defect. Inlet VSD involves the interventricular septum at the level of the atrioventricular valve plane and is most commonly encountered as part of an atrioventricular canal defect.

Rarely, a PDA may be encountered in an adult due to persistence of the embryologic communication between the proximal descending aorta at the aortic isthmus and the pulmonary trunk near its junction with the left pulmonary artery.

A PAVM is a direct communication between a pulmonary artery and a pulmonary vein without an intervening capillary bed. The majority of PAVMs are simple, meaning that there is one feeding artery and one draining vein. Complex PAVMs with multiple feeding arteries and/or veins may also be encountered. Occasionally, the communication occurs across multiple tiny vascular channels, creating a telangiectatic appearance. The resultant right-to-left shunt may produce hypoxia.

How to Approach the Image

In cases of restrictive ASD or VSD, the chest radiograph may be completely normal. Shunts that are nonrestrictive to flow result in pulmonary overcirculation, which manifests with increased vascular markings extending to the lung periphery and upper lobes (shunt vascularity) (Fig. 94.1). ASD results in increased right atrial volume (due to left-to-right shunting) and subsequently increased right ventricular volume with resultant right atrial and right ventricular enlargement with normal-sized left-sided cardiac chambers. VSD results in right ventricular, pulmonary artery and left atrial enlargement with the right atrium and left ventricle remaining normal in size, at least early in the disease. PDA shunts do not cross cardiac chambers, which are usually of normal size with enlargement of the pulmonary trunk and left greater than right pulmonary arteries. Chronic or severe pulmonary hypertension manifests with rapid tapering of size from the central to peripheral pulmonary arteries (pruning), although this finding is not specific for shunt lesions. Atherosclerosis manifesting as mural calcification of the central pulmonary arteries is more commonly encountered in long-standing shunts than in other causes of pulmonary hypertension.

PAVMs are often undetectable at radiography, but they may occasionally manifest as a solitary pulmonary nodule. Feeding arteries and draining veins may manifest as tubular opacities extending to and from the nodule. Most patients are screened using contrast-enhanced CT. Multiplanar thin maximum projection images created and viewed on a three-dimensional workstation are optimal for visualization of abnormal vascular communications. A pre-contrast CT is useful to avoid confusing a calcified granuloma with feeding artery from a PAVM.

What Not to Miss

The diagnosis of a septal defect requires visualization of a communication between the affected chambers. One must be careful to look at the septae and the region of a PDA,

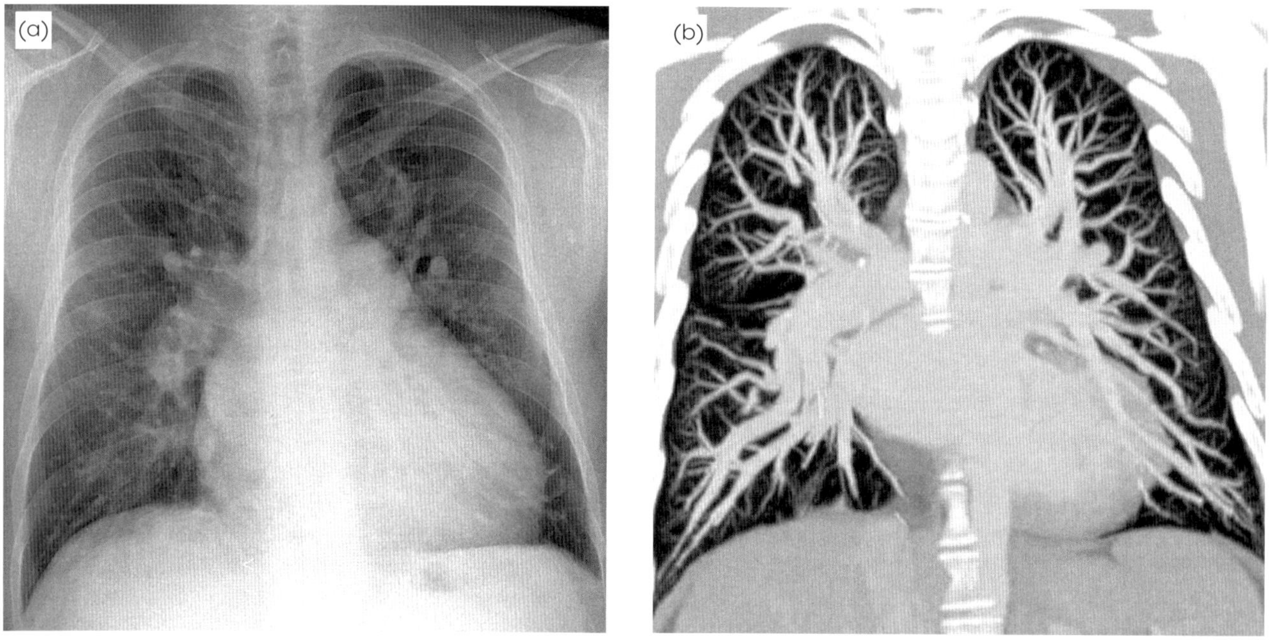

Figure 94.1. Shunt vascularity and pulmonary artery pruning. (a) Posteroanterior chest radiograph of a patient with a VSD shows enlargement of the pulmonary trunk and central pulmonary arteries with rapid peripheral vessel tapering (pruning) consistent with pulmonary hypertension. (b) Coronal maximum intensity projection contrast-enhanced chest CT of the same patient shows enlarged pulmonary arteries, greater than expected vascular markings in the upper lobes, and vascular markings in the lung periphery (shunt vascularity).

especially when shunt vascularity CT or chamber enlargement is seen. However, when the images are acquired with a slice thickness of 5 mm or greater, a normal septum may be volume-averaged with adjacent blood pool and simulate a septal defect.

For a PAVM, identification of a feeding artery and draining vein is diagnostic but may be mimicked by conditions in which feeding arteries are not associated with draining veins, such as the following:

- Granuloma
- Angioinvasive fungal infection
- Vascular metastases
- Pulmonary venous collaterals (as in fibrosing mediastinitis)

Differential Diagnosis

- Pulmonary hypertension
  - Parenchymal lung disease (fibrosis, emphysema)
  - Chronic thromboembolic disease
  - Left heart disease

PAVM manifests as a solitary pulmonary nodule on radiography. Additional considerations include the following:

- Lung cancer
- Granuloma
- Hamartoma
- Metastasis
- Carcinoid
- PDA
- Ductus aneurysm
- Post-traumatic aortic pseudoaneurysm

Imaging Findings

Atrial Septal Defect

- Right atrial, right ventricular, and pulmonary artery enlargement
- Absence of septal tissue at the fossa ovalis in ostium secundum defects
- High communication between left and right atrium at junction with superior vena cava in superior sinus venosus defects
- Absence of septal tissue just proximal to the atrioventricular valve plane in ostium primum defects
- Dephasing jets across defects on cine bright blood MRI (Fig. 94.2)
- Patent foramen ovale can exhibit differential contrast enhancement occurring at an obliquity to the interatrial septum on CT or separation of membranes and dephasing on cine bright blood MRI

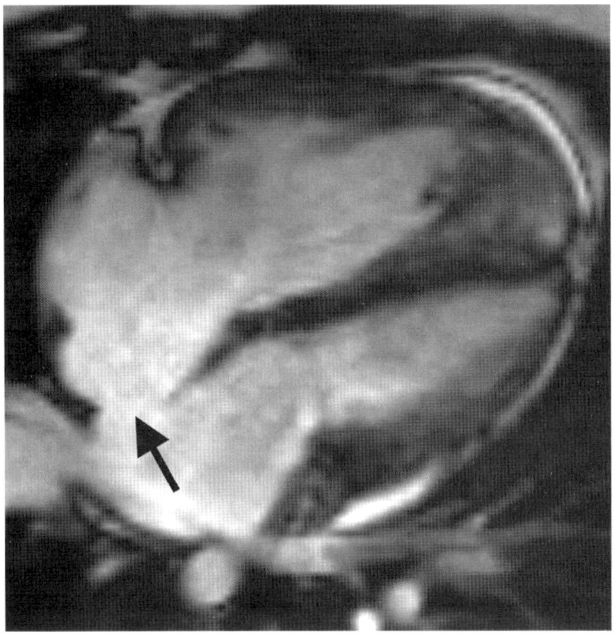

Figure 94.2. ASD. Bright blood four-chamber long-axis MR image demonstrates widening of the fossa ovalis (arrow) with absence of septal tissue consistent with an ostium secundum ASD. Note right atrial and right ventricular enlargement and right ventricular hypertrophy.

Ventricular Septal Defect

- Right ventricular, pulmonary artery, and left atrial enlargement
- Absence of interventricular septal tissue immediately beneath the aortic valve plane in perimembranous defects with differential contrast flow across the defect on CT or dephasing across the defect on cine bright blood MR
- Occasionally, perimembranous VSD will heal spontaneously, forming an aneurysm or "windsock" by redundant tissue derived from the septal leaflet of the tricuspid valve
- Tubular channels across the muscular interventricular septum filled with contrast on CT or with dephasing across the defect on cine bright blood MRI (Figs. 94.3 and 94.4)
- Look for evidence of prior infarction, such as delayed gadolinium enhancement on MRI or myocardial fat deposition on CT in muscular defects (Fig. 94.5)
- Absence of septal tissue above the crista supraventricularis in the right ventricular infundibulum (outlet VSD) or just below the atrioventricular valve plane (inlet VSD)

Patent Ductus Arteriosus

- Enlarged pulmonary trunk and asymmetric left greater than right pulmonary artery enlargement
- Channel between the aortic isthmus and the pulmonary artery (usually the main or left pulmonary artery)

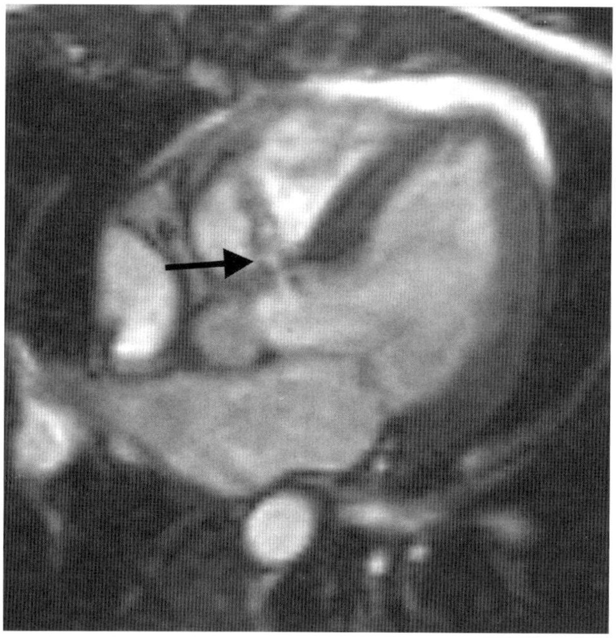

Figure 94.3. VSD. Bright blood four-chamber long-axis MR image of a patient with a perimembranous VSD demonstrates a dark dephasing jet arising immediately proximal and inferior to the aortic valve in the left ventricular outflow tract (arrow) extending into the right ventricle.

Note that in the setting of long-standing shunts and pulmonary hypertension from any of the previously mentioned defects, the following can be seen:

- Shunt vascularity
- Pulmonary artery pruning
- Pulmonary artery atherosclerosis

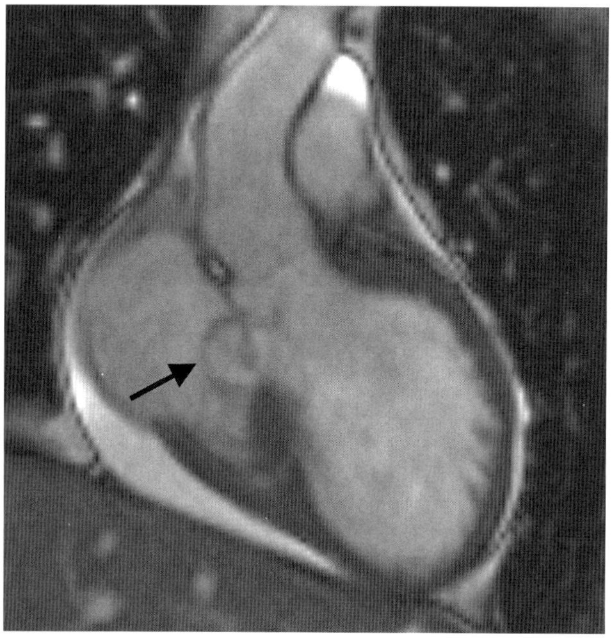

Figure 94.4. VSD. Oblique coronal bright blood MR image demonstrates a focal contained outpouching bulging rightward at the level of the membranous interventricular septum corresponding to the windsock of a healed VSD (arrow).

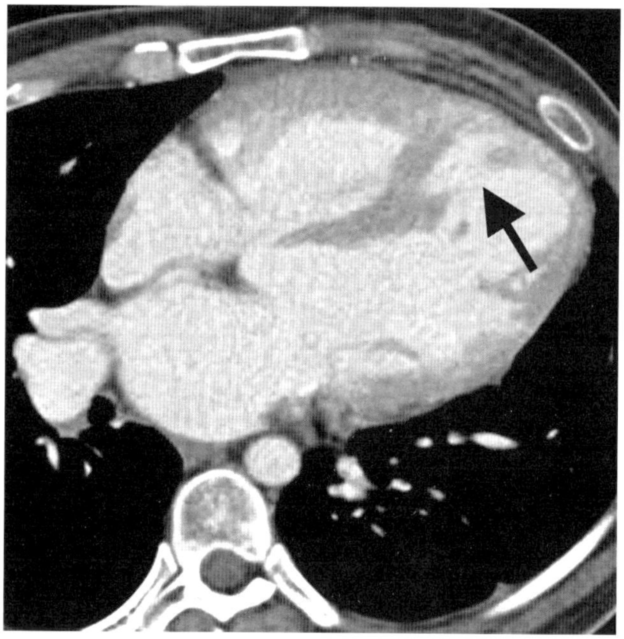

Figure 94.5. VSD. Oblique axial contrast-enhanced chest CT demonstrates a large congenital apical muscular ventricular septal defect (arrow). Note right ventricular enlargement and hypertrophy.

- Right ventricular hypertrophy
- Right ventricular and atrial enlargement

Pulmonary Arteriovenous Malformation

- Solitary or multiple pulmonary nodules with or without feeding vessels on radiography (Fig. 94.6)
- Feeding artery or arteries and draining vein or veins best seen on CT
- Focal ground-glass opacities associated with feeding arteries and draining veins (telangiectatic AVM)
- In HHT, may also see the following:
  - Visceral AVMs in liver, spleen, pancreas, small bowel, stomach, and kidneys
  - Enlargement of celiac axis and hepatic artery, which should raise suspicion for hepatic malformations

Clinical Issues

- Management of intracardiac shunt lesions is largely dependent on the degree of shunting and the presence or absence of paradoxical embolic events.
- With either cardiac catheterization or flow quantification cardiac MRI, the forward flow in the pulmonic system across the pulmonic valve (Q_p) and forward flow in the arterial system across the aortic valve (Q_s) can be measured. Nonrestrictive defects (Q_p:Q_s > 1.5:1) require closure.
- Ostium secundum ASD is most commonly treated via percutaneous occluder device placement, with surgery being reserved for large defects (>40 mm) or small residual septal rims.
- Ostium primum and sinus venosus defects are treated surgically.

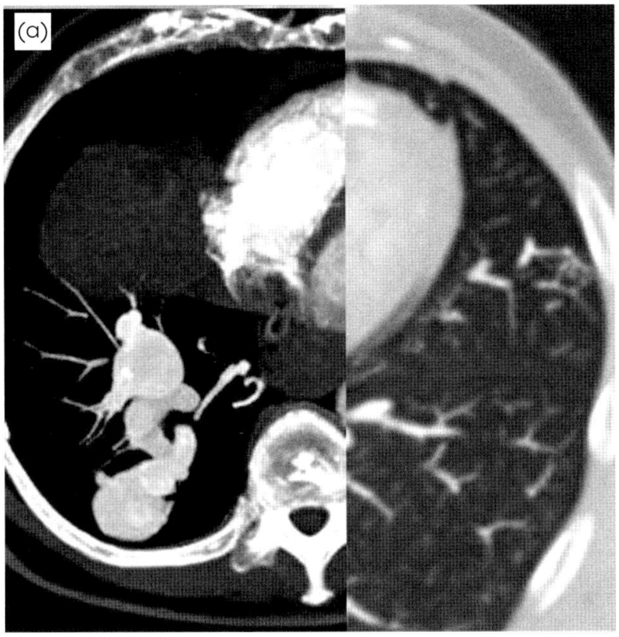

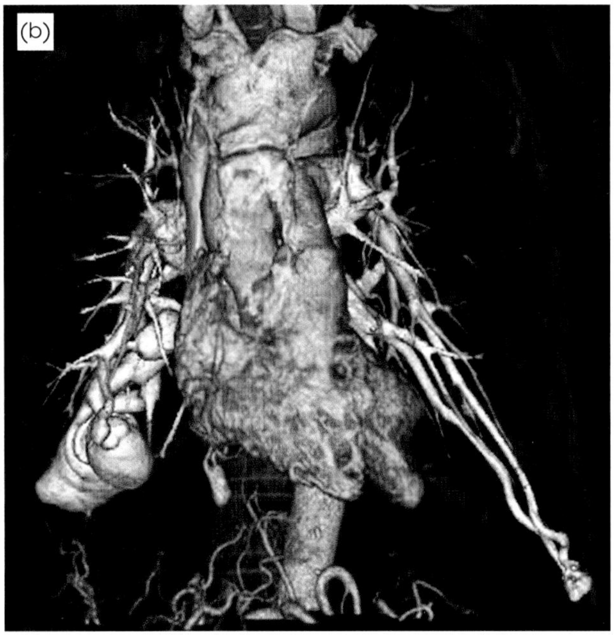

Figure 94.6. Pulmonary arteriovenous malformations. (a) Composite image with contrast-enhanced chest CT from two different patients shows a large enhancing vascular nidus in the right lower lobe filled by a large pulmonary arterial branch (left) and a small ground-glass or telangiectatic nidus with an associated feeding artery and draining vein in the lingula (right). (b) Volume-rendered three-dimensional CT image demonstrates bilateral, right larger than left, arteriovenous malformations in a patient with hereditary hemorrhagic telangiectasia.

- All types of nonrestrictive VSD are considered surgical lesions.
- Restrictive perimembranous VSD may be surgically corrected if there is evidence of aortic insufficiency, which can be seen with high-velocity flow from left to right underneath the right or noncoronary sinus of the aortic valve leading to a suction (Venturi) effect on the affected cusp.
- PDA is commonly managed by percutaneous occluder device placement and, less commonly, by surgical ligation.
- If irreversible pulmonary hypertension has developed in the setting of any long-standing cardiac shunt, closure of the defect is contraindicated because the defect is acting as a "pop-off" mechanism allowing for a degree of compensation for the dramatically elevated pulmonary pressures.
- Due to the risk of systemic embolic event, PAVMs with feeding arteries 3 mm or greater are targeted for embolization.

Key Points

- Ostium secundum defects are the most common cardiac shunt lesion and most common form of ASD in adults.
- Perimembranous VSD is the most common type of VSD in adults, with muscular defects second in frequency.
- Sinus venosus ASD, ostium primum ASD, outlet VSD, and inlet VSD have strong associations with other forms of congenital heart defects.
- Ostium secundum ASD, patent foramen ovale, and PDA are often treated percutaneously.
- Pulmonary AVMs are most commonly encountered in patients with HHT.
- The feeding artery size, not size of the nidus, is the most important factor in management of PAVM because lesions with feeding arteries greater than 3 mm are coil embolized.

Suggested Reading

Berko NS, Haramati LB. Simple cardiac shunts in adults. *Semin Roentgenol.* 2012 Jul;47(3):277–288.

Cottin V, Dupuis-Girod S, Lesca G, Cordier JF. Pulmonary vascular manifestations of hereditary hemorrhagic telangiectasia (Rendu–Osler disease). *Respiration.* 2007;74(4):361–378.

Cummings KW, Bhalla S. Multidetector computed tomographic pulmonary angiography: Beyond acute pulmonary embolism. *Radiol Clin North Am.* 2010 Jan;48(1):51–65.

Wang ZJ, Reddy GP, Gotway MB, Yeh BM, Higgins CB. Cardiovascular shunts: MR imaging evaluation. *RadioGraphics.* 2003 Oct;23(Spec No):S181–S194.

Section XVIII

Diseases of the Chest Wall and Diaphragm

CHAPTER 95

Diseases of the Chest Wall and Diaphragm

Sanjeev Bhalla

Introduction

The chest wall consists of osseous structures, fascial planes, nerves, muscles, vessels, and fat that surround the parietal pleura. The diaphragm is the main muscular division between the thorax and abdomen, and it is the key muscle of respiration.

Diseases of the Chest Wall and Diaphragm

Chest wall conditions can be categorized as masses, fluid collections, and congenital abnormalities. The variety of masses encountered in the chest wall is reflective of the tissue of origin. These include masses of fat origin (lipoma and liposarcoma), muscle origin (rhabdomyosarcoma, leiomyosarcoma, and metastases), osseous origin (osteochondroma, fibrous dysplasia, aneurysmal bone cyst, giant cell tumor, osteosarcoma, plasmacytoma, and metastases), neurogenic origin (nerve sheath tumor and its malignant counterparts), vascular origin (hemangioma and angiosarcoma), and mixed tissue origin (elastofibroma dorsi, desmoid tumor, undifferentiated pleomorphic sarcoma (formerly malignant fibrous histiocytomas), Ewing sarcoma, and synovial cell sarcoma). Fluid collections of the chest wall may be diffuse or mimic a mass, including hematoma, infection, and edema. Congenital lesions other than masses usually manifest as absence of normal structures (such as with Poland syndrome) or with anomalies of innervation that may result in asymmetric musculature or a winged scapula (Fig. 95.1).

A variety of diaphramatic conditions manifest as thoracic imaging abnormalities and can be categorized as masses, defects, and anomalies of function. Masses of the diaphragm are rare, and are typically pleural metastases that invade the diaphragm (see Chapter 32). Rarely, a primary tumor of the diaphragm may arise (usually a

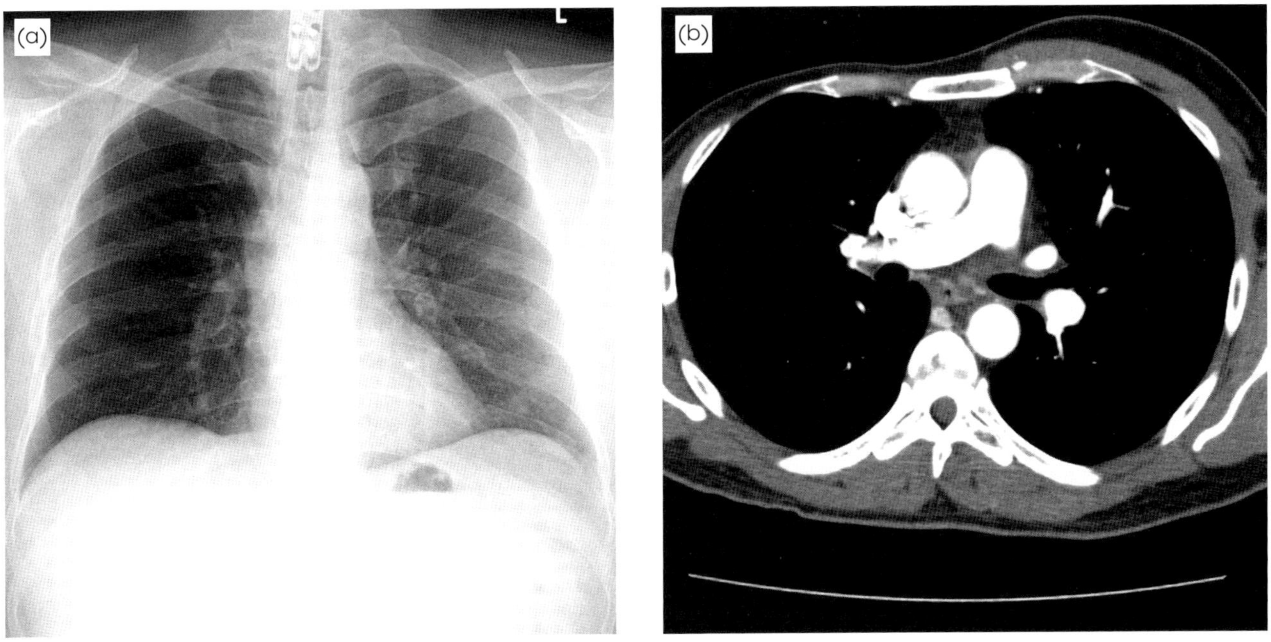

Figure 95.1. Poland syndrome. (a) Posteroanterior chest radiograph of a 25-year-old man with congenital absence of the right pectoralis muscles (Poland syndrome) shows a hyperlucent right lung with symmetric bilateral lung volumes and vascularity. (b) Contrast-enhanced chest CT of the same patient shows absence of the right musculature, which is diagnostic of Poland syndrome.

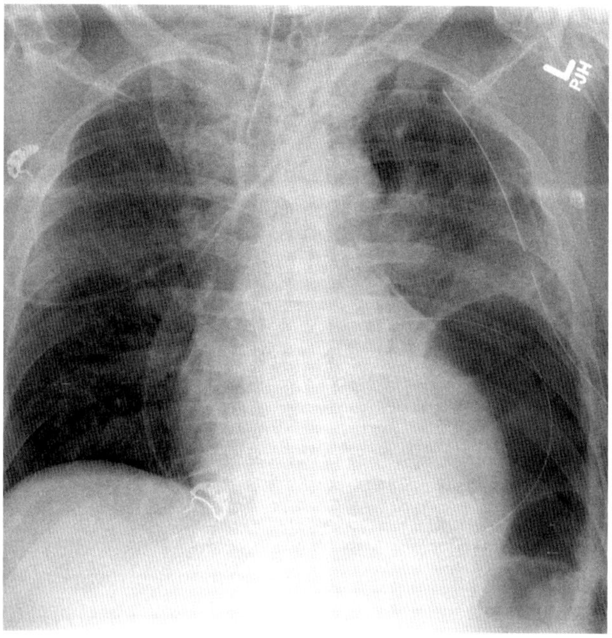

Figure 95.2. Traumatic diaphragmatic hernia or rupture. Anteroposterior portable chest radiograph of a 28-year-old woman involved in a motor vehicle accident shows apparent elevation of the left hemidiaphragm with an unusual location of the nasogastric tube, a medial left pneumothorax, and subcutaneous gas typical of diaphragmatic rupture.

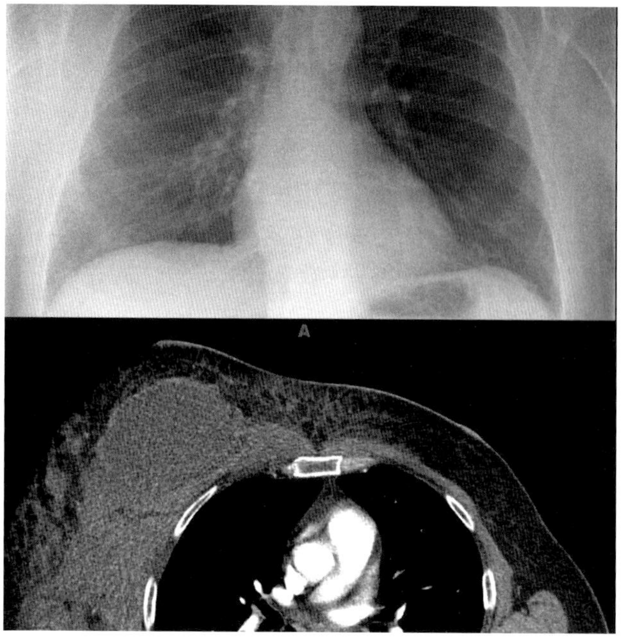

Figure 95.3. Chest wall hematoma. Composite image with anteroposterior chest radiograph (top) and contrast-enhanced chest CT (bottom) of a 45-year-old man with right chest pain shows increased opacity of the right hemithorax (top) compared to the left secondary to a large right anterior chest wall hematoma.

sarcoma). Defects of the diaphragm are far more common. Their significance depends on location. Hiatal hernias are frequent and occur centrally at the level of the esophageal hiatus. Morgagni hernias occur anteriorly and usually on the right, and may mimic anterior fat-containing mediastinal masses. The diagnosis is confirmed by documenting intrathoracic extension of abdominal vessels and organs through the defect. Bochdalek hernias occur posteriorly and often result in herniation of retroperitoneal fat, but sometimes kidney or bowel, into the chest. Far more concerning is post-traumatic diaphragmatic rupture, which typically occurs on the left (Fig. 95.2). These lesions have a high risk of infarction of herniated bowel and are usually surgically corrected. Focal muscular diaphragmatic thinning resulting in a wide contour bulge, known as eventration, is commonly encountered, typically as an incidental finding. When the entire hemidiaphragm is elevated, concern must be raised regarding ipsilateral phrenic nerve paralysis. A subpulmonic effusion may mimic an elevated diaphragm. Helpful findings of a subpulmonic effusion on radiography include lateral displacement of the peak of the hemidiaphragm, increased distance from a bowel loop to the base of the aerated lung, and fluid tracking in the fissure (sometimes called the thorn sign).

Approach to Chest Wall and Diaphragmatic Disorders

The approach to the chest wall lesion will be guided by three main considerations: the patient's age, the acuity of the process, and the center of origin. Symptoms can also be helpful because infection, hematoma, and malignant lesions are more often associated with chest pain (Fig. 95.3). Younger patients (<20 years) are more likely to present with a primary chest wall mass. If the lesion is chronic and exhibits with phleboliths on imaging, hemangioma may be suspected and confirmed on cross-sectional imaging. Benign lesions include osteochondroma and fibrous dysplasia. More aggressive lesions include metastatic neuroblastoma, rhabdomyosarcoma, and Ewing sarcoma.

In patients aged 20–40 years, desmoid tumors are fairly common. These tend to mimic an enlarged muscle on CT but exhibit variable signal intensity on MRI. In patients of this age group, primary tumors of the chest wall may be as common as metastases, including sarcomas and benign lesions such as fibrous dysplasia. Occasionally, chest wall infection may mimic a mass. Although classically seen in tuberculous empyema with involvement of the adjacent chest wall (empyema necessitans), this finding may also be seen with other infections, most notably actinomycosis and nocardia.

In patients older than age 40 years, chest wall lesions must be assumed to be metastases or related to multiple myeloma until proven otherwise. Often, isolated lesions are biopsied because of their ease of access. One notable benign lesion in older patients is the elastofibroma dorsi. This benign, fibrofatty lesion is almost always encountered in the dorsal soft tissues between the inferior scapula and the posterior ribs. Knowledge of the classic imaging features of these lesions is important to avoid unnecessary surgery because they often show increased uptake on FDG PET.

Another lesion of note is the nerve sheath neoplasm (usually a schwannoma). These lesions are usually rounded or elliptical with low attenuation on CT and may exhibit increased uptake on FDG PET. MRI may show a characteristic high-T2 signal with targetoid enhancement.

The approach to diaphragmatic abnormalities should be based on the presence or absence of bilaterality of involvement, stability over time, and whether involvement is focal or diffuse. Bilateral diaphragmatic elevation is often indicative of a shallow inspiration or underlying ascites. When an elevated hemidiaphragm is seen on multiple imaging studies over time, phrenic nerve palsy becomes a concern. Paralysis must be differentiated from eventration. When the contour abnormality is focal, usually a hernia is present, although rarely a mass may account for the focal contour bulge. Although CT is often the next step, MRI with the newer sequences including real-time imaging has become a more commonly used problem-solving modality.

Suggested Reading

Nam SJ, Kim S, Lim BJ, Yoon CS, Kim TH, Suh JS, et al. Imaging of primary chest wall tumors with radiologic–pathologic correlation. *RadioGraphics*. 2011 May–Jun;31(3):749–770.

Nason LK, Walker CM, McNeeley MF, Burivong W, Fligner CL, Godwin JD. Imaging of the diaphragm: Anatomy and function. *RadioGraphics*. 2012 Mar–Apr;32(2):E51–E70.

CHAPTER 96

Chest Wall Abnormalities

Clinton E. Jokerst, Kristopher W. Cummings, and Andrew J. Bierhals

Definition

The chest wall consists of the thoracic cage and related supporting tissues. The thoracic cage is made up of the ribs, sternum, costal cartilages, and thoracic vertebral bodies. It is supported by chest wall musculature, fascia, and subcutaneous tissues and is bounded externally by the skin, internally by the pleura, and inferiorly by the diaphragm. The chest wall is predominantly composed of bone, muscle, and fat. Aberrations in these tissues constitute most chest wall abnormalities. The chest wall also contains nerves, lymph nodes, blood vessels, and breast tissue, all of which can give rise to chest wall lesions.

Clinical Features

Chest wall abnormalities may manifest as either masses or absence of normal tissues or structures. Such abnormalities may be evident on visual inspection or physical exam. The chest wall is plastic and able to expand to ensure normal respiration. Conditions that affect the plasticity of the chest wall can lead to difficulty breathing and may manifest as restrictive patterns on incentive spirometry. Because of the constant motion of the chest wall and relatively high density of nerves, many chest wall lesions cause pain. Given the high incidence of symptoms, many chest wall lesions are found by the patient rather than discovered incidentally on imaging.

Anatomy and Physiology

The chest wall is a symmetric space. Evaluation of unilateral abnormalities is aided by comparison to the contralateral side. The chest wall has both structural and functional roles. Structurally, it protects vital organs such as the heart, lungs, and liver. It also provides a flexible skeletal framework for the upper extremities. To meet these structural demands, the chest wall must have some rigidity. The chest wall must also be flexible because its expansion plays a vital role in respiration.

The thoracic cage is primarily made up of 12 paired ribs. Running under each rib is an intercostal nerve accompanied by an intercostal artery and vein. The location of the intercostal artery beneath the rib accounts for the inferior rib notching seen in patients with aortic coarctation and enlarged intercostal collaterals. The course of the intercostal nerve accounts for the horizontal orientation of chest wall schwannomas that arise from these nerves. Contrast this to the craniocaudal orientation of ganglioneuromas that arise from the sympathetic trunk, a vertically oriented structure that runs along the lateral margins of the vertebral bodies. Costal cartilage is located anteriorly spanning the gap between the ribs and sternum, which explains why most chondral lesions arise in the anterior chest wall (Fig. 96.1). Chest wall lesions that extend into the thoracic cavity may exhibit the incomplete border sign on chest radiography. This sign is helpful in distinguishing intrapulmonary versus extrapulmonary masses.

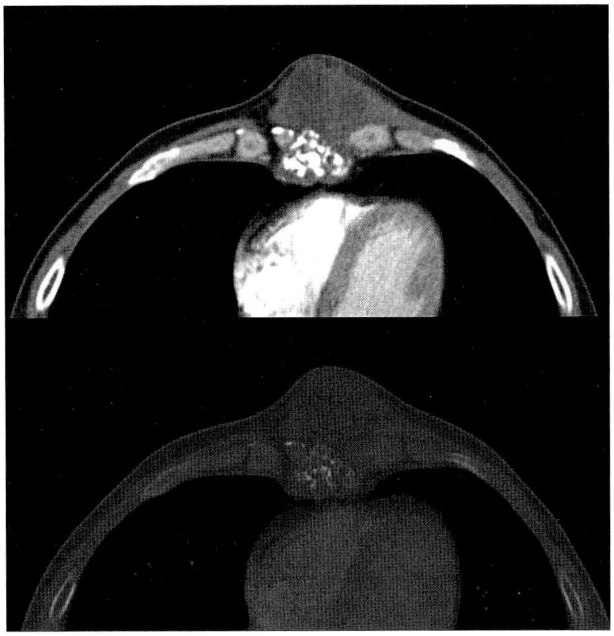

Figure 96.1. Chondrosarcoma. Composite image with contrast-enhanced chest CT in soft tissue (top) and bone (bottom) window of a 63-year-old man with a palpable chest wall chondrosarcoma shows a sternal mass with a large soft tissue component and a characteristic pattern of "rings and arcs" calcification, likely arising from costal cartilage.

How to Approach the Image

When faced with a chest wall abnormality, there are two decision points that the radiologist can navigate to narrow the differential diagnosis. The first is whether the process is bone/cartilage-centered or centered in the soft tissues.

Bone/cartilage-centered processes have their own unique differential diagnoses depending on associated imaging findings. The second is whether the process is mass-like/neoplastic, stems from an absence or malformation of normal structures, or is *other* such as trauma. Once these decision points have been addressed, additional factors such as clinical history and demographic information can be used to further narrow the differential diagnosis.

What Not to Miss

Because chest wall masses are usually easily palpated, it is incumbent upon the radiologist to ensure that any mass felt by the patient or physician be adequately imaged. The use of radiopaque marker for CT (usually a metallic pellet) or a vitamin E capsule can ensure that the mass felt on exam is covered by the diagnostic study. This often allows for detection of the process that can be subtle and easily overlooked. It is also key that the radiologist not misdiagnose a tumefactive process such as a hematoma or infection as a mass. One such infection is empyema necessitans, in which the pleural infection invades chest wall. This process can be seen with empyema secondary to tuberculosis, actinomycosis, and nocardiosis. An understanding of the time course is key because these latter conditions tend to develop rapidly.

Differential Diagnosis

Bone/Cartilage-Centered Lesions

Neoplastic

- Metastases: Most common malignant chest wall neoplasm.
- Chondrosarcoma: Usually affects the elderly; commonly involves costal cartilage/anterior chest wall.
- Osteosarcoma: Usually affects younger patients (unless related to prior radiation therapy) (Fig. 96.2); rare.
- Plasmacytoma and multiple myeloma: A plasmacytoma is a plasma cell neoplasm that may arise in the soft tissues or bone. Myeloma refers to a more systemic plasma cell neoplastic process that is usually multiple and less well-defined. Both may present in the chest wall.
- Ewing sarcoma family of tumors: Most common chest wall sarcomas in children and young adults.
- Fibrous dysplasia: Common benign osseous chest wall lesion (Fig. 96.3).

Malformations/Absent Tissue

- Pectus deformities: Pectus excavatum is approximately four times more common than pectus carinatum; pectus excavatum is more common in male patients. Both have an association with Marfan syndrome.
- Clagett window: For refractory empyema; window created in chest wall to allow for continuous drainage of pleural space.

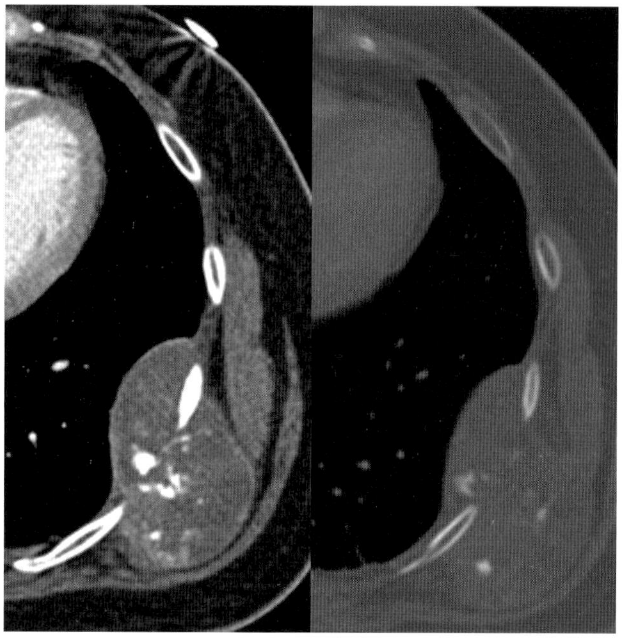

Figure 96.2. Osteosarcoma. Contrast-enhanced CT in a 63-year-old woman with a left osteosarcoma. The lesion is centered in the chest wall of the posterolateral hemithorax. The bone windows show an osseous matrix, in keeping with the diagnosis.

Other

- Flail chest: At least three contiguous ribs fractured in two or more separate locations; flail segment moves paradoxically during respiration.

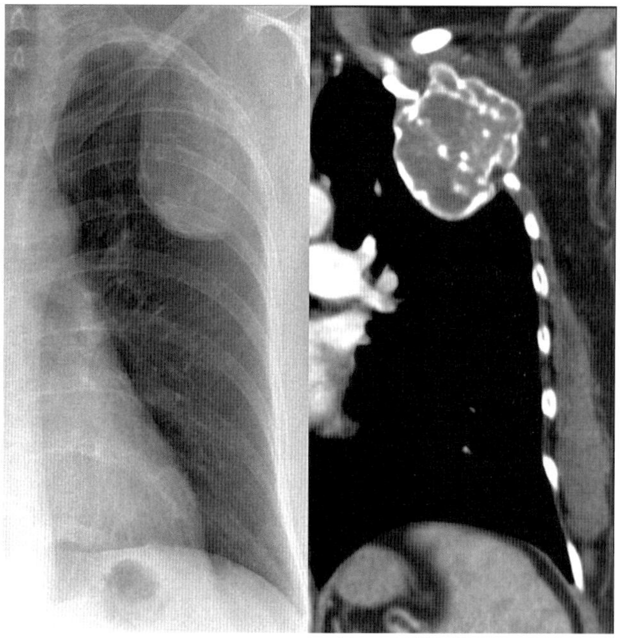

Figure 96.3. Fibrous dysplasia. Composite image with posteroanterior (PA) chest radiograph (left) and coronal contrast-enhanced chest CT (right) of a 39-year-old woman with chest discomfort shows a left chest wall mass that exhibits the incomplete border sign consistent with an extrapulmonary location, expands the second rib, and contains coarse calcifications. CT demonstrates an expansile left second rib mass with intrinsic ground-glass matrix consistent with fibrous dysplasia.

- Sternoclavicular dislocation: Anterior more common; dislocation more often associated with vascular injury.
- Sternal dehiscence: Look for malaligned sternal wires.

Soft Tissue-Centered Lesions

Neoplastic

- Breast cancer: Aside from nonmelanoma skin cancer, it is the most common cancer in women; it is 100 times less common in men.
- Lipoma: Most common benign chest wall neoplasm.
- Soft tissue sarcomas: Heterogeneous group of tumors; often affects middle-aged subjects; can be associated with prior radiation.
- Nerve sheath tumors: Common in type 1 neurofibromatosis.
- Desmoid: Young patients; locally aggressive fibroblast tumor (Fig. 96.4).
- Elastofibroma dorsi: Soft tissue nonenoplastic mass more common in women; classic location medial to the inferior scapula.
- Hemangioma/lymphangioma: Benign and more commonly seen in younger patients, especially infants.

Malformations/Absent Tissue

- Mastectomy: Radical mastectomy involves removing the pectoralis muscles; modified radical mastectomy spares the pectoralis muscles.
- Poland syndrome: Congenital unilateral absence of the pectoralis muscles; rarely associated with ipsilateral limb anomalies.

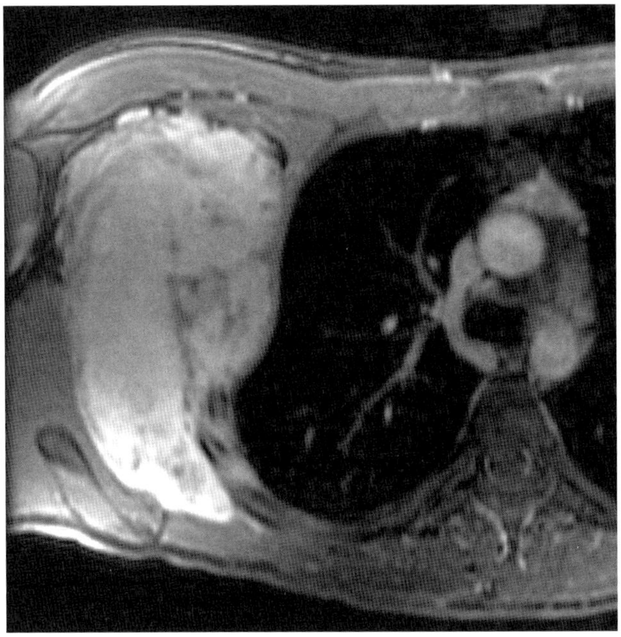

Figure 96.4. Desmoid. Contrast-enhanced T1-weighted MR image of a 20-year- old weightlifter with a chest wall mass extending into the right axilla which was resected; pathology demonstrated fibromatosis consistent with a desmoid tumor

Imaging Findings

Metastases

- Multiple masses; may be osteolytic, osteoblastic, or mixed lesions (depends on primary tumor)

Chondrosarcoma

- Slowly growing anterior chest wall mass that usually originates in the anterior cartilage
- Peripheral “rings and arcs” pattern of calcification characteristic of chondroid matrix

Osteosarcoma

- Usually manifests as a painful chest wall tumor in younger patients or those with a history of prior radiation therapy
- Central dense calcification typical of osseous matrix
- May have fluid–fluid levels on CT or MR

Plasmacytoma/Myeloma

- Expansile, lytic lesion in patients older than age 40 years
- May be solitary (plasmacytoma) or multifocal (myeloma)

Ewing Sarcoma Family of Tumors

- Includes primitive neuroectodermal tumors and Askin tumors
- Permeative, noncalcified invasive mass that can be centered in bone or in soft tissues; nonspecific appearance

Fibrous Dysplasia

- Expansile lesion with peripheral trabeculation and internal “ground-glass” matrix optimally evaluated with CT; may be monostotic or polyostotic

Pectus Deformities

- Pectus excavatum: Consists of a sunken sternum, Haller index greater than 2.5 (>3.25 considered severe) (Figs. 96.5 and 96.6)
- Pectus carinatum: Consists of protuberance of the sternum, Haller index usually less than 2.5 (Fig. 96.7)

Breast Cancer

- Primary tumor better evaluated with combination of mammography, ultrasound, and sometimes MRI
- CT for evaluation of associated lymphadenopathy, especially involving internal mammary lymph nodes

Lipoma

- Encapsulated fat
- Presence of significant soft tissue component worrisome for possible liposarcoma

Soft Tissue Sarcomas

- Large soft tissue mass without calcifications, often a large amount of central necrosis

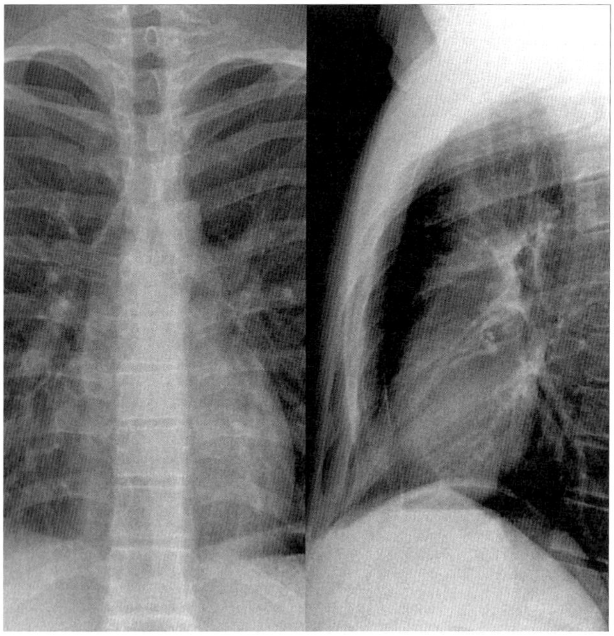

Figure 96.5. Pectus excavatum. Composite image with PA (left) and lateral (right) chest radiographs of a 16-year-old boy with pectus excavatum shows an indistinct right heart border on the PA chest radiograph and posterior displacement of the inferior sternum on the lateral radiograph.

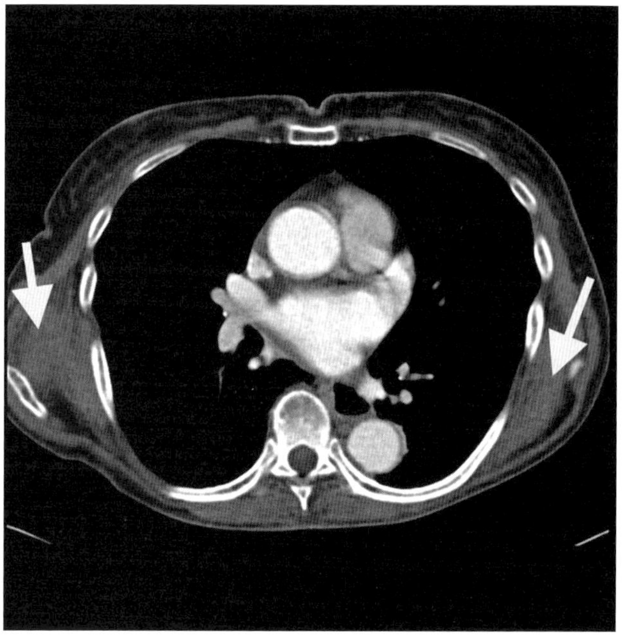

Figure 96.7. Contrast-enhanced chest CT of a 26-year-old woman with a palpable right chest wall "lump" shows bilateral masses (arrows) located under the inferior aspects of the scapulae with admixed muscle and fascicular fat pathognomonic of elastofibroma dorsi. This can be overlooked due to its frequent symmetry.

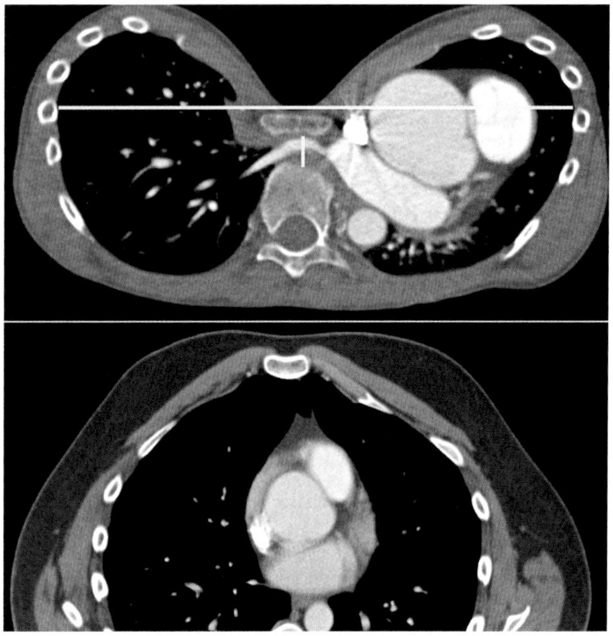

Figure 96.6. Composite image of Pectus excavatum and carinatum. Contrast-enhanced CT of a 14-year-old boy above with Loeys–Dietz syndrome and severe pectus excavatum ("funnel chest"). Note the large ascending aortic aneurysm. Haller index is the ratio of the lateral thoracic dimension to the minimum anteroposterior thoracic dimension, indicated by the blue lines on this patient's CT. A Haller index greater than 3.25 is considered severe; this patient's index is approximately 15, consistent with a very severe pectus excavatum. Contrast-enhanced CT of a 26-year-old man (bottom) with Marfan Syndrome demonstrates pectus carinatum ("pigeon chest").

- Pleomorphic undifferentiated sarcoma (formerly malignant fibrous histiocytoma) is most common subtype; also the most common radiation-induced sarcoma
- Liposarcoma often identifiable due to presence of fat in addition to soft tissue; increasing proportion of soft tissue:fat correlates with increasing tumor grade

Desmoid/Fibromatosis

- Large chest wall tumor that often arises in sites of prior injury/scar in younger patients
- Ill-defined margins and heterogeneous enhancement
- Often mimics skeletal muscle on CT but easily discernible on MRI with increased T2 signal and enhancement on T1 images

Elastofibroma Dorsi

- Often bilateral, characteristic location under distal scapula
- Usually low in attenuation on CT with alternating layers of fat and fibrous soft tissue; these layers better seen on MRI (Fig. 96.7)

Clinical Issues

- Chest wall sarcomas are often locally invasive and can be quite large at the time of presentation. The treatment of choice is complete excision, which can be

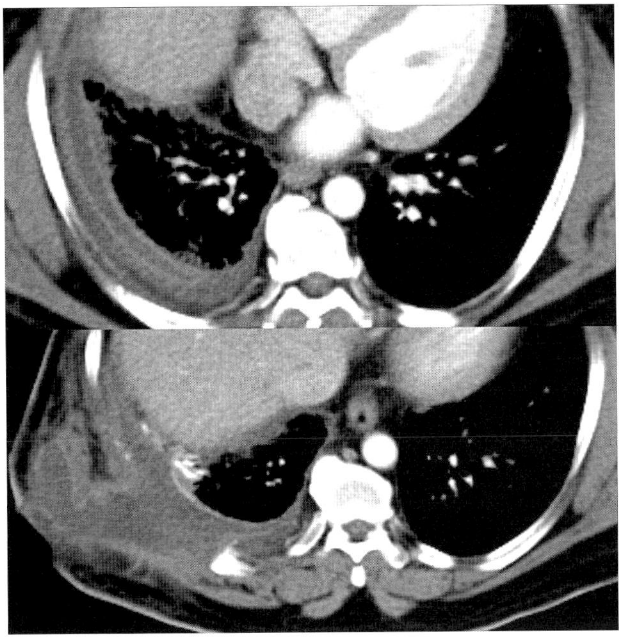

Figure 96.8. Contrast-enhanced chest CT of a 42-year-old man with fever and malaise shows a right empyema manifesting as a loculated pleural effusion with enhancement of the pleural surfaces and involvement of the adjacent chest wall consistent with empyema necessitans.

difficult with larger tumors. Adjuvant chemotherapy and/or radiation therapy may be necessary.

- Some benign chest wall lesions may warrant excision. Fibromatosis/desmoids are often locally invasive and require complete excision to prevent local recurrence. Some benign tumors may be excised for cosmetic reasons or because they bother the patient/interfere with chest wall or extremity function.
- Pectus deformities are often repaired for cosmetic reasons; however, in some instances, pectus excavatum is severe enough to interfere with cardiac or respiratory function. Pectus carinatum is almost never associated with cardiopulmonary dysfunction. In addition, the radiologist must look for findings such as aortic root dilatation and dural ectasia that might point to an underlying connective tissue disorder.

Key Points

- Characterization of a chest wall abnormality as a bone/cartilage-centered process or a soft tissue-centered process together with knowledge of clinical and demographic information allows the formulation of a focused differential diagnosis and guides further imaging.
- In general, CT is the imaging modality of choice for bone-centered lesions because of its excellent spatial resolution and ability to characterize calcifications/matrix.
- CT is also the modality of choice when evaluating chest wall trauma due to its availability, spatial resolution, and speed. In addition to superior characterization of osseous injuries such as fractures and dislocations, CT is excellent for demonstrating associated vascular and pulmonary injuries and pleural processes (Fig. 96.8).
- In general, MRI is the imaging modality of choice for soft tissue-centered lesions because of its superior soft tissue characterization and ability to demonstrate invasion of adjacent structures such as nerves, spinal canal, and vessels.
- MRI can also be helpful when evaluating chest wall infections. Its ability to demonstrate marrow edema makes it sensitive for osteomyelitis, and the addition of contrast allows for subtraction imaging, which can show the extent of devascularized bone.
- The chest wall has both functional and structural roles, and it is important to remember that chest wall abnormalities may interfere with either or both of these.

Suggested Reading

Nam SF, Kim S, Lim BF, et al. Imaging of primary chest wall tumors with radiologic–pathologic correlation. *RadioGraphics*. 2011;31:749–770.

Tateishi U, Gladish GW, Kusumoto M, et al. Chest wall tumors: Radiologic findings and pathologic correlation: Part 1. Benign tumors. *RadioGraphics*. 2003;23:1477–1490.

Tateishi U, Gladish GW, Kusumoto M, et al. Chest wall tumors: Radiologic findings and pathologic correlation: Part 2. Malignant tumors. *RadioGraphics*. 2003;23:1491–1508.

CHAPTER 97

Diaphragmatic Abnormalities

Nadeem Parkar and Andrew J. Bierhals

Definition

The diaphragm is the primary muscle of respiration and a physical barrier that separates the thorax from the abdomen. It consists of peripheral muscle fibers that originate from the entire circumference of the lower thoracic inlet and converge into a central tendon.

Clinical Features

Diaphragm dysfunction is an underappreciated cause of dyspnea due to a variety of entities, including tumor, trauma, surgery, and infection. Diaphragmatic paralysis is the absence of craniocaudal excursion on quiet and deep breathing, and paradoxical motion on sniffing. Diaphragmatic weakness is reduced or delayed excursion on deep breathing with or without paradoxical motion on sniffing. Eventration is congenital thinning of a segment of diaphragmatic muscle and is typically asymptomatic. The most common causes of unilateral diaphragmatic paralysis are phrenic nerve compression or invasion by neoplasm (Fig. 97.1) and phrenic nerve injury from prior surgery. Diaphragmatic injuries occur in 0.8–8% of patients with blunt abdominal trauma, and they may be missed due to being clinically silent or overshadowed by associated injuries.

Anatomy and Physiology

The diaphragm develops during weeks 4–12 of embryogenesis and has four components: the transverse septum, which becomes the central tendon; the pleuroperitoneal folds; the esophageal mesentery; and the muscular body wall. Defective fusion of the transverse septum to the lateral body wall leads to Morgagni hernia (10% of congenital diaphragmatic hernias (CDH)). It occurs more frequently on the right and usually affects the anteromedial right hemidiaphragm. Posterior (Bochdalek) hernias constitute 90% of CDH and are more common on the left. They can be

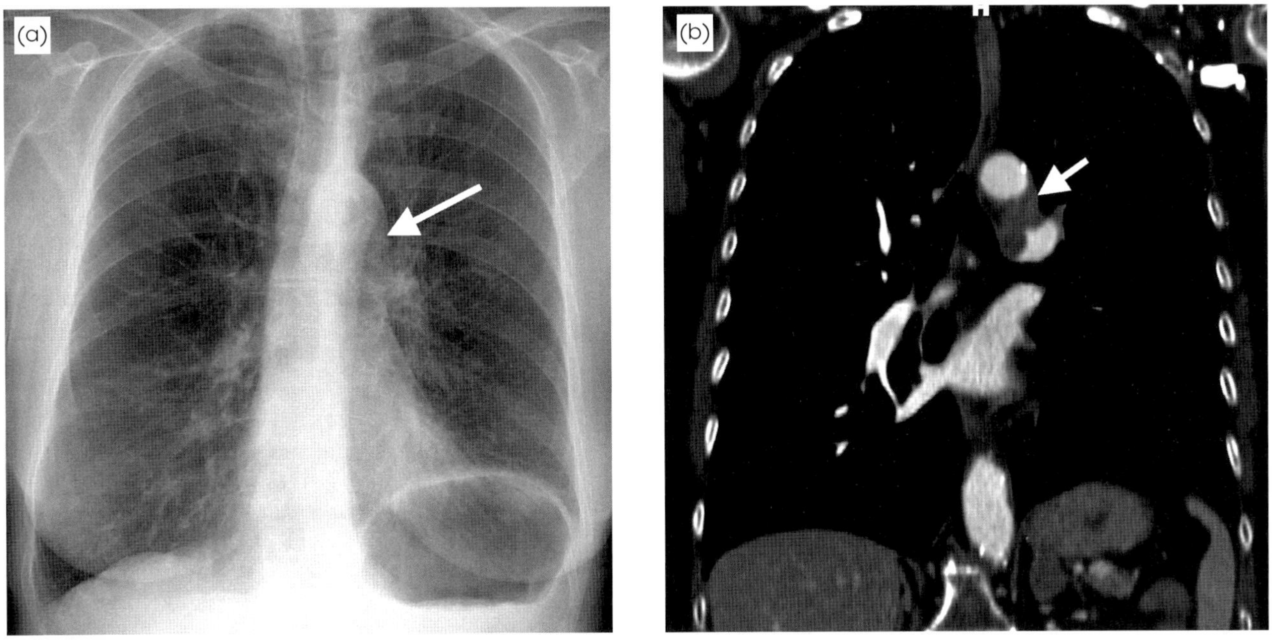

Figure 97.1. Elevated left hemidiaphragm from phrenic nerve invasion by lymphadenopathy. (a) Posteroanterior (PA) chest radiograph shows an elevated left hemidiaphragm. Note the convex bulge in the aortopulmonary window (arrow). (b) Subsequent CT confirmed a soft tissue mass in this region (arrow), which was found to represent nodal metastasis.

seen in neonates, who tend to be symptomatic, and as an incidental finding in older patients being scanned for other reasons. In neonates, it represents a developmental defect of the pleuroperitoneal folds or failure of fusion of the folds and transverse septum with the intercostal muscles. This defect can result in symptomatic herniation of bowel. In older patients, a remnant of the pleuroperitoneal canal may reopen or become larger and result in asymptomatic herniation of fat.

The diaphragm is innervated by the right and left phrenic nerves, which originate from the cervical nerves C3–C5. The right phrenic nerve runs lateral to the right brachiocephalic vein and superior vena cava. The left phrenic nerve runs along the lateral aspect of the aortic arch. Both phrenic nerves then course anterior to the hila and continue inferiorly along the pericardium.

Three main diaphragmatic hiatuses allow normal structures to course between the thorax and the abdomen. The inferior vena cava (IVC) hiatus in the midportion of the central tendon contains the IVC and right phrenic nerve branches. The esophageal hiatus passes through the right diaphragmatic crus and contains the esophagus, vagus nerve, and sympathetic nerve branches. The aortic hiatus contains the aorta, thoracic duct, and azygous and hemiazygous veins.

Eventration refers to congenital thinning of the muscle, which may be seen as a focal wide-mouthed bulge. It may become more pronounced with increasing intra-abdominal pressure, usually as a result of abdominal obesity.

How to Approach the Image

The right hemidiaphragm is normally slightly higher than the left. A diaphragmatic abnormality may be suggested by hemidiaphragm elevation on radiography. The shape of diaphragmatic elevation is important in suggesting the correct diagnosis. Elevation of both hemidiaphragms is usually due to shallow inspiration, but it can also be due to ascites or peritoneal mass effect. Unilateral hemidiaphragm elevation may be due to phrenic nerve malfunction from prior injury or neoplastic invasion. Focal elevation with a broad neck is usually due to eventration. When the neck is narrow, a hernia must be considered. The anatomic location of the herniation allows characterization as Morgagni, Bochdalek, or post-traumatic hernia. The latter is often confirmed by the presence of other imaging findings of trauma.

What Not to Miss

Pleural masses and mediastinal masses (especially anterior mediastinal masses) can mimic an elevated diaphragm or hernia on a frontal radiograph. Ideally, one would have a two-view radiograph to distinguish the diaphragmatic process from the other masses. Visualization of bowel near the abnormal contour can be very helpful in confirming the diaphragmatic abnormality. A subpulmonic effusion can also mimic an elevated hemidiaphragm. An effusion may displace the diaphragmatic peak laterally. A secondary view (e.g., a decubitus radiograph) might be helpful to confirm an effusion.

Diaphragmatic injuries may be easily overlooked post trauma. An elevated hemidiaphragm in the setting of trauma should raise the suspicion of a diaphragmatic injury. In the setting of trauma, care must be taken to prevent confusion with a subplumonic pleural effusion or hemothorax.

Differential Diagnosis

Diaphragmatic Paralysis from Phrenic Nerve Invasion or Injury

- Tumor invading the phrenic nerve from direct extension
  - Metastatic disease from primary lung cancer
  - Primary phrenic nerve tumors rare but may be seen in neurofibromatosis
- Injury following cardiac surgery in up to 20% of cases (Fig. 97.1)

Traumatic Diaphragmatic Rupture

- More common on the left side than the right, probably because of the protective effects of the liver and easier identification of left-sided injuries on imaging (Fig. 97.2)

Congenital Diaphragmatic Hernia

- Bochdalek hernia is the most common diaphragmatic hernia in adults (97.3).
- Morgagni hernia is a rare congenital diaphragmatic defect (Fig. 97.4).

Eventration

Hiatus Hernia

- Herniation of the stomach through the esophageal hiatus due to stretching, weakening, or tearing of the phrenoesophageal membrane that decreases the stability of the gastroesophageal (GE) junction and allows upward displacement of the esophagus and stomach (Fig. 97.5).
- Sliding hiatus hernia is more common and is characterized by the location of the GE junction above the hiatus.
- Paraesophageal hiatus hernia is characterized by herniation of all or part of the stomach alongside the esophagus and a normally located GE junction.

Hemidiaphragmatic Inversion from Large Pleural Effusion

- Unusual complication of large pleural effusion.

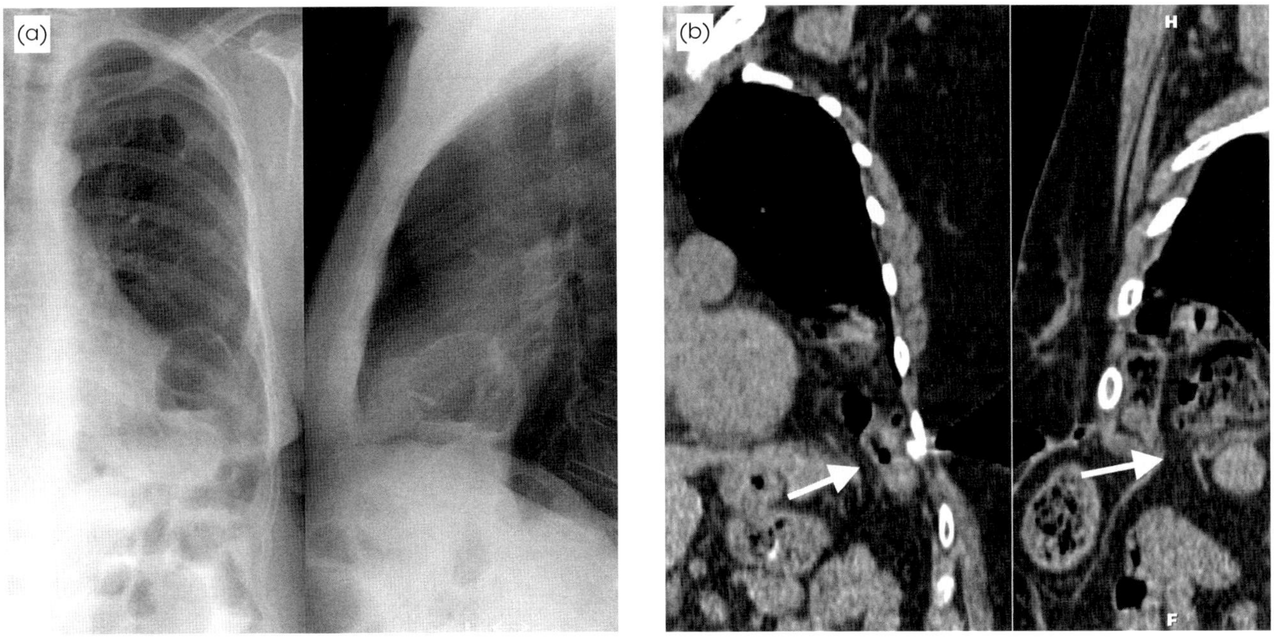

Figure 97.2. Traumatic diaphragm rupture. (a) Composite image with PA (left) and lateral (right) chest radiographs shows an intrathoracic bowel loop with an air-fluid level. (b) Composite image with coronal (left) and sagittal (right) chest CT shows a diaphragmatic defect and herniated bowel. Note the collar sign.

- Hemidiaphragms move in opposite directions during respiration with gas moving from one lung to another (Pendelluft respiration).
- Both ventilation and perfusion are diminished on the affected side due to the increased dead space and tension on the pulmonary vasculature.

Imaging Findings

Diaphragmatic Paralysis from Phrenic Nerve Invasion or Injury

- Radiography
  - Diaphragmatic elevation

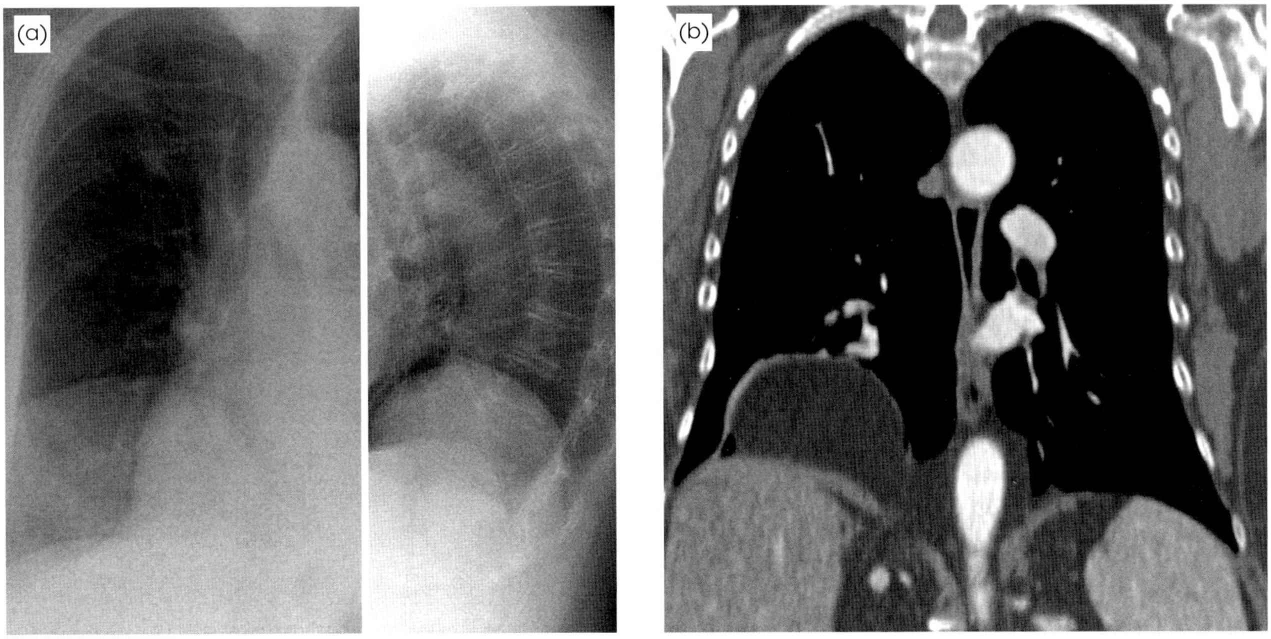

Figure 97.3. Bochdalek hernia. (a) Composite image with PA (left) and lateral (right) chest radiographs shows a rounded mass along the posterior right hemidiaphragm. (b) Contrast-enhanced coronal chest CT shows a fat-containing Bochdalek hernia.

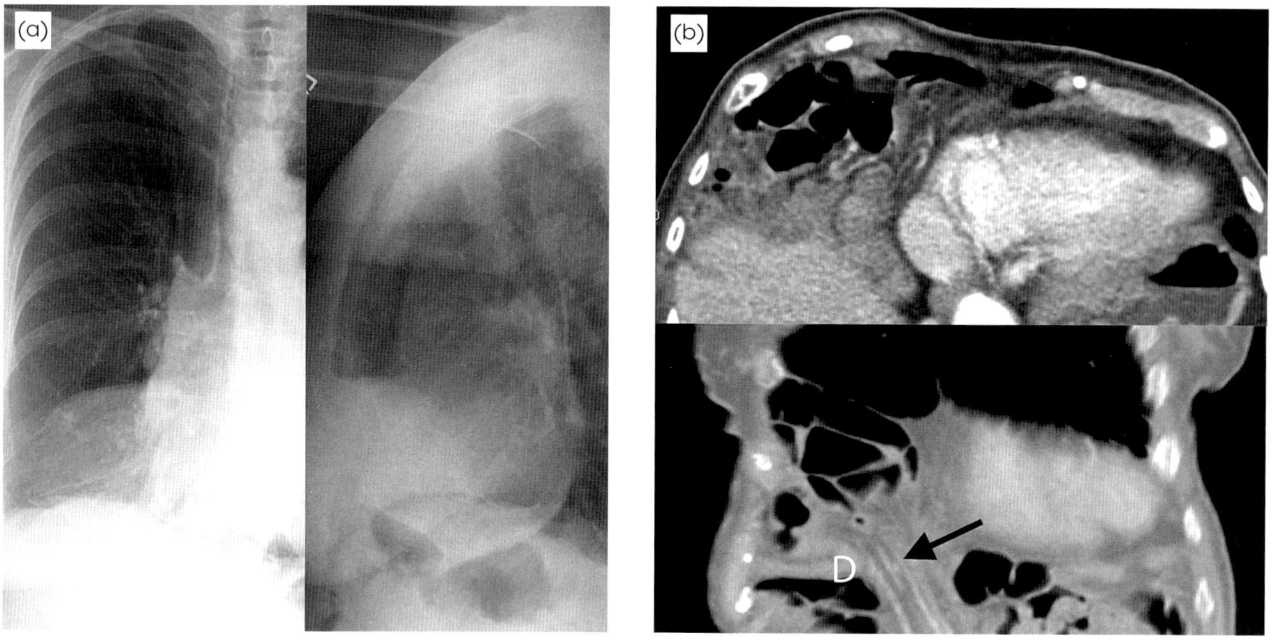

Figure 97.4. Morgagni hernia. (a) Composite image with PA (left) and lateral (right) chest radiographs shows a right cardiophrenic angle mass that is somewhat lucent. (b) Composite image with axial (top) and coronal (bottom) chest CT performed a few years later shows herniated bowel and vessels (arrow) traversing the diaphragmatic defect. Note the diaphragm edge (D).

- Ipsilateral hilar/mediastinal lymphadenopathy or lung mass
- CT
  - Confirmation of hilar/mediastinal lymphadenopathy or lung mass
  - Hemidiaphragm elevation best evaluated on coronal reformatted images or the topogram
- Fluoroscopy
  - Functional imaging for diagnosing diaphragmatic dysfunction.

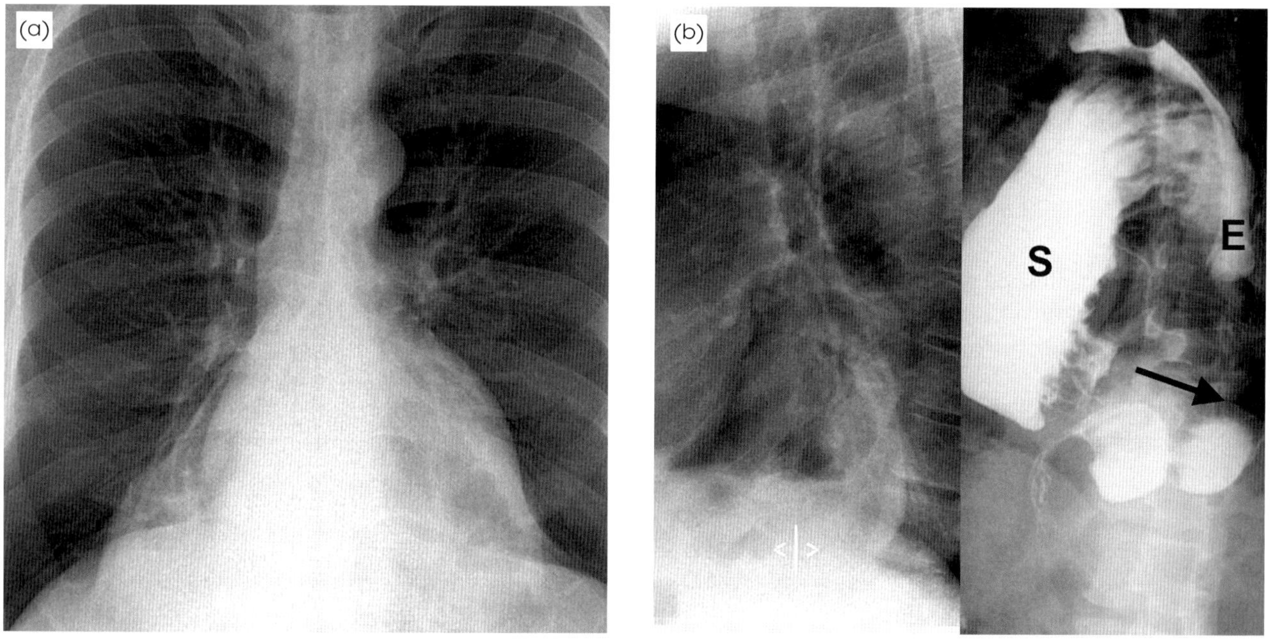

Figure 97.5. Large hiatus hernia in a 70-year-old man. (a) Frontal radiograph shows a mass overlying the heart, with internal lucency indicative of bowel. (b) Composite image with a lateral radiograph (left) and oblique from an upper gastrointestinal series (right) shows that the mass corresponds to a large hiatus hernia. The stomach (S) is rotated so that the greater curvature is above the lesser curvature. The esophagus (E) and relationship with the diaphragm (arrow) are also seen.

- Absence of craniocaudal excursion on quiet and deep breathing and paradoxical motion on sniffing.
- Reduced or delayed excursion on deep breathing with or without paradoxical motion on sniffing indicates diaphragmatic weakness
- MRI
  - Increasingly used for evaluation of diaphragmatic function
  - Real-time images allow for assessment of function with deep inspiration and rapid sniffing; features similar to those of the fluoroscopy, but adjacent organs (e.g., liver) are seen

Traumatic Diaphragmatic Rupture
- Radiography
  - Often subtle and nonspecific findings
  - Apparent hemidiaphragm elevation with elevated gastric bubble
  - Rarely, a focal contour bulge
- CT
  - Sensitivity of 71–90% and specificity of 98–100% for the detection of traumatic rupture on multidetector CT assisted by multiplanar reformatted images

Direct CT Signs
- Segmental diaphragmatic defect sign: Focal and abrupt loss of diaphragmatic continuity; free edge of the disrupted diaphragm demarcates the defect and may appear thickened because of muscle retraction or hemorrhage
- Dangling diaphragm sign: Free edge of torn diaphragm curls inward from its normal course toward the center of the body, forming a curvilinear structure at a near right angle to the chest wall
- Absent diaphragm sign: Absence of a part of the hemidiaphragm in areas where the diaphragm is expected to be well demonstrated (where it is outlined by air or fat)

Indirect CT Signs Related to Herniation
- Herniation through a defect sign: Abdominal organs or peritoneal fat passing into the pleural space
- Collar sign: Waist-like constriction of the herniated structure at the site of the diaphragmatic rupture, especially with liver herniation on the right side
- Dependent viscera sign: Direct contact between herniated abdominal organs and the posterior chest wall without interposed lung

Congenital Diaphragmatic Hernia
- Bochdalek hernia: Discontinuity of posterior diaphragm with protrusion of peritoneal or retroperitoneal fat and, less commonly, bowel or solid organs through the defect into the thoracic cavity producing focal posterior bulge on radiography and confirmed on chest CT
- Morgagni hernia: Soft tissue mass, typically in the right cardiophrenic angle, that may contain bowel. Detection of displaced curvilinear omental vessels within the lesion or coursing across the diaphragmatic defect is diagnostic and best seen on reformatted CT images or MRI

Eventration
- Radiography: Elevation of a portion of the radiograph while the remaining portion is of normal height
- CT: Sharp transition at the edge of the eventration
- Often better seen on coronal or sagittal reconstructions

Hiatal Hernia
- Radiography
  - Variable size of herniated portion of stomach
  - Gastric bubble demonstrated above the diaphragm on frontal view and posterior to the heart on lateral view
  - Middle mediastinal mass that produces lateral displacement of the inferior third of the azygoesophageal recess on frontal chest radiographs
  - Visualization of gastric air–fluid level on frontal or lateral radiographs
- Esophagram
  - Characterization of sliding and paraesophageal hernias
  - B ring demarcates the GE junction, which is above the diaphragm in the sliding hernia and below the diaphragm in the paraesophageal hernia
- CT and MRI
  - Gastric folds passing through esophageal hiatus
  - Evaluation of complications, including volvulus

Inverted Hemidiaphragm from Large Pleural Effusion
- Radiography
  - Best appreciated on the left; opaque left hemithorax with displacement of stomach and splenic flexure inferiorly on frontal radiograph and anteriorly on lateral
- CT
  - Altered relationship of pleural effusion and peritoneal space with the pleural effusion now being central to the peritoneal contents
  - Often better seen on coronal or sagittal reconstructions

Clinical Issues
- The presence of phrenic nerve invasion changes the T status of lung cancer staging.

- Blunt diaphragmatic rupture requires prompt surgical management due to the increased risk of strangulation of the herniated viscera.
- Elevated abdominal pressures force abdominal organs into the pleural space through diaphragmatic defect.
- Positive pressure ventilation may mask blunt diaphragmatic rupture by reducing the pleural pressure gradient and preventing herniation.
- Treatment of diaphragmatic paralysis depends on the cause of the dysfunction and the severity of the symptoms. Plication and phrenic nerve stimulation are options.
- Differentiation between sliding and paraesophageal hiatus hernias is important due to a higher risk of gastric volvulus in the latter.
- Pleural effusions resulting in hemidiaphragm inversion require urgent drainage because they can cause profound dyspnea.

Key Points

- Phrenic nerve invasion by tumor may occur anywhere along the course of the nerve and produce diaphragmatic paralysis.
- Phrenic nerve invasion by tumor impacts lung cancer staging.
- Phrenic nerve injury during surgery may also produce paralysis.
- The prospective diagnosis of traumatic diaphragmatic injury requires a high index of suspicion in every case of thoracoabdominal trauma with hemidiaphragmatic elevation and knowledge of the direct and indirect signs of diaphragmatic rupture.
- Blunt diaphragmatic injury is more common on the left.
- A location-based approach to congenital diaphragmatic defects allows distinction among Morgagni (anteromedial), Bochdalek (posterolateral), and hiatus (central) hernias.
- Diaphragmatic inversion is an unusual complication of large pleural effusion resulting in diaphragmatic dysfunction that impairs respiration.

Suggested Reading

Bhalla SB, Javidan CN, Cummings KW, Bierhals AB. *Chest imaging cases*. New York, NY: Oxford University Press; 2012.

Celli BR. Respiratory management of diaphragm paralysis. *Semin Respir Crit Care Med.* 2002;23:275–280.

Desir A, Ghaye B. CT of blunt diaphragmatic rupture. *RadioGraphics.* 2012;32:477–498.

Dorffner R, Eibenberger K, Youssefzadeh S, et al. Diaphragmatic dysfunction after heart or lung transplantation. *J Heart Lung Transplant.* 1997;16:566–569.

Nason LK, Walker CM, Godwin JD. RadioGraphics. 2012;32: E51–E70.

Sandstrom CK, Stern EJ. Diaphragmatic hernias: A spectrum of radiographic appearances. *Curr Probl Diagn Radiol.* 2011 May–Jun;40(3):95–115.

Index

Note: Page numbers followed by *f* indicate a related image on the specified page.